Series Editor: Richard Riegelman

Global Health 101 FOURTH EDITION

Richard Skolnik, MPA

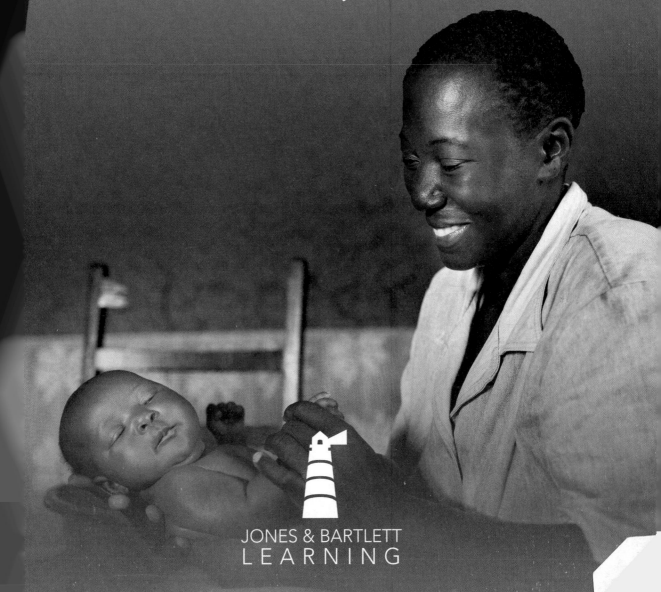

JONES & BARTLETT
LEARNING

World Headquarters
Jones & Bartlett Learning
5 Wall Street
Burlington, MA 01803
978-443-5000
info@jblearning.com
www.jblearning.com

Jones & Bartlett Learning books and products are available through most bookstores and online booksellers. To contact Jones & Bartlett Learning directly, call 800-832-0034, fax 978-443-8000, or visit our website, www.jblearning.com.

Production Credits

VP, Product Management: Amanda Martin
Director of Product Management: Cathy Esperti
Product Manager: Sophie Fleck Teague
Product Specialist: Sara Bempkins
Senior Project Specialist: Alex Schab
Digital Project Specialist: Rachel Reyes
Senior Marketing Manager: Susanne Walker
Production Services Manager: Colleen Lamy
Manufacturing and Inventory Control Supervisor: Amy Bacus

Composition: codeMantra U.S LLC
Cover Design: Kristin E. Parker
Text Design: Kristin E. Parker
Senior Media Development Editor: Shannon Sheehan
Rights Specialist: Maria Leon Maimone
Cover Image (Title Page, Part Opener, Chapter Opener):
 Courtesy of Mark Tuschman
Printing and Binding: LSC Communications
Cover Printing: LSC Communications

16095-6

Library of Congress Cataloging-in-Publication Data
Names: Skolnik, Richard L., author.
Title: Global health 101 / Richard Skolnik.
Other titles: Global health one hundred one | Global health one hundred and one
Description: 4th edition. | Burlington, Massachusetts : Jones & Bartlett Learning, [2020] | Includes bibliographical references and index.
Identifiers: LCCN 2019014106 | ISBN 9781284145380 (paperback)
Subjects: | MESH: Global Health | Health Services Accessibility | Global Burden of Disease
Classification: LCC RA441 | NLM WA 530.1 | DDC 362.1--dc23
LC record available at https://lccn.loc.gov/2019014106
6048

Printed in the United States of America

25 24 23 22 21   10 9 8 7 6 5 4

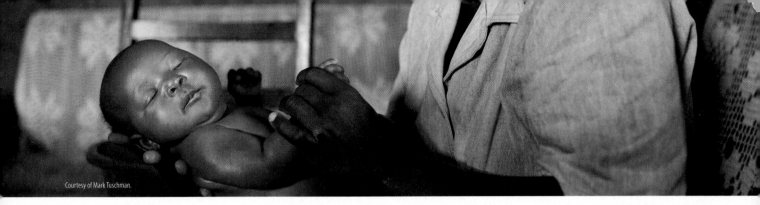

Courtesy of Mark Tuschman.

Brief Contents

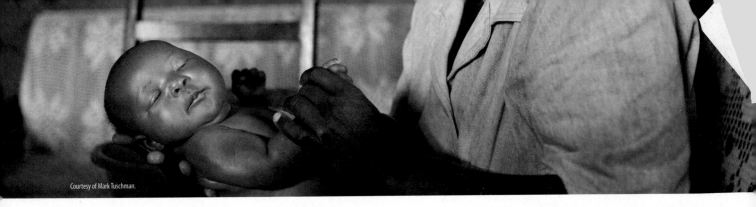
Courtesy of Mark Tuschman.

Contents

PART I Principles, Measurements, and the Health–Development Link 1

Chapter 1 The Principles and Goals of Global Health 3

Chapter 2 Health Determinants, Measurements, and the Status of Health Globally 19

Chapter 3 The Global Burden of Disease 33

BONUS CHAPTERS IN THE COMPANION EBOOK

Chapter 20   Working in Global Health

Chapter 21   Profiles of Global Health Actors

To access the eBook, simply redeem the access code found at the front of this book at **www.jblearning.com**

THE ESSENTIAL PUBLIC HEALTH SERIES

From the impact of AIDS to the cost of health care, this unique series will introduce you to the full range of issues that impact the public's health.

Current and Forthcoming Titles in The Essential Public Health Series:

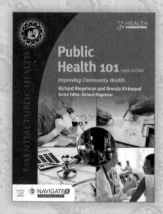
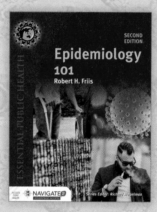
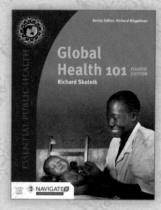
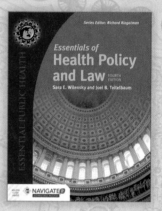

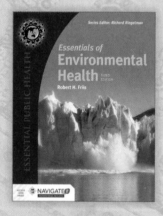
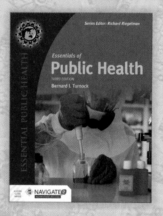
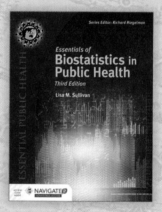

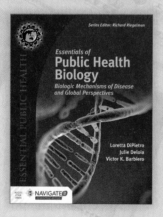
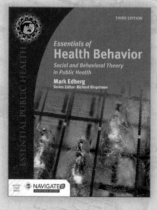
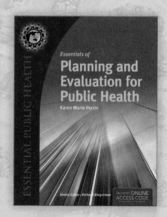

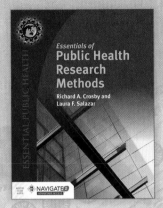
Essentials of
Public Health Research Methods
Richard A. Crosby and Laura F. Salazar

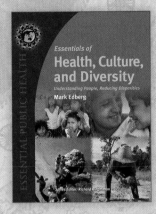
Essentials of
Health, Culture, and Diversity
Understanding People, Reducing Disparities
Mark Edberg

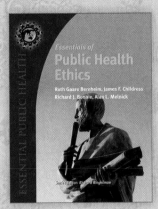
Essentials of
Public Health Ethics
Ruth Gaare Bernheim, James F. Childress
Richard J. Bonnie, Alan L. Melnick
Series Editor: Richard Riegelman

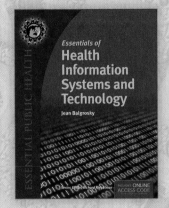
Essentials of
Health Information Systems and Technology
Jean Balgrosky

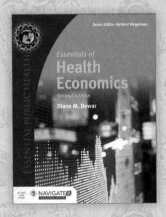
Series Editor: Richard Riegelman
Essentials of
Health Economics
Second Edition
Diane M. Dewar

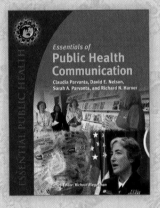
Essentials of
Public Health Communication
Claudia Parvanta, David E. Nelson,
Sarah A. Parvanta, and Richard N. Harner
Series Editor: Richard Riegelman

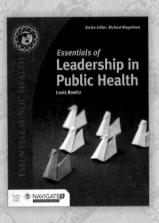
Series Editor: Richard Riegelman
Essentials of
Leadership in Public Health
Louis Rowitz

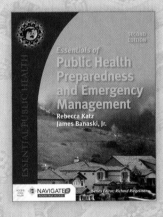
SECOND EDITION
Essentials of
Public Health Preparedness and Emergency Management
Rebecca Katz
James Banaski, Jr.
Series Editor: Richard Riegelman

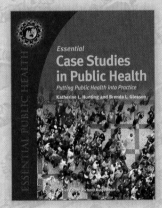
Essential
Case Studies in Public Health
Putting Public Health into Practice
Katherine L. Hunting and Brenda L. Gleason
Series Editor: Richard Riegelman

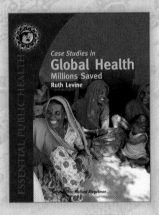
Case Studies in
Global Health
Millions Saved
Ruth Levine
Series Editor: Richard Riegelman

ABOUT THE EDITOR

Richard K. Riegelman, MD, MPH, PhD, is Professor of Epidemiology-Biostatistics, Medicine, and Health Policy, and Founding Dean of The George Washington University Milken Institute School of Public Health in Washington, DC. He has taken a lead role in developing the Educated Citizen and Public Health initiative which has brought together arts and sciences and public health education associations to implement the Institute of Medicine of the National Academies' recommendation that "...all undergraduates should have access to education in public health." Dr. Riegelman also led the development of The George Washington's undergraduate major and minor and currently teaches "Public Health 101" and "Epidemiology 101" to undergraduates.

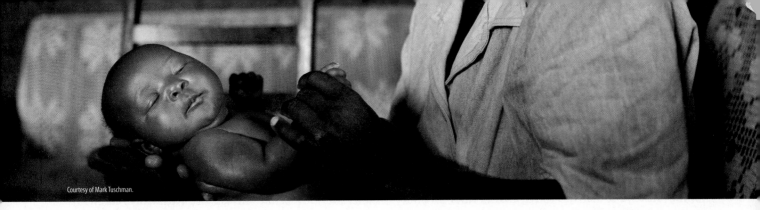

Foreword

I am delighted to write this foreword for the new *Fourth Edition* of *Global Health 101*. I am following in the steps of illustrious predecessors, but unlike them am not a clinician, scientist, or epidemiologist but rather an economist and health systems researcher. In these introductory comments I will therefore focus on those aspects of global health I know best, namely the importance of introducing to students the economic aspects of global health and the economic dimensions of health systems.

Health economics, and health systems research, are relative newcomers amongst the disciplines and subject areas considered relevant to global health. Normally, the development of health economics is dated to the late 1960s, and health systems research is even more recent. But global health has a number of important economic dimensions. Health and national and global economies are intertwined, with influence in both directions. Health is both influenced by economic development, and an important determinant of economic development. At the micro level, households can be driven into poverty by the costs of ill health and of obtaining health care, but conversely good health can help households flourish. With respect to the health system, its size renders it of national and global economic significance – whether assessed as a share of national and global income spent on health care, or burden on household budgets, or proportion of the total workforce employed in the health system.

Economics also provides important tools for decision makers. Its analytical methods can guide priority setting, and help improve resource allocation. It provides insights on the critical question of how best to finance a health system, and understanding incentive structures in the health system can help determine how to improve its efficiency and equity.

Global Health 101, I am pleased to see, has ensured that these critical dimensions of global health are not overlooked. It has an important chapter on Health, Education, Poverty, and the Economy, which addresses the health – development link. It also introduces the use of cost-effectiveness analysis and cost-benefit analysis to help set health priorities. More broadly, across the text it draws on the exceptional range of evidence and recommendations included in the recently completed nine-volume study: *Disease Control Priorities, Third Edition (DCP3)* and its related *Lancet* articles, where cost-effectiveness analysis is extensively used to help derive recommendations on priority interventions and platforms.

New material has also been included in this edition on universal health coverage. Most of the rich world has benefited for decades from health systems that provide everyone with financial risk protection and access to health care. With the declaration of the United Nations General Assembly in 2012 on Universal Coverage, the importance of a health system that benefits everyone has risen on global and national policy agendas. This edition includes substantial additional information about the quest for universal health coverage, including greater treatment of universal health coverage as an organizing principle for health systems. It also includes the most recent evidence-based recommendations, drawn from *DCP3*, on an essential package of interventions for universal health coverage for low-income countries, and how low- and middle-income countries can move toward universal health coverage in cost-effective, feasible, sustainable, and equitable ways.

Richard's passion for teaching and learning illuminates the entire text. He ensures that the human dimension of global health is never forgotten, while still conveying the necessary technical instruction. I am sure that this updated edition will maintain the reputation of this textbook as an indispensable guide for both those who want a basic introduction to global health and those who want a sound foundation on which to build further, in-depth study.

Dame Anne Jane Mills, DCMG, CBE, FRS, FMedSci

Professor Dame Anne Mills is Deputy Director & Provost at The London School of Hygiene & Tropical Medicine (LSHTM) and a worldwide authority on health economics, with a particular focus on how to create efficient and equitable health systems in low- and middle-income countries. Her specific areas of expertise include contracting-out health services, health insurance, the role of the private sector, and evaluation of malaria control interventions and delivery approaches. Her ground-breaking work includes research on the economic impact of malaria and the most cost-effective ways to control the disease in Africa and Asia. She is heavily engaged in supporting capacity building in low- and middle-income countries in the areas of health economics and health systems research, and has trained many generations of masters and doctoral students.

Anne joined the LSHTM as a lecturer in 1979 after working at the Ministry of Health in Malawi as an economist, and has worked at the School ever since. She has held the position of President of the International Health Economics Association, was the Chair of the Board of the Alliance for Health Policy and Systems Research for its first 10 years, and was a founding Board member of Health Systems Global. She received a CBE for services to medicine in 2006, and is an elected Fellow of the US Academy of Medicine, the UK Academy of Medical Sciences and the Royal Society. In 2015, she was awarded a DCMG in recognition of her services to international health.

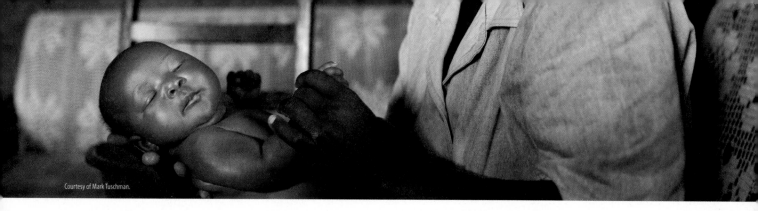
Courtesy of Mark Tuschman.

Editor's Preface

In the prologue to the previous editions, I wrote, "The issues of global health have finally arrived in the consciousness of the developed world through a unique union of efforts by former presidents, software pioneers, and rock stars. It is now time that students have a textbook ... that systematically leads them through the issues of global health from basic principles, to the burden of disease, to examples of successful efforts to improve lives and livelihoods." *Global Health 101* has fulfilled these expectations and more. It has become the classic textbook of global health and is now being used in a wide range of countries.

What can students and faculty expect from the *Fourth Edition* of *Global Health 101*? The *Fourth Edition* builds on the strengths of the *Third Edition*. Like the *Third Edition*, the *Fourth Edition* is written in a single voice, has a consistent format, and includes core chapters that are organized around a common set of questions about the burden of disease and what can be done to address it. The *Fourth Edition* also contains an extensive array of case studies, including a large number of new case studies.

In addition to updating and expanding many of the chapters, the *Fourth Edition* includes new emphasis on universal health coverage. The quest for universal health coverage includes treatment of universal health coverage as an organizing principle for health systems. It includes the most recent evidence-based recommendations on how low- and middle-income countries can move toward universal health coverage in cost-effective, doable, sustainable, and fairly distributed ways. Evidence-based recommendations on an essential package of services for low-income countries are also included.

The chapter on ethics and global health now includes information on best practices in ethical priority setting in global health. This chapter has been expanded with the assistance of the leading global authority on ethical priority setting. The notion of ethical and fair priority setting is now embedded throughout the book.

Issues of quality of care in low- and middle-income countries have recently received increased attention. How they might be addressed is discussed more extensively than before in the health systems chapter of this edition. They are also embedded throughout the book and highlighted as a central issue in global health.

The *Fourth Edition* also includes, for the first time, photos, many from an award-winning photographer. The photos are used in a manner that illustrate key themes in the book. In addition, the photos have not only a caption but also study questions linked to the caption.

As students you'll enjoy and learn from the engaging videos, expand your knowledge using the web links, and test your understandings using the interactive questions and answers. The expanded chapters on careers in global health has additional profiles, including profiles of women and global health actors from outside of medicine and public health. These profiles bring to life opportunities in this growing and dynamic field.

For faculty, the book's website provides an abundance of additional resources to help broaden and deepen students' understanding of global health. Whether you are taking a global health course as part of general education, a major or minor in public health or global health, as part of your health professions education, or as part of your interest in international affairs, you will find the *Fourth Edition* an exhilarating experience that opens your mind and your heart to the world of global health.

Richard Riegelman, MD, MPH, PhD
Essential Public Health Series Editor

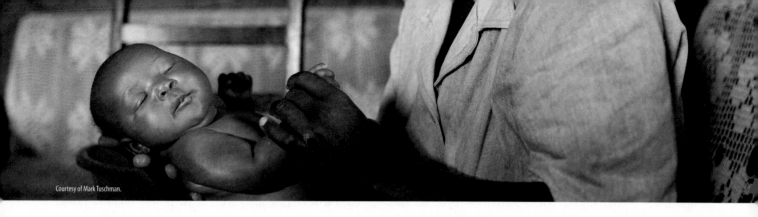

Courtesy of Mark Tuschman.

Author's Preface

THE IMPORTANCE OF GLOBAL HEALTH

Why should we care about the health of other people, especially that of people in other countries? For a number of critical reasons, the health of people everywhere must be an important concern for all of us.

First, diseases do not respect boundaries and globalization has increased the speed with which diseases can cross boundaries. Human immunodeficiency virus (HIV) has spread worldwide. A person with tuberculosis can infect 15 people a year. The West Nile Virus came from Egypt but occurs today in many countries. There is an important risk of a worldwide epidemic of influenza. Clearly, the health of each of us increasingly depends on the health of others.

Second, there is an ethical dimension to the health and well-being of other people. Many children in poor countries get sick and die needlessly of nutrition-related causes or from diseases that are preventable and curable. Many adults in poor countries die because they lack access to medicines that are typically available to people in rich countries. Is this just? Is this fair? Are we prepared to accept such deaths without collectively taking steps to prevent them?

Third, health is closely linked with economic and social development in an increasingly interdependent world. Children who suffer from undernutrition may not reach their full mental potential and may not enroll in or stay in school. Sick children from low- and middle-income countries are less likely than healthy children to become productive adults who can contribute to the economic standing of their family, community, or country. Adults who suffer from HIV/AIDS, tuberculosis, malaria, and other diseases lose income while they are sick and out of work, which contributes in many ways to keeping their families in an endless cycle of poverty. Clearly, improving health enables individuals, their families, and their communities to realize more of their full social and economic potential than would otherwise be the case.

Finally, the health and well-being of people everywhere have important implications for global security and freedom. High rates of HIV/AIDS have contributed to destabilizing some countries, as more teachers and health workers died than were trained, and as insufficient numbers of rural workers grew and harvested crops. Outbreaks of other diseases, such as cholera, the plague, SARS (Severe Acute Respiratory Syndrome), and Ebola, for example, threaten people's ability to engage freely in economic pursuits and can have devastating economic and social consequences. An outbreak of cholera in 1991 cost Peru about $1 billion, the plague in 1994 cost India about $2 billion, and SARS in Asia in 2003 cost the economies of Asia a staggering $18 billion in lost economic activity.

Indeed, these factors have increased interest in global health universally. The aim of this book, therefore, is to examine the most critical global health topics in a clear and engaging manner. The book will provide the reader with an overview of the importance of global health in the context of development, examine the most important global health issues and their economic and social consequences, and discuss some of the steps that are being taken to address these concerns. It will also provide numerous "success stories" as examples of effectively dealing with important global health problems.

This book is intended to provide an introduction to global health for all students. This includes students who have never studied public health before and who will not take additional public health courses in the future. However, it also includes those students, whether they have studied public health before or not, who may wish to pursue additional studies in public health later.

This approach of the book closely follows undergraduate global health courses that I taught at The George Washington University in Washington, DC and at Yale University in New Haven, Connecticut. The text seeks to "speak" to the reader in a manner one would find in an exciting and motivating classroom.

There are very few introductory materials on global health available that are compherensive, clear, and written in a consistent format. Hopefully, this book will help to close that gap by providing a foundation for enhanced studies in public health, global health, and economic and social development.

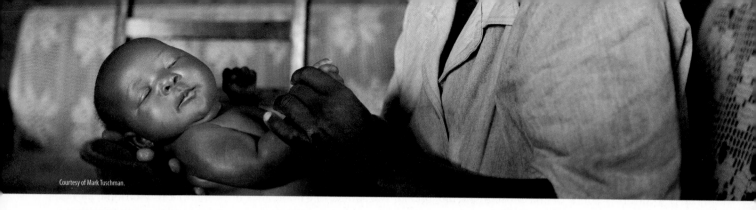

Courtesy of Mark Tuschman.

About the Text

THE ORGANIZATION OF THIS TEXT

The book aims to assist students in gaining the understanding of global health needed to be able to address five questions from an evidence-based and interdisciplinary perspective:

What is the problem? This relates to what people get sick, disabled, and die from and how that varies, by age, sex, income and a number of other factors. It particularly concerns preventable illness and death.

Who gets the problem? This concerns the most affected population groups. For example, are they rich or poor? The educated or not educated? The majority or minority ethnic groups?

Why do they get this problem? What are the determinants of their morbidity and mortality? Are they, for example, social determinants, such as poverty and discrimination against their community? Or, are they more discrete risk factors, such as tobacco smoking?

Why should we care about this problem? What is the relationship between these concerns and the opportunity of people, communities, and nations to realize their full social and economic potential?

What can be done to address the problem? What does the best evidence say can be done to address the problem at least cost, as fast as possible, and in doable, sustainable, and fair ways?

This book is organized in several parts. **PART I** introduces the reader to the basic principles of global health, key measures of health, and the concepts of the health and the development link. Chapter 1 introduces readers to some key principles, themes, and goals of global health. Chapter 2 examines the determinants of health, how health is measured, and the health status of the world. Chapter 3 reviews the global burden of disease and risk factors. Chapter 4 looks at the links between health and development, touching upon the connections between health and education, equity, and poverty.

PART II reviews cross-cutting themes in global health. Chapter 5 examines human rights and ethical issues in global health, with special attention to ethical priority setting. Chapter 6 reviews the purpose and goals of health systems, how different countries have organized their health systems, and the quest for universal health coverage. The chapter also reviews the key challenges that health systems face, the costs and consequences of those challenges, and how some countries have addressed health system challenges. Culture plays an extremely important part in health and Chapter 7 examines the links between culture and health. This chapter reviews the importance of culture to health, how health is perceived in different groups, the manner in which different culture groups seek health care and engage in health practices, and how one can promote changes in health behavior.

PART III reviews the most important causes of illness, disability, and death, particularly in low- and middle-income countries. The chapters in this part of the book examine environmental issues, nutrition, women's health, child health, and the health of adolescents and young adults. The book then reviews communicable diseases, noncommunicable diseases, and unintentional injuries.

PART IV examines how cooperative action can address global health issues and how intersectoral action is needed to deal with the most important health and global health issues. Chapter 16 reviews the impact on health of conflicts, natural disasters, and other health emergencies. Chapter 17 examines how different actors in the global health field work both individually and cooperatively to address key global health problems. Chapter 18 reviews how science and technology have helped to improve public health and how further advances in science and technology could help to address some of the most important global health challenges that remain. Chapter 19 examines intersectoral approaches to addressing global health priorities.

PART V focuses on careers in the global health field. Chapter 20 examines the types of careers in global health; the skills, knowledge, and experience needed to pursue these careers; and how you can get those skills, knowledge, and experience. The book ends with Chapter 21, which includes profiles of 22 actors in the global health field whose personal stories are meant to inspire you, as well as provide guidance about pursuing a career in global health if that is your interest.

Each of the chapters, other than those on working in global health and on profiles of global health actors, follows a similar outline. The chapters begin with vignettes that relate to the topic to be covered and which are intended to make the topic "real" for the reader. Some of these vignettes are not true in the literal sense. However, each of them are based on real events that occur regularly in the countries discussed in this book. Most chapters then explain key concepts, terms, and definitions. The chapters that deal with cross-cutting issues in the second and fourth parts of the book then examine the importance of the topic to enhancing global health, some key challenges in further improving global health, and what can be done to address those challenges.

The chapters that focus on health conditions look at the burden of disease related to these conditions; who is most affected by these issues; major risk factors for these burdens; and, the costs and consequences of these issues for individuals, communities, and the world. These chapters then examine the future challenges in each of these areas and what we have learned about how to deal with these health burdens in the most cost-effective, doable, sustainable, and fair ways.

All of the chapters, except Chapter 19 on intersectoral approaches, contain "case studies" that are meant to briefly introduce you to and illustrate important global health topics, actors, and organizations. There are more than 75 case studies overall. Some of these are explanatory, such as the case that examines the "One Health" approach. Some deal with well-known cases that have already proven to be models for global health efforts. Others, however, are based on experiences that

show good promise, both for success and for providing lessons, but which have not yet proven themselves.

Each chapter concludes with a summary of the main messages in the chapter and a set of study questions that can assist the reader in reviewing the materials included in the chapter. Each chapter also contains endnotes with citations for the data that are used in the book. The book does not contain any additional lists of reference materials. Those wishing to explore topics in greater depth will find ample suggestions for additional reading in the endnotes and on the website associated with the book.

The reader should note that the chapters are not in order of importance. Nutrition, for example, is fundamental to all health concerns. However, it only makes sense to cover nutrition in this book after establishing the context for studying global health and after covering some cross-cutting global health issues. In addition, you will note that there is no chapter called "globalization and health." Rather, you will find that the relationships between globalization and health are integrated into all of the chapters. Some students may also wish to read Chapter 16 on global health policy, actors, and actions before they cover many of the other chapters. This may help them understand at an earlier stage how different actors have organized themselves to address key global health issues.

THE PERSPECTIVE OF THE BOOK

The book will take a global perspective to all that it covers. Although the book includes many country case studies, topics will be examined from the perspective of the world as a whole. The book also pays particular attention to the links between poverty and health and the relationship between health, equity, and health disparities. Special attention will also be given to gender and ethnicity and their relation to health. Another theme that runs through the book is the connection between health and social and economic development.

The book follows the point of view that health is a human right. The book is written with the presumption that governments have an obligation to try to ensure that all of their people have access to an affordable package of healthcare services and that all people should be protected from the costs of ill health. The book is also based on the premise, however, that the development of a health system by any country is inextricably linked to the value system and the political structure of that country.

The book covers key global health topics, including those that affect high-income countries. However, the book pays particular attention to low- and middle-income countries and to poor people within them. The rationale for this is that improving health status indicators within and across countries can only be accomplished if the health of the poor and other disadvantaged groups is improved. The idea of social justice is at the core of public health.

WHAT'S NEW TO THIS EDITION?

Almost every table and figure in *Global Health 101, Fourth Edition* has been updated. Whenever possible, data has been shown for 2016 or later. This edition takes account of the most recent major data sources on global health and the burden of disease, including the Global Burden of Disease and Risk Factors study (GBD). This edition of the book also takes account of the exceptional range of evidence and recommendations included in the recently completed nine-volume study: *Disease Control Priorities, Third Edition (DCP3)* and its related *Lancet* articles. This edition also uses the most up-to-date data and studies from the World Health Organization (WHO), UNAIDS, and the World Bank. Information provided by a range of *Lancet* Commissions is also used extensively. For the first time, much of the data on health status and the burden of disease is shown not only by region, but also by country income group.

Sustainable Development Goals

Each core chapter has a table that relates the chapter topic to the Sustainable Development Goals.

The Burden of Disease and Risk Factors

Understanding the burden of disease and related risk factors is a starting point for the book. All of the chapters on health issues are based on updated data on the burden of disease and related risk factors. Most of the data is for 2016 or later and comes from the GBD. This data is complemented by data from the World Bank, UNAIDS, and WHO that is also for 2016 or later. The burden of disease and risk factors is now discussed in its own chapter, rather than in combination with a discussion of the determinants of health and health status.

Universal Health Coverage (UHC)

This edition includes substantial additional information about "the quest for universal health coverage." This includes, for example, more treatment of universal health coverage as an organizing principle for health systems. It also includes the most recent evidence-based recommendations on what an essential package of UHC for low-income countries would include and how low- and middle-income countries can move toward UHC in cost-effective, doable, sustainable, and fair ways. The book also embeds many of the recommendations for addressing particular health conditions in the notion of high-quality primary health care and universal health coverage.

Quality of Care

There are enormous issues in the quality of care in most countries, but especially in low- and middle-income countries. This was highlighted in a recent *Lancet* commission on quality. Issues of quality and how they might be addressed are discussed more extensively than before in the health systems chapter of this edition. They are also embedded throughout the book and highlighted as a central issue in global health.

Ethics and Global Health

The chapter on ethics and global health has been expanded to include considerable additional information about best practices in "ethical priority setting in global health." This chapter has been expanded with the assistance of the leading global authority on ethical priority setting. The notion of ethical and fair priority setting is now embedded throughout the book.

Women's Health

The chapter on women's health has been expanded to include even more information about women's health broadly and what can be done to address women's health issues that go beyond reproductive and sexual health. This chapter also builds on the latest recommendations from *DCP3* and other up-to-date findings. Gender and equity issues run throughout the book.

Children's Health

This edition of *Global Health 101* builds on the recent recommendations of *DCP3* and a range of other global studies. It also includes an update on the history and progress of the global program on immunization that is unique among the textbooks on global health.

Adolescent Health

The chapter on adolescent health has been updated and expanded. Consistent with the growing global trend, the chapter also now includes 20-24 year old young adults, in addition to adolescents aged 10-19.

Nutrition and Global Health

The nutrition chapter has been enhanced to include additional and updated information about undernutrition and overweight and obesity. The findings on overweight and obesity are associated with the most recent recommendations about the prevention and control of a range of noncommunicable diseases.

Communicable Diseases

This edition of *Global Health 101* contains considerable updated information to its already very extensive chapter on communicable diseases. This includes enhancements on topics related to anti-microbial resistance and pandemic preparedness. Approaches to addressing TB and malaria, among other diseases, have changed substantially since the *Third Edition* and the new approaches are clearly outlined. The chapter on communicable diseases takes extensive account of the findings from *DCP3* and the latest recommendations of WHO and UNAIDS on measures to address HIV, TB, malaria, diarrhea, and selected neglected tropical diseases.

Noncommunicable diseases (NCDs)

The world is now paying dramatically more attention to NCDs than ever before. *Global Health 101, Fourth Edition* includes a substantial amount of updated and additional information on NCDs, including the most recent recommendations about packages for addressing NCDs and the platforms from which to do so, as suggested by *DCP3*, WHO, and other global studies.

Science and Technology for Global Health

The information on science and technology has been revised to focus on a range of public goods in global health and how science and technology can be used to make them available.

Complex Humanitarian Emergencies

The chapter on complex emergencies has been updated and enhanced with comments on the coordination of emergencies.

Intersectoral Approaches

A bonus chapter for the *Third Edition* on intersectoral approaches to enhancing global health is an integral part of this edition.

Working in Global Health

Two chapters cover careers in global health, as in the *Third Edition*. The chapter on "Working in Global Health" has been updated. The chapter on Profiles of "Global Health Actors" includes several new profiles and more profiles than before of women who are involved in global health. It also includes more profiles than earlier of global health actors from outside the fields of medicine and public health. These two chapters are available in the Navigate 2 Advantage platform, accessible by redeeming the code found on the card at the front of the book.

Case Studies

As in the *Third Edition*, the *Fourth Edition* of *Global Health 101* offers a number of case studies at the end of almost every chapter, to illustrate the main points of that chapter. The *Fourth Edition* includes over 75 cases. There are 47 case studies in the printed text found at the end of each chapter. An additional 30 case studies are available online through the Navigate 2 Advantage platform.

Photos

The *Fourth Edition* of *Global Health 101* includes photos for the first time. To enhance teaching and learning, the photos are captioned in a unique way that raises questions for study and thinking. As an example, a picture might be labelled: "This photo shows a woman seeking a TB test in a clinic in Pakistan. What type of communications and other efforts might be needed to encourage such women to present for a test for a highly stigmatized disease in male-dominated countries like Pakistan?" Most of the photos come from an award-winning photographer, Mark Tuschman, and help to make "real" the topics covered in the book.

Blog on Teaching Global Health

The author will continue to prepare a blog on teaching global health. The blog will contain information about resources for teaching global health. It will also include lessons that the author has learned from his teaching Global Health at the undergraduate level, to graduate students of public health, and to graduate students of business.

PEDAGOGICAL FEATURES

Learning Objectives

Learning Objectives at the start of each chapter give you a preview of what topics will be covered in the pages to follow.

▸ Vignettes

By 2005, polio was on the verge of being eradicated. That year, however, rumors circulated in northern Nigeria that the polio vaccine was causing sterility. In response to these rumors, some community leaders discouraged people from immunizing their children. Within months, polio cases began to appear in the area. Shortly thereafter, polio cases spread from northern Nigeria to Sudan, Yemen, and Indonesia. The global campaign to eradicate polio had been dealt a major blow, stemming partly from rumors in one country about the alleged side effects of the vaccine.[1]

Getachew is a 20-year-old Ethiopian with HIV. He was recently placed on antiretroviral therapy for his infection. He is already gaining weight and feeling much stronger than before. Getachew is one of about 1.2 million people in Ethiopia who are living with HIV.[2] He is also one of about 37 million people in the world who are HIV positive.[3] In Botswana, Lesotho, and Swaziland, more than 20 percent of all adults are HIV-positive.[4]

Laurie lives in Portsmouth, Virginia, in the United States. She is 50 years old and has always been healthy. Last weekend, she woke up with a headache, a high fever, and a very stiff neck. Laurie was so sick that she went to the emergency room of the local hospital. The physicians diagnosed Laurie as having meningitis, an inflammation of the membrane around the brain and spinal cord,[5] that was caused by West Nile virus. This virus originated in Egypt in the 1930s and is transmitted by mosquitoes. Today, the virus can be found in much of the world.[6]

Vignettes

Based on events that occur regularly in countries across the globe, each chapter begins with several vignettes that bring to life the topic to be covered.

Tables and Figures

Colorful, clear, easy-to-read tables and figures that engage you in visualizing and understanding key data.

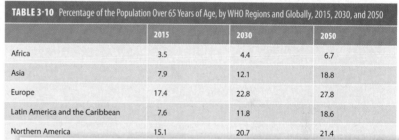

TABLE 3-10 Percentage of the Population Over 65 Years of Age, by WHO Regions and Globally, 2015, 2030, and 2050

	2015	2030	2050
Africa	3.5	4.4	6.7
Asia	7.9	12.1	18.8
Europe	17.4	22.8	27.8
Latin America and the Caribbean	7.6	11.8	18.6
Northern America	15.1	20.7	21.4

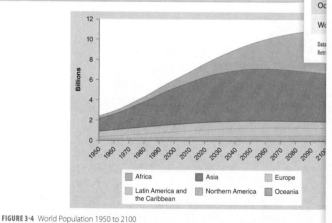

FIGURE 3-4 World Population 1950 to 2100

Modified from United Nations, Department of Economic and Social Affairs, Population Division. (2017). *World population prospects: The 2017 revision, key findings and advance tables* (Working Paper No. ESA/P/WP/248). New https://esa.un.org/unpd/wpp/Publications/Files/WPP2017_KeyFindings.pdf

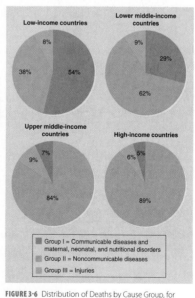

FIGURE 3-6 Distribution of Deaths by Cause Group, for World Bank Country Income Groups

Data from Institute of Health Metrics and Evaluation (IHME). (n.d.). GBD Compare: Viz Hub. Retrieved from https://vizhub.healthdata.org/gbd-compare/

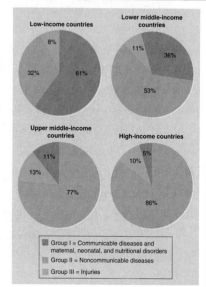

FIGURE 3-7 Distribution of DALYs by Cause Group, for World Bank Country Income Groups

Data from Institute of Health Metrics and Evaluation (IHME). (n.d.). GBD Compare: Viz Hub. Retrieved from https://vizhub.healthdata.org/gbd-compare/

Before starting our review of global health in greater detail, it will be helpful to define health, public health, and global health. Most of us think of "health" from our individual perspective as "not being sick." The World Health Organization (WHO), however, set out a broader definition of health in 1948 that is still widely used:

Key Terms

Throughout the text, key terms are highlighted in an orange, bold font and are defined in the glossary at the back of the book, for easy reference and review.

Award-Winning Photographs

The *Fourth Edition* offers stunning new photos throughout the text, many from the award-winning photographer, Mark Tushman. Each with captions and discussion questions, these photos bring Global Health to life and illustrate key concepts and themes to provide a more meaningful learning experience.

TABLE 3-5   Leading Causes of Death in Children Under 5 by World Bank Country Income Group, 2016

Rank	Low-Income	Lower Middle-Income	Upper Middle-Income	High-Income
1	Malaria	Lower respiratory infections	Neonatal preterm birth	Congenital defects
2	Lower respiratory infections	Neonatal preterm birth	Congenital defects	Neonatal preterm birth
3	Diarrheal diseases	Neonatal encephalopathy	Lower respiratory infections	Other neonatal disorders
4	Neonatal encephalopathy	Malaria	Neonatal encephalopathy	Neonatal encephalopathy
5	Neonatal preterm birth	Diarrheal diseases	Other neonatal disorders	Sudden infant death syndrome (SIDS)
6	Protein-energy malnutrition	Congenital defects	Neonatal sepsis	Neonatal sepsis
7	Neonatal sepsis	Other neonatal disorders	HIV/AIDS	Lower respiratory infections
8	Congenital defects	Neonatal sepsis	Diarrheal diseases	Road injuries
9	Other neonatal disorders	Meningitis	Road injuries	Endocrine, metabolic, blood, and immune disorders
10	Meningitis	Protein-energy malnutrition	Drowning	Mechanical forces

Data from Institute of Health Metrics and Evaluation (IHME). (n.d.). GBD Compare: Viz Hub. Retrieved from https://vizhub.healthdata.org/gbd-compare/

Nutritional issues are also prominent in the lowest-income countries, and road traffic injuries and drowning are important causes of death in the low- and ... this age group, the ... ath occurs as one ... untries and con- ... ries. In these two ... portance of road ... ncers among the ... income countries ... leading causes of

... causes of deaths ... 9, by World Bank

... e from Table 3-7.

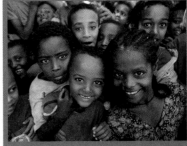

PHOTO 3-2   This picture depicts a group of older Ethiopian children. What health conditions are likely to be the most

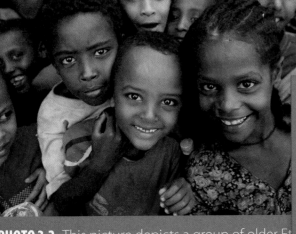

PHOTO 3-2   This picture depicts a group of older Et... children. What health conditions are likely to be th... important causes of death for children 8 to 10 yea... in Ethiopia? How would that vary between better... places and lower-resource places within Ethiopia?

Courtesy of Mark Tuschman.

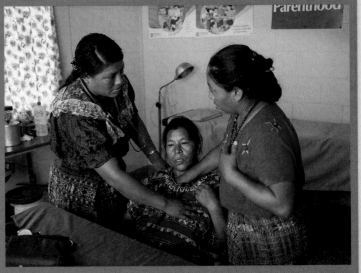

PHOTO 3-3   An indigenous woman in Guatemala is shown here being examined by healthcare workers in a local clinic. What are the most important burdens of disease for women like the one shown? What are the most important risk factors for those burdens? Why is it so important to consider the health of women broadly and not just focus on their reproductive health?

Courtesy of Mark Tuschman.

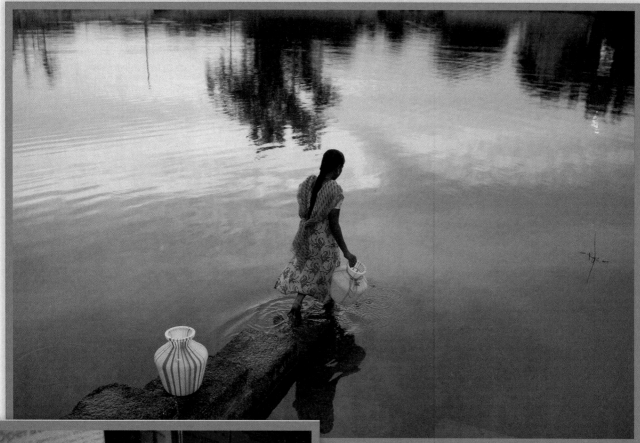

...isk factor for ill health in many low- and lower middle-income ...ater for household use from an open source. What risks does ...hat is likely to be the most cost-effective way of addressing ...ves?

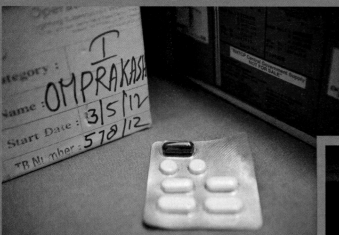

PHOTO 13-2 People with active TB disease need to t... four drugs daily for the first 2 months of treatment and two drugs daily for 4 months after that. This ph... shows the pills a patient in India has to take daily fo... first 2 months of treatment. This large pill burden is ... disincentive to completing treatment. What measu... have countries taken to try to ensure their TB patie... take all of their medicines?

© Andrew Aitchison/Corbis Historical/Getty Images.

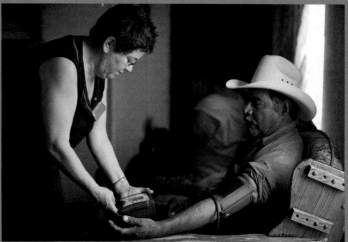

PHOTO 3-1 A healthcare worker is pictured here, taking the blood pressure of a man in a health center in Mexico. Why is this so important? What risks does high blood pressure pose? What are some of the most important risk factors for having hypertension?

Courtesy of Mark Tuschman.

Case Studies

More than 75 case studies are offered in the *Fourth Edition* of *Global Health 101*. These case studies bring issues to life. Most follow a consistent format that walks you through the background, the intervention, the impact, and the cost and benefits.

Situated at the end of each chapter, the printed textbook offers 47 case studies that help you relate to the topics learned in the chapter. An additional 30 bonus case studies are offered on the Navigate 2 Advantage platform giving you further opportunity to understand the concepts learned through the text.

▶ Case Study: Smallpox Eradication—The Most Famous Success Story

It is fitting to end the main part of this introductory chapter with a summary of the most famous public health success story of all: the case of smallpox eradication. This effort was not only a great triumph of public health but also a great accomplishment for humanity. In addition, the history of smallpox eradication is well known to everyone who works in public health, and it provides many lessons that can be applied to other public health efforts.

Background

In 1966, smallpox ravaged over 50 countries, affecting 10 million to 15 million people, of whom almost 2 million died each year.[32] At the time, smallpox killed as many as 30 percent of those infected. Those who survived could suffer from deep-pitted scars and blindness as a result of their illness.[33]

veillance and searching, WHO declared smallpox the first disease in history to have been eradicated. Smallpox had previously been eliminated in Latin America in 1971 and in Asia in 1975.[34]

The Intervention

Although a vaccine against smallpox was created by Edward Jenner in 1798, eradication of smallpox became a practical goal only in the 1950s, when the vaccine could be mass produced and stored without refrigeration. A later breakthrough came in the form of the bifurcated needle, a marvel of simple technology that dramatically reduced costs by allowing needles to be reused endlessly after sterilization and by requiring a far smaller amount of vaccine per patient than had previously been the case. The needle also made vaccination easy, thereby reducing the time and effort required to train villagers in its use.

In 1959, WHO adopted a proposal to eradicate smallpox through compulsory vaccination, but the program languished until 1965, when the United States stepped in with technical and financial support. A Smallpox Eradication Unit was established at WHO, headed by Dr. D. A. Henderson of the Centers for Disease Control and Prevention (CDC) in the United States. As part of the smallpox eradication program, all WHO member countries were required to manage program funds effectively, report smallpox cases, encourage research on smallpox, and maintain flexibility in the implementation of the smallpox program to suit local conditions.

The Smallpox Eradication Unit proved to be a small but committed team, supplying vaccines and specimen kits to those countries that still had smallpox. Although wars and civil unrest caused disruptions in the program's progress, momentum was always regained with new methods and extra resources that focused on containing outbreaks by speedily seeking out new cases with motorized teams, isolating new cases, and vaccinating everyone in the vicinity of the

Costs and Benefits

The annual cost of the eradication campaign between 1967 and 1979 was $23 million U.S. dollars (from here on, the dollar sign will refer to U.S. dollars unless otherwise stated). For the whole campaign, international donors provided $98 million, and $200 million came from the endemic countries.[31] The United States saves the total of all its contributions every 26 days because it no longer needs to spend money on vaccination or treatment, making smallpox eradication one of the best-value health accomplishments ever achieved.[35] Estimates for

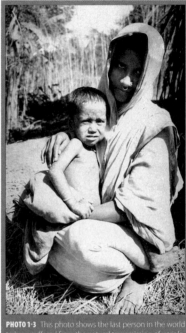

PHOTO 1-3 This photo shows the last person in the world to have suffered from the natural transmission of *variola major*, a 3-year-old girl in Bangladesh named Rahima Banu. This occurred in late 1975. In 1977, Ali Maow Maalin, a Somali, was the last person to have naturally acquired smallpox caused by *variola minor*. Why was smallpox chosen for eradication? What factors were behind the success of the eradication effort? Are there diseases today that are good candidates for eradication?
Stanley O. Foster M.D., M.P.H. World Health Organization/CDC. Centers for Disease Control and Prevention. (2016). *History of smallpox.* Retrieved from https://www.cdc.gov/smallpox/history/history.html

Study Questions

Each chapter ends with study questions so you can check your knowledge of the concepts presented while also applying critical and analytical thinking skills.

Study Questions

1. What are some examples of important progress in improving health worldwide over the last 50 years?
2. What are some of the global health challenges that remain to be addressed?
3. How might one define *health, public health,* and *global health*?
4. What are some examples of public health activities?
5. What are some examples of global health issues?
6. What are the key differences between the approach of medicine and the approach of public health?
7. What are some of the most important challenges to health globally?
8. Why should everyone be concerned with critical global health issues?
9. What are the Sustainable Development Goals and how do they relate to health?
10. What were some of the keys to the eradication of smallpox? What lessons does the smallpox eradication program suggest for other health programs?

References

Interested in learning more? Use the references listed at the end of each chapter to go online (or to the library), to read the information from its original source.

References

1. World Health Organization. (2004, August 24). *New polio cases confirmed in Guinea, Mali and the Sudan.* Retrieved from http://www.who.int/mediacentre/news/releases/2004/pr57/en
2. UNICEF Ethiopia. (n.d.). *Introduction—HIV/AIDS.* Retrieved from https://www.unicef.org/ethiopia/hiv_aids.html
3. UNAIDS. (n.d.). *Global HIV & AIDS statistics—2018 fact sheet.* Retrieved from http://www.unaids.org/en/resources/fact-sheet
4. WorldAtlas.com. (2017). *Countries with the highest rates of HIV/AIDS.* Retrieved from https://www.worldatlas.com/articles/countries-with-the-highest-rates-of-hiv-aids.html
5. Centers for Disease Control and Prevention. (2018). *Meningococcal disease.* Retrieved from http://www.cdc.gov/meningococcal/
6. World Health Organization. (2011). *West Nile virus.* Retrieved from http://www.who.int/mediacentre/factsheets/fs354/en/
7. International Diabetes Federation. (2017). *IDF Diabetes Atlas* (8th Ed.). Retrieved from http://www.diabetesatlas.org/IDF_Diabetes_Atlas_8e_interactive_EN/
8. WorldAtlas.com. (2018). *Countries with the highest rates of diabetes.* Retrieved from https://www.worldatlas.com/articles/countries-with-the-highest-rates-of-diabetes.html
9. Statista. (n.d.). *Countries with the highest prevalence of diabetes worldwide, 2017.* Retrieved from https://www.statista.com/statistics/241814/countries-with-highest-number-of-diabetics/
10. World Health Organization. (2014). Dengue, countries or areas at risk, 2013 [Map]. Retrieved from http://gamapserver.who.int/mapLibrary/Files/Maps/Global_DengueTransmission_ITHRiskMap.png
11. World Health Organization. (n.d.). *Dengue control—Epidemiology.* Retrieved from https://www.who.int/denguecontrol/epidemiology/en/.
12. The World Bank. (n.d.). *Data: Life expectancy at birth, total (years).* Retrieved from https://data.worldbank.org/indicator/SP.DYN.LE00.IN?view=chart
13. World Health Organization. (1946). *Preamble to the Constitution of the World Health Organization 1946, as adopted by the International Health Conference, New York,* 19 June–22 July 1946. Retrieved from http://gb/bd/PDF/bd47/EN/constitution-en.pd
14. Merson, M. H., Black, R. E., & Mills, A. (2 *public health: Diseases, programs, sys* (p. xvii). Gaithersburg, MD: Aspen Publis
15. American Public Health Association. (2 *the ethical practice of public health.* Retr www.apha.org/-/media/files/pdf/mem /ethics_brochure.ashx
16. Harvard School of Public Health. (n.d.). *I medicine and public health.* Retrieved fro .harvard.edu/about/public-health-medici
17. Last, J. M. (2001). *A dictionary of epidemic* York, NY: Oxford University Press.
18. Institute of Medicine. (1998). *America global health: Protecting our people, enha and advancing our international interests* National Academy Press.
19. Merson, M. H., Black, R. E., & Mills, A. (2 *public health: Diseases, programs, sys* (p. xix). Gaithersburg, MD: Aspen Publis
20. Koplan, J. P., Bond, T. C., Merson, M. Rodriguez, M. H., Sewankambo, N. K., (2009). Towards a common definition of *Lancet, 373*(9679), 1993–1995.
21. Fried, L. P., Bentley, M. E., Buekens, P., J. J., Klag, M. J., & Spencer, H. C. (2010 public health. *The Lancet, 375*(9714), 535–
22. American Veterinary Medical Foundatic *One Health—It's all connected.* Retrieved .avma.org/KB/Resources/Reference/Pages
23. Whitmee, S., Haines, A., Beyrer, C., Bolt de Souza Dias, B. F., ... Yach, D. (2015). Sa health in the Anthropocene epoch: Repor Foundation-Lancet Commission on pla *Lancet, 386*(10007), 1973–2028. doi: http /S0140-6736(15)60901-1
24. The World Bank. (n.d.). *World Ba lending groups.* Retrieved from h .worldbank.org/knowledgebase/artic -bank-country-and-lending-groups

Case Studies Included in the Printed Textbook

1. Smallpox Eradication—The Most Famous Success Story (Chapter 1)

2. The Million Deaths Study (Chapter 3)

3. Health Equity and Lesbian, Gay, Bisexual and Transgender People (Chapter 4)

4. The Challenge of Guinea Worm in Asia and Sub-Saharan Africa (Chapter 4)

5. Ethical Priority Setting in Norway (Chapter 5)

6. Pharmaceuticals (Chapter 6)

7. Essential Surgery (Chapter 6)

8. Improving Health Outcomes in Rwanda through Pay-for-Performance Schemes (Chapter 6)

9. Health for All in Thailand through the Universal Coverage Scheme (Chapter 6)

10. Breastfeeding in Burundi (Chapter 7)

11. Polio Vaccination in India (Chapter 7)

12. Ebola and Culture (Chapter 7)

13. Handwashing with Soap in Senegal (Chapter 8)

14. Total Sanitation and Sanitation Marketing: East Java, Indonesia (Chapter 8)

15. Concrete Floors for Child Health (Chapter 8)

16. Climate Change and Health (Chapter 8)

17. South Korea's Promotion of and Adherence to a Traditional Diet (Chapter 9)

18. Brazil: The Agita São Paulo Program Uses Physical Activity to Promote Health (Chapter 9)

19. Finland Uses Labels to Reduce Salt Consumption (Chapter 9)

20. Tamil Nadu State, India Nutrition Project (Chapter 9)

21. The Challenge of Iodine Deficiency Disease in China (Chapter 9)

22. Maternal Mortality in Sri Lanka (Chapter 10)

23. Reducing Fertility in Bangladesh (Chapter 10)

24. Eliminating Polio in Latin America and the Caribbean (Chapter 11)

25. Measles—Progress and Challenges (Chapter 11)

26. Reducing Child Mortality in Nepal Through Vitamin A (Chapter 11)

27. Cash Transfer Program for Adolescent Girls in Malawi (Chapter 12)

28. One Health (Chapter 13)

29. The West African Ebola Outbreak of 2014 and 2015 (Chapter 13)

30. Preventing HIV/AIDS and Sexually Transmitted Infections in Thailand (Chapter13)

31. Controlling TB in China (Chapter 13)

32. Controlling Trachoma in Morocco (Chapter 13)

33. Dementia (Chapter 14)

34. Oral Health (Chapter 14)

35. The Challenge of Curbing Tobacco Use in Poland (Chapter 14)

36. Saving Lives Through Helmet Laws in Vietnam (Chapter 15)

37. The Genocide in Rwanda (Chapter 16)

38. Haiti's 2010 Earthquake (Chapter 16)

39. Healthcare in the Syrian Civil War (Chapter 16)

40. The TB Alliance (Chapter 17)

41. Innovative Financing Mechanisms for Global Health: UNITAID (Chapter 17)

42. Onchocerciasis (Chapter 17)

43. mHealth: Using Mobile Technology to Improve the Health of the Poor in Poor Countries (Chapter 18)

44. New Diagnostics for TB: Xpert MTB/RIF (Chapter 18)

45. Saving Women's Lives: The Nonpneumatic Antishock Garment (Chapter 18)

46. Advance Market Commitments (Chapter 18)

47. International Finance Facility for Immunisation (Chapter 18)

Bonus Case Studies Available in the Navigate 2 Advantage Platform

Redeem the access code (found on the card at the front of the book) at **www.jblearning.com** to gain access to these 30 additional case studies:

1. The State of Kerala (Chapter 2)
2. Brazil's Programa Saúde da Família (Chapter 6)
3. Improving Provincial Health – Argentina's Plan Nacer (Chapter 6)
4. Birthing Services in Peru (Chapter 7)
5. Conditional Cash Transfers in Mexico (Chapter 7)
6. Care Groups (Chapter 7)
7. Arsenicosis in Bangladesh (Chapter 8)
8. Nepal Addresses Micronutrient Deficiencies (Chapter 9)
9. Rapid Results Initiative for Food Fortification in Kenya (Chapter 9)
10. Childhood Nutrition Supplementation and Adult Productivity in Guatemala (Chapter 9)
11. Addressing Female Genital Mutilation in Senegal (Chapter 10)
12. Reducing Maternal Mortality in Tamil Nadu, India (Chapter 10)
13. The Global Polio Eradication Initiative (Chapter 11)
14. HealthWise South Africa: A Life Skills Course for Adolescents (Chapter 12)
15. Chikungunya Fever (Chapter 13)
16. Cryptococcosis: A New Leading Cause of Death in Patients with HIV (Chapter 13)
17. A Comprehensive Approach to Tuberculosis: Operation ASHA and the Last-Mile Pipeline (Chapter 13)
18. The Long-Term Costs and Financing of HIV/AIDS (Chapter 13)
19. Controlling Chagas Disease in the Southern Cone of South America (Chapter 13)
20. The Economic Costs of Noncommunicable Diseases in the Pacific Islands (Chapter 14)
21. Mental Disorders—The Unacceptable Gap Between Their Burden and the Lack of Attention Paid to Them (Chapter 14)
22. Cataract Blindness Control in India (Chapter 14)
23. Motorcycle Helmet Use in Taiwan (Chapter 15)
24. Rumble Strips and Speed Bumps in Ghana (Chapter 15)
25. Preventing Childhood Drowning in Bangladesh (Chapter 15)
26. The Earthquake in Pakistan (Chapter 16)
27. Myanmar: Cyclone Nargis (Chapter 16)
28. Prioritizing Gavi Assistance and Sustaining Country Vaccine Programs (Chapter 17)
29. Eliminating Borders: Using Telemedicine to Connect the Medical Community in India (Chapter 18)
30. The Human Hookworm Vaccine Initiative (Chapter 18)

ADDITIONAL MATERIALS AVAILABLE ONLINE

Additional resources are available in the Navigate 2 Advantage platform to help you learn the material and prepare for assessments.

Simply redeem the access code found on the card at the front of the book at www.jblearning.com and get access to the following:

Comprehensive eBook

Looking for the book in digital format? You can find it here along with practice quizzes at the end of each chapter and links to external resources for further reading. Our eBook reader also offers features such as bookmarking, highlighting, and voice notes.

Bonus Case Studies

30 additional case studies are available on the Navigate 2 Advantage platform. Learn about events such as the recent earthquake in Pakistan and topics such as birthing services in Peru or new technologies such as telemedicine in India. These additional case studies will give you further understanding of the concepts learned through the text and prepare you for written assessments.

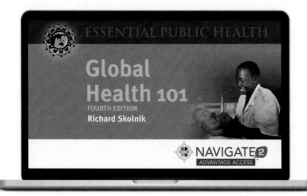

Bonus Chapters

Interested in pursuing a career in global health? These two bonus chapters will introduce you to the various professional opportunities in this exciting field as well as profiles of real world actors making strides in improving the health of people across the globe.

Chapter 20: Careers in Global Health

YOU'LL LEARN ABOUT:

- The wide variety of professional opportunities
- The skills, knowledge, and experience required to take advantage of those opportunities
- Some of the different routes to a career in global health
- Key resources for information about careers in global health
- Articulating career goals in the global health field, as appropriate to the readers interests.

Chapter 21: Profiles of Global health Actors

YOU'LL LEARN ABOUT:

- A range of global health careers
- The array of people involved in global health
- The factors that have inspired people to work in global health and the diverse ways they entered the field
- The types of mentors one might find in global health
- Key lessons from experiences in global health work

Redeem Your Access Code at **www.jblearning.com**

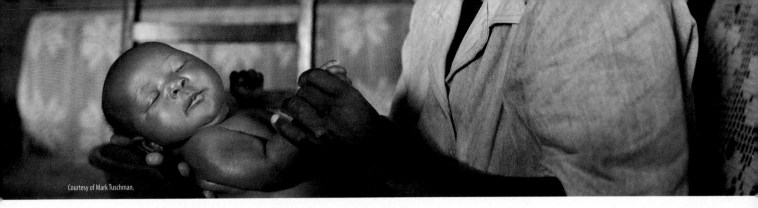

Courtesy of Mark Tuschman.

Acknowledgments

A range of people assisted with the development of the first, second, and third editions of this book. I remain very grateful to them.

This edition would also not have been possible without the help of the people noted here.

Rachel Strodel and Diksha Brahmbhatt served as the primary research assistants for this edition. They gathered resources and data, and prepared tables, figures, and several case studies. They also reviewed each round of the text that I prepared and helped me put the many different components of the book together. The book would have been impossible to write or produce without their help.

Tessa Snyder and Mary Gaul assisted in the development and production of the many materials on the book's website. Their assistance was invaluable.

Ole Norheim coauthored the ethics chapter, for which I am very grateful. Aviva Musicus coauthored the nutrition chapter, for which I am also very thankful.

Several friends assisted me in preparing technical elements of the book, for which I am also very appreciative. These include Madhukar Pai of McGill University and Mario Raviglione, the former director of the TB program at WHO. They also include Peter Hotez and Maria Elena Botazzi of the School of Tropical Medicine of the Baylor College of Medicine. Several of the *DCP3* series editors and staff were also helpful in many ways, including Rachel Nugent, Sue Horton, Dean Jamison, David Watkins, Brie Adderley, Kristen Danforth, and Tiffany Wilk. Staff of the Institute of Health Metrics and Evaluation assisted me on several occasions to make the best use of their data. Susan Sawyer and George Patton of the University of Melbourne were very helpful to my work on adolescent health. Jim Levinson has responded over the years to many requests for information on nutrition and this has also been helpful to my preparing the book. Bob Black's work has both inspired and informed me and I am grateful for his always being responsive to my questions.

Rosa Shapiro-Thompson was a research assistant for the development of the chapter on complex humanitarian emergencies. Lindsey Hiebert, who was the research assistant for the *Third Edition*, kindly assisted with a number of matters in this edition as well.

I am also very grateful to the people who let me profile them in Chapter 21.

My sincere thanks go, as well, to Anne Mills for so kindly writing the preface to the book.

In addition, I am enormously grateful to Dick Reigelman for his continuous encouragement, excellent ideas, and remarkable support to my preparing the book.

I also welcome the opportunity to collaborate in this edition with Mark Tuschman, whose photos are always exceptional and add much to the book.

The staff of Jones & Bartlett Learning, including Sophie Teague, Carter McAlister, and Alex Schab, among others were always helpful and always a delight to work with.

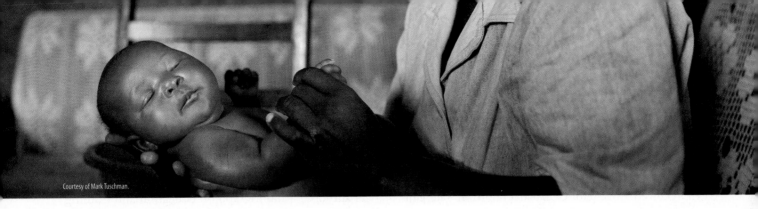

About the Author

Richard Skolnik has worked for more than 40 years in education, health, and development and is one of the world's most experienced teachers of global health.

Richard worked at the World Bank from 1976 to 2001, last serving as the Director for Health and Education for the South Asia region. His health work at the World Bank focused on health systems development, family planning and reproductive health, child health, the control of communicable diseases, and nutrition in low-income countries. He was also deeply engaged with tuberculosis, HIV, leprosy, and cataract blindness control projects in India.

Richard has also participated extensively in policy-making and program development at the international level. Richard coordinated the World Bank's work on TB for 5 years, was deeply involved in the establishment of STOP TB, represented the World Bank to the Global Polio Eradication Initiative, served on a number of WHO working groups on TB, and served three rounds on the Technical Review Panel of the Global Fund. Richard led two evaluations of the International AIDS Vaccine Initiative and also led an evaluation of the Global Alliance to Eliminate Leprosy. Richard also worked with the Results for Development Institute on the long-run financing of HIV programs in Cambodia, India, and Nigeria.

In addition, Richard has served on advisory groups and faculty for the Harvard Humanitarian Initiative, the development of a women's health program at Harvard University, and the Global Health Leadership Institute at Yale University. He was also a member of an expert panel that reviewed the Framework Program of the Fogarty Center of the United States National Institutes of Health. He also served 3 years on the advisory board for the College of Health and Human Services at George Mason University. He recently served on the editorial advisory committee for *Disease Control Priorities in Developing Countries, Third Edition*. Richard has given scores of guest lectures and in 2011 was the commencement speaker for the College of Health and Human Services at George Mason University.

From 2001 to 2004 and from 2009 until 2011, Richard was a lecturer in the Department of Global Health at The George Washington University (GWU), where he taught four courses per year of an introductory global health course for undergraduates. At GWU, Richard also supervised final research projects for master of public health (MPH) students. Richard was an Undergraduate Public Health Teacher of the Year at The George Washington University and was asked in 2009 to deliver a lecture in the GWU "Last Lecture" series. He also served as the Director of the Center for Global Health at George Washington.

In 2005 and 2006, Richard was the Executive Director of the Harvard School of Public Health PEPFAR program for AIDS treatment in Botswana, Nigeria, and Tanzania. In 2007 and 2008, he was the Vice President for International Programs at the Population Reference Bureau (PRB).

From 2012 to 2016, Richard was a Lecturer in the Health Policy and Management Department at the Yale School of Public Health and from 2013 until 2016 he was also a Lecturer in the Practice of Management at the Yale School of Management. At Yale, Richard taught an introductory global health course twice a year to undergraduate students. He also taught a once-a-year upper level undergraduate course called "Case Studies in Global Health." Richard also taught an introduction to global health for graduate MPH students and a global health course to students in the healthcare stream of the Executive MBA program of the Yale School of Management. Richard also developed for Yale a massive open online course, *Essentials of Global Health*, which is on Coursera.

Richard attended high school in Dayton, Ohio. He received a bachelor of arts degree from Yale University and a master of public affairs degree from the Woodrow Wilson School of Princeton University. At Yale, he participated in the Experimental Five-Year BA Program, under which he spent 1 year teaching high school biology in Laoag City, Philippines, living with the same family with whom he had lived

as an exchange student in 1966. Upon graduation from Yale, Richard was selected for a fellowship by the Yale–China Association and spent 2 years teaching at The Chinese University of Hong Kong. In the summer between his 2 years at the Woodrow Wilson School, Richard was a research fellow at the Institute of Southeast Asian Studies in Singapore, where he authored a monograph on education and training in Singapore. Richard has worked on health issues in Africa, Latin America and the Caribbean, the Middle East and North Africa, South Asia, and South-East Asia. He has also studied and learned to varying degrees Cantonese, French, Ilocano, Mandarin, Spanish, and Tagalog.

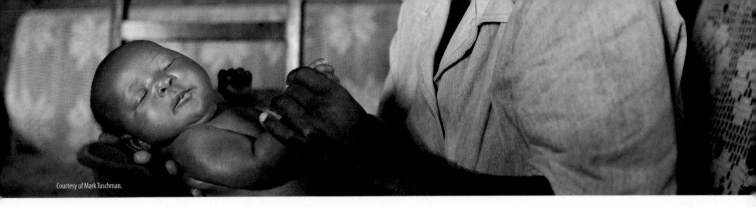

Courtesy of Mark Tuschman.

Abbreviations

Term	Definition
ACT	artemisinin combination therapy
ADB	Asian Development Bank
ADL	adenolymphangitis
AfDB	African Development Bank
AIDS	acquired immune deficiency syndrome
AMC	Advance Market Commitments
APOC	African Programme for Onchocerciasis Control
ARI	acute respiratory infection
ART	antiretroviral therapy
AZT	zidovudine
BCG	Bacillus Calmette-Guérin (the tuberculosis vaccine)
BMI	body mass index
BOD	burden of disease
CCT	conditional cash transfer
CDC	The U.S. Centers for Disease Control and Prevention
CFR	case fatality ratio
CHC	community health center
CHE	complex humanitarian emergency
CLTS	community-led total sanitation
CMR	crude mortality rate
COPD	chronic obstructive pulmonary disease
CRC	Convention on the Rights of the Child
CVD	cardiovascular disease
DALY	disability-adjusted life year
DANIDA	Danish International Development Agency
DCP3	*Disease Control Priorities, Third Edition*
DEC	diethylcarbamazine citrate
DFID	Department for International Development of the United Kingdom
DHS	Demographic and Health Survey
DRC	Democratic Republic of the Congo
DTP	diphtheria, tetanus, and pertussis
ECCE	extracapsular cataract extraction
EPI	Expanded Program on Immunization
EU	European Union
EVD	Ebola virus disease
FAO	Food and Agriculture Organization of the United Nations
FDA	Food and Drug Administration (United States)
FGM	female genital mutilation
FSU	Former Soviet Union
Gavi	The Vaccine Alliance
GBD	Global Burden of Disease Study
GDM	gestational diabetes mellitus
GDP	gross domestic product
GIS	geographic information system
GNI	gross national income
GNP	gross national product

GOARN	Global Outbreak and Response Network
GOBI	growth monitoring, oral rehydration, breastfeeding, and immunization
GPEI	Global Polio Eradication Initiative
HALE	health-adjusted life expectancy
HDL	high-density lipoprotein
Hib	Haemophilus influenzae type b
HIV	human immunodeficiency virus
HPV	human papillomavirus
HSV	herpes simplex virus
IASC	Interagency Standing Committee
IBRD	International Bank for Reconstruction and Development (World Bank)
ICCE	intracapsular cataract extraction
ICCPR	International Covenant on Civil and Political Rights
ICESCR	International Covenant on Economic, Cultural, and Social Rights
IDA	International Development Association (the "soft" lending window of the World Bank)
IDB	Inter-American Development Bank
IDD	iodine deficiency disorder
IDF	International Diabetes Federation
IDP	internally displaced person
IEC	information, education, and communication
IFFIm	International Financing Facility for Immunisation
IHD	ischemic heart disease
IHME	Institute of Health Metrics and Evaluation
IHR	International Health Regulations
ILO	International Labor Organization
IMCI	integrated management of childhood illness
IMF	International Monetary Fund
IMR	infant mortality rate
INCOSUR	Southern Cone Initiative to Eliminate Chagas
IPT	intermittent preventive treatment
IPV	injectable polio vaccine
IQ	intelligence quotient
IRB	institutional review board
ITI	International Trachoma Initiative
ITN	insecticide-treated bednet
IUD	intrauterine device
LDL	low-density lipoprotein
LGBT	Lesbian, gay, bisexual, and transgender
LMICs	low- and middle-income countries
MCH	maternal and child health
MDG	Millennium Development Goal
MDR	multidrug resistant
MERS	Middle-East respiratory syndrome
MI	The Micronutrient Initiative (now Nutrition International)
MMR	maternal mortality rate
MSF	Doctors Without Borders (Médicins Sans Frontières in French)
NAACP	National Association for the Advancement of Colored People
NCD	noncommunicable disease
NGO	nongovernmental organization
NHS	National Health Service (United Kingdom)
NID	National Immunization Day
NIH	National Institutes of Health (United States)
NNMR	neonatal mortality rate
NTD	neglected tropical disease
OCHA	Office for the Coordination of Humanitarian Affairs
OCP	Onchocerciasis Control Program
OPV	oral polio vaccine
ORS	oral rehydration solution
ORT	oral rehydration therapy
PAHO	Pan American Health Organization
PDP	product development partnership
PEPFAR	President's Emergency Plan for AIDS Relief
PHC	primary health care

PHS	Public Health Services (United States)	SARS	severe acute respiratory infection
PMTCT	prevention of mother-to-child transmission	SDG	sustainable development goal
PPP	public–private partnership	SIDA	Swedish International Development Cooperation Agency
PTSD	post-traumatic stress disorder	SSB	sugar-sweetened beverage
QALY	quality-adjusted life year	STI	sexually transmitted infection
RBM	Roll Back Malaria	SUS	Sistema Único de Saúde (Unified Health System, Brazil)
RDT	rapid diagnostic kit	TB	tuberculosis
REC	Research Ethics Committee	TBA	traditional birth attendant
ROC	Republic of the Congo	TDR	Special Program for Research and Training in Tropical Diseases (WHO)
RR	rifampicin resistant	TFR	total fertility rate
RTI	road traffic injury	TRIPS	Agreement on Trade-R
SAFE	surgery, antibiotics, face washing, environmental change		
SAM	severe acute malnutrition		

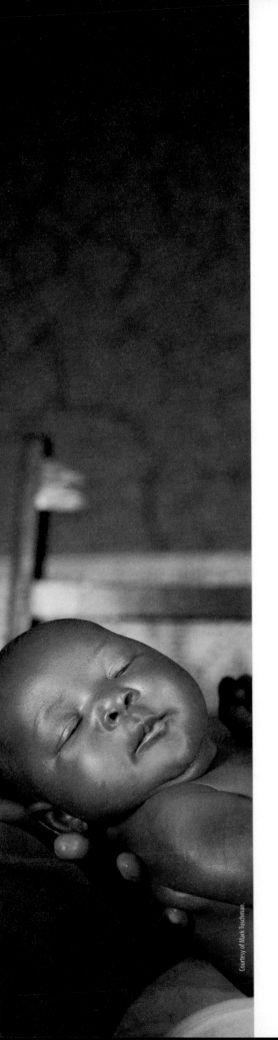

PART I

Principles, Measurements, and the Health– Development Link

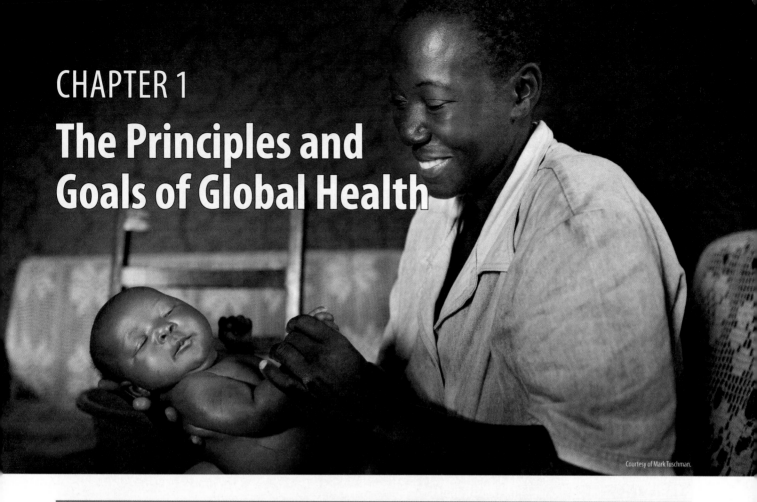

CHAPTER 1

The Principles and Goals of Global Health

LEARNING OBJECTIVES

By the end of this chapter, the reader will be able to do the following:

- Define the terms *health*, *public health*, and *global health*
- Discuss some examples of public health efforts
- Discuss some examples of global health activities
- Describe some of the guiding principles of public health work
- Describe the Sustainable Development Goals and their relation to global health
- Briefly discuss the global effort to eradicate smallpox

▶ Vignettes

By 2005, polio was on the verge of being eradicated. That year, however, rumors circulated in northern Nigeria that the polio vaccine was causing sterility. In response to these rumors, some community leaders discouraged people from immunizing their children. Within months, polio cases began to appear in the area. Shortly thereafter, polio cases spread from northern Nigeria to Sudan, Yemen, and Indonesia. The global campaign to eradicate polio had been dealt a major blow, stemming partly from rumors in one country about the alleged side effects of the vaccine.[1]

Getachew is a 20-year-old Ethiopian with HIV. He was recently placed on antiretroviral therapy for his infection. He is already gaining weight and feeling much

stronger than before. Getachew is one of about 1.2 million people in Ethiopia who are living with HIV.[2] He is also one of about 37 million people in the world who are HIV positive.[3] In Botswana, Lesotho, and Swaziland, more than 20 percent of all adults are HIV-positive.[4]

Laurie lives in Portsmouth, Virginia, in the United States. She is 50 years old and has always been healthy. Last weekend, she woke up with a headache, a high fever, and a very stiff neck. Laurie was so sick that she went to the emergency room of the local hospital. The physicians diagnosed Laurie as having meningitis, an inflammation of the membrane around the brain and spinal cord,[5] that was caused by West Nile virus. This virus originated in Egypt in the 1930s and is transmitted by mosquitoes. Today, the virus can be found in much of the world.[6]

Jim Smith is a high school student in London, England. Early in the school year, he had a fever and cough that would not go away. He did not feel like eating. He slept badly and woke up every morning in a sweat. Jim had tuberculosis (TB). Although many people think that TB has been eliminated from high-income countries, it has not.

Nirupama is a 50-year-old woman who lives in Chennai, India. Niru, as her friends call her, has diabetes. She is dependent on a regular supply of insulin, which she picks up monthly at a government clinic. Although she is only 50, she has already suffered from some of the circulatory complications of diabetes. There is a common perception that diabetes is a disease that affects only people in high-income countries. This, however, is not the case. Rather, the prevalence of diabetes is growing rapidly in low- and middle-income countries. India now has the largest number of people with diabetes among such countries.[7] Large proportions of populations in other low- and middle-income countries also suffer from this disease. More than one-third of the adults in the Marshall Islands have diabetes,[8] which is highest rate for any country in the world.[9]

▶ Why Study Global Health?

Over the last 50 years, the world has made significant progress in improving human health. Some of this progress is reflected in **TABLE 1-1**.

As shown in Table 1-1, never before have so many people lived for so long. Never before have so few young children died each year, or so few women died each year of maternal causes. There has also been enormous progress against vaccine-preventable diseases and against neglected tropical diseases, such as many parasitic infections. In addition, the consumption of tobacco, a major risk factor for noncommunicable diseases, has decreased in many countries. One reason to study global health is to gain a better understanding of the progress made so far in addressing global health problems.

Another reason to study global health, however, is to better understand the most important global

---

TABLE 1-1 Selected Progress in Global Health

- Global life expectancy increased 37% from 1960 to 2016.[1]

- The rate of child mortality fell 62% from 1990 to 2016.[2]

- Nearly 3 billion children have been vaccinated against polio, with only 22 cases of wild poliovirus cases reported in 2017.[3]

- There were 44% fewer maternal deaths in 2015 than in 1990.[4]

- Fifty-three million tuberculosis deaths were averted from 2000 to 2016 through successful diagnosis and treatment.[5]

- There were 900,000 fewer deaths due to HIV/AIDS in 2016 compared to 2005.[6]

- The number of Guinea worm cases has decreased over 99.9%, from 3.5 million in 1986 to 30 in 2017.[7]

- The global prevalence of tobacco smoking decreased from 24% in 2007 to 21% in 2015, despite population growth.[8]

---

[1]Modified from The World Bank. (n.d.). *Life expectancy at birth, total (years)*. Retrieved from https://data.worldbank.org/indicator/SP.DYN.LE00.IN

[2]UNICEF, World Health Organization, World Bank Group, & United Nations. (2017). *Levels and trends in child mortality: Report 2017*. Retrieved from http://data.unicef.org/resources/levels-trends-child-mortality/

[3]Gardner, T. J., Diop, O. M., Jorba, J., Chavan, S., Ahmed, J., & Anand, A. (2018). *Surveillance to track progress toward polio eradication—Worldwide, 2016–2017. MMWR, 67, 418–423.* doi: http://dx.doi.org/10.15585/mmwr.mm6714a3

[4]World Health Organization, UNICEF, UNFPA, World Bank Group, & the United Nations Population Division. (2015). *Trends in maternal mortality: 1990 to 2015*. Geneva, Switzerland: World Health Organization. Retrieved from http://apps.who.int/iris/bitstream/handle/10665/194254/9789241565141_eng.pdf?sequence=1

[5]World Health Organization. (2017). *Global tuberculosis report 2017*. Geneva, Switzerland: World Health OrganizationAuthor. Retrieved from http://apps.who.int/iris/bitstream/handle/10665/259366/9789241565516-eng.pdf?sequence=1

[6]UNAIDS. (2017). *Ending AIDS: Progress toward the 90-90-90 targets*. Geneva, Switzerland: Author. Retrieved from http://www.unaids.org/en/resources/documents/2017/20170720_Global_AIDS_update_2017

[7]The Carter Center. (2018, May 3). *Guinea Worm case totals*. Retrieved from https://www.cartercenter.org/health/guinea_worm/case-totals.html

[8]World Health Organization. (2017). *WHO report on the global tobacco epidemic, 2017: Monitoring tobacco use and prevention policies*. Geneva, Switzerland: Author. Retrieved from http://apps.who.int/iris/bitstream/handle/10665/255874/9789241512824-eng.pdf?sequence=1

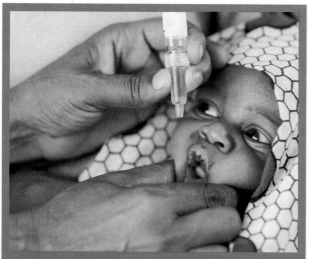

PHOTO 1-1 A child is shown here receiving polio vaccine. Although challenges to polio eradication remain, the world has made an enormous amount of progress in reducing the burden of polio. What have been some of the reasons for the success of this effort? What can be done to address the remaining challenges to eradication?
© Ranplett/E+/Getty Images.

of neonatal, maternal, and nutritional causes and of communicable diseases. It also speaks to the growing burden of noncommunicable diseases and an earlier onset of these conditions in low- and middle-income countries than in high-income countries. In addition, many countries continue to face a substantial burden of injuries, especially from road traffic accidents.

As the world becomes more globalized, the health of people everywhere must be of concern to all of us. This is particularly important because many diseases—such as TB, HIV/AIDS, and polio—are not limited by political boundaries. Prior to 1960, dengue fever was concentrated largely in Southeast Asia and the coast of South America. However, cases are now seen in five continents, as shown in **FIGURE 1-1**.[10,11]

The "avian flu" first appeared in East Asia, but it, too, is spreading to other regions. As described in the vignette at the beginning of this chapter, no one in Laurie's neighborhood ever thought of getting West Nile virus 20 years ago. Recently, the Chikungunya and Zika viruses have also been spreading globally.

There are also exceptional disparities in the health of some groups compared to the health of others. Life expectancy in Japan, for example, is 84 years, but it is only 52 years in Sierra Leone.[12] In addition, there are a number of lifesaving technologies, such as the

health challenges that remain and learn how to address them rapidly, effectively, efficiently, and fairly. **TABLE 1-2** describes some of the "unfinished agenda"

TABLE 1-2 Some of the Unfinished Agenda in Global Health

- There were 5.6 million under-5 child deaths in 2016.[1]

- Almost half of all under-5 child deaths are related to malnutrition.[1]

- There were 435,000 malaria deaths in 2017.[2]

- 1.3 million HIV-negative people died from tuberculosis in 2017, in addition to 300,000 people with HIV.[3]

- 1.8 million people became infected with HIV in 2017.[4]

- In 2017, there were 940,000 deaths caused by AIDS.[4]

- There were 303,000 maternal deaths in 2015.[5]

- Approximately 1 billion people are infected with roundworm.[6]

- The prevalence of diabetes has doubled since 1980.[7]

[1] Modified from UNICEF, World Health Organization, World Bank Group, & United Nations. (2017). *Levels and trends in child mortality: Report 2017*. Retrieved from http://data.unicef.org/resources/levels-trends-child-mortality/

[2] World Health Organization. (2018). *Malaria*. Retrived from https://www.who.int/en/news-room/fact-sheets/detail/malaria.

[3] World Health Organization. (2018). Tuberculosis. *Global Tuberculosis Report 2018*. Retrieved from https://www.who.int/tb/publications/factsheet_global.pdf?ua=1.

[4] UNAIDS. (2018, July). *Fact sheet—Latest statistics on the status of the AIDS epidemic*. Retrieved from http://www.unaids.org/en/resources/fact-sheet

[5] World Health Organization, UNICEF, UNFPA, World Bank Group, and the United Nations Population Division. (2015). *Trends in maternal mortality: 1990 to 2015*. Geneva, Switzerland: World Health Organization. http://apps.who.int/iris/bitstream/handle/10665/194254/9789241565141_eng.pdf?sequence=1

[6] Centers for Disease Control and Prevention. (2018, February). *Parasites–Ascariasis*. Retrieved from https://www.cdc.gov/parasites/ascariasis/index.html

[7] World Health Organization. (2016). *Global report on diabetes*. Geneva, Switzerland: Author. Retrieved from http://www.who.int/diabetes/global-report/en/

hepatitis B vaccine, that have been widely used in high-income countries for many years that are not yet disseminated as widely in low-income countries. These points raise important ethical and humanitarian concerns about disparities in access to health services and in health status.

The important link between health and development is another reason to pay particular attention to global health. Poor health of mothers is linked to poor health of babies and the failure of children to reach their full mental and physical potential. In addition, ill health of children can delay their entry into school and can affect their attendance, their academic performance, and, therefore, their future economic prospects. Countries with major health problems, such as high rates of malaria or HIV, have difficulty attracting the investments needed to develop their economies. Moreover, having large numbers of undernourished, unhealthy, and ill-educated people in any country can be destabilizing and poses health, economic, and security threats to all countries.

The intersectoral nature of many global health concerns and the need for different actors to work together to address them are additional reasons why we should be concerned with global health. Although locally relevant solutions are needed to address most health problems, some health issues can be solved only with a global approach. In addition, some problems, such as ensuring access to drugs to treat HIV/AIDS, may require more financial resources than some individual countries can provide. Still other global health issues require technical cooperation across countries because few countries have the technical capacity to deal with them. Global cooperation might be needed, for example, to establish standards for drug safety, to set protocols for the treatment of certain health problems, or to develop an HIV vaccine that could serve the needs of low-income countries.

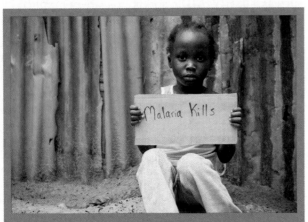

PHOTO 1-2 Despite very good progress against malaria, it is estimated that over 700,000 people died of malaria in 2016. Most of these deaths were among young children in Africa. What can be done to further reduce the burden of malaria?
© Himarkley/E+/Getty Images.

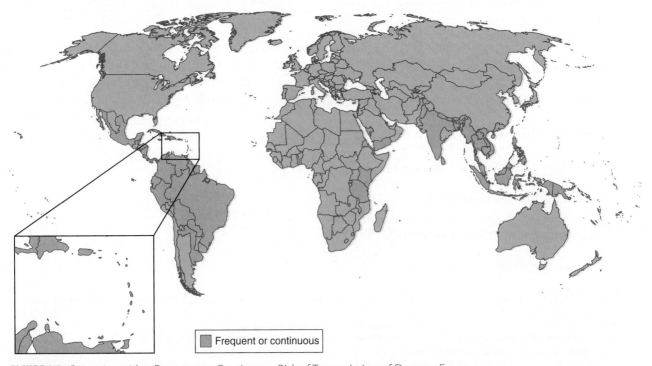

■ Frequent or continuous

FIGURE 1-1 Countries with a Frequent or Continuous Risk of Transmission of Dengue Fever

Reproduced from Sharp, T. M., Perez-Padilla, J., & Waterman, S. H. (2017). *Infectious diseases related to travel: Dengue*. Retrieved from https://wwwnc.cdc.gov/travel/yellowbook/2018/infectious-diseases -related-to-travel/dengue

The concepts and concerns of global health are also becoming increasingly prominent worldwide. The spread of HIV, the SARS scare in the early 2000s, the fear of the avian flu, and outbreaks of Ebola virus in West Africa and the Democratic Republic of the Congo have all brought attention to global health. The advocacy efforts of Doctors Without Borders, the establishment of the Millennium and Sustainable Development Goals, and the philanthropy of the Bill & Melinda Gates Foundation have also dramatically raised awareness about global health. The topic has become so important that there is a push in many universities throughout the world to ensure that all students have a basic understanding of key global health issues.

▶ Health, Public Health, and Global Health

Health

Before starting our review of global health in greater detail, it will be helpful to define health, public health, and global health. Most of us think of "health" from our individual perspective as "not being sick." The World Health Organization (WHO), however, set out a broader definition of health in 1948 that is still widely used:

> Health is a state of complete physical, mental and social well-being and not merely the absence of disease or infirmity.[13]

This is the definition of health used in this text.

Public Health

Although the WHO concept of health refers first to individuals, this book is mostly about public health

and the health of populations. C.E.A. Winslow, considered to be the founder of modern public health in the United States, formulated a definition of public health in 1923 that is still commonly used today:

> The science and the art of preventing disease, prolonging life, and promoting physical health and mental health and efficiency through organized community efforts toward a sanitary environment; the control of community infections; the education of the individual in principles of personal hygiene; the organization of medical and nursing service for the early diagnosis and treatment of disease; and the development of the social machinery to ensure to every individual in the community a standard of living adequate for the maintenance of health.[14]

According to Winslow's definition, some examples of public health activities would include the development of a campaign to promote child immunization in a particular country, an effort to get people in a city to use seat belts when they drive, and actions to get people in a specific setting to eat healthier foods and to stop smoking tobacco. In addition, most levels of government also carry out certain public health functions. These include the management of public health clinics, the operation of public health laboratories, the inspection of public eating establishments, and the maintenance of disease surveillance systems. Other examples are shown in **TABLE 1-3**.

There are a number of guiding principles to the practice of public health that have been articulated, for example, by the American Public Health Association in its public health code of ethics.[15] These principles focus on prevention of disease, respect for the rights of individuals, and a commitment to developing public health efforts in conjunction with communities.

TABLE 1-3 Selected Examples of Public Health Activities

- The promotion of handwashing
- The promotion of bicycle and motorcycle helmets
- The promotion of knowledge about HIV/AIDS
- Large-scale screening for diabetes and hypertension
- Large-scale screening of the eyesight of schoolchildren
- Mass dosing of children against worms
- The operation of a supplementary feeding program for poorly nourished young children
- The taxation of tobacco and alcohol
- The regulation of industrial pollution
- The regulation of food labeling

They also highlight the need to pay particular attention to disenfranchised people and communities and the importance of evidence-based public health interventions. In addition, they note the importance of taking account of a wide range of disciplines and appreciation for the values, beliefs, and cultures of diverse groups. Finally, they put considerable emphasis on engaging in public health practice in a way that "enhances the physical and social environment" and that builds on collaborations across public health sectors and actors.[15]

Many people confuse "public health" and "medicine," although they have quite different approaches. **TABLE 1-4** outlines these differences.[16] To a large extent, the biggest difference between the medical approach and the public health approach is the focus in public health on the health of populations rather than on the health of individuals. Exaggerating somewhat for effect, we could say, for example, that a physician cares for an individual patient whom he or she immunizes against a particular disease, whereas a public health specialist is likely to focus on how one ensures that the whole community gets vaccinated. A physician will counsel an individual patient on the need to exercise and avoid obesity; a public health specialist will work with a program meant to help a community stay sufficiently active to avoid obesity. In addition, there are branches of public health, such as **epidemiology**, that focus on studying patterns and causes of disease in specific populations and the application of this information to controlling health problems.[17] Finally, we should note the exceptional attention that public health approaches pay to the prevention of health problems.

Global Health

What exactly is *global health*? The U.S. Institute of Medicine defined global health as "health problems, issues, and concerns that transcend national boundaries and may best be addressed by cooperative actions."[18]

Another group defined what we would now call global health as "the application of the principles of public health to health problems and challenges that transcend national boundaries and to the complex array of global and local forces that affect them."[19]

The discussion of the definition of global health has continued. Two groups of distinguished public health scholars and practitioners offered additional commentaries on this matter. One group suggested that we should define global health as follows:

> An area for study, research, and practice that places a priority on improving health and achieving equity in health for all people worldwide. Global health emphasizes transnational health issues, determinants, and solutions; involves many disciplines within and beyond the health sciences and promotes interdisciplinary collaboration; and is a synthesis of population based prevention with individual-level clinical care.[20]

In response to this suggestion, however, another panel suggested that one should not distinguish between global health and public health more broadly. They also suggested that the key principles of both are the same: a focus on the public good, belief in a global perspective, a scientific and interdisciplinary approach, the need for multilevel approaches to

TABLE 1-4 Approaches of Public Health and Medicine

Differentiating Factors	Public Health	Medicine
Focus	Population	Individual
Ethical basis	Public service	Personal service
Emphasis	Disease prevention and health promotion for communities	Disease diagnosis, treatment, and care for individuals
Interventions	Broad spectrum that may target the environment, human behavior, lifestyle, and medical care	Emphasis on medical care

Modified with permission from Harvard School of Public Health. (n.d.). *About HSPH: Distinctions between public health and medicine.* Retrieved from http://www.hsph.harvard.edu/about/public-health-medicine/

interventions, and the need for comprehensive frameworks for health policies and financing.[21]

The study and practice of global health today reflects many of the above comments. Global health implies a global perspective on public health problems. It suggests issues that people face in common, such as the impact of a growing and aging worldwide population on health or the potential risks of climate change to health. The topic also relates in important ways to problems that require cooperative action. An important part of global health also covers the growing problem everywhere of noncommunicable diseases, as well as the "unfinished agenda" of the health needs of the poor in low-income countries. In practical terms, as a new student to global health, it may be best not to worry much about the definition of global health, but rather to see the topic as an important part of public health, which itself has many areas of critical importance.

Some examples of important global health concerns include the factors that contribute to women dying of pregnancy-related causes in so many countries; the exceptional amount of undernutrition among young children, especially in South Asia and Africa; and the burden of different communicable and noncommunicable diseases worldwide and what can be done to control those diseases. The impact of the environment on health globally and the effects of natural disasters and conflicts are also important to global health. The impact of climate change on health is also becoming an important global health concern. Other significant global health issues include how countries can organize and manage their health systems to enable the healthiest population possible given the resources available, the search for new technologies to address important global health problems, and how different actors can work together to solve health problems that no country or actor can solve on their own. Another global health matter of importance is the relationship between globalization and the health of different communities. Some additional global health issues are shown in **TABLE 1-5**.

▶ One Health and Planetary Health

While this text focuses on *global health*, it will also deal in a number of sections with the concept of "One Health." The American Veterinary Medical Foundation defined One Health as follows:

> The integrative effort of multiple disciplines working locally, nationally, and globally to attain optimal health for people, animals, and the environment.[22]

Learners should note that the One Health approach is getting increasing attention among those working in global health.

A related concept is referred to as Planetary Health. A report of a commission of the Rockefeller Foundation and *The Lancet* noted the following:

> Planetary health is the achievement of the highest attainable standard of health, wellbeing, and equity worldwide through judicious attention to the human systems—political, economic, and social—that shape the future of humanity and the Earth's natural systems that define the safe environmental limits within which humanity can flourish. Put simply, planetary health is the health of human civilisation and the state of the natural systems on which it depends.[23]

It may be helpful to think of One Health as focusing on the interconnectedness of animal, human, and environmental health; whereas Planetary Health has a greater focus on the health of the environment and the connections between that and human and animal well-being.

▶ Critical Global Health Concepts

In order to understand and help address key global health issues, there are a number of concepts with which one must be familiar. Some of the most important include the following:

- The determinants and social determinants of health
- The key risk factors for different health conditions
- The global burden of disease

TABLE 1-5 Selected Additional Examples of Global Health Issues

- Emerging and re-emerging infectious diseases
- Antimicrobial resistance
- Eradication of polio
- TB
- Malaria
- HIV
- The increasing prevalence of diabetes and heart disease globally

- The measurement of health status
- The demographic and epidemiologic transitions
- The organization and functions of health systems
- Links among health, education, development, poverty, and equity

Building on these concepts, those interested in global health also need to understand how key health issues, such as the following, affect different parts of the world and the world as a whole:

- Environmental health
- Nutrition
- Reproductive health
- The health of children, adolescents, and young adults
- Communicable diseases
- Noncommunicable diseases
- Injuries

Finally, it is important to understand global health issues that are generally addressed through cooperation. Some of these concern conflicts, natural disasters, and humanitarian emergencies. Others relate to the mechanisms by which different actors in global health activities work together to solve global health problems. Harnessing the power of science and technology for global health also requires cooperation. Many health issues require the action of agencies beyond the health sector, and it is critical to understand how intersectoral approaches are needed to address much of the burden of disease in any country.

▶ The Organization of Data in This Text

This is a text about global health that has a particular focus on the "health–development link." Thus, data are organized wherever possible by the seven World Bank regions:

- East Asia and Pacific
- Europe and Central Asia
- Latin America and the Caribbean
- Middle East and North Africa
- North America
- South Asia
- Sub-Saharan Africa

The World Bank regions are shown in **FIGURE 1-2**.

As you consider data by World Bank region, it is important to remember that the region that encompasses Europe contains a number of countries that are not high-income, whereas the region of North America includes only high-income countries.

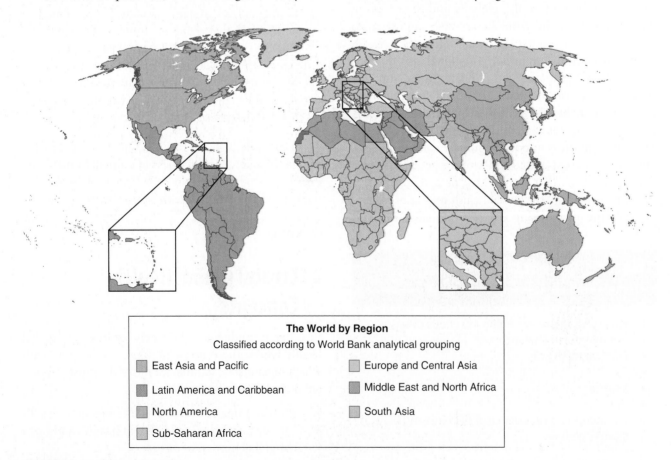

The World by Region
Classified according to World Bank analytical grouping

- East Asia and Pacific
- Latin America and Caribbean
- North America
- Sub-Saharan Africa

- Europe and Central Asia
- Middle East and North Africa
- South Asia

FIGURE 1-2 World Bank Regions

Data from The World Bank. (n.d.). World Bank country and lending groups. Retrieved from https://datahelpdesk.worldbank.org/knowledgebase/articles/906519-world-bank-country-and-lending-groups

Some critical data are organized only by the regions of WHO. WHO regions cover all countries. Those regions are as follows:

- Africa
- The Americas
- Southeast Asia
- Europe
- Eastern Mediterranean
- Western Pacific

FIGURE 1-3 shows the WHO regions.

This text presents considerable data in terms of the income level of different countries. The World Bank classifies countries into four income groups, based on estimates of their gross national income (GNI) per capita:

- Low-income economies
- Lower middle-income economies
- Upper middle-income economies
- High-income economies

For the World Bank's 2019 fiscal year, country income groups are defined as follows:

- Low-income economies: GNI per capita of $995 or less in 2017
- Lower middle-income economies: GNI per capita between $996 and $3,895

- Upper middle-income economies: GNI per capita between $3,896 and $12,055
- High-income economies: GNI per capita of $12,056 or more[24]

TABLE 1-6 shows a representative sample of countries organized by World Bank country income group.

This text contains considerable information on the burden of disease and attributable risk factors. This information is drawn largely from the *Global Burden of Diseases, Injuries, and Risk Factors Study, 2016* (*GBD 2016*), which was prepared by the Institute of Health Metrics and Evaluation (IHME).[25] Much of the data from that study is presented on the extensive burden of disease website of the IHME.[26] Findings of the study have also been published in a series of articles in *The Lancet*.[27] This text will refer to the study and all of its related parts as *The Global Burden of Disease Study 2016*, *GBD 2016*, or *GBD*.

The burden of disease data from the IHME study are complemented as needed by data published by other organizations such as UNICEF, WHO, and the World Bank. The data are also supplemented when necessary by data from earlier burden of disease studies and from data published in *Disease Control Priorities in Developing Countries*, *Second Edition* and *Third Edition*.[28,29]

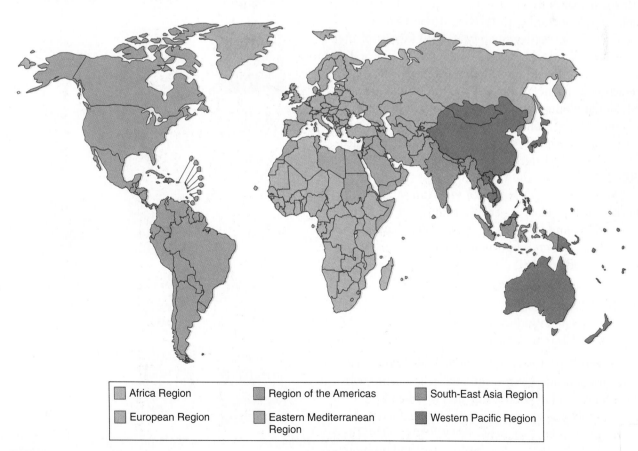

| Africa Region | Region of the Americas | South-East Asia Region |
| European Region | Eastern Mediterranean Region | Western Pacific Region |

FIGURE 1-3 WHO Regions

Data from World Health Organization. (n.d.). WHO regional offices. Retrieved from http://www.who.int/about/regions/en/

TABLE 1-6 World Bank Country Income Groups, 2018–2019, Selected Representative Countries

Low-Income	Lower Middle-Income	Upper Middle-Income	High-Income
Afghanistan	Bangladesh	Botswana	Argentina
Ethiopia	Bolivia	Costa Rica	Belgium
Haiti	Cameroon	Jamaica	Canada
Mozambique	Egypt	South Africa	Denmark
Nepal	India	Turkey	Italy
Zimbabwe	Morocco	Venezuela	Netherlands
	Philippines		Portugal
	Swaziland		Singapore

Data from the The World Bank. (n.d.). World Bank country and lending groups. Retrieved from http://data.worldbank.org/about/country-and-lending-groups

▶ The Sustainable Development Goals

This text makes frequent reference to the 17 Sustainable Development Goals (SDGs). These were formulated by the global community in 2015 as part of the 2030 Agenda for Sustainable Development.[30] The SDGs build on the Millennium Development Goals (MDGs), which were formulated in 2000 at the United Nations Millennium Summit and were articulated in the Millennium Declaration.[31] There were 8 MDGs and 15 core targets that related to them. The countries that signed the declaration pledged to meet the MDGs by 2015. **FIGURE 1-4** portrays the 17 SDGs.

Some of the SDGs have a very direct link with health, such as Goal 3—ensure healthy life and promote well-being for all at all ages. Others have a less direct but still very important link with the achievement of good health:

- Goal 1: No poverty
- Goal 2: Zero hunger
- Goal 4: Quality education
- Goal 6: Clean water and sanitation

In addition, it is easy to see how all of the goals have an important, even if indirect, relationship with the achievement of good health and well-being.

Most of the goals also have an associated set of specific targets that are to be achieved by 2020 or 2030. The targets for Goal 3—to ensure healthy lives and promote well-being for all at all ages—are shown in **TABLE 1-7**.

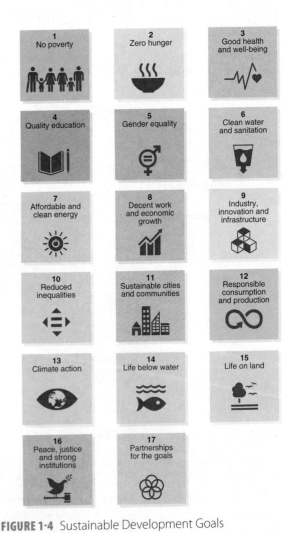

FIGURE 1-4 Sustainable Development Goals

United Nations Sustainable Development Goals Knowledge Platform. (n.d.). Sustainable Development Goals. © United Nations. Reprinted with the permission of the United Nations.

TABLE 1-7 Targets for Sustainable Development Goal 3

- By 2030, end the epidemics of AIDS, tuberculosis, malaria, and neglected tropical diseases, and combat hepatitis, waterborne diseases, and other communicable diseases.

- By 2030, reduce by one-third premature mortality from noncommunicable diseases through prevention and treatment and promote mental health and well-being.

- Strengthen the prevention and treatment of substance abuse, including narcotic drug abuse and harmful use of alcohol.

- By 2020, halve the number of global deaths and injuries from road traffic accidents.

- By 2030, ensure universal access to sexual and reproductive healthcare services, including for family planning, information and education, and the integration of reproductive health into national strategies and programs.

- Achieve universal health coverage, including financial risk protection, access to quality essential healthcare services and access to safe, effective, quality, and affordable essential medicines and vaccines for all.

- By 2030, substantially reduce the number of deaths and illnesses from hazardous chemicals and air, water, and soil pollution and contamination.

- Strengthen the implementation of the World Health Organization Framework Convention on Tobacco Control in all countries, as appropriate.

- Support the research and development of vaccines and medicines for the communicable and noncommunicable diseases that primarily affect developing countries, provide access to affordable essential medicines and vaccines, in accordance with the Doha Declaration on the TRIPS Agreement and Public Health, which affirms the right of developing countries to use to the full the provisions in the Agreement on Trade-Related Aspects of Intellectual Property Rights regarding flexibilities to protect public health, and, in particular, provide access to medicines for all.

- Substantially increase health financing and the recruitment, development, training, and retention of the health workforce in developing countries, especially in least developed countries and small island developing states.

- Strengthen the capacity of all countries, in particular developing countries, for early warning, risk reduction, and management of national and global health risks.

United Nations Sustainable Development Goals Knowledge Platform. (n.d.). Sustainable Development Goals. © United Nations. Reprinted with the permission of the United Nations.

▶ Case Study: Smallpox Eradication—The Most Famous Success Story

It is fitting to end the main part of this introductory chapter with a summary of the most famous public health success story of all: the case of smallpox eradication. This effort was not only a great triumph of public health but also a great accomplishment for humanity. In addition, the history of smallpox eradication is well known to everyone who works in public health, and it provides many lessons that can be applied to other public health efforts.

Background

In 1966, smallpox ravaged over 50 countries, affecting 10 million to 15 million people, of whom almost 2 million died each year.[32] At the time, smallpox killed as many as 30 percent of those infected. Those w survived could suffer from deep-pitted scars blindness as a result of their illness.[33]

The Intervention

Although a vaccine against smallpox was created by Edward Jenner in 1798, eradication of smallpox became a practical goal only in the 1950s, when the vaccine could be mass produced and stored without refrigeration. A later breakthrough came in the form of the bifurcated needle, a marvel of simple technology that dramatically reduced costs by allowing needles to be reused endlessly after sterilization and by requiring a far smaller amount of vaccine per patient than had previously been the case. The needle also made vaccination easy, thereby reducing the time and effort required to train villagers in its use.

In 1959, WHO adopted a proposal to eradicate smallpox through compulsory vaccination, but the program languished until 1965, when the United States stepped in with technical and financial support. A Smallpox Eradication Unit was established at WHO, headed by Dr. D. A. Henderson of the Centers for Disease Control and Prevention (CDC) in the United States. As part of the smallpox eradication program, all WHO member countries were required to manage program funds effectively, report smallpox cases, encourage research on smallpox, and maintain flexibility in the implementation of the smallpox program to suit local conditions.

The Smallpox Eradication Unit proved to be a small but committed team, supplying vaccines and specimen kits to those countries that still had smallpox. Although wars and civil unrest caused disruptions in the program's progress, momentum was always regained with new methods and extra resources that focused on containing outbreaks by speedily seeking out new cases with motorized teams, isolating new cases, and vaccinating everyone in the vicinity of the new cases.

This military-style approach proved effective even in the most difficult circumstances. It also took practical account of the facts that (1) it would have been extraordinarily difficult to immunize the whole world against smallpox, and (2) the transmission of the smallpox virus could be stopped by focusing vaccination efforts around new cases.

The Impact

In 1977, the last endemic case of smallpox in the world was recorded in Somalia. In 1980, after additional surveillance and searching, WHO declared smallpox the first disease in history to have been eradicated. Smallpox had previously been eliminated in Latin America in 1971 and in Asia in 1975.[34]

Costs and Benefits

The annual cost of the eradication campaign between 1967 and 1979 was $23 million U.S. dollars (from here on, the dollar sign will refer to U.S. dollars unless otherwise stated). For the whole campaign, international donors provided $98 million, and $200 million came from the endemic countries.[31] The United States saves the total of all its contributions every 26 days because it no longer needs to spend money on vaccination or treatment, making smallpox eradication one of the best-value health accomplishments ever achieved.[35] Estimates for

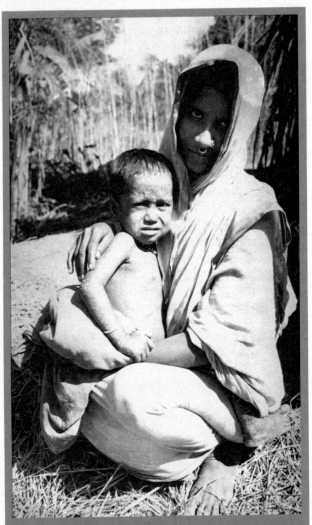

PHOTO 1-3 This photo shows the last person in the world to have suffered from the natural transmission of *variola major*, a 3-year-old girl in Bangladesh named Rahima Banu. This occurred in late 1975. In 1977, Ali Maow Maalin, a Somali, was the last person to have naturally acquired smallpox caused by *variola minor*. Why was smallpox chosen for eradication? What factors were behind the success of the eradication effort? Are there diseases today that are good candidates for eradication?

Stanley O. Foster M.D., M.P.H., World Health Organization/CDC. Centers for Disease Control and Prevention. (2016). *History of smallpox.* Retrieved from https://www.cdc.gov/smallpox/history/history.html

economic loss due to smallpox being endemic in a low- or middle-income country are available only for India. Based on these, it has been estimated that low- and middle-income countries as a whole suffered economic losses related to smallpox of about $1 billion each year at the start of the intensified campaign.[36]

Lessons Learned

The success of the smallpox eradication program can be attributed to the political commitment and leadership exemplified in the partnership between WHO and the U.S. Centers for Disease Control and Prevention. Success in individual countries hinged on having someone who was responsible, preferably solely, for the eradication effort. In addition, small WHO teams made frequent field trips to review progress, and a small number of committed people working in the program were able to motivate large numbers of staff. Moreover, in the days before the internet and email, the program managers held a monthly meeting in which they exchanged information about the progress of the campaign and the lessons learned from working on it in different countries.

No two national campaigns were alike, and flexibility was an essential asset in the design of this program. The plan for eradicating smallpox used existing healthcare systems and enabled many countries to improve their health services. This benefited immunization programs more generally and also offset the cost of the initial smallpox campaign.

Monitoring standards were established across the program to constantly evaluate progress against agreed benchmarks. Community participation provided strategic lessons for later community-based projects. The value of publicity was highlighted when news about the program's progress triggered large donations in 1974 to complete eradication in five remaining countries. An important discovery made during the campaign was that immunization programs could vaccinate people against more than one disease at a time. This helped to pave the way for routine immunization.

The eradication of smallpox continues to inspire efforts against other diseases, but it must be remembered that the particular features of smallpox made it a prime candidate for eradication. The disease was passed directly between people, without an intervening carrier, so there were no reservoirs; the distinctive rash of smallpox made diagnosis easy; survivors gained lifetime immunity; and the severity of symptoms, once the disease became infectious, made patients take to their beds and infect few others. Good vaccination coverage could therefore disrupt transmission entirely. Unfortunately, almost 30 years after eradication, funds are still allocated to precautionary measures against the disease because of the continuing threat of smallpox being used as an agent of bioterrorism.

▶ Central Messages of This Text

Because this is the introductory chapter of the text, it does not end with a summary, as the other chapters do. Rather, it is more valuable to end this chapter by highlighting some of the central messages of the text as a whole. They are listed without citations or recitation of the evidence behind them. That evidence is provided and cited in the chapters that follow. It is very important to keep these messages in mind while reading the rest of the text.

- Most countries regard health as a human right. Toward this aim, they seek to achieve a system of universal health coverage. This is a package of health services linked to mechanisms to protect people from the costs of healthcare services. Universal health coverage is well developed in most high-income countries. Most low-income countries do not yet have well-developed systems of universal health coverage.
- There are strong links among health, human development, labor productivity, and economic development.
- Health status is determined by a variety of factors, including age, culture, income, education, knowledge of healthy behaviors, social status, sex, genetic makeup, and access to health services. The economic and social conditions under which people live, as well as government policies, also have an important influence on people's health.
- Given the wide range in the determinants of health, it is fundamental to think and act broadly in health policy—in some respects more like a minister of finance must think and act, rather than how a minister of health would act.
- There has been enormous progress in improving health status over the last 50 years in many countries. This is reflected in the substantial increases these countries have witnessed in that period, for example, in life expectancy and the substantial reductions in the deaths of children under 5 years of age.
- Some of this progress has come about as a result of overall economic development and improvements in income. However, much of it is due to

improvements in public hygiene, better water supply and sanitation, and better education. Increased nutritional status has also had a large impact on improvements in health status. Technical progress in some areas, such as the development and dissemination of vaccines against childhood diseases and antibiotics, has also improved human health.

- There are proven packages of investments that can address a range of issues related to neonatal, maternal, and child health and communicable diseases. However, they have not yet been taken to sufficient scale in many low- and middle-income countries.

- There is an increasing amount of evidence about measures that can be taken, on a large scale, to reduce the risk of and address noncommunicable diseases in cost-effective ways. However, many low- and middle-income countries are only now beginning to take steps to reduce the burden of noncommunicable diseases. Many high-income countries have also failed to address these issues effectively at scale.

- The progress in improving health status has been very uneven. Hundreds of millions of people, especially poor people in low- and middle-income countries, continue to get sick, be disabled by, or die from preventable causes of disease. In many countries, the nutritional status and health status of lower-income people have improved only slowly. In addition, HIV/AIDS caused a decline in health, nutritional status, and life expectancy in a number of countries in sub-Saharan Africa and the former Soviet Union.

- There are enormous disparities in health status and access to health services both within and across countries. Wealthier people in most countries have better health status and better access to health services than poorer people. In general, urban dwellers and ethnic majorities enjoy better health status than rural people and disadvantaged ethnic minorities. In addition, women face a number of unique challenges to their health, as do lesbian, gay, bisexual, and transgender (LGBT) people, prisoners, and other marginalized people.

- There are exceptional gaps in the quality of health services everywhere, but especially in low- and middle-income countries. Poor-quality health services not only fail to achieve their aims but they are also dangerous to people's health. Major attention needs to be paid to ensuring that health servces are of appropriate quality.

- Countries do not need to be high-income to enjoy good health status. By contrast, there are a number of examples, such as China, Costa Rica, Cuba, Kerala state in India, and Sri Lanka, that make clear that low-income countries or low-income areas within countries can help their people achieve good health, even in the absence of extensive financial resources to do so. However, this requires strong political will and a focus on public hygiene, education, and low-cost but high-yield investments in nutrition and health.

- In this light, when considering health policy, one must always seek value for money and ask: "If we only had $100 to spend, how should we spend it to achieve the maximum health for our people, at least cost, and in doable, sustainable, and fair ways?"

- The burden of disease is evolving in light of economic and social changes, aging populations, and scientific and technical progress, among other things. The burden of disease is predominantly communicable, maternal, neonatal, and nutritional only in sub-Saharan Africa. In all other regions, the burden of disease is predominantly noncommunicable. In the absence of new communicable disease threats of major importance, the burden of disease is expected to shift universally toward noncommunicable disease. Climate change could also have an important impact on health.

- Some global health issues can be solved only through the cooperation of various actors in global health. This could include, for example, the eradication of polio.

- An important part of health status is determined by an individual's and family's own knowledge of health and hygiene. People and communities have tremendous abilities to enhance their own health status.

- Nonetheless, political circumstances, the quality of governance, and the level of government commitment to equity all have an important bearing on the health of a people.

- The world is increasingly becoming interconnected at a rapid pace. For both security and humanitarian reasons, each of us should be concerned about the health of everyone else.

- Taking account of these points, we could say, in many respects, that low-income countries should focus on "burying old people, instead of young people, making the transition as fast as possible, and doing so at least cost and in fair ways."

- Taking account of these points, we could also say, in many respects, that the health goals for all countries are to enable the maximum health for their people, in fairly distributed ways, at least cost.

Study Questions

1. What are some examples of important progress in improving health worldwide over the last 50 years?
2. What are some of the global health challenges that remain to be addressed?
3. How might one define *health*, *public health*, and *global health*?
4. What are some examples of public health activities?
5. What are some examples of global health issues?
6. What are the key differences between the approach of medicine and the approach of public health?
7. What are some of the most important challenges to health globally?
8. Why should everyone be concerned about critical global health issues?
9. What are the Sustainable Development Goals, and how do they relate to health?
10. What were some of the keys to the eradication of smallpox? What lessons does the smallpox eradication program suggest for other global health programs?

References

1. World Health Organization. (2004, August 24). *New polio cases confirmed in Guinea, Mali and the Sudan.* Retrieved from http://www.who.int/mediacentre/news/releases/2004/pr57/en
2. UNICEF Ethiopia. (n.d.). *Introduction—HIV/AIDS.* Retrieved from https://www.unicef.org/ethiopia/hiv_aids.html
3. UNAIDS. (n.d.). *Global HIV & AIDS statistics—2018 fact sheet.* Retrieved from http://www.unaids.org/en/resources/fact-sheet
4. WorldAtlas.com. (2017). *Countries with the highest rates of HIV/AIDS.* Retrieved from https://www.worldatlas.com/articles/countries-with-the-highest-rates-of-hiv-aids.html
5. Centers for Disease Control and Prevention. (2018). *Meningococcal disease.* Retrieved from http://www.cdc.gov/meningococcal/
6. World Health Organization. (2011). *West Nile virus.* Retrieved from http://www.who.int/mediacentre/factsheets/fs354/en/
7. International Diabetes Federation. (2017). *IDF Diabetes Atlas* (8th Ed.). Retrieved from http://www.diabetesatlas.org/IDF_Diabetes_Atlas_8e_interactive_EN/
8. WorldAtlas.com. (2018). *Countries with the highest rates of diabetes.* Retrieved from https://www.worldatlas.com/articles/countries-with-the-highest-rates-of-diabetes.html
9. Statista. (n.d.). *Countries with the highest prevalence of diabetes worldwide, 2017.* Retrieved from https://www.statista.com/statistics/241814/countries-with-highest-number-of-diabetics/
10. World Health Organization. (2014). Dengue, countries or areas at risk, 2013 [Map]. Retrieved from http://gamapserver.who.int/mapLibrary/Files/Maps/Global_DengueTransmission_ITHRiskMap.png
11. World Health Organization. (n.d.). *Dengue control—Epidemiology.* Retrieved from https://www.who.int/denguecontrol/epidemiology/en/.
12. The World Bank. (n.d.). *Data: Life expectancy at birth, total (years).* Retrieved from https://data.worldbank.org/indicator/SP.DYN.LE00.IN?view=chart
13. World Health Organization. (1946). *Preamble to the Constitution of the World Health Organization 1946, as adopted by the International Health Conference, New York, 19 June–22 July 1946.* Retrieved from http://apps.who.int/gb/bd/PDF/bd47/EN/constitution-en.pdf
14. Merson, M. H., Black, R. E., & Mills, A. (2001). *International public health: Diseases, programs, systems, and policies* (p. xvii). Gaithersburg, MD: Aspen Publishers.
15. American Public Health Association. (2002). *Principles of the ethical practice of public health.* Retrieved from https://www.apha.org/-/media/files/pdf/membergroups/ethics/ethics_brochure.ashx
16. Harvard School of Public Health. (n.d.). *Distinctions between medicine and public health.* Retrieved from http://www.hsph.harvard.edu/about/public-health-medicine/
17. Last, J. M. (2001). *A dictionary of epidemiology* (4th ed.). New York, NY: Oxford University Press.
18. Institute of Medicine. (1998). *America's vital interest in global health: Protecting our people, enhancing our economy, and advancing our international interests.* Washington, DC: National Academy Press.
19. Merson, M. H., Black, R. E., & Mills, A. (2001). *International public health: Diseases, programs, systems, and policies* (p. xix). Gaithersburg, MD: Aspen Publishers.
20. Koplan, J. P., Bond, T. C., Merson, M. H., Reddy, K. S., Rodriguez, M. H., Sewankambo, N. K., & Wasserheit, J. N. (2009). Towards a common definition of global health. *The Lancet, 373*(9679), 1993–1995.
21. Fried, L. P., Bentley, M. E., Buekens, P., Burke, D. S., Frenk, J. J., Klag, M. J., & Spencer, H. C. (2010). Global health is public health. *The Lancet, 375*(9714), 535–537.
22. American Veterinary Medical Foundation (AVMA). (n.d.). *One Health—It's all connected.* Retrieved from https://www.avma.org/KB/Resources/Reference/Pages/One-Health.aspx
23. Whitmee, S., Haines, A., Beyrer, C., Boltz, F., Capon, A. G., de Souza Dias, B. F., . . . Yach, D. (2015). Safeguarding human health in the Anthropocene epoch: Report of The Rockefeller Foundation–Lancet Commission on planetary health. *The Lancet, 386*(10007), 1973–2028. doi: https://doi.org/10.1016/S0140-6736(15)60901-1
24. The World Bank. (n.d.). World Bank country and lending groups. Retrieved from https://datahelpdesk.worldbank.org/knowledgebase/articles/906519-world-bank-country-and-lending-groups

25. Global Health Data Exchange (GHDx). (n.d.). *Global burden of disease study 2016: Data resources.* Retrieved from http://ghdx.healthdata.org/gbd-2016

26. Institute of Health Metrics and Evaluation (IHME). (n.d.). GBD Compare: Viz Hub. Retrieved from https://vizhub.healthdata.org/gbd-compare/

27. Life, death, and disability, 2016 [Editorial]. (2017). *The Lancet, 390*(10100), 1083. Retrieved from https://www.thelancet.com/journals/lancet/article/PIIS0140-6736(17)32465-0/fulltext

28. Jamison, D. E. A. (Ed.). (2006). *Disease control priorities in developing countries* (2nd ed.). New York, NY: Oxford University Press and the World Bank.

29. Jamison, D. T., Nugent, R., Gelband, H., Horton, S., Jha, P., & Laxminarayan, R. (Eds.). (2018). *Disease control priorities: Improving health and reducing poverty* (3rd ed., Vol. 9). Washington, DC: The World Bank.

30. United Nations. (n.d.). Sustainable Development Goals. Retrieved from https://www.un.org/sustainabledevelopment/

31. United Nations. (2000). *55/2: United Nations millennium declaration.* Retrieved from http://www.un.org/millennium/declaration/ares552e.htm

32. Center for Global Development. (n.d.). *Case 1: Eradicating smallpox.* Retrieved from http://www.cgdev.org/page/case-1-eradicating-smallpox

33. Roberts, M. (2005, July 3). How doctors killed off smallpox. *BBC News.* Retrieved from http://news.bbc.co.uk/1/hi/health/4072392.stm

34. Fenner, F. (1988). *Smallpox and its eradication.* Geneva, Switzerland: World Health Organization.

35. Levine, R., & the What Works Working Group. (2007). *Case studies in global health: Millions saved.* Sudbury, MA: Jones and Bartlett.

36. Brilliant, L. B. (1985). *The management of smallpox eradication in India.* Ann Arbor: University of Michigan Press.

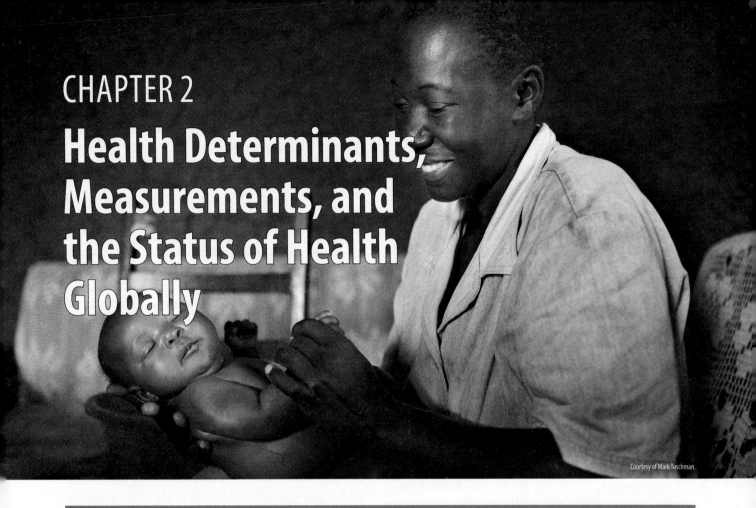

CHAPTER 2
Health Determinants, Measurements, and the Status of Health Globally

LEARNING OBJECTIVES

By the end of this chapter, the reader will be able to do the following:

- Describe the determinants of health
- Define the most important health indicators and key terms related to measuring health status and the burden of disease
- Discuss the status of health globally and how it varies by country income group, region, and age group

▶ Vignettes

Maria is a poor woman who lives in the highlands of Peru. She is from an ethnic group called Quechua. In Peru, poor people tend to live in the mountains and be indigenous, be less educated, and have worse health status than other people. In Eastern Europe, the same issues occur among ethnic groups that are of lower socioeconomic status, such as the Roma people. In the United States, there are also enormous health disparities, as seen in the health status of African Americans and Native Americans, compared to white Americans. If we want to understand and address differences in health status among different groups, how do we measure health status? Do we measure it by age? By gender? By socioeconomic status? By level of education? By ethnicity? By location?

Yevgeny is a 56-year-old Russian male. Life expectancy in Russia in 1985 was about 64 years for males and 74 years for females. It then fell to about 59 years for males and 72 years for females in 2001,[1] before rising again to 67 for males[2] and 77 for females[3] in 2016. What does life expectancy at birth measure? What are the factors contributing to the earlier decline in life expectancy at birth in Russia? What has happened to trends in life expectancy in other countries? Which countries have the longest and shortest life expectancies, and why?

Sarah is a 27-year-old woman in northern Nigeria. While women in high-income countries very rarely die of pregnancy-related causes and have a maternal mortality ratio of about 10 per 100,000 live births, the maternal mortality ratio for women in low-income countries like Sarah is about 500 per 100,000 live births.[4] This is 50 times higher than that in the best-off country income group. What does the maternal mortality ratio suggest about a country? What does it say about the status of women in that country? What does it indicate about the access of women to obstetric and emergency obstetric care of appropriate quality?

Abdul is a 4-year-old in northern India. For every 1,000 children born in South Asia in 2016, about 50 will die before their fifth birthday. The rate of child death is even higher in sub-Saharan Africa. In the cohort of 1,000 children born there in 2016, almost 80 will die before they are five. These two regions have the worst child mortality rates.[5]

▸ The Importance of Measuring Health Status

If we want to understand the most important global health issues and what can be done to address them, then we must understand what factors have the most influence on health status, as well as how health status is measured.

This chapter, therefore, covers two distinct but closely related topics. The first section concerns what are called *the determinants of health*. That section examines the most important factors that relate to people's health status. The second section reviews some of the most important indicators of health status and how they are used.

▸ The Determinants and Social Determinants of Health

Why are some people healthy and some people not healthy? When asked this question, many of us will respond that good health depends on access to health services. Yet, as you will learn, whether or not people are healthy depends on a large number of factors, many of which are interconnected, and most of which go considerably beyond access to health services.

The World Health Organization (WHO) defines the **determinants of health** as the "range of personal, social, economic and environmental factors which determine the health status of individuals or populations."[6] WHO defines the social determinants of health as the "conditions in which people are born, grow, live, work and age."[7]

There has been considerable writing about the determinants and social determinants of health, which different organizations depict in a range of ways. The next section builds on the work of a number of actors and agencies. It briefly discusses the determinants and social determinants of health and how they influence health. It is essential to understand these concepts if one wants to understand why people are healthy or not and what can be done to address different health conditions in different settings. **FIGURE 2-1** shows one way of depicting the determinants of health.

The first group of factors that helps to determine health relates to the personal and inborn features of individuals. These include genetic makeup, sex, and age. Our genetic makeup contributes to what diseases we get and how healthy we are. One can inherit, for example, a genetic marker for a particular disease, such as Huntington's disease, which is a neurological disorder. One can also inherit the genetic component of a disease that has multiple causes, such as breast cancer. Sex also has an important relationship with health. Males and females are physically different, for example, and may get different diseases. Females face the risks involved in childbearing. They also get cervical and uterine cancers that males do not. Females have higher rates of certain health conditions, such as thyroid and breast cancers. For similar reasons, age is also an important determinant of health. Young children in low- and middle-income countries often die of diarrheal disease, whereas older people are much more likely to die of heart disease, to cite one of many examples of the relationship between health and age.

Individual lifestyle factors, including people's own health practices and behaviors, are also important determinants of health. Being able to identify when you or a family member is ill and needs health care can be critical to good health. One's health also depends greatly on how one eats, or if one smokes tobacco, drinks too much alcohol, or drives safely. We also know that being active physically and getting exercise regularly is better for one's health than is being sedentary.

The extent to which people receive social support from family, friends, and community also has an important link with health.[8] The stronger the social networks and the stronger the support that people get from those networks, the healthier people will be. Of course, culture is also an extremely important determinant of health.[9]

Living and working conditions also exert an enormous influence on health. These include, for example, housing, access to safe water and sanitation, access to nutritious food, and access to health services. Crowded housing, for example, is a risk factor for the transmission of tuberculosis. The lack of safe water and sanitation, coupled with poor hygiene in many settings, is one of the major risk factors for the diarrheal disease that is associated with so much illness and death in young children. Nutrition is central to health,

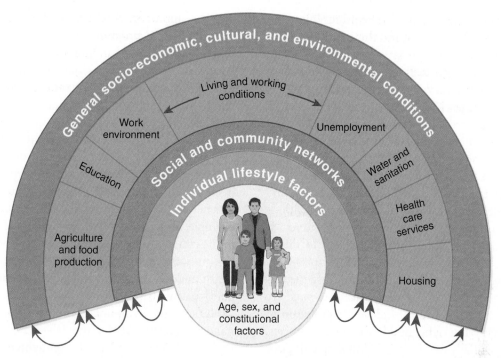

FIGURE 2-1 The Determinants of Health

Reproduced from Dahlgren, G., & Whitehead, M. (1991). *Policies and strategies to promote social equity in health*. Stockholm, Sweden: Institute for Futures Studies. Retrieved from http://www.iffs.se/media/1326/20080109110739filmZ8UVQv2wQFShMRF6cuT.pdf

beginning at conception, and families have to be able to access appropriate foods to promote good health. Of course, even if other factors are such important determinants of health, one's health *does* depend on access to appropriate healthcare services. Even if one is born and raised healthy and engages in good health behaviors, access to health services of appropriate quality is important to maintaining good health. To address the risk of dying from a complication of pregnancy, for example, one must have access to health services that can carry out an emergency cesarean section if necessary. Even if the mother has had the suggested level of prenatal care and has prepared well in all other respects for the pregnancy, in the end, certain complications can only be addressed in a healthcare setting.

A range of socioeconomic factors, including culture, education, and socioeconomic status, are important determinants of health. The broader environment is also a critical health determinant. Socioeconomic status refers to a person's economic, social, and work status. It is highly correlated with educational attainment. People with higher educational attainment have better economic opportunities, higher socioeconomic status, and more control over their lives than people of lower educational status. As one's socioeconomic status improves, so does his or her health.[10]

More specifically, education is a powerful determinant of health for several reasons. First, it brings with it knowledge of good health practices. Second, it provides opportunities for gaining skills, getting

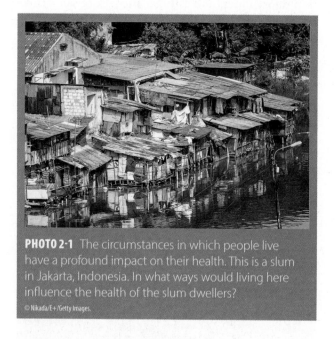

PHOTO 2-1 The circumstances in which people live have a profound impact on their health. This is a slum in Jakarta, Indonesia. In what ways would living here influence the health of the slum dwellers?
© Nikada/E+/Getty Images.

better employment, raising one's income, and enhancing one's social status, all of which are also related to health. Studies have shown, for example, that the single best predictor of the birthweight of a baby is the level of educational attainment of the mother.[11] Most of us already know that throughout the world there is an extremely strong and positive correlation between the level of education and all key health indicators. People who are better educated eat better, smoke less, have less obesity, have fewer children, and take better care of their children's health than do people with less education. It is not a surprise, therefore, that they and their children live longer and healthier lives than do less well-educated people and their children.

Culture also exerts a profound impact on health. Culture shapes how one feels about health and illness, how one uses health services, and the health practices in which one engages. In addition, the gender roles that are ascribed to women in many societies also have an important impact on health. In some settings, women may be treated more poorly than men and this, in turn, may mean that women have less income, less education, and fewer opportunities to engage in employment. All of these militate against their good health.

The environment, both indoor and outdoor, is a powerful determinant of health. Related to this is the safety of the environment in which people work. Although many people know about the consequences of outdoor air pollution for health, fewer people are aware of the consequences of indoor air pollution to health. In many low- and middle-income countries, families, and usually women, cook indoors with poor ventilation, thereby creating an indoor environment that may be full of smoke and that increases the risk of respiratory illness and asthma. The lack of safe drinking water and sanitation is a major contributor to ill health in poor countries. In addition, many people in those same countries work in environments that are unhealthy. Because they lack skills, socioeconomic status, and opportunities, they may work without sufficient protection from hazardous chemicals, in polluted air, or in circumstances that expose them to occupational accidents.

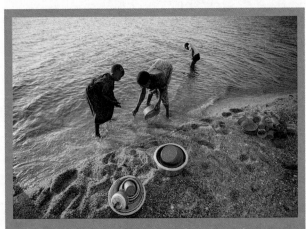

PHOTO 2-2 The lack of access to safe water and sanitation causes people to seek water from unsafe sources and is a major risk factor for child deaths. Children are shown here washing their dishes in a river. What can be done to improve access to safe water and sanitary disposal of human waste in resource-poor environments?
Courtesy of Mark Tuschman.

The approach that governments take to different policies and programs in the health sector and in other sectors also has an important bearing on people's health. People living in a country that promotes high educational attainment, for example, will be healthier than people in a country that does not promote widespread education of appropriate quality because better-educated people engage in healthier behaviors. A country that has universal health insurance is likely to have healthier people than a country that does not insure its entire population because the uninsured may lack needed health services. The same would be true, for example, for a country that promoted safe water supply for its entire population, compared to one that did not.

As we think about the determinants of health, we should be aware that increasing attention is being paid to the social determinants of health. In 2005, WHO created a Commission on the Social Determinants of Health. WHO published the commission's report in 2008. The report highlighted some of the following themes[12]:

- Health status is improving in some places in the world but not in others.
- There are enormous differences in the health status of individuals within countries, as well as across countries.
- The health differences within countries are closely linked with social disadvantage.
- Many of these differences should be considered avoidable, and they relate to the way in which people live and work and the health systems that should serve them.
- People's life circumstances, and therefore their health, are profoundly related to political, social, and economic forces.
- Countries need to ensure that these forces are oriented toward improving the life circumstances of the poor, thereby enabling them to enjoy a healthier life as well. The global community should also work toward this end.

We should also note the importance to health of child development, including the ways in which families nourish and care for infants and young children, beginning at conception. Being born premature or of low birthweight can have important negative consequences on health over the life course. There is a strong correlation between the nutritional status of infants and young children and the extent to which they meet their biological and intellectual potential, enroll in school, or stay in school. In addition, poor nutritional status in infancy and early childhood may be linked with a number of noncommunicable diseases later in life, including diabetes and heart disease.[13] There is also considerable evidence that a range of stressors, including poverty, abuse, and discrimination, have a powerful impact on the health of children that may continue through adulthood.[14]

Finally, as we think about the determinants and social determinants of health, it is important to consider how, directly and indirectly, different factors influence health. One framework for such consideration is shown in **FIGURE 2-2**. This framework places the determinants of health into three categories based on the directness of their influence on health: root causes at the macro/societal level; underlying causes at the meso/community level; and proximal causes at the immediate/interpersonal level. Viewing the determinants of health in this manner should also be helpful in assessing why health conditions exist and what can be done to address them.

▶ Key Health Indicators

It is critical that we use data and evidence to understand and address key global health issues. Some types of health data concern the health status of people and communities, such as measures of life expectancy and infant and child mortality, as discussed further hereafter. Some concern health services, such as the number of nurses and doctors per capita in a country or the indicators of coverage for certain health services, such as immunization. Other data concern the financing of health, such as the amount of public expenditure on health or the share of national income represented by health expenditure.

There are a number of very important uses of data on health status.[15] We need data, for example, to know from what health conditions people suffer. We also need to know the extent to which these conditions cause people to be sick, be disabled, or die. We need data to carry out disease surveillance. This helps us understand if particular health problems such as cancer, influenza, polio, or malaria are occurring, where they are infecting people, who is getting infected, and what might be done to address these conditions. Other forms of data also help us to understand the burden of different health conditions, the relative importance of them to different societies, and the importance that should be given to dealing with them.

If we are to use data in the previously mentioned ways, then it is important that we use a consistent set of

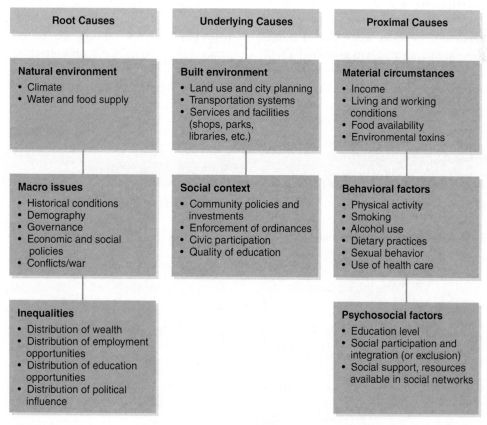

FIGURE 2-2 Selected Examples of Root, Underlying, and Immediate Determinants of Health

Modified with permission from Bouwman, L., Wentink, C., & Ormond, M. (2017, April 6). Global Health, W3 Tutorial 3: Determinants [Powerpoint Slides], Based on Northridge.

indicators to measure health status. In this way, we can make comparisons across people in the same country or across different countries. There are, in fact, a number of indicators that are used most commonly by those who work in global health and in development work. These are listed and defined in **TABLE 2-1**.

The section that follows will examine these key indicators of health status in two ways, first by World Bank region and second by country income group. The graphics will reflect a number of points quite starkly:

- There is a very strong correlation between country income group and health status. The lower the income group, the lower the status; the higher the income group, the higher the status.
- In all cases, sub-Saharan Africa has the worst health indicators of all World Bank regions, and South Asia has the second worst health indicators.

You will understand better as you progress in your study of global health that part of the relatively low health status of sub-Saharan Africa and South Asia *is* related to the fact that these are the two regions with the lowest per capita income. However, as you will read about here and elsewhere, their relatively low health status also has to do with government policies and programs, the lack of safe water and sanitation, low levels of education, and a number of other factors.

It is also important to understand that country income level does not have to determine a country's health status. Rather, as you will also read about throughout this text and elsewhere, resource-poor countries that make wise policy choices in fair ways

can enable better health for their people than their income level might suggest. This has certainly been the case for a number of countries whose development history is well known, such as Cuba, Sri Lanka, and China. Thus, it will be essential as you think about key issues in global health to always keep in mind questions about which policies can help to achieve the best health for any population at the least cost and in fair, doable, and sustainable ways. In light of all this, let us now turn to exploring the specific health indicators.

Among the most commonly used indicators of health status is **life expectancy at birth**. Life expectancy at birth is "the average number of additional years a newborn baby can be expected to live if current mortality trends were to continue for the rest of that person's life."[16(p58)] In other words, it measures how long a person born today can expect to live, if there were no change in their lifetime in the present rate of death for people of different ages. The higher the life expectancy at birth, the better the health status of a country. In the United States, a high-income country, life expectancy at birth in 2016 was about 79 years; in Jordan, a middle-income country, life expectancy was 74 years; in Sierra Leone, a very low-income country, life expectancy was 52 years.[17]

FIGURE 2-3 shows life expectancy at birth by country income level. This figure shows an exceptional correlation between country income group and life expectancy. It also shows the range of life expectancy across country income groups, from 63 years in low-income countries to 29 percent higher, or 81 years, in high-income countries.

TABLE 2-1 Key Health Status Indicators
Infant mortality rate: The number of deaths of infants under age 1 per 1,000 live births in a given year
Life expectancy at birth: The average number of years a newborn baby could expect to live if current mortality trends were to continue for the rest of the newborn's life
Maternal mortality ratio: The number of women who die as a result of pregnancy and childbirth complications per 100,000 live births in a given year
Neonatal mortality rate: The number of deaths of infants under 28 days of age in a given year per 1,000 live births in that year
Under-5 mortality rate (child mortality rate): The probability that a newborn baby will die before reaching age 5, expressed as a number per 1,000 live births

Modified from Soubbotina, T. P. (2004). Glossary. In *Beyond economic growth: An introduction to sustainable development*. Washington, DC: The World Bank. Retrieved from http://documents .worldbank.org/curated/en/454041468780615049/Beyond-economic-growth-an-introduction-to-sustainable-development

FIGURE 2-4 shows life expectancy by World Bank region. It reflects the points noted previously, with sub-Saharan Africa and South Asia having the lowest life expectancy. It is also important to note that the region with the highest life expectancy has a life expectancy that is 19 years, or about 30 percent, greater than the region with the lowest life expectancy.

The **maternal mortality ratio** is a measure of the risk of death that is associated with childbirth. Because these deaths are more rare than infant and child deaths, the maternal mortality ratio is measured as "the number of women who die as a result of pregnancy and childbirth complications per 100,000 live births in a given year."[16(p28)] The rarity of maternal deaths and the fact that they largely occur in low-income settings also contribute to maternal mortality being quite difficult to measure. Very few women die in childbirth in rich countries; for example, the maternal mortality ratio in Sweden in 2016 was 4 per 100,000 live births. On the other hand, in very poor countries, in which women have low status and where there are few facilities for dealing with obstetric emergencies, the ratios can be over 700 per 100,000 live births, as they were in 2016, for example, in the Central African Republic, Liberia, Nigeria, Somalia, and South Sudan. In the worst-off country for maternal health, Sierra Leone, the maternal mortality ratio is estimated to be 1,360 per 100,000 live births.[18]

FIGURE 2-5 gives the maternal mortality ratio by country income group, and **FIGURE 2-6** shows the same data by World Bank region.

As suggested earlier, the pattern of the maternal mortality ratio, by both country income group

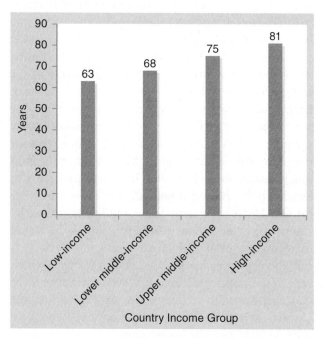

FIGURE 2-3 Life Expectancy at Birth by World Bank Country Income Group, 2016

Data from The World Bank. (n.d.). Data: Life expectancy at birth, total (years). Retrieved from https://data.worldbank.org/indicator/SP.DYN.LE00.IN?end=2016&locations=XD-XT-XN-XM&start=2016&view=bar

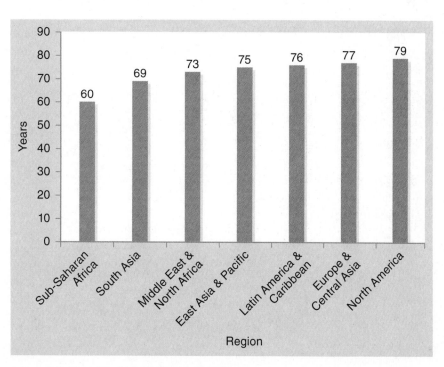

FIGURE 2-4 Life Expectancy at Birth by World Bank Region, 2016

Data from The World Bank. (n.d.). Data: Life expectancy at birth, total (years). Retrieved from https://data.worldbank.org/indicator/SP.DYN.LE00.IN?end=2016&locations=Z4-ZG-8S-ZJ-Z7-ZQ&start=2016&view=bar

and region, is similar to that for life expectancy. However, the differences among regions and country income groups are even greater. The low-income group, with the worst maternal mortality ratio, has a 50 times greater ratio than the high-income group. Sub-Saharan Africa has a ratio that is 42 times greater than in North America. Many people believe that the maternal mortality ratio is the indicator that is most sensitive to a country's overall development status and best reflects the place of women in different societies.

Another important and widely used indicator is the **infant mortality rate**. The infant mortality rate is "the number of deaths of infants under age 1 per 1,000 live births in a given year."[16(p28)] This rate is expressed in deaths per 1,000 live births. In other words, it measures how many children younger than 1 year of age will die for every 1,000 who were born alive that year. Each country seeks as low a rate of infant mortality as possible, but we will see that the rate varies largely with the income status of a country. Afghanistan, for example, had an infant mortality rate in 2016 of 53 infant deaths for every 1,000 live births, whereas in Sweden only about 2 infants die for every 1,000 live births.[19] **FIGURE 2-7** shows the infant mortality rate by country income group. **FIGURE 2-8** shows the infant mortality rate by World Bank region.

There are no surprises for these data either, which vary in the same directions as life expectancy and the maternal mortality ratio. In this case, however, the highest rates of infant mortality are both about 10 times greater than the lowest rates.

Although the infant mortality rate is a powerful indicator of the health status of a country, most children younger than 1 year of age who die actually die in the first month of life. Thus, the **neonatal mortality**

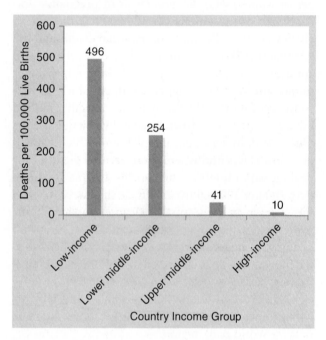

FIGURE 2-5 Maternal Mortality Ratio by World Bank Country Income Group, 2015

Data from The World Bank. (n.d.). Data: Maternal mortality ratio (modeled estimate, per 100,000 live births). Retrieved from https://data.worldbank.org/indicator/SH.STA.MMRT?end=2014&locations=XM-XD-XT-XN&start=2014&view=bar

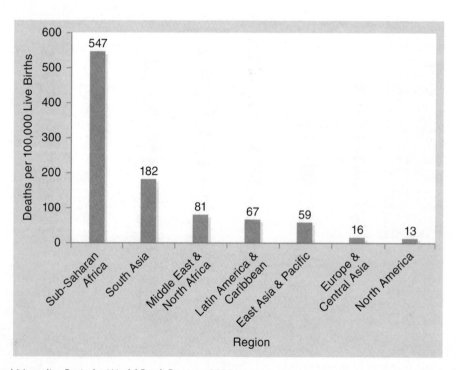

FIGURE 2-6 Maternal Mortality Ratio by World Bank Region, 2015

Data from World Bank. (n.d.). Data: Maternal mortality ratio (modeled estimate, per 1,000 live births). Retrieved from https://data.worldbank.org/indicator/SH.STA.MMRT?end=2015&locations=Z4-8S-ZG-Z7-XU-ZJ-ZQ&start=2015&view=bar

rate is also an important health status indicator. This rate measures "the number of deaths to infants younger than 28 days of age in a given year, per 1,000 live births in that year."[16(p60)] Like the infant mortality rate, this rate will generally vary directly with the level of income of different countries. Poorer countries will usually have a much higher neonatal mortality rate than richer countries. Sierra Leone, among the poorest countries in the world, had a neonatal mortality rate of 33 per 1,000 live births in 2016. In Norway, one of the highest-income countries in the world, the rate that year was 2 per 1,000 live births.[20] The neonatal mortality rate by country income group is given in **FIGURE 2-9**, and the data by World Bank region are portrayed in **FIGURE 2-10**.

The poorest countries have a neonatal mortality rate that is 9 times that of the best-off countries. The two regions with the worst rates have neonatal mortality rates that are 7 times higher than the region with the best rate.

The under-5 child mortality rate is also called the **child mortality rate**. This is "the probability that a newborn will die before reaching age five, expressed as a number per 1,000 live births."[16] Like the infant mortality rate, this rate is expressed per 1,000 live births. This rate also varies largely with the wealth of a country. In the highest-income countries, the rate is generally about 3 to 5 per 1,000 live births. However, in some of the poorest countries, such as Chad, the rate can be over 125 per 1,000 live births.[21] The under-5 child mortality rate is depicted in **FIGURE 2-11** by country income group and in **FIGURE 2-12** by World Bank region.

As expected, the relative standing of different regions in under-5 child mortality, as shown in

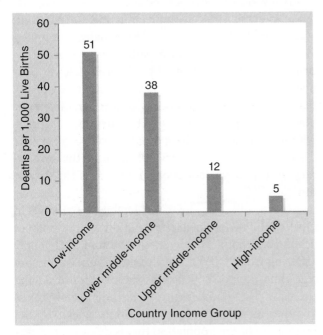

FIGURE 2-7 Infant Mortality Rate by World Bank Country Income Group, 2016

Data from The World Bank. (n.d.). Data: Mortality rate, infant (per 1,000 live births). Retrieved from https://data.worldbank.org/indicator/SP.DYN.IMRT.IN?locations=XD-XT-XN-XM

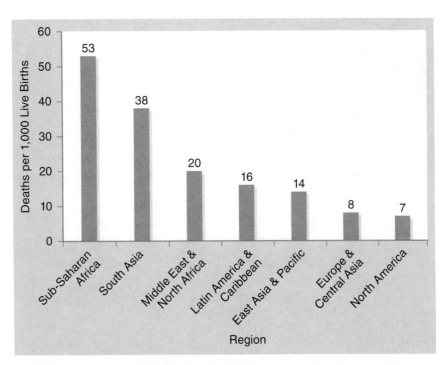

FIGURE 2-8 Infant Mortality Rate by World Bank Region, 2016

Data from The World Bank. (n.d.). Data: Mortality rate, infant (per 1,000 live births). Retrieved from https://data.worldbank.org/indicator/SP.DYN.IMRT.IN?end=2016&locations=Z4-ZG-8S-ZJ-Z7-ZQ-XU&start=2016&view=bar

the figures, looks very similar to that for neonatal mortality and for infant mortality. In both cases for under-5 child mortality, however, the highest rates are about 15 times the lowest rates. To a large extent, this reflects the fact that in high-income countries the risks for young child death post-infancy are relatively few, but in the least well-off regions, especially in sub-Saharan Africa, there are substantial risks to child health not only for neonates and infants but also between a child's first and fifth years. This is illustrated in **FIGURE 2-13**.

A few other concepts and definitions are important to understand as we think about measuring health status. The first is **morbidity**. Essentially, this means sickness or any departure, subjective or objective, from a psychological or physiological state of well-being. Second is **mortality**, which refers to death. A **death rate** is the number of deaths per 1,000 population in a given year.[16(p25)] The third is **disability**. Although some conditions cause people to get sick or die, they might also cause people to suffer the "temporary or long-term reduction in a person's capacity to function."[22(p51)]

There will also be considerable discussion in most readings on global health of the **prevalence** of health conditions. This refers to the number of people suffering from a certain health condition over a specific time period. It measures the chances of having a disease. For global health work, one usually refers to **point prevalence** of a condition, which is "the proportion of the population that is diseased at a single point in time."[16(p31)] Let's say, for example, that the point prevalence of HIV/AIDS among adults in South Africa was estimated to be 18.9 on the last day of 2016.

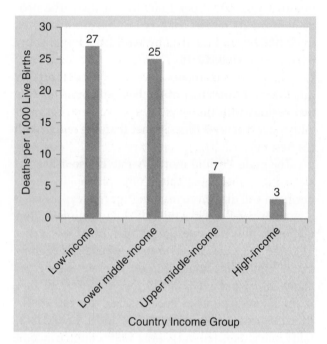

FIGURE 2-9 Neonatal Mortality Rate by World Bank Country Income Group, 2016

Data from The World Bank. (n.d.). Data: Mortality rate, neonatal (per 1,000 live births). Retrieved from https://data.worldbank .org/indicator/SH.DYN.NMRT?end=2016&locations=XD-XT-XN-XM&start=2016&view=bar

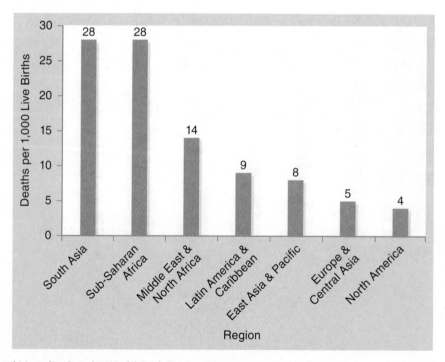

FIGURE 2-10 Neonatal Mortality Rate by World Bank Region, 2016

Data from The World Bank. (n.d.). Data: Mortality rate, neonatal (per 1,000 live births). Retrieved from https://data.worldbank.org/indicator/SH.DYN.NMRT?end=2016&locations=Z4-Z7-XU-ZG-8S-ZQ-ZJ&start=2016&view=bar

This means that 18.9 percent of all adults between the ages of 15 and 49 in South Africa were estimated that day to be HIV-positive.[23]

The **incidence rate** is also a very commonly used term. This measures how many people get a disease, for a specified number of people at risk, for a given period of time.[16] The denominator for the rate usually depends on how commonly the disease occurs in a year and is often per 1,000 or per 100,000 people. In India, for example, the incidence rate for tuberculosis (TB) in 2016 was 211 per 100,000 people.[24] This means that for every 100,000 people in India, 211 got active TB disease in 2016.

Many people confuse incidence rate and prevalence rate. It may be convenient to think of prevalence as the pool of people with a disease at a particular time and incidence as the flow of new cases of people with that disease into that pool. You should note, of course, that the size of the pool will vary as new cases flow into the pool and old cases flow out, as they die or are cured.

We will also speak about **primary prevention**, **secondary prevention**, and **tertiary prevention**. These are defined as follows:

Primary prevention: Intervening before health effects occur, through measures such as vaccinations, altering risky behaviors (poor eating habits, tobacco use, etc.), and banning substances known to be associated with a disease or health condition.

Secondary prevention: Screening to identify diseases in the earliest stages, before the onset of signs and symptoms, through measures such as mammography and regular blood pressure testing.

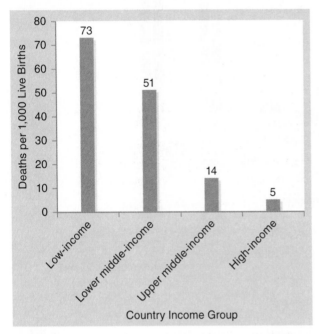

FIGURE 2-11 Under-5 Mortality Rate by World Bank Country Income Group, 2016

Data from The World Bank. (n.d.). Data: Mortality rate, under-5 (per 1,000 live births). Retrieved from https://data.worldbank.org/indicator/SH.DYN.MORT?end=2016&locations=Z4-Z7-ZJ-ZG-8S-XU-ZQ&start=2016&view=bar

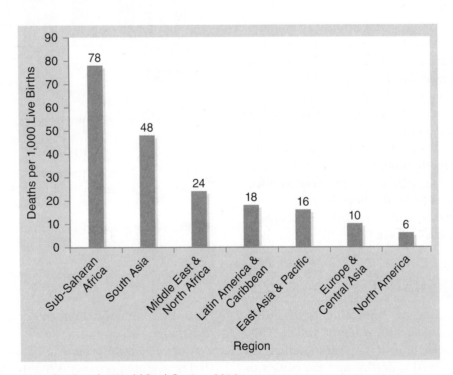

FIGURE 2-12 Under-5 Mortality Rate by World Bank Region, 2016

Data from The World Bank. (n.d.). Data: Mortality rate, under-5 (per 1,000 live births). Retrieved from https://data.worldbank.org/indicator/SH.DYN.MORT?end=2016&locations=Z4-Z7-ZJ-ZG-8S-XU-ZQ&start=2016&view=bar

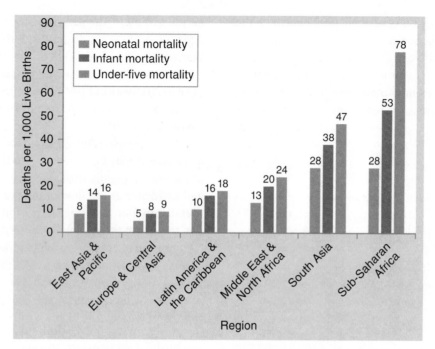

FIGURE 2-13 Under-5, Infant, and Neonatal Mortality Rate, by World Bank Region, 2016

Data from the World Bank. Data. *Mortality rate, infant (per 1,000 live births), Mortality rate, under-5 (per 1,000 live births), Mortality rate, neonatal (per 1,000 live births).* Retrieved from https://data.worldbank.org/

Tertiary prevention: Managing disease post diagnosis to slow or stop disease progression through measures such as chemotherapy, rehabilitation, and screening for complications.[25]

Finally, one needs to be familiar with how diseases get classified. When you read about health, there will be discussions of **communicable diseases**, **noncommunicable diseases**, and **injuries**. Communicable diseases are also called infectious diseases. These are illnesses that are caused by a particular infectious agent and that spread directly or indirectly from people to people, animals to people, or people to animals.[22] Examples of communicable diseases include influenza, measles, and HIV. Noncommunicable diseases are illnesses that are not spread by any infectious agent, such as hypertension, coronary heart disease, and diabetes, even though they might have an infectious cause, such as cervical cancer. Injuries include, among other things, road traffic injuries, falls, drownings, poisonings, and violence.[26]

▶ Vital Registration

The quality of data on population and health depends in many ways on the extent to which countries maintain a system of vital registration that can accurately record births, deaths, and the causes of death. Unfortunately, this is not the case in many low- and lower middle-income countries.[27] They

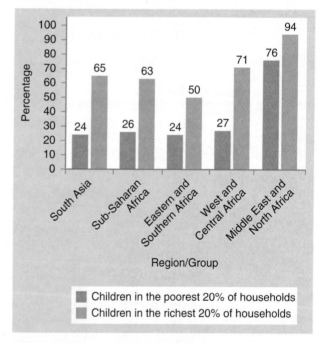

FIGURE 2-14 Percentage of Children Under 5 Whose Births Have Been Registered, by Income Quintile for Selected UNICEF Regions, 2005–2012

Data from UNICEF. (2013). *Every child's birth right: Inequities and trends in birth registration.* Retrieved from http://www.unicef.org/media/files/Embargoed_11_Dec_Birth_Registration_report_low_res.pdf

generally have only rudimentary systems for vital registration, which cannot fulfill either their statistical or their legal purposes. In addition, access to vital registration systems is highly inequitable, with higher-income groups enjoying much better access than less well-off people (**FIGURE 2-14**). UNICEF estimates that about 25 percent of all of the births in the world are never registered.[28]

There are also cultural barriers to timely vital registration because people in many countries wait until a child is a certain age before registering the birth. Coupled with the lack of access to vital registration, this means the existence of some children is never officially known because they die before their births are registered. There are also enormous difficulties with accurate indications of causes of death in countries that have weak health systems and a limited number of well-trained physicians. This is especially so for causes of death of adults.

The former director-general of WHO, Lee Jong-Wook, noted in a speech to his colleagues: "To make people count, we first need to be able to count people."[29(p1569)] To overcome the lack of effective vital registration systems in many low- and middle-income countries, a number of tools, such as surveys and projection models, have been developed. Some, like the Demographic and Health Surveys, have become an important source of information about health, population, nutrition, and HIV in low-income countries.

In the longer term, however, the world would be better served by helping countries further develop their own vital registration systems. This would allow countries and their development partners to more accurately gauge the nature of key demographic and health issues and the progress made toward resolving them. Moving in this direction will require assessments of vital registration systems. It will also require programs to improve the organization and functioning of vital registration departments. This will have to include, among other things, strengthening their methods to improve the quality of vital statistics, including for the causes of death, and enhancing their approach to publishing data.[27]

▶ Main Messages

To understand the most important global health issues, we must understand the determinants of health, how health status is measured, and how health status varies by country income group, region, age, and sex. There are a number of factors that influence health status, including genetic makeup, sex, and age. Social and cultural issues and health behaviors are also closely linked to health status. The determinants of health also include education, nutritional status, and socioeconomic status. The environment is also a powerful determinant of health, as is access to health services, and the policy approaches that countries take to their health sectors and to investments that could influence the health of their people. Increasing attention is being paid to the social determinants of health. Some determinants have a more direct influence than others, whose influence is more indirect.

There are a number of uses of health data, including measuring health status, carrying out disease surveillance, making decisions about investments in health, and assessing the performance of health programs. Those working in health use a common set of indicators to measure health status, including life expectancy, infant and neonatal mortality, under-5 child mortality, and the maternal mortality ratio. Vital registration systems are weak in low-income countries and need to be strengthened to improve the quality of health data.

There has been progress in all regions of the world in increasing life expectancy over the last several decades. In addition, the pace of those increases has been exceptionally rapid in East Asia and the Pacific. However, it is clear that the basic health indicators are much worse in sub-Saharan Africa than in any other region and that these indicators also lag substantially in South Asia.

Study Questions

1. What do we mean when we talk about "the determinants of health"?
2. Which determinants have a more direct and which have a less direct impact on people's health?
3. Why are the social determinants of health considered to be so important?
4. What are the factors that have most determined your personal health?
5. What are the factors that would most determine the health of a poor person in a low-income country?
6. If you could pick only one indicator to describe the health status of a low-income country, which indicator would you use and why?
7. In your own country, what population groups have the best health indicators and why?
8. In your country, what population groups have the worst health status and why?
9. What might prevent a country from having an effective vital registration system, and how could such systems be strengthened?
10. How much credence should you put in data on key global health indicators?

References

1. World Health Organization. (2004). A global emergency: A combined response. In *The world health report 2004—Changing history* (pp. 1–10). Geneva, Switzerland: Author.

2. The World Bank. (n.d.). Data: Life expectancy at birth, males (years). Retrieved from https://data.worldbank.org /indicator/SP.DYN.LE00.MA.IN?view=map

3. The World Bank. (n.d.). Data: Life expectancy at birth, females (years). Retrieved from https://data.worldbank.org /indicator/SP.DYN.LE00.FE.IN?view=map

4. The World Bank. (2015). Data: Maternal mortality ratio (modeled estimate, per 100,000 live births). Retrieved from https://data.worldbank.org/indicator/SH.STA.MMRT?end =2014&locations=XM-XD-XT-XN&start=2014&view=bar

5. The World Bank. (n.d.). Data: Mortality rate, under-5 (per 1,000 live births). Retrieved from https://data.worldbank .org/indicator/SH.DYN.MORT?end=2016&locations=Z4 -Z7-ZJ-ZG-8S-XU-ZQ&start=2016&view=bar

6. World Health Organization. (1998). Determinants of health. In *Health promotion glossary* (p. 6). Retrieved from http://www.who.int/healthpromotion/about/HPR%20 Glossary%201998.pdf?ua=1

7. World Health Organization. (n.d.). *About social determinants of health*. Retrieved from http://www.who.int /social_determinants/sdh_definition/en/

8. Reblin, M., & Uchino, B. N. (2008). Social and emotional support and its implication for health. *Current Opinion in Psychiatry, 21*(2), 201.

9. Public Health Agency of Canada. (2018). *Social determinants of health and health inequalities*. Retrieved from http://www .phac-aspc.gc.ca/ph-sp/determinants/index-eng.php

10. Centers for Disease Control and Prevention. (2014). *Social determinants of health: Definitions*. Retrieved http://www .cdc.gov/socialdeterminants/Definitions.html

11. Hobcraft, J. (1993). Women's education, child welfare and child survival: A review of the evidence. *Health Transition Review, 3*(2), 159–173.

12. World Health Organization. (2008). *Commission on social determinants of health. Closing the gap in a generation.* Retrieved from http://www.who.int/social_determinants /thecommission/finalreport/en/index.html

13. The World Bank. (2006). *Repositioning nutrition as central to development—A strategy for large-scale action.* Washington, DC: Author.

14. Shonkoff, J. P., Garner, A. S., The Committee on Psychosocial Aspects of Child and Family Health, Committee on Early Childhood, Adoption, and Dependent Care, & Section on Developmental and Behavioral Pediatrics. (2012). The lifelong effects of early childhood adversity and toxic stress. *Pediatrics, 129*(1), e232–e246.

15. Basch, P. (2001). *Textbook of international health* (2nd ed.). New York, NY: Oxford University Press.

16. Haupt, A., & Kane, T. T. (2004). *Population handbook.* Washington, DC: Population Reference Bureau.

17. The World Bank. (n.d.). Data: Life expectancy at birth, total (years). Retrieved from https://data.worldbank.org /indicator/SP.DYN.LE00.IN

18. The World Bank. (2015). Data: Maternal mortality ratio (modeled estimate, per 100,000 live births). Retrieved from https://data.worldbank.org/indicator/SH.STA.MMRT

19. The World Bank. (n.d.). Data: Mortality rate, infant (per 1,000 live births). Retrieved from https://data.worldbank .org/indicator/SP.DYN.IMRT.IN

20. The World Bank. (n.d.). Data: Mortality rate, neonatal (per 1,000 live births). Retrieved from https://data.worldbank .org/indicator/SH.DYN.NMRT

21. The World Bank. (n.d.). Data: Mortality rate, under-5 (per 1,000 live births). Retrieved from http://data.worldbank.org /indicator/SH.DYN.MORT

22. Last, J. M. (2001). *A dictionary of epidemiology* (4th ed.). New York, NY: Oxford University Press.

23. The World Bank. (n.d.). Data: Prevalence of HIV, total (% of population ages 15–49). Retrieved from https://data .worldbank.org/indicator/SH.DYN.AIDS.ZS?view=chart

24. The World Bank. (n.d.). Data: Incidence of tuberculosis (per 100,000 people). Retrieved from https://data.worldbank .org/indicator/SH.TBS.INCD

25. U.S. Centers for Disease Control and Prevention. (n.d.). *Prevention: Picture of America.* Retrieved from https:// www.cdc.gov/pictureofamerica/pdfs/picture_of_america _prevention.pdf

26. Lopez, A. D., Mathers, C. D., & Murray, C. J. L. (2006). The burden of disease and mortality by condition: Data, methods, and results for 2001. In A. D. Lopez, C. D. Mathers, M. Ezzati, D. T. Jamison, & C. J. L. Murray (Eds.), *Global burden of disease and risk factors* (pp. 45–240). New York, NY: Oxford University Press.

27. Setel, P. W., Macfarlane, S. B., Szreter, S., Mikkelsen, L., Jha, P., Stout, S., & AbouZahr, C. (2007). A scandal of invisibility: Making everyone count by counting everyone. *The Lancet, 370*(9598), 1569–1577.

28. UNICEF. (2017). Birth registration. Retrieved from https:// data.unicef.org/topic/child-protection/birth-registration/

29. World Health Organization. (2003). *Address to WHO staff.* Geneva, Switzerland: Author. Retrieved from http://www .who.int/dg/lee/speeches/2003/21_07/en/

CHAPTER 3

The Global Burden of Disease

Courtesy of Mark Tuschman.

LEARNING OBJECTIVES

By the end of this chapter, the reader will be able to do the following:

- Discuss the concepts of health-adjusted life expectancy (HALE), disability-adjusted life years (DALYs), and the burden of disease
- Describe the leading causes of disability, deaths, and DALYs by region, country income group, age, and sex
- Describe the leading risk factors for disability, deaths, and DALYs by region, country income group, age, and sex
- Discuss the demographic and epidemiologic transitions

▶ Vignettes

Princess is a 3-year-old girl who lives near the town of Kenema in Sierra Leone. Although Sierra Leone has made some progress in reducing young child death, the country remains very poor, still suffers from the ravages of its earlier civil war, and continues to have a very weak health system. Access to safe water and sanitation and good knowledge of hygiene are also limited. The burden of malaria has gone down, but the disease is still very prevalent. What are the leading causes of death for young children like Princess? What are the most important risk factors for those causes? Is there good evidence about what can be done in cost-effective and fair ways to reduce the burden of deaths among young children in Sierra Leone and similar countries?

Aisha is a 50-year-old woman who lives in the northern part of Nigeria. She is from a lower middle-class family, in an area that is still quite poor. Aisha has been feeling unwell and recently visited the outpatient clinic at the regional hospital. The check-up and tests the doctors carried out indicated that she has high blood pressure, high cholesterol, and diabetes. The doctors prescribed medicines for her to reduce her blood pressure and cholesterol and another drug to lower her blood sugar. As Aisha returned home, she thought about how people's health had changed in the last decade in her town. Earlier, she rarely heard about the conditions with which she had been diagnosed. Now, however, it seemed like many of her friends had been diagnosed with the same problems.

Jose is a 30-year-old man in Bolivia. He is from an indigenous, relatively poor community in the highlands. Two decades ago, Jose's community still faced many child deaths, especially from pneumonia and diarrhea. The community also had a substantial burden of undernutrition and tuberculosis (TB). To what extent have such causes of death declined in Jose's community? If so, what are the leading causes of death now? Is there a "convergence" between the leading causes of death in Jose's community and the lowland communities populated mostly by people of European descent?

Shireen is a 22-year-old woman in Bangladesh. She is just starting a family. Her mother and grandmother have given her advice about when to have her first child and where to get and how to use family planning methods. They have also suggested that she should have only two children and that she should space them 3 or more years apart. A community health worker has been in touch with Shireen regularly and has made the same suggestions as her mother and grandmother. In Bangladesh in 1960, women had on average more than six children and the median age of the population was around 19 years of age. In 2016, women had on average just over two children and the median age of the population was around 26 years of age.[1] What causes these shifts? Do they occur consistently as countries develop socially and economically? What will the age distribution of the population look like in Bangladesh in 25 years and why?

▶ Measuring the Burden of Disease

The World Health Organization (WHO) defines health as "a state of complete physical, mental and social well-being and not merely the absence of disease or infirmity."[2] Those who work on global health have attempted for a number of years to construct a single indicator that could be used to compare how far different countries are from the state of good health. Ideally, such an index would take account of morbidity, mortality, and disability; allow one to calculate the index by age, by gender, and by region; and allow one to make comparisons of health status across regions within a country and across countries.[3] This kind of index would measure what is generally referred to as the burden of disease.

One such indicator is health-adjusted life expectancy, or HALE. This is a health expectancy measure. HALE is the number of years a person of a given age can expect to live in good health, taking account of mortality and disability.[4(p9)] This can also be seen as "the equivalent number of years in full health that a newborn can expect to live, based on current

rates of ill health and mortality."[5] To calculate HALE, "the years of ill health are weighted according to severity and subtracted from the overall life expectancy."[6]

TABLE 3-1 shows life expectancy at birth in 2016 for a number of low-, middle-, and high-income countries and how it compares with HALEs for those countries in the same year, for males and females. In principle, each country should strive to help its people live as long *and* as healthy as possible. In that case, health-adjusted life expectancy and life expectancy at birth would converge at a relatively high number.

The composite indicator of health status that is most commonly used in global health work is called the disability-adjusted life year, or DALY. This indicator was first used in conjunction with the *1993 World Development Report* of the World Bank and is a health gap measure. It is now used consistently in burden of disease studies. In the simplest terms, a DALY is "the sum of years lost due to premature death (YLLs) and years lived with disability (YLDs). DALYs are also defined as years of healthy life lost."[5(p9)]

The calculation of years lost to premature death is based on the difference between the age at which one dies and one's life expectancy at that age. To make this calculation, those involved in the key studies on the global burden of disease have constructed a reference standard life table that takes account of the highest life expectancy at birth globally. For the 2016 study, this was set at 86.6 years.[7] This life table is used to calculate premature death for all countries in the study.

One might ask why the study is not based on life tables for each individual country. In very simple terms, one could respond by noting that, in principle, any death before the life expectancy of the people who live the longest globally is "premature." One might also add that in order to make the world a healthier place, a goal must be to have people live "as long as possible," rather than live only as long as they live now.

FIGURE 3-1 illustrates the calculation of years of life lost due to premature death for three different scenarios.

As noted in Figure 3-1, if a newborn were to die in Liberia, for example, that newborn would have suffered 87 years of life lost due to premature death. Life expectancy at 40 according to the reference life tables is 87, or 47 more years. Thus, if a 40-year-old woman in Malawi were to die in a car accident, she would have suffered 47 years of life lost due to premature death. Life expectancy at 60 years of age according to the standard reference life table is 88, or 28 more years. Thus, if a French male were to die of a heart attack at age 60, he would have suffered 28 years of life lost.

The value for years lived with disability is calculated by weighting these years by a disability index.

TABLE 3-1 Life Expectancy at Birth and Health-Adjusted Life Expectancy by Sex, Selected Countries, 2016		
	Life Expectancy/Health-Adjusted Life Expectancy	**Life Expectancy/Health-Adjusted Life Expectancy**
Country	**Males**	**Females**
Afghanistan	56.9/49.1	59.2/50.0
Bangladesh	70.5/61.7	75.1/64.0
Bolivia	72.2/63.5	74.3/64.6
Brazil	71.6/63.0	79.0/68.1
Cambodia	65.7/58.0	71.6/62.1
Cameroon	58.3/51.3	62.0/53.8
China	73.4/66.0	79.9/70.1
Costa Rica	78.5/69.5	83.6/72.9
Cuba	76.7/67.8	81.3/70.7
Denmark	78.8/68.9	82.9/70.8
Ethiopia	64.7/57.2	66.5/58.7
Ghana	64.5/56.9	67.5/59.0
India	66.9/58.2	70.3/59.7
Indonesia	69.8/61.8	73.7/64.2
Jordan	74.7/64.6	78.0/65.7
Malaysia	73.2/64.8	78.0/68.1
Nepal	69.7/60.9	71.9/61.8
Niger	60.6/53.4	62.8/54.7
Nigeria	63.7/55.5	66.4/57.2
Peru	77.8/68.6	81.6/71.0
Philippines	66.6/59.1	73.9/64.5
Sri Lanka	73.7/65.1	81.1/70.5
Turkey	75.8/65.9	82.3/69.2
United States of America	76.5/66.3	81.2/69.0
Vietnam	70.9/63.3	78.1/68.4

Data from Institute of Health Metrics and Evaluation (IHME). (n.d.). GBD Compare: Viz Hub. Retrieved from https://vizhub.healthdata.org/gbd-compare/

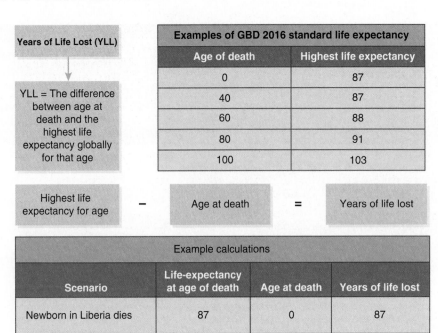

FIGURE 3-1 Calculating Years of Life Lost (YLLs) Due to Premature Death

Adapted with permission from Session 6, Module 2 of Essentials of Global Health, Coursera/Yale University, 2016. Data from Institute of Health Metrics and Evaluation (IHME). (n.d.). Global Burden of Disease Study 2016 (GBD 2016) data resources: GBD 2016 reference life table. Retrieved from http://ghdx.healthdata.org/gbd-2016

For the Global Burden of Disease Study 2010, 14,000 people were surveyed directly and 16,000 people were involved via the internet in establishing disability weights.[7] The disability weights used in the 2016 study were based on the 2010 weights, supplemented by data gathered from additional surveys done for the 2013 GBD study.[8] The study authors also made some additional refinements to these weights, especially as they related to the severity of different health conditions.[9]

FIGURE 3-2 illustrates the disability weights for five different conditions. It also shows model calculations of years of life lived with disability (YLDs) for three scenarios of people living with disability.

As noted in Figure 3-2, let's say that a person in Tanzania lives 30 years with a disability that has been given a weight of 0.10. In this case the person suffers 3 years of life lived with disability, equal to the number of years lived with disability, multiplied by the weight of that disability. If a person in France lived 20 years with a disability that has a weight of 0.25, then that person would have suffered the equivalent of 5 years lived with disability. If a person in Sri Lanka lived 10 years with a disability that has a weight of 0.5, then that person would have suffered 5 years of life lived with disability.

As noted earlier, a DALY is the sum of years of life lost due to premature death (YLL) and years of life lost due to disability (YLD). **FIGURE 3-3** illustrates the calculation of a DALY for two different scenarios.

As you can see in Figure 3-3, Person A dies at 50 years of age of drug-resistant tuberculosis, after living 3 years with this condition. In this case, the person's life expectancy at 50 was 87. Thus the person suffered a loss of 37 years of life due to premature death. The disability weight for multidrug-resistant TB is 0.333. Thus, the person would have suffered 1 year of life lived with disability. The total DALYs for this person would be 37 plus 1, or 38.

Person B dies at 65 after living 10 years with moderate disability brought on by a stroke. This person died 23 years prematurely. This person also suffered about 3 years of life lived with disability. The total DALYs associated with this person would be 23 YLLs, plus 3 YLDs, or about 26 years.

A society that has more premature death, illness, and disability has more DALYs per person in the population than a society that is healthier and has less premature death, illness, and disability. One of the goals of health policy is to avert these DALYs in the most cost-efficient and fair manner possible. If, for example, a society has many hundreds of thousands of DALYs due to malaria that are not diagnosed and treated in a timely and proper manner, what steps can be taken to avert those DALYs at the lowest cost and in the fairest ways?

An important point to remember when considering DALYs, compared to measuring deaths, is that DALYs take account of periods in which people are

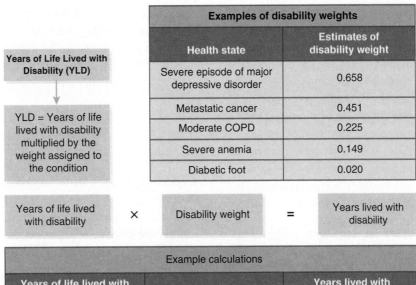

FIGURE 3-2 Calculating Years Lived with Disability (YLDs)

Adapted with permission from Session 6, Module 2 of Essentials of Global Health, Coursera/Yale University, 2016. Data from Salomon, J. A, Haagsma, J. A., Davis, A., de Noordhout, C. M., Polinder, S., Havelaar, A. H., . . . Vos, T. (2015). Disability weights for the Global Burden of Disease 2013 study. *Lancet Global Health, 3*(11), e712–e723.

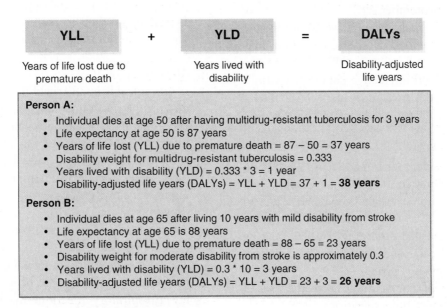

FIGURE 3-3 Calculating Disability-Adjusted Life Years (DALYs)

Adapted with permission from Session 6, Module 2 of Essentials of Global Health, Coursera/Yale University, 2016.

living with disability. By doing this, DALYs and other composite indicators try to give a better estimate of the true health of a population instead of measuring deaths alone. This is easy to understand. Contrary to most popular belief, mental health problems, for example, *are* associated with an important number of

deaths. However, they may also cause an enormous amount of disability. Several parasitic infections, such as schistosomiasis, cause very few deaths but large amounts of illness and disability. If we measured the health of a population with an important burden of schistosomiasis and mental illness only by measuring deaths, we would miss a major component of morbidity and disability and would seriously overestimate the health of that population. The next section elaborates on the concept of DALYs and how DALYs compare to deaths for a number of health conditions.

A number of critiques of DALYs have been written.[10] Nonetheless, this text repeatedly refers to DALYs because this measure is so extensively used in global health work. In addition, a considerable amount of important analysis has been carried out that is based on the use of DALYs for measuring overall health status and assessing the most cost-effective approaches to dealing with various health problems.

▶ Burden of Disease Data

As you start a review of global health, it is important to get a clear picture of the leading causes of illness, disability, and death in the world. It is also very important to understand how they vary by age, sex, ethnicity, and socioeconomic status, both within and across countries. Additionally, it is essential to understand how these causes have varied over time and how they might change in the future. These topics are examined next.

Much of the data that follows on the burden of disease and risk factors is based on the findings of the Global Burden of Disease Study 2016, published in *The Lancet* in September 2017.[11] The Institute of Health Metrics and Evaluation (IHME) coordinated that study. Those interested in the study methods may wish to consult the study directly.[12] This chapter also heavily uses data from interactive data visualizations that the IHME has posted on its website.[13] The reader should note that, while some data refer to "deaths" and some data refer to "DALYs," references to the "burden of disease" refer to DALYs.

Wherever possible, data are shown by World Bank region or World Bank country income group. However, readers should be aware that the IHME data can be categorized into a range of regional groupings and by groups that are listed according to their ranking on a composite "social and economic development index" developed by the IHME.

Earlier burden of disease studies placed causes of deaths and DALYs into three categories:

Group I—Communicable, maternal, and perinatal conditions (meaning in the first week after birth) and nutritional disorders

Group II—Noncommunicable diseases

Group III—Injuries, including, among other things, road traffic accidents, falls, self-inflicted injuries, and violence

The Global Burden of Disease Study 2016 does not use the groupings as they had been used earlier. Nonetheless, such groupings can be valuable to those who are new to the study of the burden of disease. Thus, they are used occasionally here.

Overview of Patterns and Trends in the Burden of Disease

Understanding the patterns and trends in the burden of disease is central to understanding and dealing with key issues in global health. Some of the main findings of the burden of disease studies are summarized here[14-17]:

- People in much of the world are living longer than before.
- Globally, women live longer than men by about 5 years on average.
- In the last 4 decades, there have been significant declines in communicable, maternal, neonatal, and nutritional causes of death.
- Globally, mortality rates have decreased for all age groups, with very substantial decreases for children under 5 years of age.
- Nonetheless, there are substantial differences in the rate of mortality decrease across countries.
- The years of life lost due to premature death are increasing for diabetes, some cancers, and, in some places, for drug use disorders, conflict, and terrorism.
- The burden of disease is predominantly noncommunicable in all World Bank regions and for all World Bank country income groups, except sub-Saharan Africa and low-income countries.
- Over the last few decades, the burden of disease has shifted increasingly toward noncommunicable diseases in all World Bank regions and for all country income groups.
- This shift has been fueled by, among other things, a reduction in communicable diseases and the aging of populations.
- The 10 leading causes of total YLLs in 2016 were ischemic heart disease, cerebrovascular disease, lower respiratory infections, diarrheal diseases, road injuries, malaria, neonatal preterm birth complications, HIV/AIDS, chronic obstructive pulmonary disease, and neonatal encephalopathy due to birth asphyxia and trauma.
- As life expectancies increase, death rates decline, and populations age, there is an increase in the number of years people live with disability, and this has increased as a share of the total burden of disease.

- Globally, low back pain, migraine, age-related and other hearing loss, iron-deficiency anemia, and major depressive disorder were the five leading causes of years lived with disability in 2016.
- Globally, the top 10 risk factors for the burden of disease are high blood pressure, smoking, low birthweight and short gestation, high fasting plasma glucose, high body mass index, ambient particulate matter, alcohol use, high total cholesterol, child growth failure, and household air pollution.
- There are a number of countries in which life expectancy is greater than one might predict on the basis of social and economic development. These countries could provide some useful lessons for other countries that have not made such progress in health.

The Leading Causes of Deaths and DALYs

TABLE 3-2 shows the 10 leading causes of death and the 10 leading causes of DALYs by country income group for 2016. Both deaths and DALYs are ranked in order of importance.

TABLE 3-3 shows the 10 leading causes of deaths and DALYs by region.

These tables and figures raise a number of key points concerning deaths and DALYs for all age groups and males and females globally:

- The low-income countries have a unique pattern of deaths and DALYs, compared to other country income groups, that is still dominated by Group I causes. While about 61 percent of the total DALYs were associated with Group I causes in low-income countries, about 86 percent of total DALYs were associated with noncommunicable diseases (NCDs) in high-income countries.
- The pattern of deaths and DALYs in lower middle-income countries has some resemblance to that in the low-income countries but also has similarities with the upper middle-income and high-income countries. In lower middle-income countries about 36 percent of total DALYs were associated with Group I causes, compared to 61 percent in low-income countries and 11 percent in upper middle-income countries.
- There is a great deal of convergence in the causes of deaths and DALYs in the upper

TABLE 3-2 Leading Causes of Deaths and DALYs, by World Bank Country Income Group, 2016

High-Income Countries

Rank	Cause	
	Deaths	**DALYs**
1	Ischemic heart disease	Ischemic heart disease
2	Alzheimer's disease and other dementias	Low back and neck pain
3	Stroke	Stroke
4	Tracheal, bronchus, and lung cancer	Tracheal, bronchus, and lung cancer
5	COPD	Sense organ diseases
6	Lower respiratory infections	Alzheimer's disease and other dementias
7	Colorectal cancer	Skin diseases
8	Chronic kidney disease	Diabetes
9	Diabetes	Depressive disorders
10	Other cardiovascular and circulatory diseases	Migraine

(continues)

TABLE 3-2 Leading Causes of Deaths and DALYs, by World Bank Country Income Group, 2016   *(continued)*

Upper Middle-Income Countries

	Cause	
Rank	**Deaths**	**DALYs**
1	Ischemic heart disease	Ischemic heart disease
2	Stroke	Stroke
3	COPD	Low back and neck pain
4	Alzheimer's disease and other dementias	Road injuries
5	Tracheal, bronchus, and lung cancer	Sense organ diseases
6	Road injuries	COPD
7	Liver cancer	Diabetes
8	Lower respiratory infections	Skin diseases
9	Stomach cancer	Tracheal, bronchus, and lung cancer
10	Diabetes	Depressive disorders

Lower Middle-Income Countries

	Cause	
Rank	**Deaths**	**DALYs**
1	Ischemic heart disease	Ischemic heart disease
2	Stroke	Lower respiratory infections
3	Diarrheal diseases	Diarrheal diseases
4	COPD	Stroke
5	Lower respiratory infections	Neonatal preterm birth
6	Tuberculosis	COPD
7	Diabetes	Malaria
8	Road injuries	Road injuries
9	Chronic kidney disease	Neonatal encephalopathy
10	HIV/AIDS	Low back and neck pain

	Cause	
Low-Income Countries		
Rank	**Deaths**	**DALYs**
1	Lower respiratory infections	Malaria
2	Ischemic heart disease	Lower respiratory infections
3	Diarrheal diseases	Diarrheal diseases
4	Malaria	HIV/AIDS
5	HIV/AIDS	Neonatal encephalopathy
6	Tuberculosis	Neonatal preterm birth
7	Stroke	Tuberculosis
8	Neonatal encephalopathy	Protein-energy malnutrition
9	Neonatal preterm birth	Meningitis
10	Protein-energy malnutrition	Congenital defects

Data from Institute of Health Metrics and Evaluation (IHME). (n.d.). GBD Compare: Viz Hub. Retrieved from https://vizhub.healthdata.org/gbd-compare/

TABLE 3-3 Leading Causes of Deaths and DALYs, by World Bank Region, 2016

	Cause	
North America		
Rank	**Deaths**	**DALYs**
1	Ischemic heart disease	Ischemic heart disease
2	Alzheimer's disease and other dementias	Drug use disorders
3	Tracheal, bronchus, and lung cancer	Low back pain
4	Stroke	COPD
5	COPD	Diabetes
6	Lower respiratory infections	Tracheal, bronchus, and lung cancer
7	Chronic kidney disease	Stroke
8	Colorectal cancer	Headache disorders
9	Diabetes	Alzheimer's disease and other dementias
10	Drug use disorders	Depressive disorders

(continues)

TABLE 3-3 Leading Causes of Deaths and DALYs, by World Bank Region, 2016   *(continued)*

East Asia & Pacific

Rank	Cause	
	Deaths	**DALYs**
1	Stroke	Stroke
2	Ischemic heart disease	Ischemic heart disease
3	COPD	COPD
4	Tracheal, bronchus, and lung cancer	Neonatal disorders
5	Alzheimer's disease and other dementias	Road injuries
6	Lower respiratory infections	Diabetes
7	Liver cancer	Tracheal, bronchus, and lung cancer
8	Stomach cancer	Low back pain
9	Road injuries	Lower respiratory infections
10	Diabetes	Liver cancer

Latin America & Caribbean

Rank	Cause	
	Deaths	**DALYs**
1	Ischemic heart disease	Ischemic heart disease
2	Stroke	Neonatal disorders
3	Lower respiratory infections	Interpersonal violence
4	Alzheimer's disease and other dementias	Diabetes
5	Diabetes	Road injuries
6	Chronic kidney disease	Low back pain
7	Interpersonal violence	Stroke
8	COPD	Lower respiratory infections
9	Cirrhosis	Headache disorders
10	Road injuries	Congenital defects

	Cause	
Europe & Central Asia		
Rank	**Deaths**	**DALYs**
1	Ischemic heart disease	Ischemic heart disease
2	Stroke	Stroke
3	Alzheimer's disease and other dementias	Low back pain
4	Tracheal, bronchus, and lung cancer	Tracheal, bronchus, and lung cancer
5	COPD	Headache disorders
6	Colorectal cancer	Diabetes
7	Lower respiratory infections	Falls
8	Cirrhosis	COPD
9	Cardiomyopathy	Alzheimer's disease and other dementias
10	Hypertensive heart disease	Neonatal disorders

	Cause	
Middle East & North Africa		
Rank	**Deaths**	**DALYs**
1	Ischemic heart disease	Ischemic heart disease
2	Stroke	Neonatal disorders
3	Road injuries	Conflict and terrorism
4	Conflict and terrorism	Road injuries
5	Neonatal disorders	Congenital defects
6	Alzheimer's disease and other dementias	Stroke
7	Lower respiratory infections	Low back pain
8	Cirrhosis	Headache disorders
9	Diabetes	Diabetes
10	Hypertensive heart disease	Drug use disorders

(continues)

TABLE 3-3 Leading Causes of Deaths and DALYs, by World Bank Region, 2016   *(continued)*

South Asia

Rank	Cause	
	Deaths	**DALYs**
1	Ischemic heart disease	Neonatal disorders
2	COPD	Ischemic heart disease
3	Stroke	Lower respiratory infections
4	Diarrheal diseases	Diarrheal diseases
5	Neonatal disorders	COPD
6	Lower respiratory infections	Stroke
7	Tuberculosis	Tuberculosis
8	Diabetes	Congenital defects
9	Road injuries	Road injuries
10	Asthma	Dietary iron deficiency

Sub-Saharan Africa

Rank	Cause	
	Deaths	**DALYs**
1	HIV/AIDS	Neonatal disorders
2	Neonatal disorders	Lower respiratory infections
3	Lower respiratory infections	HIV/AIDS
4	Diarrheal diseases	Malaria
5	Malaria	Diarrheal diseases
6	Tuberculosis	Congenital defects
7	Ischemic heart disease	Tuberculosis
8	Stroke	Meningitis
9	Congenital defects	Protein-energy malnutrition
10	Road injuries	Road injuries

Data from Institute of Health Metrics and Evaluation (IHME). (n.d.). GBD Compare: Viz Hub. Retrieved from https://vizhub.healthdata.org/gbd-compare/

middle-income and high-income countries, both dominated by noncommunicable causes. About 77 percent of total DALYs were associated with noncommunicable diseases in upper middle-income countries, compared with 86 percent in high-income countries.

- Injuries are important causes of deaths and DALYs. They make up between 8 percent and 11 percent of total DALYs, depending on the region.
- The only Group I cause in the top 10 causes of death in upper middle-income and high-income countries is lower respiratory infections. While these are associated mostly with young child deaths in lower-income countries, they are associated mostly with deaths in older people in higher-income countries.
- It is important to note the significance in most of the country income groups of DALYs attributable to low back and neck pain, sense organ diseases, skin diseases, and depressive disorders.

In general, the higher the level of income of the countries in a region, the more likely it is that the leading causes of deaths and DALYs will be noncommunicable. The lower the level of income, the more likely it is that communicable diseases will be important. What is most essential to note is the extent to which the burden of disease in the sub-Saharan Africa region remains dominated by Group I causes and the continuing importance of these causes in the South Asia region, as well. Of course, these are in the face of a growing burden, even in these regions, of noncommunicable diseases.

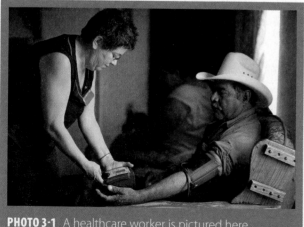

PHOTO 3-1 A healthcare worker is pictured here, taking the blood pressure of a man in a health center in Mexico. Why is this so important? What risks does high blood pressure pose? What are some of the most important risk factors for having hypertension?

Courtesy of Mark Tuschman.

Trends in the Causes of Deaths and DALYs, 1990–2016

TABLE 3-4 indicates changes that have occurred between 1990 and 2016 in the leading causes of deaths and DALYs globally.

The table indicates the important extent to which the burden of deaths globally, when considering all age groups and both sexes, has shifted toward non-communicable diseases. The trend has been similar for DALYs, with some significant shifts from communicable diseases and other Group I causes to noncommunicable diseases and injuries. In light of longer lives and aging populations, low back and neck pain and sensory organ disorders also appear in the list of 10 leading causes of DALYs in 2016, which was not the case in 1990. HIV/AIDS appears in 2016 and not in 1990 because the burden of HIV/AIDS was still relatively small in 1990.

Causes of Death by Age

TABLE 3-5 shows the leading causes of death for children aged 0 to 5 years by country income group.

The leading causes of deaths of under-5 children in low-income countries are dominated by communicable diseases—malaria, diarrhea, and lower respiratory infections. Conditions of the newborn and protein-energy malnutrition are also among the 10 leading causes of death of this age group in low-income countries. The leading causes of death among children under 5 years of age in lower middle-income countries does not differ significantly from the causes in low-income countries. As we move to upper middle-income countries, we see causes outside of Group I, including road injuries and drowning. The leading causes of death in high-income countries include congenital defects and neonatal conditions, as in the other country income groups. They also include lower respiratory conditions, which is an important cause of death for young children in all country income groups. However, in the high-income countries, 4 of the 10 leading causes of death in this age group are different from the leading causes in the other country income groups: sudden infant death syndrome, road injuries, endocrine and blood disorders, and mechanical forces.

TABLE 3-6 shows the leading causes of death for children ages 5 to 14 by country income group.

It is striking how the leading causes of death of children ages 5 to 14 in low- and lower middle-income countries are dominated by preventable or treatable communicable diseases, such as malaria, HIV/AIDS, lower respiratory diseases, and tuberculosis.

TABLE 3-4 Changes in the Leading Causes of Deaths and DALYs Globally, 1990 and 2016

Leading Causes of Deaths

1990		2016	
Rank	**Cause**	**Rank**	**Cause**
1	Ischemic heart disease	1	Ischemic heart disease
2	Stroke	2	Stroke
3	Lower respiratory infections	3	COPD
4	Diarrheal diseases	4	Alzheimer's disease and other dementias
5	COPD	5	Lower respiratory infections
6	Tuberculosis	6	Tracheal, bronchus, and lung cancer
7	Neonatal preterm birth	7	Diarrheal diseases
8	Road injuries	8	Diabetes
9	Lung cancer	9	Road injuries
10	Alzheimer's disease and other dementias	10	Tuberculosis

Leading Causes of DALYs

1990		2016	
Rank	**Cause**	**Rank**	**Cause**
1	Lower respiratory infections	1	Ischemic heart disease
2	Diarrheal diseases	2	Stroke
3	Ischemic heart disease	3	Lower respiratory infections
4	Neonatal preterm birth	4	Low back and neck pain
5	Stroke	5	Diarrheal diseases
6	Measles	6	Road injuries
7	Congenital defects	7	Sense organ diseases
8	Neonatal encephalopathy	8	COPD
9	Tuberculosis	9	Neonatal preterm birth
10	Road injuries	10	HIV/AIDS

Data from Institute of Health Metrics and Evaluation (IHME). (n.d.). GBD Compare: Viz Hub. Retrieved from https://vizhub.healthdata.org/gbd-compare/

TABLE 3-5 Leading Causes of Death in Children Under 5 by World Bank Country Income Group, 2016

Rank	Low-Income	Lower Middle-Income	Upper Middle-Income	High-Income
1	Malaria	Lower respiratory infections	Neonatal preterm birth	Congenital defects
2	Lower respiratory infections	Neonatal preterm birth	Congenital defects	Neonatal preterm birth
3	Diarrheal diseases	Neonatal encephalopathy	Lower respiratory infections	Other neonatal disorders
4	Neonatal encephalopathy	Malaria	Neonatal encephalopathy	Neonatal encephalopathy
5	Neonatal preterm birth	Diarrheal diseases	Other neonatal disorders	Sudden infant death syndrome (SIDS)
6	Protein-energy malnutrition	Congenital defects	Neonatal sepsis	Neonatal sepsis
7	Neonatal sepsis	Other neonatal disorders	HIV/AIDS	Lower respiratory infections
8	Congenital defects	Neonatal sepsis	Diarrheal diseases	Road injuries
9	Other neonatal disorders	Meningitis	Road injuries	Endocrine, metabolic, blood, and immune disorders
10	Meningitis	Protein-energy malnutrition	Drowning	Mechanical forces

Data from Institute of Health Metrics and Evaluation (IHME). (n.d.). GBD Compare: Viz Hub. Retrieved from https://vizhub.healthdata.org/gbd-compare/

Nutritional issues are also prominent in the lowest-income countries, and road traffic injuries and drowning are important causes of death in the low- and lower middle-income countries. In this age group, the significant shift in the causes of death occurs as one moves to upper middle-income countries and continues across the high-income countries. In these two country income groups, we see the importance of road injuries, drowning, violence, and cancers among the leading causes of death. In the high-income countries alone, self-harm is also among the 10 leading causes of death in this age group.

TABLE 3-7 examines the leading causes of deaths and DALYs for the age group 15 to 49, by World Bank country income group.

A number of key points emerge from Table 3-7. The leading causes of death in low-income countries are strikingly different from those in the higher country income groups and still include a number of communicable diseases beyond lower respiratory

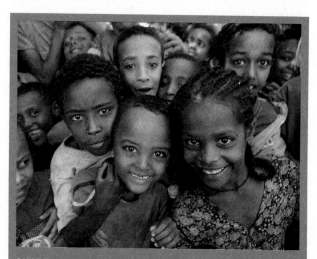

PHOTO 3-2 This picture depicts a group of older Ethiopian children. What health conditions are likely to be the most important causes of death for children 8 to 10 years old in Ethiopia? How would that vary between better-off places and lower-resource places within Ethiopia?
Courtesy of Mark Tuschman.

TABLE 3-6 Leading Causes of Death in Children Ages 5–14 by World Bank Country Income Group, 2016

Rank	Low-Income Countries	Lower Middle-Income Countries	Upper Middle-Income Countries	High-Income Countries
1	Malaria	Intestinal infectious diseases	Road injuries	Road injuries
2	HIV/AIDS	Malaria	Drowning	Congenital defects
3	Diarrheal diseases	Diarrheal diseases	Leukemia	Brain cancer
4	Lower respiratory infections	Lower respiratory infections	Congenital defects	Leukemia
5	Meningitis	Road injuries	Lower respiratory infections	Other neoplasms
6	Road injuries	Drowning	Interpersonal violence	Drowning
7	Drowning	HIV/AIDS	Brain cancer	Self-harm
8	Protein-energy malnutrition	Meningitis	Conflict and terror	Interpersonal violence
9	Intestinal infectious diseases	Congenital defects	Other neoplasms	Endocrine, metabolic, blood, and immune disorders
10	Tuberculosis	Conflict and terrorism	Falls	Lower respiratory infections

Data from Institute of Health Metrics and Evaluation (IHME). (n.d.). GBD Compare: Viz Hub. Retrieved from https://vizhub.healthdata.org/gbd-compare/

infections, such as HIV/AIDS, tuberculosis, diarrheal disease, malaria, and meningitis. The leading causes of DALYs in this country income group, however, also include a number of conditions that are mostly linked with disability, including low back and neck pain, skin disease, depressive disorders, and migraines.

The leading cause of death in lower middle-income countries is ischemic heart disease. However, the leading causes also include a number of communicable diseases beyond the lower respiratory infections one would expect, such as HIV/AIDS, tuberculosis, and diarrheal diseases. The importance of road injuries, self-harm, and interpersonal violence is also striking for this group. The leading causes of DALYs in this country income group look quite similar to those for low-income countries but also include dietary iron deficiency.

The leading causes of deaths in upper middle-income countries suggest some important shifts compared to low- and lower middle-income countries. Like in the lower middle-income countries, the leading causes of death in this country income group include HIV/AIDS, interpersonal violence, and self-harm. However, in this country income group we also see the importance of cancers, as well as falls. The leading causes of DALYs in this country income group are similar to those for the lower middle-income country group.

The leading causes of death in the high-income countries suggest substantial shifts from the lower-income groups. Self-harm, road injuries, ischemic heart disease, and stroke are important in this group, as in lower middle-income and upper middle-income countries. However, we also see here the emergence of breast, lung, and colorectal cancers, as well as drug use and alcohol use disorders. The leading causes of DALYs in the high-income countries do include ischemic heart disease and road injuries, as one might expect. However, the prominence of several mental disorders, including depressive disorders and anxiety disorders, as well as drug use disorders and self-harm, is striking.

Causes of Deaths and DALYs by Sex

It is also important to examine deaths and DALYs by sex, as shown in **TABLE 3-8**.

TABLE 3-7 Leading Causes of Deaths and DALYs, Ages 15–49, by World Bank Country Income Group, 2016

Low-Income Countries

Cause

Rank	Deaths	DALYs
1	HIV/AIDS	HIV/AIDS
2	Tuberculosis	Tuberculosis
3	Road injuries	Road injuries
4	Diarrheal diseases	Diarrheal diseases
5	Lower respiratory infections	Low back and neck pain
6	Ischemic heart disease	Skin diseases
7	Stroke	Lower respiratory infections
8	Interpersonal violence	Depressive disorders
9	Malaria	Migraine
10	Meningitis	Ischemic heart disease

Lower Middle-Income Countries

Cause

Rank	Deaths	DALYs
1	Ischemic heart disease	Road injuries
2	HIV/AIDS	Ischemic heart disease
3	Road injuries	HIV/AIDS
4	Tuberculosis	Low back and neck pain
5	Self-harm	Migraine
6	Stroke	Tuberculosis
7	Diarrheal diseases	Self-harm
8	Chronic kidney disease	Skin diseases
9	Interpersonal violence	Dietary iron deficiency
10	Lower respiratory infections	Depressive disorders

(continues)

TABLE 3-7 Leading Causes of Deaths and DALYs, Ages 15–49, by World Bank Country Income Group, 2016 *(continued)*

Upper Middle-Income Countries

Cause

Rank	Deaths	DALYs
1	Road injuries	Road injuries
2	Ischemic heart disease	Low back and neck pain
3	HIV/AIDS	HIV/AIDS
4	Interpersonal violence	Skin diseases
5	Stroke	Migraine
6	Self-harm	Ischemic heart disease
7	Liver cancer	Interpersonal violence
8	Tracheal, bronchus, and lung cancer	Depressive disorders
9	Lower respiratory infections	Stroke
10	Falls	Self-harm

High-Income Countries

Cause

Rank	Deaths	DALYs
1	Self-harm	Low back and neck pain
2	Road injuries	Migraine
3	Ischemic heart disease	Skin diseases
4	Drug use disorders	Drug use disorders
5	Stroke	Depressive disorders
6	Interpersonal violence	Self-harm
7	Breast cancer	Road injuries
8	Tracheal, bronchus, and lung cancer	Anxiety disorders
9	Colorectal cancer	Other musculoskeletal disorders
10	Alcohol use disorders	Ischemic heart disease

TABLE 3-8 Leading Causes of Deaths and DALYs by Sex, by World Bank Country Income Group, 2016

Females

Low-Income Countries

Cause

Rank	Deaths	DALYs
1	Lower respiratory infections	Malaria
2	Ischemic heart disease	Lower respiratory infections
3	Diarrheal diseases	Diarrheal diseases
4	Stroke	HIV/AIDS
5	Malaria	Neonatal encephalopathy
6	HIV/AIDS	Neonatal preterm birth
7	Tuberculosis	Tuberculosis
8	COPD	Protein-energy malnutrition
9	Neonatal encephalopathy	Congenital defects
10	Neonatal preterm birth	Meningitis

Lower Middle-Income Countries

Cause

Rank	Deaths	DALYs
1	Ischemic heart disease	Ischemic heart disease
2	Stroke	Diarrheal diseases
3	Diarrheal diseases	Lower respiratory infections
4	Lower respiratory infections	Stroke
5	COPD	Dietary iron deficiency
6	Diabetes	Neonatal preterm birth
7	Tuberculosis	Malaria
8	Alzheimer's disease and other dementias	Low back and neck pain
9	Malaria	Sense organ diseases
10	Chronic kidney disease	COPD

(continues)

TABLE 3-8 Leading Causes of Deaths and DALYs by Sex, by World Bank Country Income Group, 2016   *(continued)*

Females

Upper Middle-Income Countries

Cause

Rank	Deaths	DALYs
1	Ischemic heart disease	Ischemic heart disease
2	Stroke	Stroke
3	Alzheimer's disease and other dementias	Low back and neck pain
4	COPD	Sense organ diseases
5	Diabetes	Depressive disorders
6	Tracheal, bronchus, and lung cancer	Diabetes
7	Lower respiratory infections	Skin diseases
8	Hypertensive heart disease	Migraine
9	Chronic kidney disease	COPD
10	Breast cancer	Road injuries

High-Income Countries

Cause

Rank	Deaths	DALYs
1	Ischemic heart disease	Low back and neck pain
2	Alzheimer's disease and other dementias	Ischemic heart disease
3	Stroke	Alzheimer's disease and other dementias
4	Tracheal, bronchus, and lung cancer	Stroke
5	COPD	Skin diseases
6	Lower respiratory infections	Sense organ diseases
7	Breast cancer	Migraine
8	Colorectal cancer	Depressive disorders
9	Chronic kidney disease	Diabetes
10	Diabetes	Tracheal, bronchus, and lung cancer

Males		
Low-Income Countries		
Cause		
Rank	**Deaths**	**DALYs**
1	Lower respiratory infections	Lower respiratory infections
2	Diarrheal diseases	Malaria
3	Ischemic heart disease	Diarrheal diseases
4	Tuberculosis	HIV/AIDS
5	HIV/AIDS	Neonatal encephalopathy
6	Malaria	Tuberculosis
7	Stroke	Neonatal preterm birth
8	Neonatal encephalopathy	Protein-energy malnutrition
9	Road injuries	Meningitis
10	Protein-energy malnutrition	Neonatal sepsis
Lower Middle-Income Countries		
Cause		
Rank	**Deaths**	**DALYs**
1	Ischemic heart disease	Ischemic heart disease
2	Stroke	Lower respiratory infections
3	COPD	Diarrheal diseases
4	Lower respiratory infections	Road injuries
5	Diarrheal diseases	Stroke
6	Tuberculosis	Neonatal preterm birth
7	Road injuries	COPD
8	Diabetes	Tuberculosis
9	Chronic kidney disease	Neonatal encephalopathy
10	HIV/AIDS	Malaria

(*continues*)

TABLE 3-8 Leading Causes of Deaths and DALYs by Sex, by World Bank Country Income Group, 2016   *(continued)*

Males

Upper Middle-Income Countries

Cause

Rank	Deaths	DALYs
1	Ischemic heart disease	Ischemic heart disease
2	Stroke	Stroke
3	COPD	Road injuries
4	Tracheal, bronchus, and lung cancer	Low back and neck pain
5	Road injuries	Tracheal, bronchus, and lung cancer
6	Liver cancer	COPD
7	Alzheimer's disease and other dementias	Sense organ diseases
8	Stomach cancer	Liver cancer
9	Lower respiratory infections	Diabetes
10	Chronic kidney disease	Interpersonal violence

High-Income Countries

Cause

Rank	Deaths	DALYs
1	Ischemic heart disease	Ischemic heart disease
2	Tracheal, bronchus, and lung cancer	Low back and neck pain
3	Stroke	Tracheal, bronchus, and lung cancer
4	Alzheimer's disease and other dementias	Stroke
5	COPD	Sense organ diseases
6	Lower respiratory infections	Diabetes
7	Colorectal cancer	Road injuries
8	Prostate cancer	Self-harm
9	Self-harm	COPD
10	Chronic kidney disease	Skin diseases

Data from Institute of Health Metrics and Evaluation (IHME). (n.d.). GBD Compare: Viz Hub. Retrieved from https://vizhub.healthdata.org/gbd-compare/

When considering the leading causes of deaths and DALYs for females, it is important to remember that much of the global health literature on females focuses on reproductive health. While this *is* an important matter, it is essential to view female health more broadly. Every maternal death is unacceptable, but the leading cause of female death globally is ischemic heart disease, with stroke also being an important cause of death. We can also see that HIV/AIDS and TB remain important causes of female death in lower-income countries. As country income levels rise, diabetes, chronic obstructive pulmonary disease (COPD), a range of cancers, chronic kidney disease, and Alzheimer's disease become increasingly important causes of death.

Because these data are for all age groups, we see a range of neonatal conditions as important causes of DALYs in the low-income country group, as well as nutritional issues. However, as country incomes rise, the leading causes of DALYs cluster increasingly around a number of noncommunicable causes, plus depressive disorders.

The leading causes of death among men of all ages do not differ greatly from the leading causes of death for women of all ages. However, COPD, road injuries, self-harm, and liver cancers are more important causes of death for men than for women, as, of course, is prostate cancer. The causes of DALYs for males of all ages follow a pattern similar to that for females.

In this case, too, diabetes, COPD, sense organ diseases, and skin diseases become increasingly important as country income levels rise. For males, however, road injuries and interpersonal violence are much more important causes of deaths and DALYs than for females.

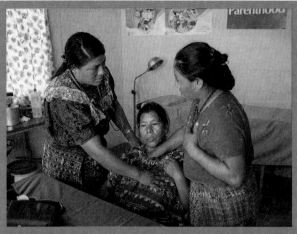

PHOTO 3-3 An indigenous woman in Guatemala is shown here being examined by healthcare workers in a local clinic. What are the most important burdens of disease for women like the one shown? What are the most important risk factors for those burdens? Why is it so important to consider the health of women broadly and not just focus on their reproductive health?

Courtesy of Mark Tuschman.

The Burden of Deaths and Disease Within Countries

As you consider causes of death and the burden of disease globally and by country income group, region, age, and sex, it is also important to consider how deaths and DALYs vary within countries by gender, ethnicity, and socioeconomic status, among other things. Generally speaking, the following statements are true:

- Rural populations will be less healthy than urban populations.
- Disadvantaged ethnic minorities will be less healthy than majority populations.
- Females will suffer a number of conditions that relate to their relatively disadvantaged social positions.
- Lower-income people will be less healthy than better-off people.
- Uneducated people will be less healthy than better-educated people.

In addition, people of lower socioeconomic status will have higher rates of communicable diseases, illness, and death related to maternal causes and malnutrition than will people of higher status. People of lower socioeconomic status will also suffer from a larger burden of disease related to smoking, alcohol, and poor diet than would be the case for better-off people. These points are fundamental to understanding global health.

Risk Factors

As we discuss the determinants of health and how health status is measured, there will be many references to **risk factors** for various health conditions. A risk factor is "an aspect or personal behavior or life-style, an environmental exposure, or an inborn or inherited characteristic, that, on the basis of epidemiologic evidence, is known to be associated with health-related condition(s) considered important to prevent."[18(p51)] Risks that relate to health can also be thought of as "a probability of an adverse outcome, or a factor that raises this probability."[19(p7)] We are all familiar with the notion of risk factors from our own lives and from encounters with health services. When we answer questions about our health history, for example, we are essentially helping to identify the most important risk factors that we face ourselves. Do our parents suffer from any health conditions that might affect our own health? Are we eating in a way that is conducive to good health? Do we get enough exercise and enough sleep? Do we smoke or drink alcohol excessively? Are there any special stresses in our life? Do we wear seat belts when we drive?

If we extend the idea of risk factors to people with fewer resources, especially in low- and lower middle-income countries, then we might add some other questions that relate more to the ways that they live. Does the family have safe water to drink? Do their house and community have appropriate sanitation? Does the family cook indoors in a way that makes the house smoky? Do the parents work in places that are safe environmentally? We might also have to ask if there is war or conflict in the country, because they are also important risk factors for illness, death, and disability.

If we are to understand how the health status of people can be enhanced, then it is very important that we understand the risk factors to which their health problems relate. **TABLE 3-9** shows the relative importance of different risk factors to deaths and DALYs for different country income groups. The burden of disease studies generally refer to these risks in three categories, behavioral, environmental and occupational, and metabolic, and it is valuable to keep this in mind as one considers risk factors.[16]

There are two points that stand out as one looks at risk factors by country income group. First, consistent with the pattern of deaths and DALYs, the low-income countries continue to face a number of risks related to Group I causes, such as the lack of safe water and sanitation, household air pollution, low birthweight, and child growth failure. Beyond this, however, there is a noteworthy convergence of key risks for deaths and DALYs across the country income groups. These risks overwhelmingly relate to high blood pressure, smoking, ambient particulate matter, and dietary risks associated with overweight and obesity.

▶ Demography and Health

There are a number of points related to population that are extremely important to people's health. These are among the most important:

- Population growth
- Population aging
- Urbanization
- The demographic divide
- The demographic transition

These factors are briefly discussed next, along with their implications for health. Other important matters related to population, such as the relationship between fertility and the health of women and children, are discussed in other chapters.

Population Growth

The population of the world was estimated in August 2018 to be about 7.6 billion[20] and is still growing. As shown in **FIGURE 3-4**, it is estimated that by 2050 the population of the world will be about 9.9 billion.[20]

As also shown in Figure 3-4, the overwhelming majority of population growth in the future will occur in low- and middle-income countries, especially in sub-Saharan Africa. This reflects the fact that fertility is falling slowly in many countries that have had high fertility rates historically, whereas many of the high-income countries already have very low fertility. In fact, some high-income countries are below **replacement fertility**. At a minimum, we should expect that increasing population growth in low-income countries will put substantial pressure on the environment, with its attendant risks for health. It will also mean that infrastructure, such as water supply and sanitation, will have to be provided to an increasing number of people in the countries that have the largest service gaps and can least afford to expand such services. This could cause these countries to face substantial impacts on health as a result. Increasing population will also make it more difficult for low-income countries to provide education and health services, with additional consequences for the health of their people in the future.

Population Aging

As shown in **TABLE 3-10**, the population of the world is aging.

This is especially true in high-income countries that have low fertility, but this is occurring in other countries as well. One impact of population aging is that it changes the ratio between the number of people that are 15 to 64 years of age, compared with the number that are 65 years of age or older. This is called the **elderly support ratio**. In Niger, with high fertility and a growing population, only 5 percent of the population in 2017 was over 65 years of age. By contrast, in

TABLE 3-9 Leading Risk Factors for Deaths and DALYs by World Bank Country Income Group, 2016

Low-Income Countries

Risk Factor

Rank	Deaths	DALYs
1	High blood pressure	Low birthweight and short gestation
2	Household air pollution	Child growth failure
3	Low birthweight and short gestation	Household air pollution
4	Child growth failure	Unsafe water
5	Unsafe sex	Unsafe sex
6	Ambient particulate matter	Unsafe sanitation
7	High fasting plasma glucose	No access to handwashing facility
8	Unsafe water	High blood pressure
9	Smoking	Ambient particulate matter
10	Unsafe sanitation	High fasting plasma glucose

Lower Middle-Income Countries

Risk Factor

Rank	Deaths	DALYs
1	High blood pressure	Low birthweight and short gestation
2	High fasting plasma glucose	High blood pressure
3	Ambient particulate matter	High fasting plasma glucose
4	Smoking	Ambient particulate matter
5	High total cholesterol	Smoking
6	Household air pollution	Child growth failure
7	High body-mass index	High body-mass index
8	Low birthweight and short gestation	Household air pollution
9	Impaired kidney function	High total cholesterol
10	Low fruit	Unsafe water

(continues)

TABLE 3-9   Leading Risk Factors for Deaths and DALYs by World Bank Country Income Group, 2016   *(continued)*

Upper Middle-Income Countries

Risk Factor

Rank	Deaths	DALYs
1	High blood pressure	High blood pressure
2	Smoking	Smoking
3	High fasting plasma glucose	High body-mass index
4	High body-mass index	High fasting plasma glucose
5	High total cholesterol	Alcohol use
6	Ambient particulate matter	High total cholesterol
7	Alcohol use	Ambient particulate matter
8	High sodium	High sodium
9	Low whole grains	Low whole grains
10	Impaired kidney function	Low fruit

High-Income Countries

Risk Factor

Rank	Deaths	DALYs
1	High blood pressure	Smoking
2	Smoking	High blood pressure
3	High body-mass index	High body-mass index
4	High fasting plasma glucose	High fasting plasma glucose
5	High total cholesterol	Alcohol use
6	Alcohol use	High total cholesterol
7	Impaired kidney function	Low whole grains
8	Low whole grains	Drug use
9	Ambient particulate matter	Impaired kidney function
10	High sodium	Low fruit

Data from Institute of Health Metrics and Evaluation (IHME). (n.d.). GBD Compare: Viz Hub. Retrieved from https://vizhub.healthdata.org/gbd-compare/

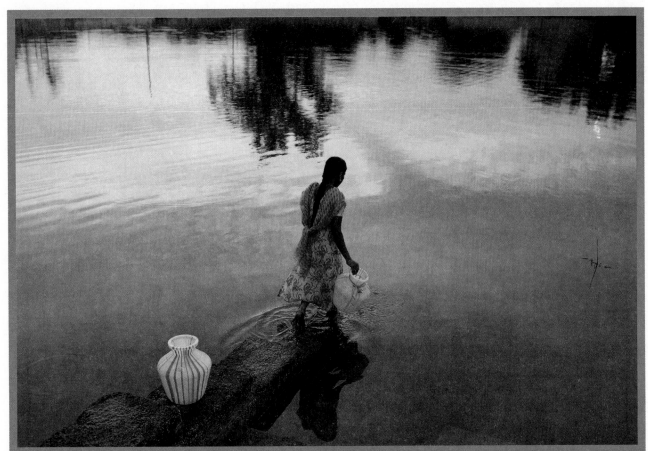

PHOTO 3-4 The lack of access to safe water remains a major risk factor for ill health in many low- and lower middle-income countries. This picture shows a woman in India retrieving water for household use from an open source. What risks does this pose to the woman, her family, and her community? What is likely to be the most cost-effective way of addressing those risks in the kind of community in which this woman lives?
Courtesy of Mark Tuschman.

Japan, with very low fertility and a shrinking population, 28 percent of the population was over 65 in 2017, as shown in Table 3-11.[21]

Population aging and the shift in the elderly support ratio have profound implications for the burden of disease and for health expenditures and how they will be financed. In the simplest terms, people will live longer and experience more years with morbidities and disabilities, largely related to noncommunicable diseases. This will raise the costs of health care. In addition, the large numbers of older adults for every working person will make it difficult for countries to finance that health care.

Urbanization

In the last 15 years, the majority of the world's population has lived in urban areas for the first time in world history. People are continuing to move from rural to urban areas, especially in low- and middle-income countries in which important shares of the population have continued to live in rural areas until recently. Continuing urbanization will also put enormous pressure on urban infrastructure, such as water and sanitation, schools, and health services, which are already in short supply in many countries. Gaps in such infrastructure, as well as the development of crowded and low-standard housing, for example, could have substantial negative consequences for health.

The Demographic Divide

Despite some convergence, there is an exceptional difference in the demographic indicators and future demographic paths of the best-off and the least-well-off countries, as suggested in the two previous sections. The highest-income countries generally have very low fertility, declining populations, and aging populations. By contrast, fertility in the lowest-income countries is generally still high, although it is declining slowly. In addition, the population is still growing in these countries and will continue to grow for some time.

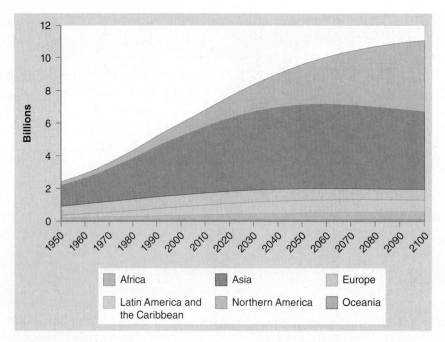

FIGURE 3-4 World Population 1950 to 2100

Modified from United Nations, Department of Economic and Social Affairs, Population Division. (2017). *World population prospects: The 2017 revision, key findings and advance tables* (Working Paper No. ESA/P/WP/248). New York, NY: United Nations. Retrieved from https://esa.un.org/unpd/wpp/Publications/Files/WPP2017_KeyFindings.pdf

TABLE 3-10 Percentage of the Population Over 65 Years of Age, by WHO Regions and Globally, 2015, 2030, and 2050

	2015	2030	2050
Africa	3.5	4.4	6.7
Asia	7.9	12.1	18.8
Europe	17.4	22.8	27.8
Latin America and the Caribbean	7.6	11.8	18.6
Northern America	15.1	20.7	21.4
Oceania	12.5	16.2	19.5
World	8.5	12.0	16.7

Data from He, W., Goodkind, D., & Kowal, P. (2016). An aging world: 2015 (U.S. Census Bureau, International Population Reports, P95/16-1).Washington, DC: U.S. Government Publishing Office. Retrieved from https://www.census.gov/content/dam/Census/library/publications/2016/demo/p95-16-1.pdf

There is also an enormous difference in the health circumstances of the high- and low-income countries. **TABLE 3-11** portrays the demographic divide.

The Demographic Transition

One important demographic trend of importance is called the **demographic transition**.[22] Simply put, this is the shift from a pattern of high fertility and high mortality to low fertility and low mortality, with population growth occurring in between.

When we look back historically at the countries that are now high-income, we can see that they had long periods when fertility was high, mortality was high, and population growth was, therefore, relatively slow, or might even have declined in the face of epidemics. Beginning around the turn of the 19th century, however, mortality in those countries began to decline as hygiene and nutrition improved and the burden of infectious diseases lessened. In most cases, this decline in mortality started before much decline in fertility. As mortality declined, the population increased and the share of the

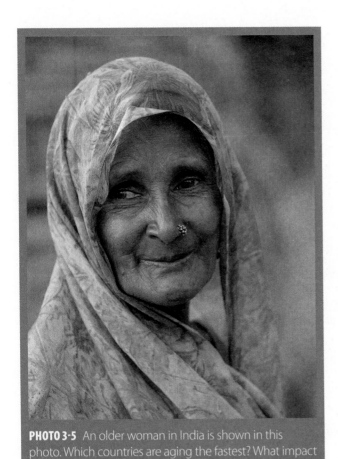

PHOTO 3-5 An older woman in India is shown in this photo. Which countries are aging the fastest? What impact is aging likely to have on the burden of disease and why?
Courtesy of Mark Tuschman.

population of younger ages also increased. Later, fertility began to decline and, as births and deaths became more equal, population growth slowed. As births and deaths stayed more equal, the share of the population that was of older ages increased. There are now some countries, as mentioned earlier, in which death rates exceed birth rates and the population is declining.

There are a number of ways to depict the demographic transition, one of which is shown in **FIGURE 3-5**.

The first "population pyramid" reflects a country with high fertility and high mortality, such as the low-income, high-fertility countries in sub-Saharan Africa. The second population pyramid is indicative of a country in which mortality has begun to decline but fertility remains high. This would be similar to the demographics one would find, for example, in a number of countries in sub-Saharan Africa that are undergoing demographic transition, or Haiti, as noted. The third pyramid reflects a population in which fertility has been reduced for a substantial period of time, in which fertility is continuing to decline, and in which there is a much larger share of older people in the population than in the first and second pyramids. This would be similar to the demographics in a number of low-fertility, aging populations in the upper middle- and high-income countries. The fourth pyramid illustrates a country, such as Japan, Russia, or

TABLE 3-11 The Demographic Divide: The Example of Nigeria and Japan		
	Nigeria	**Japan**
Population 2017 (millions)	190.9	126.7
Population 2050 (millions)	410.6	101.9
Lifetime births per woman	5.5	1.5
Births per 1,000 population	39	8
Births per 1,000 women ages 15–19	122	4
Percentage of married women ages 15–49 using modern contraception	10	44
Percentage of population below age 15	44	12
Percentage of population age 65+	3	28
Life expectancy at birth, males/females	52/54	81/87
Infant deaths per 1,000 births	69	1.9
Percentage of population ages 15–24 with HIV/AIDS, males/females	1.0/1.6	Data not available

Data from Population Reference Bureau. (2017). 2017 world population data sheet. Retrieved from https://www.prb.org/wp-content/uploads/2017/08/WPDS-2017.pdf

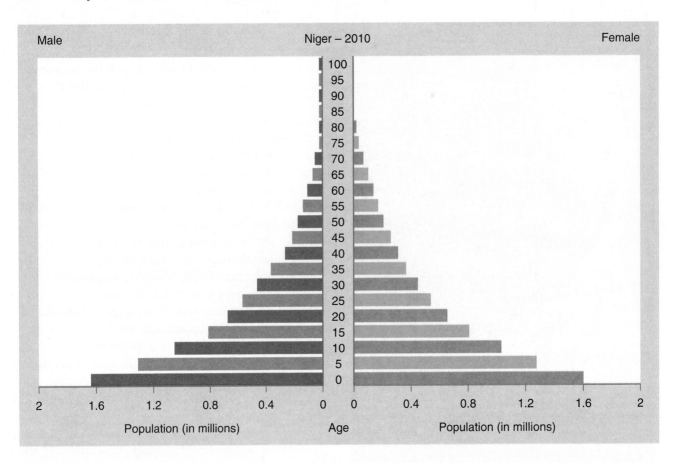

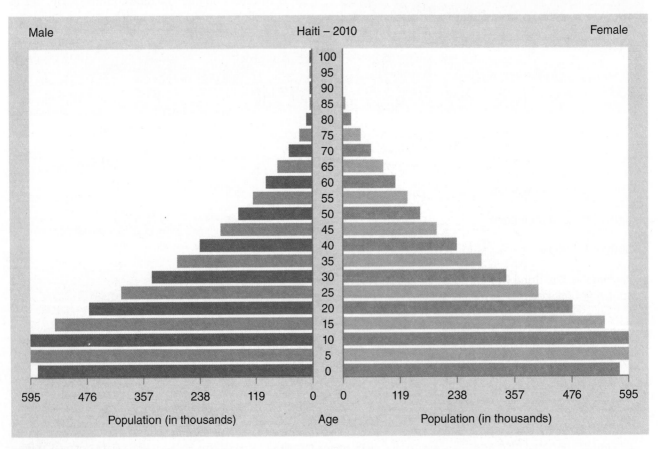

FIGURE 3-5 The Demographic Transition

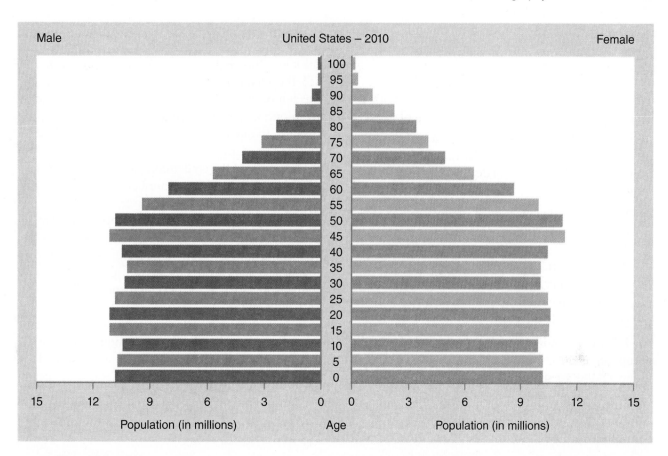

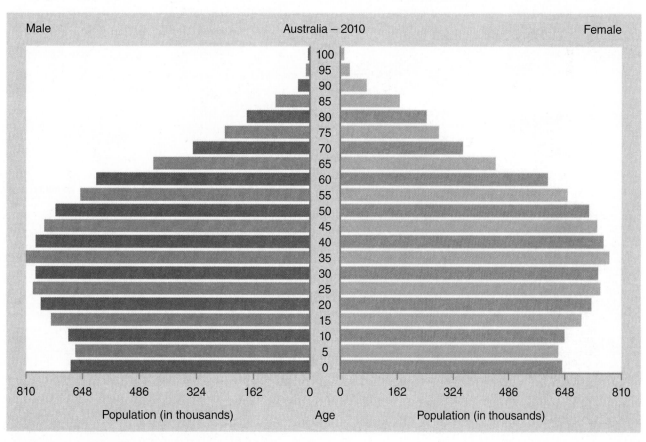

FIGURE 3-5 (CONTINUED) The Demographic Transition

Data from PopulationPyramid.net. (n.d.). Population pyramids of the world from 1950 to 2100. Retrieved from https://www.populationpyramid.net/world/2017/

Australia, in which mortality rates are low and fertility rates are very low and the population shrinks in the absence of immigration.

The Epidemiologic Transition

The **epidemiologic transition**[23] is closely related to the demographic transition, as suggested throughout the previous discussion. Historically there has been a shift in the patterns of disease that follows these trends:

- First, high and fluctuating mortality, related to very poor health conditions, epidemics, and famine
- Then, progressive declines in mortality as epidemics become less frequent
- Finally, further declines in mortality, increases in life expectancy, and the predominance of non-communicable diseases

FIGURE 3-6 shows the distribution of deaths by groups of causes, by World Bank country income group. **FIGURE 3-7** shows the distribution of DALYs.

You can see in Figures 3-6 and 3-7 how the pattern of deaths and DALYs differs between the low-, middle-, and high-income countries. You can also see the changes that will occur over time, as the burden of disease in lower-income countries moves from one with a substantial share of communicable diseases to one in which noncommunicable diseases are predominant.

The pace of the epidemiologic transition in different societies depends on a number of factors related to the determinants of health that were discussed earlier. In its early stages, the transition appears to depend primarily on improvements in hygiene, nutrition, education, and socioeconomic status. Some improvements also stem from advances in public health and in medicine, such as the development of new vaccines and antibiotics.[24]

Most of the countries that are now high-income went through epidemiologic transitions that were relatively slow, with the exception of Japan. Most low- and middle-income countries have already begun

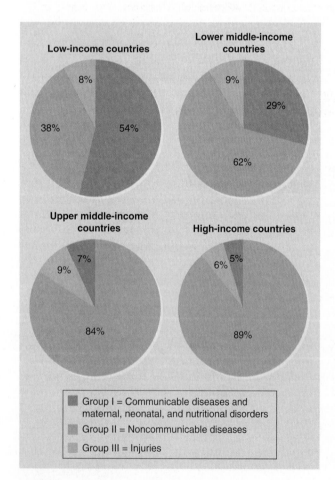

FIGURE 3-6 Distribution of Deaths by Cause Group, for World Bank Country Income Groups

Data from Institute of Health Metrics and Evaluation (IHME). (n.d.). GBD Compare: Viz Hub. Retrieved from https://vizhub.healthdata.org/gbd-compare/

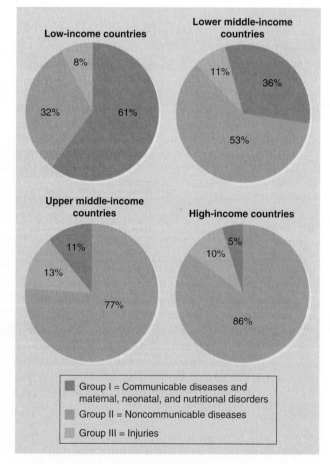

FIGURE 3-7 Distribution of DALYs by Cause Group, for World Bank Country Income Groups

Data from Institute of Health Metrics and Evaluation (IHME). (n.d.). GBD Compare: Viz Hub. Retrieved from https://vizhub.healthdata.org/gbd-compare/

their transition; however, it is still far from complete in many of them.

In fact, most low-income countries are in an ongoing epidemiologic transition, and many of them, therefore, face significant burdens of communicable and noncommunicable diseases and injuries at the same time. This strains the capacity of the health system of many of these countries. It is also expensive for countries that are resource-poor to address a substantial burden of all three of these types of conditions simultaneously.

▶ Progress in Health Status

There has been substantial progress in improving health and raising life expectancy in all parts of the world. However, those gains have not been uniform across regions or countries. Rather, life expectancy in sub-Saharan Africa and South Asia continues to substantially lag behind that in other regions. In addition, for countries that had a life expectancy in 1960 of less than 50 years, the pace of improvements in life expectancy in sub-Saharan Africa has been much slower than in any other region.

TABLE 3-12 shows life expectancy in 1960, 1990, and 2016 by World Bank region. The table also shows the percentage gain in life expectancy over three different periods, 1960 to 2016, 1960 to 1990, and 1990 to 2016.

Life expectancy grew over each period in each region; however, the increases in Europe and Central Asia were small in the period from 1990 to 2016, largely reflecting the social and economic consequences of the breakup of the former Soviet Union and the impact of changes on the health system as well. The slowdown in progress in improving life expectancy in sub-Saharan Africa between 1990 and 2016, although still very substantial, mostly reflects the negative impact on life expectancy of the HIV/AIDS epidemic, as well as slow economic progress in some countries and political conflict. The slow increase in life expectancy in the last period in North America reflects not only the high base from which it started but also the impact on life expectancy of an epidemic of substance abuse in the United States. By contrast, the dramatic increases in life expectancy from 1960 to 2016 in much of the low- and middle-income world reflects the rapid pace of economic development in many low- and middle-income countries, usually accompanied by improvements in infrastructure, nutrition, education, and health.

The factors that lead to improvements in health are complex. Additional comments are made at the end of this chapter about these factors, including the role, for example, of nutrition, education, political stability, and scientific improvements. Many other chapters also include comments on the progress in improving the health of women and children and in addressing particular causes of illness, disability, and death.

TABLE 3-12 Life Expectancy and Percentage Gain in Life Expectancy, by World Bank Region, 1960-2016

World Bank Region	Life Expectancy (Years)			Percentage Gain (1960–2016)	Percentage Gain (1960–1990)	Percentage Gain (1990–2016)
	1960	1990	2016			
East Asia & Pacific	48	69	75	56%	44%	9%
Europe & Central Asia	67	72	77	15%	7%	7%
Latin America & the Caribbean	56	68	75	34%	21%	10%
Middle East & North Africa	47	66	73	55%	40%	11%
North America	70	75	79	13%	7%	5%
South Asia	42	58	69	64%	38%	19%
Sub-Saharan Africa	40	50	60	50%	25%	20%

Data from The World Bank. (n.d.). Data: Life expectancy at birth, total (years). Retrieved from https://data.worldbank.org/indicator/SP.DYN.LE00.IN?locations=Z4-Z7-ZJ-ZQ-8S-ZG-XU-XD

The Burden of Disease: Looking Forward

The burden of disease in the future will be influenced by a number of factors that will continue to change. Some of these will relate to the determinants of health. Some will relate to the demographic forces just discussed, including population growth, population aging, and migration. The burden of disease in the future will also be driven by, among other things, the following factors:

- Economic development
- Scientific and technological change
- Climate change
- Political stability
- Emerging and re-emerging infectious diseases

These are discussed very briefly in the following sections.

Economic Development

The economies of low-income countries will need to grow if those countries are to generate the income they need to invest in improving people's health and well-being. The impact of economic development on health will depend partly on the extent to which economic growth is equitable across population groups. It will also depend on the extent to which countries are able—or choose—to use their increased income to invest in other areas that improve health, such as water, sanitation, hygiene, food security, and education. The extent and appropriateness of their investments in health, such as in low-cost, high-yielding efforts, will also be critical.

Scientific and Technological Change

Scientific and technological change has had an enormous impact on health and will continue to have an impact in the future. This is easy to understand, as one considers the development of vaccines or new drugs, such as antibiotics or antiretroviral therapy. The development of improved diagnostics for TB, for example, would have an substantial impact on the health of the world, as would the development of a vaccine against HIV or malaria. The impact of scientific and technological change on the low-income countries of today will depend to a large extent on the pace at which they are able to effectively adopt any improvements when they are developed.

Climate Change

The full extent of the impact of climate change on health is not clear; however, it is anticipated that climate change and its attendant impact on weather and rising sea levels could directly and indirectly have an important impact on health. On the indirect side, climate change could alter the nature of the food crops that can be grown in different places and food security and lead to migration from some places to others that are deemed more habitable. On the more direct side, climate change could lead to weather changes and adverse weather that harm people's health. It could also lead to the disappearance of disease vectors in some places as the weather is no longer hospitable to them, while allowing the emergence or re-emergence of disease vectors in other places.

Political Stability

In low-income countries, political stability appears to be necessary for achieving long-term gains in health. There is substantial evidence, for example, that the lack of political stability was a major impediment to progress in achieving the Millennium Development Goals in a number of countries. It is not hard to imagine, for example, how conflicts that occurred in Liberia, Sierra Leone, and the Democratic Republic of the Congo could set back health status for many years. These conflicts led directly to substantial illness, disability, and death. In addition, by causing a breakdown in infrastructure, such as water, sanitation, and electricity, as well as the erosion of health services, they also had enormous indirect impacts on health.

Emerging and Re-emerging Infectious Diseases

It is not possible to predict if and when new diseases will emerge or diseases already known will re-emerge. It is also not possible to know how well individual countries and the world will do in recognizing such problems as they arise and addressing them quickly and effectively. What is clear is that pandemic flu, for example, could have a major impact on future disease patterns. It is also clear, for example, that if the growth of drug resistance for, say, malaria, outpaced our ability to produce safe and effective drugs to fight malaria, this, too, could have a substantial impact on the burden of disease.

The Development Challenge of Improving Health

One of the key development challenges facing policymakers in low-income countries is how they can speed the demographic and epidemiologic transitions at the lowest possible cost. How can Niger, for example, improve its health status as rapidly as possible, at the least possible cost, and in the fairest ways? Will it be possible for the people of Niger to enjoy the health status of a middle-income country, even if Niger remains a low-income country?

FIGURE 3-8 shows national income of a sample of countries, plotted against life expectancy at birth for females in those countries. From this figure, one can see that, generally, the health of a country does increase as national income rises. However, one can also see that there are some countries, such as Bangladesh, Jordan, Peru, China, and Malaysia, that have achieved higher average life expectancies at birth for females than one would have predicted for countries at their level of income. At the same time, one has to ask why a country like Pakistan, with a similar per capita national income to Bangladesh and Cambodia, has lower female life expectancy than those countries have.

To a large extent, countries that have done better than one might expect in increasing life expectancy at birth for females (and males) achieved their health gains as a result of the following:

- Investing effectively and efficiently in areas that address key risk factors and determinants of health, including water, sanitation and hygiene, nutrition, and education
- Investing effectively and efficiently in relatively low-cost but high-impact health services, such as vaccination and the control of communicable diseases
- Taking a community-based approach to primary health care

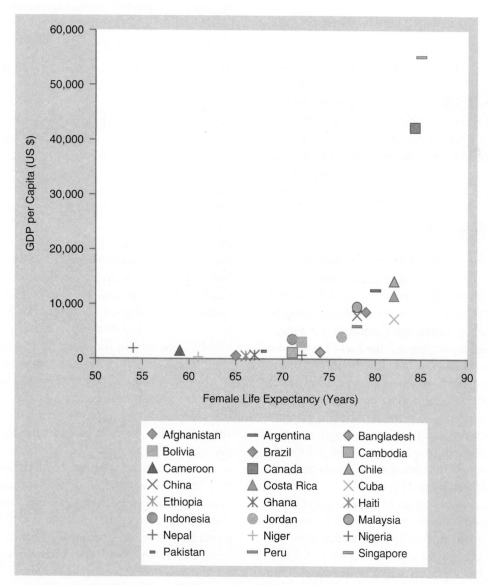

FIGURE 3-8 Gross Domestic Product per Capita and Female Life Expectancy at Birth, Selected Countries

Data from The World Bank. (n.d.). Life expectancy at birth, female (years) and GDP per capita (current US$). Retrieved from https://data.worldbank.org/

Indeed, in the long run, economic progress *will* help to bring down fertility, reduce mortality from communicable diseases, and help to produce a healthier population. However, at the present rates of progress in improving health in most low-income countries, these changes will take a very long time to occur. One considerable public policy challenge for these countries and their governments, therefore, is how they can short-circuit this process and reach reduced levels of fertility, lower mortality, and better health for their people, even as they remain relatively low-income.

▶ Case Study

One case study follows. It deals with an effort, called the Million Death Study, to gather valid data on deaths in India at a sustainable cost and in ways that are replicable.

The Aims of the Million Death Study

The Centre for Global Health Research, at the University of Toronto, Canada, is carrying out the Million Deaths Study in India in conjunction with the Registrar General of India. This study is one of the largest research efforts ever undertaken on the causes of premature mortality. Led by Professor Prabhat Jha, the study aims to help India improve the documentation of the underlying causes and risk factors of mortality as a basis for enhancing investments in health, reducing premature death, and improving the health of India's people.[25]

Vital statistics, such as fertility and mortality data, are crucial for identifying major health issues, identifying new health problems as they arise, making cost-effective public health investments, and evaluating the progress of public health interventions. Yet reliable mortality statistics are rare. As much as 75 percent of global deaths occur in low- and middle-income countries, and the majority of these lack medical supervision and official certification of cause of death.[26] In India, for example, 70 percent of deaths go unreported or misclassified.[27] Previous mortality estimates for India were largely based on data from the limited spectrum of deaths that occur in hospitals and were consequently biased toward causes of death that affect urban populations more than rural populations. They were also biased toward conditions that are more urgent and lead to hospitalization, rather than taking sufficient account of chronic health problems.[28] Moreover, in India and in many other middle- and low-income countries, there is a general dearth of knowledge around the causes of death, especially for middle-aged adults, and the corresponding risk factors leading to premature death.

The Study Approach

The Million Death Study seeks to assess the causes of death of 1 million people in India through monitoring 2.4 million households over two time periods: 1998 to 2003 and 2004 to 2014. The study is based on an approach called "verbal autopsy." The study uses India's Sample Registration System as its sampling framework. Twice a year, trained surveyors conduct surveys in order to identify households in which a death occurred. They then interview household members about the deaths in their families and record information on the events leading to death and the symptoms of the deceased. The verbal autopsies are sent to two independent physicians to be analyzed and ascertain the underlying cause of those deaths.[25] By early 2015, 600,000 deaths had been surveyed and 400,000 deaths had been fully coded.[29]

Key Findings to Date

The study thus far has exposed some mortality estimates and trends that deviate from those previously recognized.[27] First, the study has suggested that the top four causes of death in India are cardiovascular disease, chronic respiratory disease, TB, and cancer. Second, one of the most striking findings is related to the effects of tobacco. The average Indian smoker starts smoking later in life than in many other countries and often smokes hand-rolled locally manufactured cigarettes called bidis, which have a lower concentration of cancer-causing agents than commercially manufactured cigarettes. Nonetheless, this study showed that in India, smoking is as much a risk factor for premature death as in Europe and the United States. Moreover, study findings suggest that smoking is a risk factor for TB in India and that 40 percent of all TB deaths in middle-aged men in India can be attributed to smoking.[26] Third, the study suggests that some estimates of the burden of disease might be quite different from what was previously thought and that the burden of disease pattern varies greatly across the country. This study, for example, estimates that total malaria deaths are 10 times greater than the World Health Organization estimates, with over half of malaria deaths occurring in people ages 15 to 69 and the state of Odisha accounting for a quarter of India's annual malaria deaths.[26] On the other hand, the study suggests that mortality associated with HIV-related infections is lower than UNAIDS estimates, although the rural areas around Mumbai have a particularly high concentration of HIV-related deaths, with an annual death rate of 56 per 100,000.[26,27] The study has also led to revised estimates of the number of girls who are "missing" due to sex-selective abortion and suggested that most suicides are among young adults, rather than among adult farmers, as had previously been thought.[30]

Lessons of Experience

The Million Death Study may offer a model for improving mortality information that is reliable, high impact, low cost, and replicable in other countries. The ideal system to measure mortality would depend on a well-functioning system of vital registration. However, in the absence of such comprehensive registration programs, this study suggests that verbal autopsies can reduce inaccurate data by correctly classifying the underlying causes of 90 percent of the deaths occurring before age 70, an order of magnitude better than the limited cause of death data previously available.[28] This can help derive the probable cause of death when one has not been reported and help us to understand the leading causes of death.[25] Importantly, this approach has also been shown to be cost-effective. India added recording the causes of death and risk factors to a low-cost, preexisting sample registration system, at a cost of less than $2 per household.[29,31]

The long-term goal will always be universal civil registration of deaths with medical certification in order to minimize misclassification and misrepresentation. However, approaches such as those applied in the Million Death Study offer an interim solution for better statistics on mortality for many low- and middle-income countries.

▶ Main Messages

To understand and address the most important global health issues, we must understand the burden of disease, the risk factors for that burden, and how those vary among different population groups. Over the last several decades, the global burden of disease studies have provided the most comprehensive information on these matters.

These studies have also developed an important metric for assessing the burden of disease, the DALY. The DALY goes beyond measuring only deaths to provide an understanding of the amount of healthy life years lost due to both premature death and to years lived with disability. It is easy to understand the importance of the DALY when we consider causes of ill health that do not necessarily lead to death but that can lead to many years of disability, such as depressive disorders, musculoskeletal disorders, and the neglected tropical diseases.

The leading cause of death worldwide for both sexes and all age groups is ischemic heart disease, followed by stroke. All of the other 10 leading causes of death globally, except lower respiratory infections, HIV/AIDS, and TB, are noncommunicable diseases. The leading cause of DALYs for both sexes and all age groups globally is also ischemic heart disease when looking at both sexes combined and all age groups combined. However, the 10 leading causes of DALYs also include several diseases that especially affect large numbers of children in lower-income countries, such as diarrhea and malaria. The leading causes of DALYs also include road traffic injuries and low back pain.

The burden of disease is predominantly noncommunicable in all regions of the world except sub-Saharan Africa, and South Asia also continues to have a substantial burden of communicable disease. Over the last several decades, the burden of disease within regions and globally has continued to shift more and more toward a pattern dominated by noncommunicable diseases. Barring major outbreaks of communicable disease, this trend will continue, especially in the face of populations that are aging. This movement from a pattern of disease that is largely communicable to one that is largely noncommunicable is called the *epidemiologic transition.*

It is also important to understand the most important risk factors that are associated with deaths and DALYs. In the low-income countries, some of the most important risk factors include a range of nutritional issues, the lack of safe water or safe sanitation, indoor and ambient particulate matter pollution, and tobacco smoking. Poor diets that relate to obesity, high blood pressure, high cholesterol, and cardiovascular disease are becoming increasingly important problems as well, even in low-income countries. In the higher-income countries, the key risk factors for deaths and DALYs are overwhelmingly behavioral and have to do with what people eat, their levels of physical activity, and if they smoke tobacco, engage in excessive alcohol use, and drive safely. Ambient particulate matter pollution is also an important risk factor in the higher-income countries.

An understanding of basic demographic trends is also very helpful to understanding and addressing key global health issues. The three demographic trends that will have the most important impacts on health are the continuing increase in the global population, almost all from increases in low- and lower middle-income countries; the universal aging of populations; and the increasing urbanization of the world. Another fundamental concept that it is important to understand is the *demographic transition.* This refers to the movement over time from a pattern of high mortality and high fertility to one of low mortality and low fertility.

Study Questions

1. If you could pick only one indicator to describe the health status of a low-income country, which indicator would you use and why?

2. Why is it valuable to have composite indicators like the DALY to measure the burden of disease?

3. As countries develop economically, what are the most important changes that occur in their burden of disease?

4. Why do these changes occur?

5. How might the burden of disease differ from one region to another in a large and diverse country such as India or Nigeria?

6. How do we expect the burden of disease to evolve globally over the next 20 to 30 years?

7. What is the epidemiologic transition?

8. What is the demographic transition?

9. What are the leading causes of death of young children in low-income countries?

10. What are the leading causes of death in high-income countries, and how are they similar to and different from the causes in low-income countries?

References

1. Worldometers. (n.d.). *Bangladesh population.* Retrieved from http://www.worldometers.info/world-population/bangladesh-population/

2. Preamble to the Constitution of the World Health Organization as adopted by the International Health Conference, New York, 19–22 June, 1946; signed on 22 July 1946 by the representatives of 61 States (Official Records of the World Health Organization, no. 2, p. 100) and entered into force on 7 April 1948.

3. Merson, M. H., Black, R. E., & Mills, A. J. (2000). *International public health: Diseases, programs, systems, and policies.* Gaithersburg, MD: Aspen.

4. Institute of Health Metrics and Evaluation (IHME). (n.d.). *Frequently asked questions. What is HALE?* Retrieved from http://www.healthdata.org/gbd/faq#What%20is%20HALE?

5. Institute for Health Metrics and Evaluation (IHME). (2013). *The global burden of disease: Generating evidence, guiding policy.* Seattle, WA: Author. Retrieved from http://www.healthdata.org/sites/default/files/files/policy_report/2013/GBD_GeneratingEvidence/IHME_GBD_GeneratingEvidence_FullReport.pdf

6. World Health Organization (WHO). (n.d.). *Health status statistics: Mortality. Healthy life expectancy (HALE).* Retrieved from http://www.who.int/healthinfo/statistics/indhale/en/

7. Institute of Health Metrics and Evaluation (IHME). (n.d.). Global Burden of Disease Study 2016 (GBD 2016) data resources: GBD 2016 reference life table. Retrieved from http://ghdx.healthdata.org/gbd-2016

8. Salomon, J. A, Haagsma, J. A., Davis, A., de Noordhout, C. M., Polinder, S., Havelaar, A. H., . . . Vos, T. (2015). Disability weights for the Global Burden of Disease 2013 study. *Lancet Global Health, 3*(11), e712–e723.

9. GBD 2016 Disease and Injury Incidence and Prevalence Collaborators. (2017). Global, regional, and national incidence, prevalence, and years lived with disability for 328 diseases and injuries for195 countries, 1990–2016: A systematic analysis for the Global Burden of Disease Study 2016. *The Lancet* 390(10100):1227.

10. Voigt, K., & King, N. B. (2014). Disability weights in the global burden of disease 2010 study: two steps forward, one step back? *Bulletin of the World Health Organization* 92: 226–228.

11. GBD 2016 Collaborators. (2017). The Global Burden of Disease Study 2016. *The Lancet* 390(10100):1083–1464. Retrieved from https://www.thelancet.com/journals/lancet/issue/vol390no10100/PIIS0140-6736(17)X0041-X

12. Institute of Health Metrics and Evaluation (IHME). (n.d.). *Global Burden of Disease Study 2016 (GBD 2016) data resources.* Retrieved from http://ghdx.healthdata.org/gbd-2016

13. Institute of Health Metrics and Evaluation (IHME). (n.d). GBD Compare: Viz Hub. Retrieved from https://vizhub.healthdata.org/gbd-compare/

14. GBD 2016 Mortality Collaborators. (2017). Global, regional, and national under-5 mortality, adult mortality, age-specific mortality, and life expectancy, 1970–2016: A systematic analysis for the Global Burden of Disease Study 2016. *The Lancet* 390(10100):1084–1150.

15. GBD 2016 Causes of Death Collaborators. (2017). Global, regional, and national age-sex specific mortality for 264 causes of death, 1980–2016: A systematic analysis for the Global Burden of Disease Study 2016. *The Lancet* 390(10100): 1151–1210.

16. GBD 2016 Risk Factors Collaborators. (2017). Global, regional, and national comparative risk assessment of 84 behavioural, environmental and occupational, and metabolic risks or clusters of risks, 1990–2016: A systematic analysis for the Global Burden of Disease Study 2016. *The Lancet* 390(10100): 1345–1422.

17. GBS 2016 DALYs and HALE Collaborators. (2017). Global, regional, and national disability-adjusted life-years (DALYs) for 333 diseases and injuries and healthy life expectancy (HALE) for 195 countries and territories, 1990–2016: A systematic analysis for the Global Burden of Disease Study 2016. *The Lancet* 390(10100):1260–1344.

18. Last, J. M. (2001). *A dictionary of epidemiology* (4th ed.). New York, NY: Oxford University Press.

19. World Health Organization (WHO). (2002). *The world health report 2002: Reducing risks, promoting health life.* Retrieved from http://www.who.int/whr/2002/en/whr02_en.pdf

20. Population Reference Bureau. (2018). *2018 world population data sheet with focus on changing age structures.* Retrieved from https://www.prb.org/2018-world-population-data-sheet-with-focus-on-changing-age-structures/

21. The World Bank. (n.d.). Data: Age dependency ratio, old (% of working age population). Retrieved from https://data .worldbank.org/indicator/SP.POP.DPND.OL

22. Lee, R. (2003). The demographic transition: Three centuries of fundamental change. *Journal of Economic Perspectives* 17(4):167–190.

23. Omran, A. R. (2005). The epidemiologic transition: A theory of the epidemiology of population change. *Milbank Quarterly, 83*(4):731–757.

24. Jamison, D. T. (2006). Investing in health. In D. T. Jamison, J. G. Breman, A. R. Measham, et al. (Eds.), *Disease control priorities in developing countries* (pp. 3–34). New York, NY: Oxford University Press.

25. Jha, P., Gajalakshmi, V., Gupta, P. C., Kumar, R., Mony, P., Dhingra, N., & Peto, R. (2005). Prospective study of one million deaths in India: Rationale, design, and validation results. *PLoS Medicine* 3(2):e18. doi: 10.1371/journal.pmed.0030018

26. Westly, E. (2013, December 4). Global health: One million deaths. *Nature* 55:22–23. doi:10.1038/504022a

27. Vyawahare, M. (2014, May 22). Door by door, India strives to know about death. *New York Times*. Retrieved from http://www.nytimes.com/2014/05/23/world/asia/chasing -down-death-india-seeks-answers-on-premature-mortality .html?emc=edit_au_20140522&nl=afternoonupdate& nlid=54524785&_r=0

28. Aleksandrowicz, L., Malhotra, V., Dikshit, R., Gupta, P. C., Kumar, R., Sheth, J., . . . Jha, P. (2014). Performance criteria for verbal autopsy-based systems to estimate national causes of death: Development and application to the Indian Million Death Study. *BMC Medicine 12*(21). doi:10.1186/1741-7015-12-21

29. Jha, P. (2014). Reliable direct measurement of causes of death in low- and middle-income countries. *BMC Medicine* 12(19). doi:10.1186/1741-7015-12-19

30. Gomes, M., Begum, R., Sati, P., Dikshit, R., Gupta, P. C., Kumar, R., . . . Jha, P. (2017). Nationwide mortality studies to quantify causes of death: Relevant lessons from India's Million Death Study. *Health Affairs* 36(11):1887–1895. doi: 10.1377/hlthaff.2017.0635

31. World Health Organization (WHO). (2010). Save lives by counting the dead: Interview with Prabhat Jha. *Bulletin of the World Health Organization* 88: 161–241. Retrieved from http://www.who.int/bulletin /volumes/88/3/10-040310/en/

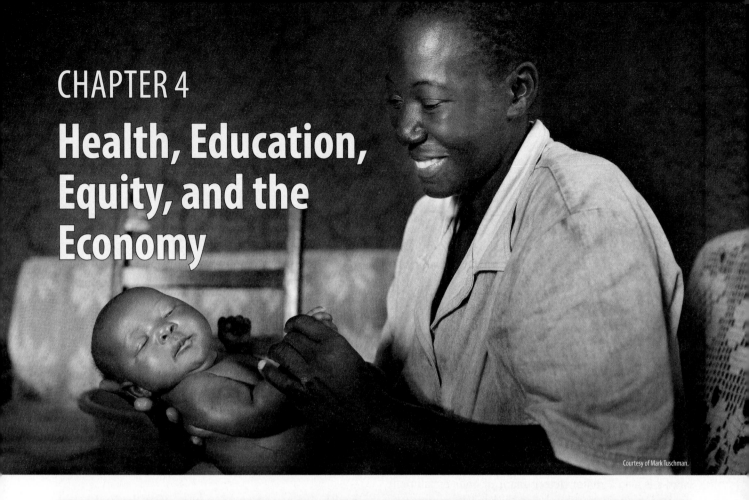

Courtesy of Mark Tuschman.

CHAPTER 4
Health, Education, Equity, and the Economy

LEARNING OBJECTIVES

By the end of this chapter, the reader will be able to do the following:

- Discuss the connections among health, education, productivity, and earnings
- Describe key relationships among health, the costs of illness, and the impact of health expenditure on poverty
- Discuss critical connections between health and equity
- Describe some relationships between expenditure on health and health outcomes
- Review the use of cost-effectiveness analysis as one tool for making investment choices in health
- Discuss the two-way relationship between health and development

▶ Vignettes

Savitha lived in a poor village in south India. When she first became sick, she visited an unlicensed "doctor." She did not recover and then went to a practitioner of Indian Systems of Medicine. After another 2 weeks of illness, she went to the outpatient clinic of the main hospital. By the time Savitha had begun to recover, she had spent the equivalent of $60 on health services and transportation to get to them. She had also missed 2 weeks of work, during which she lost another $60 of income. The total cost of this illness was about 10 percent of Savitha's annual earnings.

Mohammed was in first grade in a small town in northern Nigeria. Mohammed's family was poor. Mohammed was very small and thin for his age and

got sick more often than most children. Because of his poor health, Mohammed was unable to attend school regularly and was forced to quit school after only 1 year. Unfortunately, he could not read or write, had little knowledge of how to work with figures, and was most likely destined for a life of limited job prospects at very low pay.

Birte was born in Denmark to a middle-class family. She was exclusively breastfed until she was 6 months old, when appropriate complementary foods were introduced in a hygienic manner. Her family took her regularly for "well baby" checkups, and she received all of her scheduled childhood immunizations. Her hearing and her eyesight were checked before she enrolled in school. Birte attended school regularly, was attentive in class, and performed well there. She was able to complete secondary school and medical school and today is a physician.

ABC company was deeply invested in mining in southern Africa. The company was very concerned about the high prevalence of HIV/AIDS among its workers. This was causing losses in work days, the departure of workers, and major drops in the company's profits. The company considered leaving the region. However, the firm instead examined carefully the costs and benefits of different options for maintaining its business, including the possibility of running an HIV treatment program for its workers who were HIV-positive. In the end, the company decided that this approach would be best for its bottom line and for the communities with which it worked.

▶ Introduction

Health and economic matters are intimately linked in a number of ways. First, health is an important contributor to people's ability to be productive and to accumulate the knowledge and skills they need to be productive, known as **human capital**. Second, health status is also a major determinant of one's enrollment in and success in school, which itself is an important contributor to future earnings. Third, the costs of health care are also extremely important to individuals, especially to poor people, because large out-of-pocket expenditures can have a major impact on their financial status and can push them into poverty. Fourth, the costs of health care are also very important because health is a major item of national expenditure in all countries. Finally, the approach that different countries take to the financing and carrying out of health services raises important issues of equity and inequality.[1]

The objective of this chapter is to introduce the two-way relationship between health and development. The chapter first examines the connection between health and education. It then reviews the links between health and poverty, equity, and inequality. Lastly, the chapter explores the link between health and income at the level of individuals and the connections between health and development more broadly. As it reviews these themes, the chapter introduces some of the basic concepts of both global health and health economics.

▶ Health, Education, Productivity, and Poverty

Health and Education

Essentially, health and education are connected in three ways. First, there are intergenerational links: the

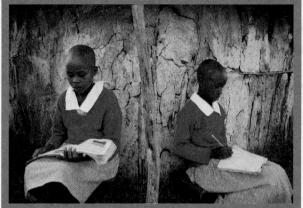

PHOTO 4-1 There has been great progress in the last 2 decades in enrolling girls in primary education, even in low-income countries. This is reflected in this photo of two Ugandan schoolgirls who are hard at work studying, albeit under rather basic conditions. It is important to ensure that children enrolled in school get an education of good quality and have a chance to go as far in education as possible. What are some of the measures that low-income and lower middle-income countries can take to achieve these aims?
Courtesy of Mark Tuschman.

health and education of parents affect the health and education of their children. Second, malnutrition and disease affect the cognitive development and school performance of children. Lastly, education enables people to better prevent and manage illness.

The global AIDS epidemic shows how the poor health of one generation can affect the schooling prospects and future earnings of the next generation. When mothers die of HIV/AIDS, for example, children are more likely to be poorly fed, malnourished, and in ill health. As a result, they are also less likely to attend school or to perform well there. During the period that a mother is sick with AIDS, it is also likely that one or more of her children will stay out of school to attend to the mother's health and the chores that the mother is no longer able to do.

Malnutrition and illness can limit schooling and school performance in a number of ways. First, families sometimes delay enrolling a sick or malnourished child in school. In addition, malnutrition and illness can reduce attendance at school and concentration when in school, thereby reducing student performance. Malnutrition and illness can also decrease cognitive development and ability. All of these factors ultimately constrain children's ability to learn in school, decrease the number of years of schooling they complete, and thereby reduce future earnings.

There is also a connection between education and health in the other direction: education is a powerful enabler of good health. We already know that education and knowledge of appropriate health behaviors are important determinants of health and, indeed, that the education of a child's mother is an important predictor of the health of a child. For example, the higher the level of education of a mother in a low- or middle-income country, the more likely she is to immunize her child, as reflected in **FIGURE 4-1** for a number of countries.[2]

The most extensive studies of the links between education and health show that the education of women has a powerful impact on child survival. One key study showed that each additional year of schooling of a woman was associated with a 7 to 9 percent reduction in the mortality of her children under 5 years of age. That same study concluded that the mortality rate of children under 5 years of age was almost 60 percent lower for the children of mothers with at least 7 years of schooling, compared to the children of mothers with no schooling.[3]

A 2010 review of the available literature on the subject also assessed the impact of the education of women on the mortality of children under 5 years of age over the period 1970 to 2009. That study also examined how the impact of a mother's education on child mortality compared with the impact of economic development on child mortality. The study focused on examining how many children died compared to how many children would have died if education and economic levels had stayed the same as they were in 1970. The study concluded that a little

more than half of the 8.2 million deaths of children under 5 years of age that were averted over this period were attributable to higher educational attainment of women of reproductive age (15 to 44 years old). The study also concluded that economic development had an important association with averting child deaths. However, the association of increased educational attainment of women of reproductive ages with averting child deaths was greater than that of economic development.[4]

Health, Productivity, and Earnings

Health has an important impact on labor productivity and earnings, separate from its link with education. First, good health increases longevity, and the longer one lives, the longer one can earn and the higher one's lifetime earnings will be. Second, a number of studies have shown that healthy workers are more productive than unhealthy workers. Among the most cited of such studies was one done on men who tapped rubber trees in Indonesia, many of whom were anemic due to hookworm infection. When the workers were treated for their infections, they became less anemic and their productivity increased by about 20 percent.[5] Third, many people cannot go to work when they are ill, and when they are absent from work, they often do not earn.

Health, the Costs of Illness, and Poverty

The costs of illness to individuals and their families can be high, can force them to lose or dispose of assets, and can cause them to fall into poverty. When people become ill in poor countries, as noted in the vignette about Savitha at the start of this chapter, they usually do seek health care, and they often seek care of different types. They frequently have to pay for treatment and for drugs, the costs of which can be a very substantial share of their income. In addition, illness often leads to a decline in earnings, because people miss work. There are also other indirect costs that people bear when they are ill, such as the costs of transportation to and from a health service provider.

Beyond the costs of either a short-term or a chronic illness, we must also remember the cost to individuals of living with the disability that comes from some health conditions. Measles or meningitis, for example, can lead to brain damage and hearing loss. Polio can lead to paralysis, and leprosy can lead to deformity. A number of mental health conditions are associated with long-term disability. The number of people with diabetes is increasing in rich and poor countries alike, and diabetes is often associated with a variety of disabilities. Long-lasting disabilities

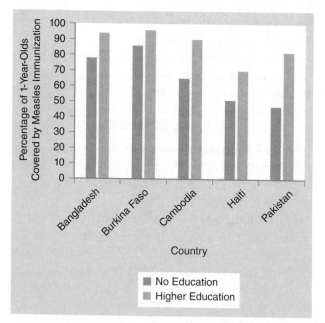

FIGURE 4-1 Percentage of 1-Year-Old Children Receiving Measles Immunization, by Mothers with No Education and Mothers with Higher Education, for Selected Countries, for Most Recent Year

generally require considerable expenditure on health services. In addition, they usually lead to a significant decline in the earnings of disabled persons and their family caretakers, compared to what they could earn if they were not disabled.

The costs of illness can be devastating for poor families. A study done in Bangladesh, for example, showed that a Bangladeshi lost the equivalent of 4 months of income from being sick with tuberculosis.[6] A review of the literature on the financial costs of tuberculosis in low- and middle-income countries found that individuals lost on average 60 percent of their annual earnings due to being sick with tuberculosis, and families lost almost 40 percent of their total household income due to such illnesses. These costs fell relatively harder on the poor and were often catastrophic.[7] Surveys done in India showed that hospitalization was a major contributor to people and families falling into poverty. Of the patients who were hospitalized at any point during a 1-year period that was studied, almost 25 percent of the people hospitalized were pushed below the official Indian poverty line because of the costs of their hospitalization, related expenditures, and lost wages. Moreover, more than 40 percent of those hospitalized borrowed money or sold assets to pay for their health care.[8] These findings were echoed in the seminal 2000 World Development Report of the World Bank, which noted that ill health is an important contributor to poverty and to the economic vulnerability that is at the foundation of poverty.[9]

▶ Health Disparities

Health disparities are an important concern of public health. As we begin to explore this issue, therefore, it is important to review some of the key terms related to health disparities.

The first key term is **health equity**. Amartya Sen, a Nobel Laureate in Economics, has suggested that we should see health equity as multidimensional:

> It includes concerns about achievement of health and the capability to achieve good health, not just the distribution of health care. But it also includes the fairness of processes and thus must attach importance to non-discrimination in the delivery of health care.[10(p665)]

Sen also suggested that health equity must be seen in the broader context of social justice issues, social structures within countries, and how countries choose to allocate their resources.[10]

A well-known British scholar of public health and the determinants of health, Margaret Whitehead, has provided a definition of **health inequity**: "differences in health that are not only unnecessary and avoidable, but also unfair and unjust."[11]

Another important term relates to inequality. The World Health Organization (WHO) defines **health inequality** as "differences in health status or in the distribution of health determinants between different population groups."[12]

Health disparities is another very commonly used term in public health and global health. The U.S. Centers for Disease Control and Prevention defines health disparities as "a type of difference in health that is closely linked with social or economic disadvantage."[13]

Although *equity* and *equality* are often used interchangeably when writing about health, in principle, *equity* concerns fairness, whereas *equality* largely refers to outcomes. Obviously, the two concepts are closely related. If a health system treats minority people in inequitable ways, such as by offering them lower coverage of key health services than it offers to others, we would expect that the minority group would have poorer health outcomes. In this case, as in many other cases, *inequity* plays an important role in the *inequality* of outcomes and the creation of health disparities.

It is essential to consider equity, inequality, and health disparities when discussing many different aspects of health care:

- Health status
- Access to health services
- Coverage of health services
- Protection from financial risks because of health costs
- The extent to which the approach to financing health is fair
- The distribution of health benefits

When thinking about these issues, one should consider the extent to which they vary across groups, why they vary, and what can be done to reduce inequity, inequality, and disparities.

In addition, when considering questions of access to and the coverage of health services, it will be important to consider such questions quite broadly. It has been suggested, for example, that one must take a multidimensional view of access that would include the following factors[14]:

- *Geographic availability:* Distance or travel time
- *Availability:* The extent to which needed services are offered in a convenient manner by staff who are properly trained to deliver them

- *Financial accessibility:* The extent to which people are able or willing to pay for services and not fall into financial distress by doing so
- *Acceptability:* The extent to which services are in line with local cultural norms and expectations

When taking an "equity, inequality, and health disparity lens" to global health concerns, it is also important to consider how they vary according to the following factors:

- Social and economic status
- Health status and whether or not the person is disabled
- Ethnicity
- Gender
- Religion
- Location
- Occupation
- Social capital
- Sexual orientation

In addition, it is important to keep in mind differences in key health issues both *across* countries and *within* countries.

When proceeding through this text, one should understand that there are enormous inequities, inequalities, and disparities in all areas of global health that are discussed. To a large extent, the pattern of inequity, inequality, and disparities can be summarized relatively easily:

- Less-well-off people, with less social and political power, will generally have worse health, poorer health services, and less protection in the financing of health services than those who are better off.
- These less-well-off groups will generally include women; indigenous people; ethnic, religious, and other minority groups; the poor; those living in rural areas; those working in the informal sector of the economy; those with limited education; and those who have relatively lower levels of social capital. Generally, disabled people, people with mental illness, and lesbian, gay, bisexual, and transgender people will also face discrimination that leads to inequities, inequalities, and disparities in health.

The following section examines some examples of the most critical concerns about health disparities and their links with inequity and inequality.

Health Disparities Across Countries

World Bank data on some of the basic indicators of health status, including life expectancy, maternal mortality, and neonatal, infant, and under-5 child mortality,

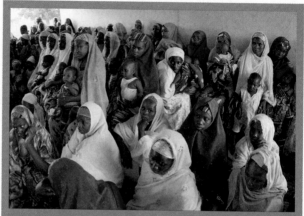

PHOTO 4-2 These families are attending a health clinic in northern Nigeria. The northern part of Nigeria has a lower per capita income, a lower level of education, and worse health indicators than the southern part of the country. What would the priority measures be for trying to enhance the health of those living in this region?

Courtesy of Mark Tuschman.

clearly portray the enormous variation across regions and countries. Life expectancy at birth in high-income countries, for example, was 80 years in 2016, which was about 27 percent higher than life expectancy at birth in low-income countries, which was 63.[15] The maternal mortality ratio in Sierra Leone was the highest in the world in 2016, at 1,360 per 100,000 live births. This was more than 450 times higher than the maternal mortality ratio of 3 per 100,000 live births that year in Greece, Iceland, and Poland.[16] The infant mortality rate in sub-Saharan Africa in 2016 was more than 10 times higher than the rate in high-income countries.[17]

Some people see these differences largely as a reflection of the status of economic development in different parts of the world. They might also believe that inequitable relationships among countries are at least partly the cause of weak economic development in poorer countries. These people would, therefore, see differences in health status at least partly as a reflection of inequity and injustice. However, some people might see health disparities both within and across countries as an indication of the lack of concern in some countries for their less-well-off people. They also believe this is inequitable and unjust.

Health Disparities Within Countries

Some countries have relatively little variation in health indicators across different population groups. This would generally be the case, for example, in Scandinavian countries and some of the other high-income nations of Europe. There are other countries, however, that have substantial variance in health indicators across population groups. These will tend to be high-income countries with disadvantaged ethnic minorities, such as Australia, Canada, or the United States, or they will be low- and middle-income countries. In 2015, for example, life expectancy for an American of Hispanic origin was 82.0, for a non-Hispanic white person it was 78.7, and it was 75.1 for a non-Hispanic black person. Thus, there was a difference of about 10 percent between the longest-lived group and the shortest-lived group.[18] Life expectancy for an aboriginal Australian or Torres Strait Islander female born between 2010 and 2012 was 73.7, compared to 83.1 for a nonindigenous female.[19]

FIGURE 4-2 shows the under-5 child mortality rate for a sample of five Indian states, including the state with the lowest rate and the state with the highest rate. The graph shows that some of the worst-performing Indian states have a child mortality rate more than four times that of one of the best-performing states. We should expect to see substantial variance in child mortality rates across geographic units in many other low- and middle-income countries as well, including countries like Brazil, Indonesia, and Nigeria. These variances remind us of the importance of looking beyond national averages and examining differences within, as well as across, countries.

Health Disparities and Location

We should expect basic health indicators to vary by location, with urban dwellers generally enjoying better access to health services, coverage, and health status than rural dwellers. We might also expect the variation between urban and rural dwellers to be greater

in low-income countries than in middle- and high-income countries.[20]

FIGURE 4-3 shows how the rate of stunting varies by location in three regions: Latin America and the Caribbean, South Asia, and sub-Saharan Africa. The gaps were most severe in Latin America and the Caribbean, with stunting of children under 5 years of age about 50 percent greater in rural areas than in urban ones.

FIGURE 4-4 shows, for select regions, how contraceptive use varies between rural and urban areas. In the East Asia and Pacific region, contraceptive prevalence rates were very high and about the same for urban and rural dwellers. In all other regions shown, however, there was a substantial gap in contraceptive

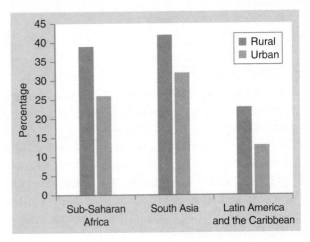

FIGURE 4-3 Percentage of Children 0 to 5 Years Who Are Stunted, by Location, for Selected Regions, Latest Data 2011–2016

Data from UNICEF. (n.d.). The state of the world's children 2017: Children in a digital world. Retrieved from https://www.unicef.org/sowc2017/

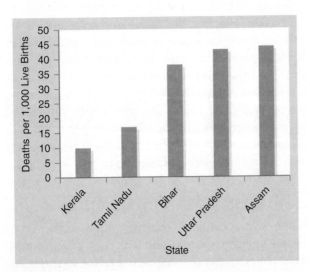

FIGURE 4-2 Infant Mortality in Selected Indian States, 2016

Data from National Institution for Transforming India. (2016). Infant Mortality Rate (IMR) (per 1000 live births). Retrieved from http://niti.gov.in/content/infant-mortality-rate-imr-1000-live-births

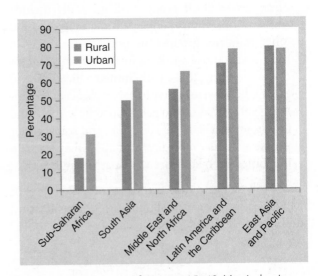

FIGURE 4-4 Percentage of Women 15–49, Married or in Union, Who Are Using Contraception, by Location, for Selected Regions

Data from UNICEF. (n.d.). Progress for children: Achieving the MDGs with equity. Retrieved from http://www.unicef.org/media/files/Progress_for_Children-No.9_EN_081710.pdf

prevalence between rural and urban dwellers, ranging from approximately a 50 percent difference in sub-Saharan Africa to about a 10 percent difference in Latin America and the Caribbean.

We should expect there to be substantial variation in access, coverage, and health status between rural and urban dwellers. Although many cities do contain large numbers of poor and slum-dwelling people, rural people generally will have lower incomes, less education, less access to health services and other health-related infrastructure, and less political voice than those who live in urban areas. Many ethnic minorities and indigenous people are also more likely to live in rural than in urban settings.

Health Disparities and Income

Much of the literature on health disparities and global health has focused on the relationship between those disparities and income. This literature has highlighted the sharp gaps in access, coverage, health status, fairness of financing, and health benefits between the less-well-off and the better-off.[20] In addition, much of this work has examined the variation of different health indicators by income quintiles, meaning divisions of the population into five equal income groups from the least-well-off to the best-off.

FIGURE 4-5 examines the extent to which births were attended by skilled personnel in South Asia and sub-Saharan Africa over the period 2011 to 2016. The figure reflects enormous gaps in both regions between the richest and the poorest income groups.

In sub-Saharan Africa, the richest 20 percent were 2.6 times more likely than the poorest 20 percent to have their birth attended by skilled personnel. In South Asia, the richest 20 percent of the population was 1.7 times more likely to have a birth attended by skilled personnel than the poorest 20 percent.

FIGURE 4-6 looks at the percentage of children who were stunted by income group for sub-Saharan Africa and South Asia around the same time as the other UNICEF data cited previously. This figure reflects almost the same level of variation between the better-off and the least-well-off as in the previous figure. Children under 5 from the lowest income group in South Asia were more than two times more likely to be stunted than children from the highest income group. Children under 5 from the lowest income group in sub-Saharan Africa were more than 2.5 times more likely to be stunted than those from the highest income group.

FIGURE 4-7 shows data from UNICEF on the coverage of measles immunization by income group for selected countries. Although the data is a bit dated, it is indicative of historic trends in immunization coverage before more recent progress in coverage in almost all low- and middle-income countries. The data in the figure clearly shows that the less well developed the immunization program in a particular country, the greater the gaps in coverage between income groups.

Although these differences by income may not be acceptable to us, they are not surprising. Income is associated with better education; better housing; better access to safe water, sanitation, hygiene, and health services; and safer work environments. It is

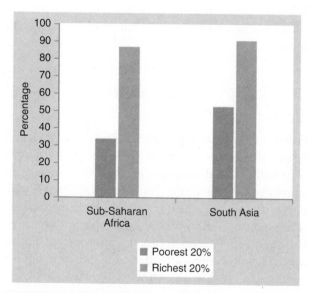

FIGURE 4-5 Percentage of Births Attended by Skilled Personnel, by Income Quintile, Latest Data 2011–2016, for Selected Regions

Data from UNICEF. (2017). The state of the world's children 2017: Children in a digital world. Retrieved from https://www.unicef .org/publications/files/SOWC_2017_ENG_WEB.pdf

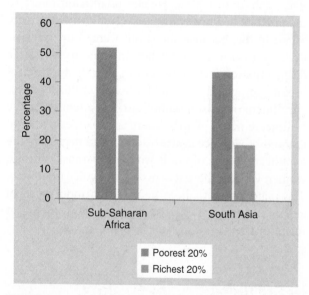

FIGURE 4-6 Percentage of Children 0 to 5 Years Who Are Stunted, by Income Quintile, Selected Regions, 2011–2016

Data from UNICEF. (2017). The state of the world's children 2017: Children in a digital world. Retrieved from https://www.unicef .org/sowc2017/

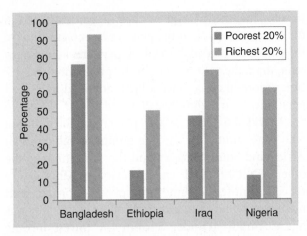

FIGURE 4-7 Coverage of Measles Immunization by Income Quintile, for Selected Countries, 2011

Restrepo-Méndez, M. C., Barros, A. J., Wong, K. L., Johnson, H. L., Pariyo, G., França, G. V., ... & Victora, C. G. (2016). Inequalities in full immunization coverage: trends in low- and middle-income countries. *Bulletin of the World Health Organization, 94*(11), 794.

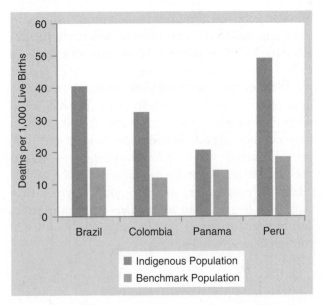

FIGURE 4-8 Infant Mortality Rates in Colombia, Panama, Peru, and Brazil, for the Indigenous Population and Benchmark Population

Note: The benchmark population is the total population for Colombia and Brazil; the total population excluding the indigenous population for Panama; and the population with Spanish as a mother tongue for Peru.

Anderson, I., Robson, B., Connolly, M., Al-Yaman, F., Bjertness, E., King, A., ... & Pesantes, M. A. (2016). Indigenous and tribal peoples' health (The Lancet–Lowitja Institute Global Collaboration): a population study. *The Lancet, 388*(10040), 131–157.

also associated mostly with dominant ethnic groups, rather than indigenous people or other minorities, as in the Americas. Higher incomes are also associated with more political power and voice.

Health Disparities and Gender

Concerning the health of women, "being born female is dangerous to your health,"[21] especially in low-income countries. Women are discriminated against in many settings in ways that are harmful to their health. This starts with sex-selective abortion and female infanticide. Sex-selective abortion refers to the abortion of fetuses that are female, generally in places with a strong son preference. This is usually heightened by desire for a small family or limits on family size, such as in China. Female infanticide refers to the practice of actively or passively allowing a female infant to die, because she is not wanted or the family feels it cannot care for her. In some settings, this discrimination is also evident in shorter duration of breastfeeding and less food for female children, lower enrollment of girls in school, and less attention to the healthcare needs of girls. There is also an exceptional amount of violence against women and neglect of the healthcare needs of adult women. In most settings, women will also have less power and voice than men. The main point to note here is the importance of keeping in mind the health concerns of women that relate to their diminished place and power in many societies.

Health Disparities and Ethnicity

There is a strong association in most countries between ethnicity and health status, access, and coverage. Examples were given previously of the large gaps between white people and African Americans in the United States and white people and Aboriginal people in Australia.

FIGURE 4-8 shows how infant mortality ratios have tended to vary in selected countries with an indigenous population. Except in Panama, we see dramatic differences in infant mortality between the indigenous groups and the remainder of the population. Given the strong association between ethnicity and power, education, and income, it is not surprising to find such a strong association between ethnicity and health status.

Health Disparities and Other Marginalized Groups

Other marginalized groups also face inequity and health disparities. Some of these might be people who suffer social isolation because they engage in stigmatized occupations. Some might be people with disabilities or deformities, such as people with physical handicaps, blind people, or people with leprosy. Prisoners often lack access to appropriate health services, and prisons are often breeding grounds for communicable diseases. Other people who are marginalized because of their sexuality or gender identity might also face inequity in health, such as lesbian, gay, bisexual, and transgender people (LGBT). This is discussed further in a policy and program brief later in this chapter.

Financial Fairness

All high-income countries, except the United States, have some type of mandatory and universal health insurance system that is meant to ensure that access to health services is not dependent on income. These systems are also meant to offer financial protection to those who participate in them. Many middle-income countries also have such insurance systems. However, most low-income countries do not have formalized health insurance systems outside of the free or low-cost provision of some health services by the public sector or nongovernmental sectors. Thus, the poor in many countries must bear substantial out-of-pocket costs for health, as discussed later. In addition, many low-income countries fail to protect their poor from potentially catastrophic health costs that higher-income individuals could afford. Moreover, the relative cost of those health services is much greater for the poor than for better-off people, which also raises important equity issues.

Another set of important equity concerns deals with the extent to which different income groups benefit from public subsidies for health services. This can be a complicated issue to assess.[8] Nonetheless, it is clear that there are many countries in which public subsidies for health are disproportionately received by better-off people. It is easy to imagine, for example, a country in which poor people use basic health services financed by the public sector that are relatively inexpensive, whereas better-off people in the urban areas disproportionately use publicly supported hospital services that are relatively expensive. Under these circumstances, better-off people, who will have higher rates of noncommunicable diseases, will get most of the expensive surgeries. Those surgeries will cost hundreds of times what basic health care costs, and the country would be providing a disproportionate share of public subsidies to the better off, rather than to the poor. There is no justification on clinical, economic, or equity grounds for this being the case.

Concluding Comments on Health Disparities

This section has only begun to introduce the many dimensions of equity, inequality, and health disparity issues in global health. When engaging in global health activities, it is critical to do the following:

- Keep equity, inequality, and disparities in mind at all times.
- Always consider the multiple dimensions of these issues.
- Be careful when using numbers that reflect averages for health indicators because they may hide variation across and within groups.
- Examine how each piece of key data on health status, access, coverage, and financing relates to different population groups, especially the poor and marginalized.

As noted earlier, much of this text is oriented toward addressing the health concerns of the poor, especially in low- and middle-income countries. Different parts of the text will offer suggestions about how those health needs can be met as quickly as possible and at the lowest possible cost. One critical point in efforts to do this, which emerges partly from concerns for health disparities, is to ensure that the poor and other marginalized groups are involved in the design, development, monitoring, and evaluation of such efforts. It is also crucial to ensure that such activities pay particular attention to monitoring the benefits that accrue to them and the distribution of those benefits to various population groups. Without paying sufficient attention to these points, it is likely that health disparity issues will not be addressed satisfactorily and that it will be difficult to monitor the extent to which the desired benefits of an investment in health go to the intended beneficiaries.[14]

▶ Health Expenditure and Health Outcomes

One of the reasons health is so important to countries is that they spend a lot of money on it. In addition, as noted earlier, they should be trying, at least in principle, to get the most for the money they spend, consistent with efforts to maximize the health of their population in fair ways. **FIGURE 4-9** shows the relationship between gross domestic product (GDP) per capita and total health expenditure as a share of GDP.

The main themes that emerge from this figure are clear:

- Most high-income countries cluster around an expenditure of 9 percent to 12 percent of their national income on health.
- Many low-income countries cluster around an expenditure of 3 percent to 6 percent of their national income on health. This can be seen for Bangladesh, Ghana, and Nigeria.
- Despite the clustering, there are countries that are outliers—they sit significantly away from the general relationship between income per capita and percentage of national income spent on health. The United States spends more than any other country on health as a share of GDP. Cambodia spends relatively more than one would expect for countries at its level of income. Sri Lanka spends relatively less than one would expect.

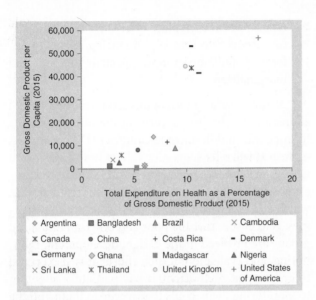

FIGURE 4-9 National Income and Total Health Expenditure, Selected Countries, 2015

Data from The World Bank. (n.d.). Data: GDP per capita (current US$), current health expenditure (% of GDP). Retrieved from https://data.worldbank.org/indicator/SH.XPD.CHEX.GD.ZS

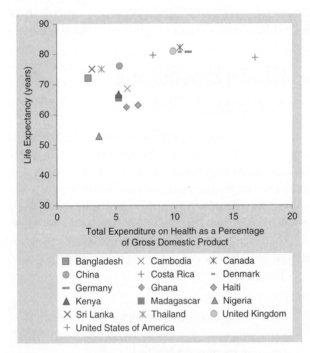

FIGURE 4-10 Life Expectancy, Compared to Total Expenditure on Health as a Share of GDP, Selected Countries, 2015

Data from The World Bank. (n.d.). Data: Life expectancy at birth, total (years) and current health expenditure (% of GDP). Retrieved from https://data.worldbank.org/indicator/SH.XPD.CHEX.GD.ZS

Having seen what countries spend on health, it is now important to ask what they get in return for that expenditure. Do countries that spend higher shares of their national income on health have better health outcomes? **FIGURE 4-10** plots life expectancy against total health expenditure as a share of GDP for selected countries.

From this figure, we can see the following:

- Some countries spend a relatively low share of their GDP on health and also have low life expectancy. This is seen in Nigeria.
- Some countries, such as Ghana and Haiti, spend a relatively high share of their GDP on health but still have relatively short life expectancies.
- Most high-income countries spend a relatively high share of their GDP on health and have high life expectancy. This can be seen in Germany and Canada.
- Some countries spend relatively little on health but still have relatively higher life expectancy than many countries that spend a higher share of GDP on health. This can be seen in Bangladesh and Thailand.
- Some high-income countries spend relatively high shares of GDP on health but still have lower life expectancy than countries that spend a lower share of GDP on health than they do. This is best shown by the United States, which is an outlier on this figure, as well as on Figure 4-9.

Why is it that some countries are outliers when considering their health outcomes related to health expenditure? First, we know that health status depends on a number of genetic, social, and economic factors, including the "social determinants of health," and those factors vary across countries. Second, health outcomes depend not only on how much countries spend per capita on health but also on the particular investments they make with that money. In colloquial terms, we could say, "What you spend the money on is as important as how much you spend." Countries that make health investments aligned with their burden of disease; that focus expenditure on evidence-based, least-cost approaches; and that seek to maximize the health of their people in fair ways will achieve their aims at lower cost than countries that do not take this approach. Countries that invest wisely in addressing the social determinants of health will also have better health outcomes at lower levels of expenditure on health than countries that fail to pay appropriate attention to the social determinants.

▶ Public and Private Expenditure on Health

Another important concept is the distinction between **public expenditure on health** and **private expenditure on health**. Public expenditure refers to expenditure by any level of government or of a government agency. Expenditure by a city, state, or national government would be public expenditure. Expenditure on health by government agencies such as a social security system, as in many countries in Latin America; the national insurance agency, as in most countries in Western Europe; or of a specialized agency, such as a national commission on HIV/AIDS, would also be considered public expenditure.

Private expenditure is expenditure that comes from sources other than governments. One such source is the money that individuals spend on health. When this money is not covered or reimbursed by an insurance program, it is also called **out-of-pocket expenditures on health**. Other sources of private expenditure on health include expenditure by nongovernmental organizations (NGOs), such as by BRAC in Bangladesh or the Self Employed Women's Association (SEWA) in India. In addition, private expenditure on health includes expenditure by the private for-profit sector. Private sector firms, for example, might contribute to the cost of health insurance or health services for their employees. They might also make contributions to the health work of other organizations.

There is some debate about what are legitimate focuses of public expenditure on health.[22] However, there is widespread agreement that public expenditure on health is warranted when the investment benefits society as a whole, such as an immunization program; when health investments promote equity; and when such expenditure provides financial protection to the poor from expenditures on health that they cannot afford.[22]

▶ The Cost-Effectiveness of Health Interventions

Most governments have a limited amount of money for health, and that money is rarely enough to finance all of the health interventions that a country would like to carry out. Thus, governments have to decide what share of their total budget will go to health and how much of the health budget will be allocated to different health interventions. They also have to consider how those investments will be carried out. All governments have to set priorities for expenditure on health, just as they have to set priorities for expenditure in other sectors.

One important tool for setting priorities for public expenditure on health is **cost-effectiveness analysis**. This is a method for comparing the cost of an investment with the amount of health that can be purchased with that investment. The cost of the investment can be thought of as the price of the investment.

The amount of health that can be purchased could be measured, for example, in deaths avoided, life years saved, or disability-adjusted life years (DALYs) averted. The cost-effectiveness of an investment in health will depend, among other things, on the incidence and prevalence of the health condition being considered; the cost of the intervention; the extent to which it can reduce morbidity, mortality, and disability; and how effectively it can be implemented.

One important example of the use of cost-effectiveness analysis is to set priorities among different ways of achieving the same health goal. Important studies were conducted, for example, on the cost-effectiveness of alternative approaches to treating tuberculosis. These studies examined the cost-effectiveness of 6 months of treatment with direct supervision of people taking their medicines compared to treatment that was not supervised. The supervised method was more expensive than the unsupervised method. However, in that study the supervised method led to a higher rate of people taking all of their medicine and being cured than the unsupervised approach. As a result, it proved to be more cost-effective than the traditional approach that had been used, as reflected in **FIGURE 4-11**.[23]

It is easy to imagine how important this type of cost-effectiveness analysis can be when considering different ways of delivering the same health services. In fact, there are many important issues in delivering health services in low-income countries in which such questions remain critical. In Haiti, for example, there is a program operated by Partners in Health. Those carrying out the program had to assess whether the services could be delivered as effectively by volunteer workers as they could be by workers who were paid for their efforts. Although it cost more to deliver the program when the workers were paid, the outcomes

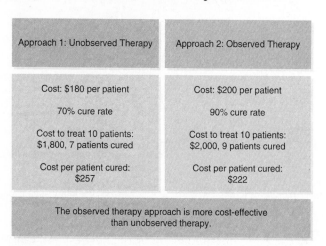

FIGURE 4-11 Unobserved Therapy vs. Observed Therapy for Tuberculosis Treatment

Note: Based on modeled and not actual data

were superior to those when the workers were not paid, and Partners in Health has continued to use the approach of paid workers.[24] Another issue of great importance has been the extent to which antiretroviral drugs for HIV or diagnosis and first-line treatment of mental disorders can be delivered effectively by nurses and community health workers instead of physicians, because physicians are in such short supply in so many countries.

The second manner in which cost-effectiveness analysis is used is to compare the costs and the gains of different health interventions so that investment choices can be made among them. For every $100, for example, that a government spends on health, what allocation of government expenditure on health will buy the most DALYs averted? What is the cost per DALY averted from different interventions? In a relatively poor country with a high burden of communicable diseases, such as tuberculosis and malaria, is it more cost-effective to invest public resources for health in communicable disease control or in coronary bypass surgery? In a richer country with little tuberculosis, will it be cost-effective to invest in vaccination against tuberculosis?

Even if we examine the first question in a somewhat exaggerated and simplistic manner, it will still help us to understand some of the value of cost-effectiveness analysis. Let us say, for example, that the cost of coronary bypass surgery in a low-income country is about $5,000. Let us also say that the costs of such surgery are covered completely by the public sector. This surgery would benefit one individual, who is aged 50 and will live an additional 20 years in perfectly good health because of the surgery. In the same country, we can assume an entire course of treatment for tuberculosis costs about $100. In addition, we can assume that people who get tuberculosis will all be 50 years of age and that they will live an additional 20 years in perfectly good health if they are treated for tuberculosis. What this means, in principle, is that if these were the only choices for the investment of $5,000 in health that a country faced, and if this were the only type of analysis that would be done to assess investment choices, then the choice would be between spending the same amount of money to save 1 life or 50 lives. In addition, the choices would be between saving 20 additional years of healthy life of the coronary bypass patient or 1,000 additional healthy years of life of the 50 tuberculosis patients.

FIGURE 4-12 illustrates the cost per DALY averted of a selected number of health interventions. These interventions would be cost-effective in most settings, as described later on in this chapter.

It is important to note that cost-effectiveness analysis is never the sole means for determining choices among investments and generally should not be used

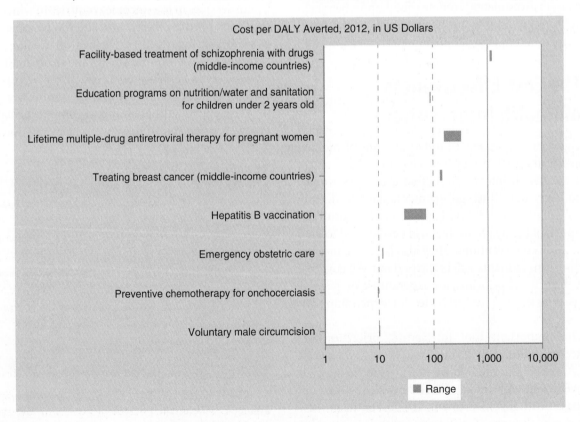

FIGURE 4-12 Cost per DALY Averted for Selected Health Interventions

Data from Horton, S., Gelband, H., Jamison, D., Levin, C., Nugent, R., & Watkins, D. (2017). Ranking 93 health interventions for low- and middle-income countries by cost-effectiveness. *PloS One*, 12(8), e0182951.

in that way.[25] However, it is one valuable tool in making choices among different investments in health. It will always be important, for example, to consider such analyses in light of a number of other factors, including the following[25]:

- Equity considerations
- The burden of disease
- The extent to which the investment serves society as a whole
- The extent to which the investment produces benefits in addition to its usual ones
- The impact of the intervention on the provision of insurance

In addition, those who set priorities for health investments will also have to take account of several factors[25]:

- The capacity to deliver the proposed services
- The links between the proposed services and other important services
- The ability to change budget priorities in favor of the proposed investment
- Any transitional costs associated with making the proposed changes in priorities

In this text, most of the cost-effectiveness assessments are calculated using DALYs averted. This is because examining the cost of life years saved from death would fail to capture reductions in morbidity and disability that are also important aims of health interventions. In addition, it is important to note that there is no unique cutoff below which interventions are considered "cost-effective" and above which they are not. WHO has, however, developed thresholds for cost-effectiveness. These are used less frequently nowadays than earlier but can still be helpful. Using this approach, investments are "highly cost-effective" if the cost per DALY averted is less than GDP per capita, "cost-effective" if the cost per DALY averted is one to three times GDP per capita, and not cost-effective if the cost is more than three times GDP per capita. In any case, it is important to group the cost-effectiveness of different interventions into ranges and to use cost-effectiveness analysis to explore the relative extent to which various interventions will lead to DALYs averted and at what cost.

▶ Cost–Benefit Analysis

Cost–benefit analysis is another tool of economic analysis, to which there will be occasional references in the text. This type of analysis can also be used to choose among investments or to select an approach to

addressing an issue that has the highest benefit-to-cost ratio. In cost–benefit analysis, one assigns a monetary value to all of the expected costs and to all of the expected benefits of an investment. Some costs and benefits will accrue in the future and they have to be discounted to show what their value would be today. Thus, one has to compare the net present value of the expected benefits to the net present value of the expected costs. Investments that yield a positive benefit-to-cost ratio are worth consideration. However, when selecting among investments one would select, in principle, the investment that would have the highest benefit-to-cost ratio. In the simplest terms, one seeks through cost–benefit analysis to determine "how much will I get back for every dollar I invest?" If each dollar invested in a vitamin A program in a low-income country yields $4 of return, than it is certainly a "good investment." By contrast, if each dollar invested in another intervention only yielded $0.80 of return, that would be an investment that should not be made because one would be "losing money" on it. This is a highly simplified statement on cost–benefit analysis, and readers are encouraged to explore this concept further if they are interested.

▶ Health and Development

An important question at the core of global health concerns the links between health and development at the individual, community, and societal levels. Does individual health produce more individual wealth and higher levels of economic development at the community and societal levels? Or are the effects in the opposite direction: Does more economic development at the societal level produce better health for individuals, communities, and societies? What we find when we examine these questions is that the effects of health and development go in both directions.

There is no question that good health promotes economic development at the societal level. First, we know that when countries have to spend money to address health problems, they cannot use that money for other purposes. Countries that have to spend substantial resources to treat malaria, for example, have less money to spend not only on other areas of health but also on schools, roads, and other investments outside of the health sector that could spur economic growth.

In addition, investment in economic activities, by local and foreign investors, is an essential ingredient to the economic growth prospects of low-income countries. Yet, as seen in one of the vignettes that opened this chapter, countries that have high burdens of disease may not appear to be good investment choices. In fact, in a study of the impact of malaria on economic development that is frequently cited, it was found that a high prevalence of malaria reduces economic growth by about 1 percent per year.[26]

There is also growing evidence of the importance of health to economic development from a number of other studies done by economists. Some have shown that higher life expectancy at birth is associated with faster economic growth rates. These studies suggest that a country with a life expectancy at birth of 77 years would be expected to grow economically 1.6 percent faster each year than a country with a life expectancy at birth of 49 years.[26] Another study showed that poor health was an important contributor to the slow pace of economic growth of countries in Africa, compared to other countries with better health.[27] Another series of studies showed that improvements in nutritional status and related health status improvements were very important historically in boosting labor productivity and spurring economic growth in the United Kingdom and Europe.[28-31]

It is also true that higher levels of economic development do promote better health at the level of both individuals and society. In fact, studies on the impact of income on the health of different societies suggest that higher income is associated with better health and longer life expectancy.[31] However, more recent analyses of this question suggest that although income growth is associated with better health indicators for a country, the effect of income alone on health indicators is less significant than previously thought. Rather, these analyses suggest that a considerable share of the improvements in health indicators stem, as noted earlier, from progress in education; from technical progress such as the development of new vaccines or new drugs; or from simple life-saving approaches, such as the use of oral rehydration for young children with diarrhea.[32]

In this light, we should ask the following question: Is income growth necessary or sufficient for enhancing health status at the individual, community, or societal levels? Over the long run, increases in income will improve health. However, they will not improve it fast enough in most settings to achieve the health status objectives that many countries have set for themselves or that are necessary to achieve the Sustainable Development Goals in the time that has been set for them. What low- and middle-income countries must do, therefore, is adopt public policy choices that will allow them to speed the achievement of their health aims, even in the face of constrained income, as Cuba, China, and Sri Lanka did historically and as the state

of Kerala in India has done. As indicated earlier, this is the approach that has been taken by the countries that have been particularly successful in meeting their health aims, even at relatively low levels of income per capita.

▶ Case Studies

Two case studies follow. The first explores in greater detail some of the health equity issues that arise for lesbian, gay, bisexual, and transgender people. Although the data on this issue are not extensive, the comments will enable further consideration of this matter as one continues to study or work in global health. The second case study examines one of the great public health success stories—the fight against Guinea worm. Those interested in more detail in the case should consult *Case Studies in Global Health: Millions Saved* and the latest information on Guinea worm from WHO, the U.S. Centers for Disease Control and Prevention (CDC), and the Carter Center.[33]

Health Equity and Lesbian, Gay, Bisexual and Transgender People

There has been an increasing global awareness of the health disparities experienced by lesbian, gay, bisexual, and transgender (LGBT) individuals.[34] Conservative estimates suggest that there are 84 million individuals, or 1.2 percent of the world's population, who identify with a sexual orientation other than heterosexual, including LGBT people.[34] Stigma and discrimination often heighten the vulnerability of these populations to experiencing health disparities, as these populations are often subject to institutionalized prejudice, social stress, social exclusion, public hatred, and violence, and consequently even possibly an internalized sense of shame about their sexuality.[35] In some low- and middle-income countries, these sociopolitical factors can be more pronounced because engaging in homosexual acts is considered a criminal offense.[36]

LGBT individuals can experience increased risk of certain health conditions because social factors such as stigma and discrimination can have a direct impact on an individual's health status. Negative social attitudes, perceived discrimination, and even violence can place stressors on the lives of these individuals that contribute to these observed health outcomes.[34] For example, lesbian, gay, and bisexual people (LGB) have a documented increased risk of mental disorders including depression, suicidal ideations, and substance dependence compared to heterosexuals in North America, Europe, and Canada.[34] Similarly, a meta-analysis of studies conducted in the United States and other high-income countries specifically found that over a period of 1 year, the risk of depression in LGB individuals was at least twice that of heterosexuals.[35] Overall, there is a lack of data on equity for LGB people in low- and middle-income countries, often because of cultural and political sensitivity. It is likely that these health inequities persist or are exacerbated in these contexts, and there is an urgent need to generate further evidence in order to better target interventions.

Recent literature has given light to the inequities faced by the global transgender community, which the United Nations Development Programme (UNDP) defines as "all people whose sense of their gender identity differs from the sex they were assigned at birth."[37] Many transgender people do not have access to the health care they need and deserve not only because of social stigma and discrimination, similar to the LGB community, but also because the appropriate services do not exist. A large-scale survey in the United Kingdom found that 17 percent of transgender people had been refused services by a doctor or nurse because of their gender identity.[37] Similar to LGB people, transgender people often have worse health outcomes because they lack access to the needed interventions. UNAIDS and WHO have noted that transgender women often experience HIV prevalence rates in excess of 60 percent, but there are few targeted interventions for them and limited research on effective interventions.[37] Moreover, transgender people often experience health conditions that do not fit directly into either men's or women's health areas, reflecting that healthcare services often fail to meet their needs or to have sufficiently sensitive healthcare workers.

Equity and MSM

Like LGBT people, men-who-have-sex-with-men (MSM) often experience inequitable health outcomes because of their social status. For example, it is estimated that HIV prevalence among MSM in South Africa is 26.8 percent, compared to 18.1 percent for the general population.[38] MSM can experience an increased risk of certain diseases or conditions because of biological or behavioral factors that can become exacerbated in contexts when their marginalized status prevents them from receiving preventive interventions or appropriate treatment.[39] MSM have elevated risks for HIV infection, for example,

because of higher probabilities of HIV transmission in receptive anal sex and because of their higher probability of engaging in risky behaviors such as extra-primary partnerships. Nonetheless, these risk factors can be mitigated with effective interventions such as targeted distribution of condoms and lubricant, as well as targeted pre-exposure prophylaxis. These interventions, however, are currently lacking in many settings.[39,40]

Although most of the current literature on inequitable outcomes for MSM is on HIV, it has been suggested that these patterns affect MSM for other health conditions as well, especially those conditions associated with mental health.[41] These differences may reflect a lack of healthcare access or fear of seeking health services for MSM. In general, research has shown that MSM who disclose their sexual orientation have better health outcomes than MSM who do not, but social stigma and discrimination often prevent this.[41] One study found that 17.6 percent of MSM in Malawi, 18.3 percent of MSM in Namibia, and 20.5 percent of MSM in Botswana were afraid to seek health services due to their sexual orientation.[42] In all three of these countries, prevention or treatment programs for this population remain limited in nature, as is the case for many other countries. The inequities in health outcomes for MSM will remain until interventions no longer neglect MSM or fail to acknowledge their unique needs.

Overall, there is a need for more comprehensive analyses of the inequities faced by LGBT people and MSM in low- and middle-income settings if more effective health services are to be available to these groups. To achieve this, it will be essential to train healthcare workers to work with greater sensitivity to and respect for these groups.[38] It will also be important to educate society more broadly about the LGBT and MSM communities in order to help reduce stigma and discrimination against them.[43]

The Challenge of Guinea Worm in Asia and Sub-Saharan Africa
Background

Dracunculiasis, or Guinea worm disease, is an ancient scourge that once afflicted much of the world. Today, it is truly a disease of the poor, persisting only in some of the world's most remote and disadvantaged regions with limited access to potable water, despite being one of the most preventable parasitic diseases. In the 1980s, an estimated 3.5 million people in 20 countries in Africa and Asia were infected with Guinea worm disease, and an estimated 120 million were at risk of becoming infected.[44]

The disease is contracted by drinking stagnant water from a well or pond that is contaminated with tiny fleas that carry Guinea worm larvae. Once inside the human, the larvae can grow up to 3 feet long. After a year, the grown female worm rises to the skin in search of a water source to release her larvae. A painful blister forms, usually in the person's lower limbs. To ease the burning pain, infected individuals frequently submerge the blister in water, causing the blister's rupture and the release of more larvae into the water. This contaminated water, when it is drunk, perpetuates the cycle of reinfection. Worms, usually as wide as a match, can take up to 12 weeks to emerge from the blister. They are coaxed out by being slowly wound around a stick a few centimeters each day. Debilitating pain from this process can linger for as long as 18 months.

Although rarely fatal, the disease takes a heavy toll by causing low productivity that makes it both a symptom and perpetrator of poverty—in Mali, it is called the "disease of the empty granary." Because water in contaminated ponds is widely consumed during peak periods of cyclical harvesting and planting, an entire community can be left debilitated and unable to work during the busiest agricultural seasons. The economic damage is severe: annual economic loss in three rice-growing states in Nigeria was calculated at $20 million.[45] Although the disease afflicts all age groups, it particularly harms children.[45] School absenteeism rises when infected children are unable to walk to school and when children forgo school to take on the agricultural and household work of sick adults. The likelihood of a child in Sudan being malnourished is more than three times higher when the adults in the child's home are infected with the disease.

The Intervention

In 1980, when the CDC first proposed an eradication campaign, the three interventions that would be required to address the disease effectively did not seem feasible: construction of expensive water sources, controlling the vector that spreads the disease through the use of larvicides in water sources, and health education campaigns promoting the filtration of water with a cloth filter, self-reporting of infections, and avoidance of recontamination of public water sources. The absence of a vaccine or cure made success seem even more improbable.

The International Drinking Water Supply and Sanitation Decade was launched the following year, however, and D. A. Henderson, who worked at the

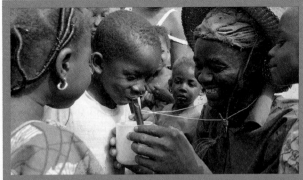

PHOTO 4-3 The Guinea Worm Eradication Program has used pipe filters to filter water, especially in areas impacted by conflict or where there is a large nomadic population. These simple but innovative devices enable people to drink water without the threat of contracting Guinea worm disease no matter where they are. Pipe filters have been displayed at museums around the world as an example of innovative design. Can you list other innovative technologies that might assist in addressing the most critical health conditions faced by the poor in low- and middle-income countries?
© The Carter Center/L. Gubb.

CDC, seized the opportunity to include the eradication of Guinea worm disease as a subgoal of the Water Decade program. Nonetheless, progress against Guinea worm disease remained slow until 1986, when three key events occurred: WHO declared eradication of Guinea worm disease a goal, public health ministers from 14 African nations met to affirm their commitment to the eradication effort, and U.S. President Jimmy Carter became a powerful advocate, personally persuading many leaders to launch national eradication efforts. He also recruited the help of two former popular heads of state of Mali and Nigeria, General Amadou Toumani Touré and General Yakubu Gowon, respectively, thereby consolidating political commitment in Africa.

Meanwhile, technical and financial resources of the donor community were marshaled, and by 1995, eradication programs had been established in 20 countries. Water sources were provided, mainly through the construction of wells—in southeast Nigeria alone, village volunteers hand-dug more than 400 wells.[46] Larvicide was added to water sources to kill the fleas. People were taught to filter drinking water using a simple cloth filter. However, these filters were found to clog up and were used as decoration items instead.[45] A newly developed nylon cloth was then donated by the Carter Center, Precision Fabrics, and DuPont. Public education campaigns, including intensive efforts during so-called worm weeks, encouraged people to use the nylon filters, avoid recontaminating ponds, and report infections.[47] Most of the eradication staff were volunteers trained by the ministries of health, but they pioneered a monthly reporting system for tracking and monitoring that is now hailed as a model for disease surveillance.[48]

The Impact

The campaign led to a 99 percent drop in Guinea worm disease prevalence. In 2005, fewer than 11,000 cases were reported, compared with an estimated 3.5 million infected people in 1986. Most remaining cases were then in Sudan, where civil conflict impeded progress against the disease over many years. By 1988, the campaign had already prevented between 9 million and 13 million cases of Guinea worm disease.[48] The Asian countries that were targeted—India, Pakistan, and Yemen—are now free of the disease.

Costs and Benefits

The total cost of the program between 1986 and 1998 was $87.5 million, with an estimated cost per case averted of $5 to $8.[48] The World Bank determined that the campaign has been highly cost-effective and cost-beneficial. In addition, the program had a very high economic rate of return, even when basing the calculation of economic benefits only on increases in agricultural productivity that accrued from people having avoided the disease.[48]

Lessons Learned

Success of the program has been attributed to three factors. The first is the exemplary coordination between major partners and donors. The second is the power of data, gathered through the monthly reporting system, to monitor national programs and to help keep countries focused and motivated on the program goals. The third is the high-level advocacy and political leadership from current and former heads of state, especially President Jimmy Carter and General Gowon, who visited and revisited villages in Nigeria to check on progress. The program drew on a truly global partnership among the CDC, UNICEF, WHO, the Carter Center, governments, NGOs, the private sector, and volunteers that was able to motivate changes in individual and community behaviors and successfully control a disease.

The Guinea Worm Eradication Campaign has continued to be successful, and the world is now nearing eradication of Guinea worm. In 2017, there were 30 cases of Guinea worm worldwide. Between January 1 and September 30 of 2018, 19 cases were reported. This included 1 case in Angola, 11 in Chad, and 7 in South Sudan.[49] When Guinea worm disease is eradicated, it will be the only human disease eradicated besides smallpox and the first human disease eradicated without the use of a vaccine.

▶ Main Messages

The aim of this chapter is to introduce some of the basic concepts concerning the health-development link. One important message of the chapter is that education and health are closely linked. Good health encourages school enrollment at the appropriate age, improves school attendance, enhances students' cognitive performance, and increases the completed years of schooling. Education and knowledge are consistently correlated with engagement in more appropriate health behaviors and living healthier lives, compared to people with less schooling. Important progress in reducing child mortality, for example, is associated with increased educational attainment for women. In addition, education promotes greater opportunities for income earning, which itself is an important determinant of health.

We also learned that health is strongly associated with productivity and earnings. Healthier people can work harder, work more hours, and work over a longer lifetime than can those who are less healthy. Related to this in many ways, we also saw that health has an important relationship with poverty. If people work fewer hours because of ill health, then there is a risk that their income status will decline, perhaps below the poverty line. In addition, there is evidence from many countries that the direct and indirect costs to individuals of obtaining health services can push people into poverty.

Equity, inequality, and health disparities are important concerns of public health. It is essential to consider these factors when discussing health status, access to health services, coverage of services, protection from financial risk, the fairness of financing health, and the distribution of health benefits.

Health is an important subject for all countries for many reasons, among the most important of which is the amount of money they spend on health. Generally, high-income countries spend more money on health per capita and as a share of GDP than do low-income countries. However, health outcomes depend not just on how much money is spent but also on how the money is used. One tool that countries use to help set priorities for health expenditure is cost-effectiveness analysis. This allows them to compare how much health they can buy for a given level of expenditure. All countries, of course, face the question of how they can maximize the health of their population for the minimum cost, in the fairest possible way, and cost-effectiveness analysis can aid in this process.

There are also many strong relationships between the health of a population and the economic development of the society in which they live. Better health does promote wealth in a variety of ways, including enhancing labor productivity, reducing the amount countries have to spend on health, and enabling a more attractive investment climate. In addition, the negative impact of some diseases on economic development, such as tuberculosis, HIV/AIDS, and malaria, can be very significant. Economic development does improve health; however, many gains in health stem from educational and technological progress, such as on vaccines. Low-income countries have to develop approaches to improving population health faster than economic development alone will allow. A number of countries have suggested the path for such an approach.

Study Questions

1. How does poor health status affect a person's income?
2. What is the relationship between health and the productivity of individuals?
3. What part does health play in promoting the education of a child?
4. What part does the education of a mother play in promoting the health of her children?
5. Why might the health of some culture groups be different from the health of others?
6. What is the relationship between a country's expenditure on health as a share of national income and its health status?
7. In your country, is expenditure on health from the public sector, private sector, or both?
8. In using cost-effectiveness analysis, why should you also take into account issues such as equity?
9. How could you ensure that public subsidies on health care appropriately benefit the poor?
10. Does "health make wealth," or does "wealth make health"?
11. What impact would the health status of a country have on the likelihood that people will invest in economic activity in that country?
12. Why did Guinea worm disease remain so prevalent for so long?

References

1. Ruger, J. P., Jamison, D. T., & Bloom, D. E. (2001). Health and the economy. In M. H. Merson, R. E. Black, & A. J. Mills (Eds.), *International public health, diseases, programs, systems, and policies* (pp. 617–666). Gaithersburg, MD: Aspen.
2. Pebley, A., Goldman, N., & Rodriguez, G. (1996). Prenatal and delivery care and childhood immunization in Guatemala: Do family and community matter? *Demography, 33,* 197–210.
3. Hobcraft, J. (1993). Women's education, child welfare and child survival: A review of the evidence. *Health Transition Review, 3*(2), 159–175.
4. Gakidou, E., Cowling, K., Lozana, R., & Murray, C. J. L. (2010). Increased educational attainment and its effect on child mortality in 175 countries between 1970 and 2009: A systematic analysis. *The Lancet, 376*(9745), 959–974.
5. Basta, S. S., Soekirman, Karyadi, D., & Scrimshaw, N. S. (1979). Iron deficiency anemia and the productivity of adult males in Indonesia. *American Journal of Clinical Nutrition, 32*(4), 916–925.
6. Croft, R. A., & Croft, R. P. (1998). Expenditure and loss of income incurred by tuberculosis patients before reaching effective treatment in Bangladesh. *International Journal of Tuberculosis and Lung Disease, 2*(3), 252–254.
7. Tanimura, T., Jaramillo, E., Weil, D., Raviglione, M., & Lonnroth, K. (2014). Financial burden for tuberculosis patients in low- and middle-income countries: A systematic review. *European Respiratory Journal, 43*(6), 1763–1775.
8. Peters, D. H., Yazbek, A. S., Sharma, R. R., Ramana, G. N. V., Pritchett, L. H., Wagstaff. (2002). *Better health systems for India's poor.* Washington, DC: The World Bank.
9. The World Bank. (2001). *World development report 2000/2001: Attacking poverty.* New York, NY: Oxford University Press.
10. Sen, A. (2002). Why health equity? *Health Economics, 11*(8), 659–666.
11. Whitehead, M. (1992). The concepts and principles of equity and health. *International Journal of Health Services, 22,* 429–445.
12. World Health Organization. (n.d.). *Health impact assessment. Glossary of terms used.* Retrieved from http://www.who.int/hia/about/glos/en/index1.html
13. Centers for Disease Control and Prevention. (n.d.). *Social determinants of health. Definitions.* Retrieved from http://www.cdc.gov/socialdeterminants/Definitions.html
14. Peters, D. H., Garg, A., Bloom, G., Walker, D. G., Brieger, W. R., & Rahman, M. H. (2008, June). Poverty and access to health care in developing countries. *Annals of the New York Academy of Sciences, 1136,* 161–171.
15. The World Bank. (n.d.). *Data: Life expectancy at birth, total (years).* Retrieved from https://data.worldbank.org/indicator/SP.DYN.LE00.IN
16. The World Bank. (n.d.). *Data: Maternal mortality ratio (modeled estimate per 100,000 live births).* Retrieved from https://data.worldbank.org/indicator/SH.STA.MMRT

17. The World Bank. (n.d.). *Data: Mortality rate, infant (per 1,000 live births)*. Retrieved from https://data.worldbank.org/indicator/SP.DYN.IMRT.IN

18. U.S. Department of Health and Human Services. (2017). *Health, United States, 2016: With chartbook on long-term trends in health* (p. 4). Retrieved from https://www.cdc.gov/nchs/data/hus/hus16.pdf#015

19. Australian Institute of Health and Welfare. (2015). Life expectancy & deaths. Retrieved from http://www.aihw.gov.au/deaths/life-expectancy/

20. Gwatkin, D. R., Rutstein, S., Johnson, K., Suliman, E., Wagstaff, A., & Amouzou, A. (2007). *Socio-economic differences in health, nutrition, and population within developing countries*. Washington, DC: The World Bank.

21. Murphy, E. M. (2003). Being born female is dangerous to your health. *American Psychologist, 58*(3), 205–210.

22. Preker, A. S., & Harding, A. (2000). *The economics of public and private roles in health care*. Washington, DC: The World Bank.

23. Murray, C. J., DeJonghe, E., Chum, H. J., Nyangulu, D. S., Salomao, A., & Styblo, K. (1991). Cost effectiveness of chemotherapy for pulmonary tuberculosis in three sub-Saharan African countries. *The Lancet, 338*(8778), 1305–1308.

24. Walton, D. A., Farmer, P. E., Lambert, W., Leandre, F., Koenig, S. P., & Mukherjee, J. S. (2004). Integrated HIV prevention and care strengthens primary health care: Lessons from rural Haiti. *Journal of Public Health Policy, 25*(2), 137–158.

25. Yazbeck, A. S. (2002). *An idiot's guide to prioritization in the health sector*. Washington, DC: The World Bank.

26. Commission on Macroeconomics and Health. (2001). *Macroeconomics and health: Investing in health for economic development*. Geneva, Switzerland: World Health Organization.

27. Bloom, D. E., & Sachs, J. (1998). Geography, demography, and economic growth in Africa. *Brookings Papers on Economic Activity, 2*, 207–295.

28. Fogel, R. (1991). *New sources and new techniques for the study of secular trends in nutritional status, health, mortality and the process of aging* (NBER Historical Working Paper No. 26). Cambridge, MA: National Bureau of Economic Research.

29. Fogel, R. (1997). New findings on secular trends in nutrition and mortality: Some implications for population theory. In M. Rosenzweig & O. Stark (Eds.), *Handbook of population and family economics* (Vol. 1a, pp. 433–481). Amsterdam, Netherlands: Elsevier Science.

30. Fogel, R. (2000). *The fourth great awakening and the future of egalitarianism*. Chicago, IL: University of Chicago Press.

31. Pritchett, L. H., & Summers, L. H. (1996). Wealthier is healthier. *Human Resources, 31*(4), 841–868.

32. Jamison, D. T., Sandbu, M., & Wang, J. (2004). *Why has infant mortality decreased at such different rates in different countries?* Bethesda, MD: Disease Control Priorities Project.

33. Levine, R., & What Works Working Group. (2007). *Case studies in global health: Millions saved*. Sudbury, MA: Jones & Bartlett.

34. Logie, C. (2012). The case for the World Health Organization's commission on the social determinants of health to address sexual orientation. *American Journal of Public Health, 102*(7), 1243–1246. doi: 10.2105/AJPH.2011.300599

35. King, M., Semlyen, J., Tai, S., Killaspy, H., Osborn, D., Popelyuk, D., & Nazareth, I. (2008). A systematic review of mental disorder, suicide, and deliberate self harm in lesbian, gay and bisexual people. *BMC Psychiatry, 8*, 70.

36. Beyrer, C., & Baral, S. D. (2011, July 7–9). *MSM, HIV and the law: The case of gay, bisexual and other men who have sex with men (MSM)*, Working Paper for the Third Meeting of the Technical Advisory Group of the Global Commission on HIV and the Law.

37. United Nations Development Programme. (2013). *Discussion paper: Transgender health and human rights*. Retrieved from http://www.undp.org/content/dam/undp/library/HIV-AIDS/Governance%20of%20HIV%20Responses/Trans%20Health%20&%20Human%20Rights.pdf

38. Avert. (n.d.). *HIV and AIDS in South Africa*. Retrieved from https://www.avert.org/professionals/hiv-around-world/sub-saharan-africa/south-africa

39. *The Lancet special issue on HIV in men who have sex with men: Summary points for policy makers*. (2012, July). Retrieved from http://www.amfar.org/uploadedFiles/_amfarorg/On_the_Hill/SummaryPtsLancet2012.pdf

40. Baral, S., Sifakis, F., Cleghorn, F., & Beyrer, C. (2007). Elevated risk for HIV infection among men who have sex with men in low- and middle-income countries 2000–2006: A systematic review. *PLoS Medicine, 4*(12), 1901–1911.

41. Centers for Disease Control and Prevention. (2010). *Gay and bisexual men's health*. Retrieved from http://www.cdc.gov/msmhealth/mental-health.htm

42. Baral, S., Trapence, G., Motimedi, F., Umar, E., Ilpinge, S., Dausab, F., & Beyrer, C. (2009). HIV prevalence, risks for HIV infection, and human rights among men who have sex with men (MSM) in Malawi, Namibia, and Botswana. *PLoS ONE, 4*, e4997.

43. Reisser, W. (2014, September 26). Free and equal: Working with the United Nations to support LGBT rights. *Dipnote: U.S. Department of State official blog*. Retrieved from https://web.archive.org/web/20161102161346/http://blogs.state.gov/stories/2014/09/26/free-and-equal-working-united-nations-support-lgbt-rights

44. Cairncross, S., Muller, R., & Zagaria, N. (2002). Dracunculiasis (Guinea worm disease) and the eradication initiative. *Clinical Microbiology Reviews, 15*(2), 223–246.

45. Hopkins, D. R. (1998). Perspectives from the dracunculiasis eradication programme. *Bulletin of the World Health Organization, 76*(Suppl. 2), 38–41.

46. Hopkins, D. R., Ruiz-Tiben, E., Diallo, N., Withers, P. C., Jr., & Maguire, J. H. (2002). Dracunculiasis eradication: And now, Sudan. *American Journal of Tropical Medicine and Hygiene, 67*(4), 415–422.

47. Hopkins, D. R. (1998). The Guinea worm eradication effort: Lessons for the future. *Emerging Infectious Diseases, 4*(3), 414–415.

48. Kim, A., Tandon, A., & Ruiz-Tiben, E. (1997). *Cost-benefit analysis of the global dracunculiasis eradication campaign*. Washington, DC: The World Bank.

49. The Carter Center. (n.d.). *Guinea worm case totals*. Retrieved from https://www.cartercenter.org/health/guinea_worm/case-totals.html

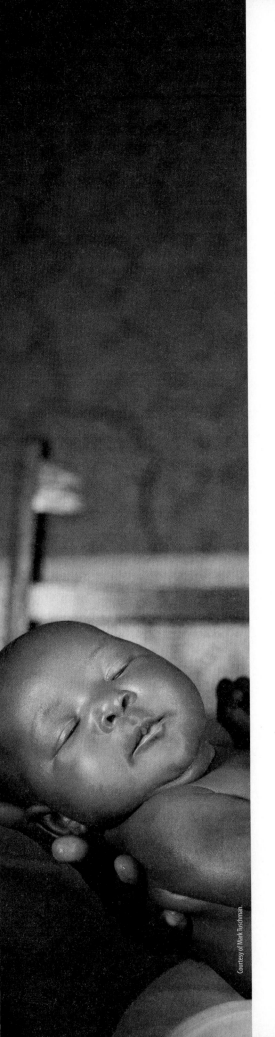

PART II

Cross-Cutting Global Health Themes

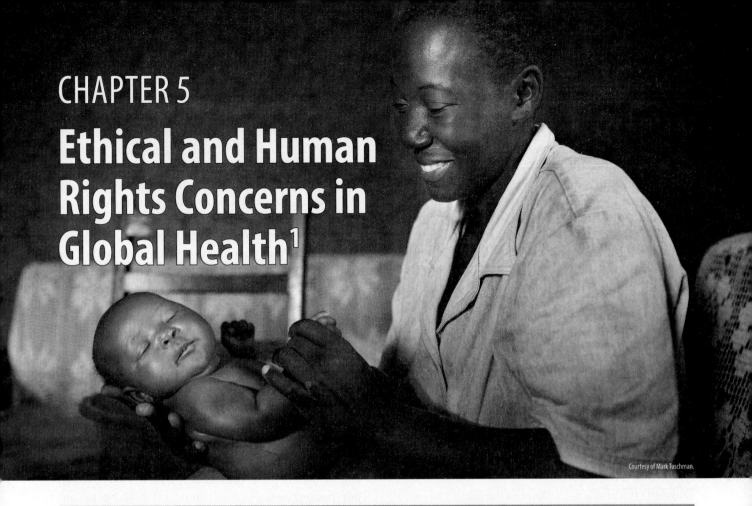

CHAPTER 5
Ethical and Human Rights Concerns in Global Health[1]

Courtesy of Mark Tuschman.

LEARNING OBJECTIVES

By the end of this chapter, the reader will be able to do the following:

- Review key ethical and human rights concerns as they relate to global health
- Discuss some of the central treaties and conventions related to human rights
- Show familiarity with the most important ethical guidelines for research with human subjects
- Discuss some historically significant cases in research with human subjects
- Identify key ethical principles for priority setting in health

▶ Vignettes

Suraiya was a 21-year-old woman in Kabul, Afghanistan. Her sister recently died in childbirth at the age of 16. Suraiya took her sister to a health center when she was having trouble during labor. However, the health center was 50 miles away from their house. In addition, partly because of the neglect of the last government and its discrimination against women, the health center was dilapidated. It had no equipment, and the midwife there was unable to save Suraiya's sister. The baby died a few days later.

John Williams was a 32-year-old office clerk who lived in a small country in sub-Saharan Africa during the early stages of the HIV/AIDS epidemic. For 3 months he had experienced weight loss, continuous fever, and chronic fatigue. He finally gathered the strength to visit the local hospital. When he got there, the staff was not welcoming. They did not treat him kindly. They did not offer to help him. They did not arrange for him to be seen by a doctor. They knew that he had HIV and did not want to treat him in their hospital.

A research team was conducting a study of malaria in villages in West Africa. When the doctors working for the study diagnosed children with severe malaria, they would provide treatment free of charge. However, sometimes the children in the study had other medical problems that needed attention. For example, many children presented with diarrheal diseases, parasitic infections, or pneumonia. Some of the doctors wanted to treat these conditions, too. Other members of the team worried that their budget would not cover the extra costs for such treatment. In any case, they said, the purpose of the study was to learn about malaria, not to provide clinical care.

The newly elected government of an Indian state won the election on a pledge to increase investment in health care. The government plans to build new primary health clinics. However, with the money available, the government can build and staff fewer clinics than are needed. Some members of the government argue that the clinics should be located in the countryside. People there are poorer than those in the cities and have less access to medical facilities. Others argue that the cities should get priority. A clinic in the urban slums serves more people than a rural clinic and is easier to staff and supply. Besides, they say, the party's electoral base is in the cities, and if they want to be re-elected to continue their good work, it is important to keep their voters happy.

▸ The Importance of Ethical and Human Rights Issues in Global Health

Difficult ethical dilemmas arise in the pursuit of global health, whether in planning health care provision, implementing public health measures, or conducting health research. It is important to address these issues, both for their own sake and because there is a strong complementarity between good ethical and human rights practices on the one hand and good health outcomes on the other.[2]

One set of important ethical issues that relate to global health concerns human rights. International conventions and treaties recognize access to health services and health information as human rights. Yet, in many countries, there are remarkable gaps in access to health services. The poor and the disenfranchised suffer from these gaps the most.

The failure to respect human rights is often associated with harm to human health. This has often been the case, for example, with diseases that are highly stigmatized, such as leprosy, tuberculosis (TB), and HIV/AIDS. If leprosy patients are not provided with the best care because some health workers are afraid to work with them, the leprosy patients cannot stop the progression of their disease. If TB patients are shunned by health workers, they may die, usually after infecting many other people.

Efforts to maintain public health while dealing with new and emerging diseases, such as Zika, a potential avian influenza, or the Ebola virus, raise another array of ethical and human rights issues. When we face a potential health threat, for example, what are the

rights of individuals compared to the rights of society to protect its members from illness? Is it acceptable to quarantine a city? Is it permissible to ban travel to and from certain places? These are real issues with which policymakers and health practitioners must wrestle.

Another set of ethical issues is associated with research with human subjects. Health research involving people is generally considered ethically challenging because, in contrast to clinical care, participants in research are put at risk for the sake of other people's health rather than their own. An important part of the research that takes place in the pursuit of global health must also deal with further ethical concerns that arise when research is conducted with poor people who do not have access to satisfactory levels of health care outside of a research study.

Finally, it is important to ensure that health investments are made in fair ways. Even in high-income countries, the resources available for health care are limited. How can choices about who should live and who should die be fair and perceived as legitimate? In low- and middle-income countries, where there are fewer resources and greater needs, difficult decisions must constantly be made about which populations and diseases should get priority. Recent developments in ethical theory can help illuminate such difficult choices.

This chapter provides an overview of some of the most important ethical issues pertaining to global health. It briefly reviews the most important charters and conventions that set the foundation for health-related human rights and shows some of the contexts in which human rights concerns arise. It summarizes some important cases and guidance documents pertaining to the ethics of international medical research and discusses how to evaluate the ethics of clinical research. It then lays out the principles that are often thought to underlie fair decisions about allocating health resources and some of the difficulties in applying them. The chapter concludes with comments on key challenges concerning ethics and human rights in global health activities.

▸ The Foundations for Health and Human Rights

The cornerstone of human rights is the International Bill of Human Rights, which is made up of the Universal Declaration of Human Rights, the International Covenant on Civil and Political Rights, and the International Covenant on Economic, Social, and Cultural Rights. These documents place obligations on governments to *respect*, *protect*, and *fulfill* the rights stated in the document; that is, to refrain from violating people's rights, to prevent others from violating them, and to actively promote the realization of people's rights.

The most significant international declaration on human rights is the Universal Declaration of Human Rights (UDHR), which was announced and adopted in 1948. The UDHR is generally regarded as the basis for most of the later treaties and documents pertaining to human rights. As a declaration, the UDHR does not have the force of law. However, it has moral force, it has influenced the development of a number of national constitutions, and its invocation by many states over the last 50 years has led some to argue that it has the status of customary international law—unwritten law that is nonetheless reflected in the practice of states.[3] With respect to health, the UDHR states in Article 25:

1. Everyone has the right to a standard of living adequate for the health and well-being of himself and of his family, including food, clothing, housing and medical care and necessary social services, and the right to security in the event of unemployment, sickness, disability, widowhood, old age or other lack of livelihood in circumstances beyond his control.

2. Motherhood and childhood are entitled to special care and assistance. All children, whether born in or out of wedlock, shall enjoy the same social protection.[4]

Since 1948, more than 20 multilateral treaties that are legally binding and that relate to health have been formulated. In 1966, two important treaties were adopted—the International Covenant on Economic, Social, and Cultural Rights (ICESCR) and the International Covenant on Civil and Political Rights (ICCPR).[5,6] These two covenants are legally binding on those states that have ratified them (166 countries in the case of the ICESCR and 170 in the case of the ICCPR).[7] The ICCPR discusses rights of equality, liberty, and security, as well as freedom of movement, religion, expression, and association.[6] The ICESCR focuses on the well-being of individuals, including their right to work in safe conditions, receive fair wages, be free from hunger, get an education, and enjoy the highest attainable standard of physical and mental health.[5]

Although increasing attention is being paid to the links between health and human rights, there is no mechanism for holding countries accountable for ensuring that they honor or even try to honor the right to health. The international mechanism now in place for reviewing compliance with treaties and conventions that include the right to health is voluntary reporting by national governments. There are also provisions in human rights treaties and conventions that recognize that resource-poor countries will not be able to help all of their people to "achieve the highest standard of health possible."[8] Instead, states are required only to "take steps" toward the progressive realization of **positive rights**. There is also no clear definition of the meaning of the "right to health" or agreed indicators for measuring progress toward fulfilling it.[9] Although considerable attention was paid to the Millennium Development Goals (MDGs) and progress toward meeting them, the discussion about the MDGs did not often take human rights explicitly into account. It will be important to see the extent to which human rights issues are considered in the implementation and monitoring of the Sustainable Development Goals.

At least 115 countries have written a right to health or health care into their constitutions.[10] In recent years, several countries have seen litigation successfully result in access to previously unavailable treatment.[11] For example, in Brazil there are thousands of court cases each year in which individual patients sue the government to receive drugs that they are not receiving through the public health system.[12] In South Africa, the Treatment Action Campaign successfully sued the national government over its failure to make the drug nevirapine widely available for HIV-infected pregnant women to prevent mother-to-child transmission.[13] In 1999, a court in Venezuela held that the Venezuelan government violated the constitutional right of its people to health by failing to guarantee access to antiretroviral therapy for people living with HIV/AIDS. The court ruled that this right is *both* part of the Venezuelan constitution and a part of the ICESCR, to which Venezuela is party.[14] More recently, a surge of successful individual litigations has created other types of challenges for health systems.[15] In Costa Rica, for example, citizens have sued for the right of access to certain medicines, many of which are new and expensive. Yet, a systematic analysis found that less than 3 percent of the successful legal cases of this type would provide access to medications that could be classified as high priority according to standard criteria.[16]

Women and children are especially vulnerable groups in many countries, and enhancing their health is central to improving the well-being of the poor. For these reasons, a number of international conventions focus on women and children.

The Convention on the Elimination of All Forms of Discrimination Against Women was adopted in 1979 by the United Nations General Assembly. It has been ratified by 83 countries. The convention commits states to legally promote equality between men and women and to eliminate discriminatory practices against women, and it affirms women's reproductive rights.[17]

Many international human rights documents, including the ICCPR, have specific clauses for protecting the rights of children. Most articles in the general human rights instruments also apply equally to both adults and children. The 1989 Convention on the Rights of the Child (CRC), however, is the first human rights document that focuses specifically on children. This document accords children—defined as "every human being below the age of 18 years"—the right to be free of discrimination, to health, and to education. In addition, it states that children must have a say in decisions affecting their lives and puts the rights of children on the same plane as the rights of adults.[18]

The CRC says the following concerning health:

States Parties recognize the right of the child to the enjoyment of the highest attainable standard of health and to facilities for the treatment of illness and rehabilitation of health. States Parties shall strive to ensure that no child is deprived of his or her right to access such health care services.[18]

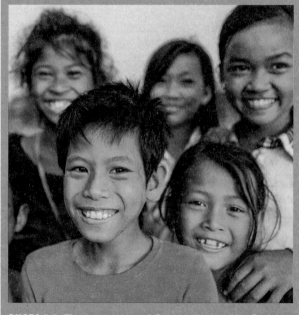

PHOTO 5-1 The International Convention on the Rights of the Child recognizes "the right of the child to the enjoyment of the highest attainable standard of health."[18] In the absence of enforcement mechanisms, can the convention really be used to promote better health among children? If so, how?

© Hadynyah/E+/Getty Images.

▶ Selected Human Rights Issues

There are many human rights issues relating to health that could be considered here. This section examines two overarching issues—the rights-based approach to health and limits to human rights—and then discusses some human rights issues related to HIV/AIDS, which illustrate many of the points previously made.

The Rights-Based Approach

Some scholars and global health advocates argue that we should adopt a human rights approach to global health.[19,20] This approach builds upon the insight that the fulfillment of people's human rights is conducive to their health and that the violation of human rights tends to be detrimental to health. For some human rights—such as the right to health or the right to an adequate standard of living—this is obvious. However, the importance of the social determinants of health, including social status, discrimination, and social exclusion, suggests that the fulfillment of civil and political rights may have an important relationship with population health.[21] Health and human rights are therefore inextricably linked.

In simple terms, if we were to apply the health and human rights approach to global health, this would mean that we would do the following:

- Assess health policies, programs, and practices in terms of their impact on human rights
- Analyze and address the health impacts resulting from violations of human rights when considering ways to improve population health
- Prioritize the fulfillment of human rights

The health and human rights approach reminds us to take an inclusive view of what is needed to promote health: it is not just a matter of having sufficient doctors and drugs, but of addressing poverty, homelessness, education, discrimination, violence, asymmetries in power, and civil and political inclusion. Moreover, in the design and implementation of global health efforts, we should pay particular attention to factors such as the participation in program design of affected people and communities, equity across groups, and the empowerment of individuals over their own lives.

Limits to Human Rights

The importance of protecting human rights related to health is widely acknowledged. Yet, there are exceptional circumstances in which someone's rights may be temporarily suspended. For instance, in order

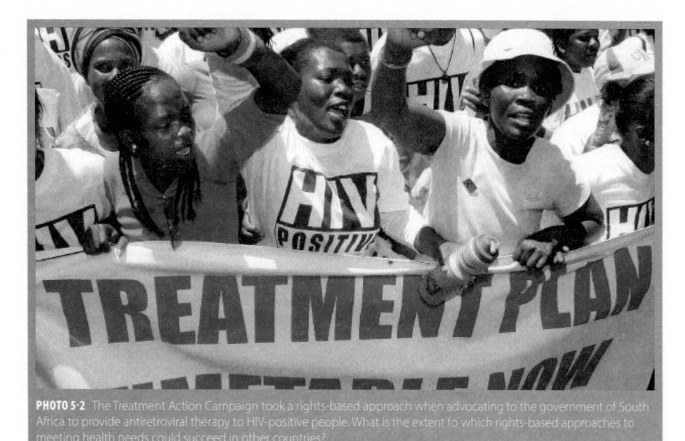

PHOTO 5-2 The Treatment Action Campaign took a rights-based approach when advocating to the government of South Africa to provide antiretroviral therapy to HIV-positive people. What is the extent to which rights-based approaches to meeting health needs could succeed in other countries?
© Mike Hutchings/Reuters.

to protect the interest of the public during an influenza epidemic or an outbreak of an emerging or re-emerging infectious disease such as the Ebola virus, a government might suspend for a certain time the right of people to leave their homes, to go to work, to travel, or to participate in mass gatherings, such as sporting events. Few people would deny the obligation of governments to make laws that permit urgent action to protect public health. However, few would also deny the tendency of autocratic governments to use the excuse of public order or the public interest to consolidate power and suppress political opposition. Consequently, any suspension of people's rights should be as narrow as possible, so that only those aspects of their rights that allow the government to achieve its legitimate goals are suspended. Furthermore, the suspension should be carried out with due process, rights should be monitored during the suspension period, and all efforts should be made to reinstate them as soon as possible.[22]

Human Rights and HIV/AIDS

As much as any health condition in history, HIV/AIDS has raised a host of human rights issues. One reason for this is that HIV/AIDS is a health condition that

was and still is stigmatized and discriminated against in many cultures. For example, many people continue to see HIV/AIDS as a self-inflicted disease caused by engaging in what they consider promiscuous behavior. This could be homosexual sex, injection drug use, having multiple sex partners, or commercial sex work. In addition, in places where people are not familiar with how the disease is spread, there is often great fear of catching the disease.

An important question that arose in many societies as HIV/AIDS became more prevalent was how to protect the rights of people who are HIV-positive to employment, schooling, and participation in social activities. When the epidemic was first recognized, there was considerable discrimination in a number of countries against HIV-positive people, some of whom lost their jobs or were not allowed to enroll in school. Such discrimination continues in some places.

Another matter, as we saw in the opening vignette with John Williams, is the access of people with HIV to health care. In at least the early stages of the HIV/AIDS epidemic in many countries, most health workers were poorly informed about HIV, not aware of how it is spread, and afraid to care for people who were HIV-positive. In fact, people living with

HIV/AIDS were frequently denied care or treated with discrimination when they did receive it.

HIV testing has raised further questions related to protecting people's well-being while respecting human rights. For many years, a cardinal principle of work on HIV has been that testing for it should be voluntary and confidential. This is to ensure that people are not forced to get tested and then discriminated against if others learn that they are HIV-positive.

This point highlights the issues of confidentiality that have also arisen in the context of HIV/AIDS. Yet, the clinical settings in some resource-poor countries with high HIV prevalence are poorly organized, inefficient, and not accustomed to treating patients and patient records confidentially. They also may not have the physical space to treat people privately and confidentially.

Related to concerns about privacy have been important questions about the disclosure of HIV status. Should the healthcare system notify spouses or sexual partners of the HIV status of patients? Should the patients do that? What are the risks? For example, if a husband is notified about the status of his wife, he may harm or reject her, or his family may force her to leave the house.

As mentioned already, a constitutional right to health has been successfully invoked in several countries in order to get access to HIV/AIDS treatment. One of the reasons why this strategy was adopted was the high market price of antiretroviral therapy (ART) in many settings at the time. At present, the goal is to place HIV-positive individuals on treatment as soon as their positive status is known. The majority of people living in these countries cannot afford the cost of such drugs, even at the reduced prices at which they are available today, compared to earlier.

Although these rights-related questions have been particularly prominent when thinking about HIV/AIDS, many of them are relevant to global health more generally. For example, many vulnerable populations and disease groups are stigmatized or discriminated against. Moreover, all patients ought to be treated with respect and their medical records kept confidential. Finally, questions about the appropriate limits that can be placed on people's rights might arise even more dramatically with other communicable diseases. For example, the isolation or quarantine of people who have drug-resistant tuberculosis or the Ebola virus forcefully raises the question of how to balance individual liberty with the safety of the public.

▶ Research with Human Subjects

Research is essential for improving global health. Not only do new health interventions need to be developed to address the world's diseases, but ways to deliver existing interventions also need to be improved. Health research, however, generates some distinctive ethical problems. Eventually, all new healthcare interventions must be tested with human beings, but most research studies are not designed to benefit the people who participate in them. Instead, they are designed to create knowledge that can help patients in the future. Medical research therefore raises special ethical concerns because research participants are put at risk for the sake of other people's health.

This section outlines some historically important cases in research ethics and surveys some of the ethical guidelines that emerged from them. It also describes the current global system of review for research ethics. Finally, it considers how to go about the ethical evaluation of clinical research.

Key Human Research Cases

A number of historical cases of research with human subjects have raised ethical concerns and subsequently have encouraged the development of guidelines for carrying out research ethically. Among the best known of these are the Nazi medical experiments, the Tuskegee study in the United States, and the "short-course" trials for the drug zidovudine (AZT) in Africa and Asia.

The Nazi Medical Experiments

In 1931 the Reich Circular on Human Experimentation laid out German regulations for the conduct of research with human beings. With a strict requirement for the consent of the subject (or the subject's legal representative) and restrictions on the risks to which children could be exposed, these regulations were ahead of their time. Yet, just a few years later, German physicians and scientists perpetrated some of the worst medical atrocities in history.

Hitler's accession to the chancellorship in 1933 began a process of Nazification of the German state and German society. This included research institutions, universities, and the medical profession. It coincided with the rise in popularity of eugenics in many countries. With the Nazi emphasis on racial purity, this eventually led to widespread forced sterilization of "undesirable groups," such as people with disabilities, people with inherited mental and physical anomalies, and ethnic minorities, as well as the eventual "euthanasia" of hundreds of thousands of "incurables."[23] The views that justified these acts were supported by the research of anthropologists and geneticists.

German medical researchers conducted many experiments on euthanasia victims, prisoners of war, and those held in Nazi concentration camps. In support of the war effort, prisoners were deliberately infected with diseases like tuberculosis and malaria. Josef Mengele, as camp doctor at the Auschwitz concentration camp, studied around 900 children in his research on twins, as a part of which he conducted operations without anesthetics, killed children's siblings, and injected children with infective agents. Anthropologists collected body parts from prisoners of war and concentration camps for the study of comparative anatomy.

Following the end of World War II, amid widespread evidence of medical research abuses by the Nazis, the Allies set up an International Scientific Commission to investigate and document these abuses. Subsequently, 23 Nazi scientists were charged with war crimes and crimes against humanity at the Nuremberg Doctors' Trial. Sixteen were convicted, of whom 7 were sentenced to death and hanged.

Most of the researchers who took part in medical research under the Nazis were not prosecuted. Indeed, many of them went on to have scientific careers in postwar Germany, and until the 1990s, specimens taken from victims of the Holocaust and euthanasia were preserved in German medical institutes.[23] Debate continues over the use of the results of the Nazi medical research. Some commentators argue that most of the experiments were poorly designed and so the data are valueless. Others contend that the research does contain valuable data, but there is disagreement over whether it would be ethical to use it.[24]

The Tuskegee Study

In 1932, the U.S. Public Health Service (PHS), in collaboration with the Tuskegee Institute, began a study of syphilis in Macon County, Alabama. One of the study's original aims was to justify the creation of syphilis treatment programs for African Americans at a time of considerable racial discrimination against this group.

Six hundred African American men took part in the study, 399 with syphilis and 201 without. The men were told by researchers that they were being treated for "bad blood," a term that was used locally to describe a number of ailments, including syphilis, anemia, and fatigue. Those participating in the study received aspirin and iron tonics to make them think that they were being treated, and their families were offered burial stipends if they agreed to autopsies.[25] In fact, the men were not being treated at all; the study's aim was simply to document the natural history of syphilis.

The Tuskegee Study of Untreated Syphilis in the Negro Male, though originally planned to last 6 months, went on for 40 years.[26] In its early years, the infected participants would not have received treatment outside of the study anyway, given the limited treatment options available for syphilis and their limited contact with doctors. However, during the late 1930s and the 1940s, the PHS repeatedly intervened to prevent them from receiving effective treatment, even when penicillin became widely available after World War II.

In July 1972, a front-page article in the *New York Times* broke the story of the Tuskegee study. In response to the ensuing public outcry, the U.S. Assistant Secretary for Health and Scientific Affairs appointed an advisory panel to review the study, and the study was swiftly brought to a close. In the summer of 1973, the National Association for the Advancement of Colored People (NAACP) filed a class-action lawsuit on behalf of the Tuskegee subjects. It was settled out of court. As part of the $9 million settlement, the U.S. government promised to give free medical and burial services to all living participants, as well as health services for wives, widows, and children who had been infected because of the study.

The impact of the Tuskegee study on human subjects research was profound. U.S. Senate hearings on human experimentation in 1973 focused further attention on the study. These hearings were followed by the creation of the National Commission for the Protection of Human Subjects of Biomedical and Behavioral Research, whose recommendations would eventually result in regulations for the protection of human research subjects in the United States.[25]

The Tuskegee study on syphilis in African-American men has had a profound impact on the development of ethical approaches to medical research on human subjects. Are the safeguards now in place sufficient to protect the rights of less powerful groups?

The "Short-Course" AZT Trials

In 1994, a study conducted by the AIDS Clinical Trials Group demonstrated the effectiveness of the antiretroviral drug zidovudine (AZT) in preventing mother-to-child transmission of HIV. The complex "076 regimen," which started with intravenous administration of AZT in the second trimester of pregnancy and continued through to treatment of the infant, reduced HIV infection by two-thirds.[27] It immediately became the standard of care in high-income countries. In most low-income countries, however, the 076 regimen was thought to be too complicated and too expensive to implement. This is despite the fact that such countries were exactly the places where the HIV epidemic was worst and where effective prevention was needed. Consequently, there was great interest in developing a cheaper intervention that would be easier to implement.

Following a meeting organized by the World Health Organization (WHO), 15 trials were set to take place in low- and middle-income countries, mostly in sub-Saharan Africa, including tests of simpler "short-course" AZT regimens. The trials provoked fierce criticism. Opponents of the trials noted that they would not be permitted to take place in high-income countries, where the 076 regimen was the standard of care. They therefore accused the sponsors of the short-course AZT trials of ethical double standards. Moreover, they claimed that the studies violated the restrictions on placebo use stated in the Declaration of Helsinki (which is discussed later in this chapter).[28] In 1997, Peter Lurie and Sidney Wolfe wrote the following in the *New England Journal of Medicine*:

> Residents of impoverished, postcolonial countries, the majority of whom are people of color, must be protected from potential exploitation in research. Otherwise, the abominable state of health care in these countries can be used to justify studies that could never pass ethical muster in the sponsoring country.[29]

Proponents of the trials defended their design. They noted that the results of the trials were likely to be valuable to the communities from which the participants were drawn. The trials were therefore not exploiting poor people for the gain of people in high-income countries. The 076 regimen would not, in any case, be available to the women enrolling in these trials, and so they were not being deprived of treatment. Finally, they argued that there were methodological reasons for using a placebo-controlled design. A study using the 076 regimen as an active control was quite likely to show that the short-course regimen was inferior. However, it would not show whether the short-course regimen was better than nothing at all. Furthermore, the background rate of mother-to-child transmission of HIV varied between populations, which meant that a comparison to placebo would be scientifically necessary.[30]

Unlike the Nazi experiments and the Tuskegee study, which were clearly unethical, the ethics of the short-course AZT trials remain controversial. Although some commentators remain convinced that they were unethical, many people think that trials like these are essential if we are to develop interventions that can help large numbers of people in low- and middle-income countries. The last revision of the Helsinki Declaration, however, does take a clear stand on issues like those raised by this trial:

> The benefits, risks, burdens and effectiveness of a new intervention must be tested against those of the best proven intervention(s), except in the following circumstances: Where no proven intervention exists, the use of placebo, or no intervention, is acceptable; or Where for compelling and scientifically sound methodological reasons the use of any intervention less effective than the best proven one, the use of placebo, or no intervention is necessary to determine the efficacy or safety of an intervention and the patients who receive any intervention less effective than the best proven one, placebo, or no intervention will not be subject to additional risks of serious or irreversible harm as a result of not receiving the best proven intervention. Extreme care must be taken to avoid abuse of this option.[31]

The debate over these trials did highlight the existence of additional ethical issues concerning research conducted in low- and middle-income countries. Along with a framework for evaluating the ethics of human subjects research, these additional issues are outlined next.

▶ Research Ethics Guidelines

The Nuremberg Code

At the close of the Nuremberg trial, the three presiding U.S. judges issued the Nuremberg Code (see **TABLE 5-1**). This was the first document to specify the ethical principles that should guide physicians engaged in human subjects research.[32] Among other principles, it states that the "voluntary consent of the human subject is absolutely essential," emphasizes that human subjects should only be involved in research if it is necessary for an important social good, and requires limits on and safeguards against risks to participants.[32] The Nuremberg Code was foundational for later research ethics guidelines and national regulations.

TABLE 5-1 The Standards of the Nuremberg Code

- Those who participate in the study must freely give their consent to do so. They must be given information on the "nature, duration, and purpose of the experiment." They should know how it will be conducted. They must not be forced or coerced in any way to participate in the experiment.
- The experiment must produce valuable benefits that cannot be gotten in other ways.
- The experiment should be based on animal studies and a knowledge of the natural history of the disease or condition being studied.
- The conduct of the research should avoid all unnecessary physical and mental suffering and injury.
- The degree of risk of the research should never exceed that related to the nature of the problem to be addressed.
- The research should be conducted in appropriate facilities that can protect research subjects from harm.
- The research must be conducted by a qualified team of researchers.
- The research subject should be able to end participation at any time.
- The study will be promptly stopped if adverse effects are seen.

Data from *Trials of War Criminals Before the Nuremberg Military Tribunals Under Control Council Law.* (1949). Washington, DC: U.S. Government Printing Office. Retrieved from http://www.hhs.gov/ohrp/archive/nurcode.html

The Declaration of Helsinki

In 1964, the World Medical Association (WMA) developed a set of ethical principles, the Declaration of Helsinki, to guide physicians conducting biomedical research with human subjects. Although the declaration targets physicians (the members of the WMA), its principles are supposed to apply equally to nonphysicians. It is the most influential and most cited set of international research ethics guidelines. The Declaration of Helsinki was revised in 1975, 1983, 1989, 1996, 2000, 2008, and 2013.[31]

Some key principles from the Declaration of Helsinki are summarized in **TABLE 5-2**.

The Belmont Report

On July 12, 1974, the U.S. National Commission for the Protection of Human Subjects of Biomedical and Behavioral Research was created via the U.S. National Research Act. The commission's mandate was to identify basic ethical principles for the conduct of biomedical and behavioral research with human subjects and to develop guidelines for researchers so that all human research would conform to the principles identified. The commission prepared what has come to be known as the Belmont Report.[33] The ethical principles of this report and their applications are outlined in **TABLE 5-3**.

▶ Evaluating the Ethics of Human Subjects Research

The Nuremberg Code, the Declaration of Helsinki, and the Belmont Report all provide ethical principles that should be used to evaluate research protocols. But how should one carry out this evaluation? A simple framework, derived from the general principles enunciated in the Belmont Report, can help us systematically think through the ethics of many proposed clinical research studies. According to this framework, a clinical research protocol must satisfy at least six conditions: (1) social value, (2) scientific validity, (3) fair subject selection, (4) acceptable risk/benefit ratio, (5) informed consent, and (6) respect for enrolled subjects.[34]

In general, research is ethically justified only if it is socially beneficial; that is, if it generates knowledge that can help people. Otherwise, it exposes participants to risks and burdens for no good reason. A study can fail to be socially beneficial in two ways. First, if the scientific questions that the study seeks to answer are not important questions; for example, if the results of the study are known beforehand, then its data are not important. This gives rise to the requirement that research must have **social value**. Second, a study can fail to be socially beneficial, even if it is trying to answer important questions, if the study methodology is inadequate to answer those questions. For example, if a study will not enroll enough participants to generate a statistically significant result, then the methodology is inadequate. If a study cannot test its hypotheses, then no matter how important they are, it cannot result in social benefit. This gives rise to the requirement that research must be **scientifically valid**.

The third requirement, **fair subject selection**, concerns the equitable distribution of the benefits and burdens of research. When considering who will be asked to enroll in a study, researchers should make sure they do not enroll members of vulnerable

TABLE 5-2 The Declaration of Helsinki: Key Principles

Scientific Validity

- Medical research involving human subjects must conform to generally accepted scientific principles and be based on a thorough knowledge of the scientific literature.

Fairness

- Groups that are underrepresented in medical research should be provided appropriate access to participation.
- Medical research with a vulnerable group is justified only if the research is responsive to the health needs or priorities of this group and the research cannot be carried out in a non-vulnerable group. In addition, this group should stand to benefit from the knowledge, practices, or interventions that result from the research.
- In advance of a clinical trial, sponsors, researchers, and host country governments should make provisions for post-trial access for all participants who still need an intervention identified as beneficial in the trial.

Risks and Benefits

- The well-being of the individual research subject must take precedence over all other interests.
- The importance of the objective of a study must outweigh the risks to the research subjects.
- Physical, mental, and social risks must be minimized.

Placebos

- A new intervention must be tested against the best current proven intervention, except when:
  - No current proven intervention exists; or
  - Where for methodological reasons the use of placebo is necessary and subjects who receive placebo will not be subject to any risk of serious or irreversible harm.

Consent

- Potential subjects must give voluntary, informed consent.
- For a potential research subject who is incompetent, the physician must seek informed consent from a legally authorized representative.
- Where possible, the physician must seek the assent and respect the dissent of an incompetent potential research subject.

Oversight and Accountability

- The research protocol must be submitted to an independent research ethics committee before the study begins.
- Every clinical trial must be registered in a publicly accessible database before recruitment begins.
- Authors have a duty to make publicly available the results of their research, including negative and inconclusive results.

Modified from World Medical Association. (2013). *WMA declaration of Helsinki: Ethical principles for medical research involving human subjects.* Retrieved from https://www.wma.net/policies-post /wma-declaration-of-helsinki-ethical-principles-for-medical-research-involving-human-subjects/

populations in risky studies simply for reasons of convenience. Similarly, privileged people should not be preferred for participation in research that promises to be beneficial. Sometimes enrollment criteria are explicit; for example, a study may exclude children or people with certain comorbidities. Other times they are more subtle; for example, a study that requires extended visits to a hospital may exclude people who cannot take time away from work or family responsibilities, and a study that advertises for participants online will exclude people who do not have access to the internet.

The requirement for an **acceptable risk/ benefit ratio** combines several concerns. First, the risks to participants should be minimized as much as possible and consistent with meeting the scientific objectives of the study. Second, there is a limit to the level of risk to which participants may be exposed. We do not think, for example, that people should be asked to risk their lives for the cause of science. Finally, the risks to participants must be balanced by the possible benefits to the participants and to society. Thus, the social value of a study is a vital part of the assessment of whether the risk/benefit ratio is acceptable.

TABLE 5-3 The Belmont Report

Basic Ethical Principle	Application of the Principle
Respect for Persons: ■ Treat individuals as autonomous persons. ■ Protect individuals with diminished autonomy.	*Informed Consent:* ■ Individuals should be allowed to make an informed, voluntary decision about what happens to them. ■ Individuals whose capacity is limited should be given the opportunity to choose to the extent that they are able.
Beneficence: ■ Maximize possible benefits. ■ Minimize possible harms.	*Assessment of Risks and Benefits:* ■ A data-based risk/benefit assessment should be made. ■ Risks to subjects should be outweighed by the sum of the benefits to subjects and the benefit to society. The interests of the subjects should be given priority. ■ Risks should be reduced to those necessary to achieve the research objective.
Justice: ■ The benefits and burdens of research must be distributed fairly.	*Selection of Subjects:* ■ There must be fair procedures and outcomes in the selection of those participating in the research.

Data from Office for Human Research Protections. (1976). *The Belmont report.* Retrieved from https://www.hhs.gov/ohrp/regulations-and-policy/belmont-report/index.html

Obtaining competent people's **informed consent** to research participation respects them by letting them choose what happens to them. Valid informed consent consists of several elements, including a description of the research that potential participants can understand and the voluntary choice to participate. Some individuals, such as children, are unable to give their own consent. They are respected by having a surrogate decision maker give permission for research enrollment on their behalf and by being involved in the decision as far as they are able.

In some cultures, there are people with the authority to make decisions on behalf of other competent adults. For example, it may be considered normal for a village elder to make decisions on behalf of the people living in the village or for a husband to make decisions on behalf of his wife. It is important that research be conducted in culturally sensitive ways. However, this does not imply that any competent adult may be enrolled in research against his or her will. The individual's informed consent should always be obtained.

Researchers still have a number of ethical duties once participants are enrolled. For example, they must respect participants' rights to withdraw from research, protect their confidentiality, and so on. These duties fall under the umbrella of **respect for enrolled subjects**.

Going through these principles in order is a helpful way of systematically evaluating the ethics of a proposed research study. However, they are not the only considerations that are ethically relevant, and the framework does not tell us how to balance conflicting principles against one another. For example, how should we decide when it is permissible to use a study design that exposes subjects to a slightly greater risk of harm in order to collect more valuable data? Thus, the framework does not constitute a checklist, but is simply a guide to some of the most important ethical considerations and an order in which to consider them.

Research in Low- and Middle-Income Countries

The controversy concerning the short-course AZT trials put a spotlight on the ethics of clinical research conducted in low- and middle-income countries. Such research is frequently sponsored by institutions or companies based in high-income countries, and it draws on a pool of potential participants who are likely to be poor, undereducated, and without access to good-quality medical care outside of their participation in the research. Consequently, some ethical issues arise much more frequently in low- and middle-income countries. Three of the most important issues are summarized here: (1) the standard of care, (2) post-trial benefits, and (3) ancillary care.

The "standard of care" discussion centers on questions concerning what level of medical care should be provided to participants in controlled clinical trials.

These trials give an experimental intervention, such as a new drug, to members of one group of participants and compare their symptoms with a similar group of people who do not receive the intervention. The comparison group, or **arm**, sometimes receives an established treatment, sometimes an inactive substance (placebo), and sometimes nothing at all. Much debate has focused on when it is permissible to give participants a placebo if an effective treatment already exists for the condition being studied. This was the question at the heart of the dispute over the short-course AZT trials. However, similar questions can arise whenever the standard of care offered in any arm of the trial is less than the standard available to patients in high-income countries with universal health care.[30]

The issue of post-trial benefits arises both with respect to participants and with respect to the community or society they come from. When research participants are also patients, they may receive treatment during a trial. But at the end of the trial their condition may not be cured. For example, participants in HIV/AIDS treatment trials may be treated with antiretroviral therapy during the trial. However, if they do not continue this treatment after the trial, their condition will start to deteriorate again. In high-income countries with universal health care this is not a problem, because participants will leave the trial and then continue to receive treatment in their communities. However, in low- and middle-income countries this may not be an option for the majority of participants. It is widely recognized that post-trial benefits to participants is an important ethical issue. What benefits should be provided and by whom has not been decided in a definitive manner. Yet, the latest revision of the Helsinki Declaration requires that sponsors, researchers, and host country governments should, in advance of a clinical trial, make provisions for post-trial access for all participants who may need an intervention identified as beneficial in the trial .[31,35,36]

Concerns have also been raised about whether other members of the communities hosting research will benefit. For example, a pharmaceutical company might test a new drug for schizophrenia on patients in Peru but either not market the drug in Peru or price it out of the reach of most of Peru's population. To some commentators, such trials seem exploitative. They argue that research should not be permitted unless the communities that host it will have access to successful interventions that result.[37,38] Other commentators argue for a broader understanding of how exploitation can be avoided. They think that communities that host research should receive a fair level of benefits from the research, but this need not be in the form of post-trial access to interventions.[39]

Ancillary care is medical care that is given to study participants but that is not required by the scientific design of the study. In the vignette at the beginning of this chapter, malaria researchers were conflicted about whether they should provide ancillary care to the children in their study, including treatment for malaria, diarrhea, parasitic infections, and pneumonia. Such dilemmas are common for researchers who are working in environments where many people lack access to health care. The researchers may be trained clinicians who could provide much-needed care. However, time and resources spent on medical care take away from those that can be spent on conducting research. There is no established way to work out how much ancillary care researchers ought to provide to participants. However, there is agreement that researchers have *at least* the following duties:

- First, researchers, like other people, have a duty to provide life-saving medical care when they can do so at a relatively low cost.
- Second, if participants are harmed by research procedures and do not have access to health care outside the trial, they should be treated for those harms.
- Third, ancillary care should be incorporated into the planning for research studies conducted in poor populations.

Some bioethicists have also tried to work out further ancillary care responsibilities on the basis of the contribution participants make and the relationship that develops between researchers and participants.[40]

Human Subjects Research Oversight Today

In the majority of countries today, it is a legal requirement for most clinical research with human subjects to undergo independent ethical review by a research ethics committee (REC). Also called an institutional review board (IRB), a research ethics board, or independent ethics committee, the REC is intended to provide a safeguard against the exploitation of human subjects in research. Many countries also have a national ethics committee, which may oversee the local RECs, review certain studies, or disseminate guidelines for research.

The regulations that govern REC review of research vary from country to country. Some RECs are regionally based, so they are responsible for all the human subjects research taking place in a particular area of the country. For example, Sweden has six regional boards for research ethics. Others are institutionally based, so they review research that is conducted by that particular institution, as well as research by other bodies that do not have their own REC. This is the situation in South Africa, for example. The U.S. system requires ethical review for research that is funded by the federal government or regulated by the U.S. Food and Drug Administration (FDA). This is important when research sponsored by the U.S. government is carried out in another country, because the research is then subject to both the U.S. and the host country regulations. In addition, institutions in the United States carry out ethical reviews of research on human subjects that is related to their institution even if such research is not supported by the federal government.

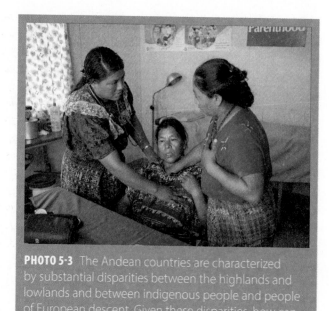

PHOTO 5-3 The Andean countries are characterized by substantial disparities between the highlands and lowlands and between indigenous people and people of European descent. Given these disparities, how can governments ensure that they invest in health in a way that is fair and seeks to maximize population health?
Courtesy of Mark Tuschman.

▶ Ethical Issues in Making Investment Choices in Health

As noted earlier, one central issue in global health is the need to make choices among investments that can enhance the health of a population. This is necessary, especially in low- and middle-income countries, because resources will always be fewer than needed to meet everyone's health needs. Sometimes a single type of scarce resource needs to be distributed. For example, there may be a limited number of kidneys or a limited amount of blood for transfusion. More commonly, government ministries have tight budgets and must decide how to allocate their funds among many options, ranging from the purchase of medicines to investments in infrastructure. These investment choices will get made, one way or another. It is better that they be made according to explicit, publicly justified criteria rather than in secret or without serious consideration of the ethical reasons for different distributions.

Cost-effectiveness analysis is one important tool for making decisions about health investments; however, it is rarely a sufficient approach to deciding what to do. Decision makers must still make value judgments about what use to make of a cost-effectiveness analysis. Consider the vignette about the Indian state discussed at the beginning of this chapter. Investing in urban clinics would likely have the greatest total impact on health—it would avert the most disability-adjusted life years (DALYs). But the poorer people in the countryside might still, quite reasonably, think that they were being unfairly treated. After all, they were already worse off than the city residents, so why should they lose out again? Health economics, although indispensable for making health investment choices, cannot replace hard decisions about what is fair.

Principles for Distributing Scarce Resources

Various ways to distribute scarce resources have been suggested. Take the problem of allocating live organs for transplant. One way to allocate organs is to have a waiting list, so that those people who are diagnosed as needing a transplant first are also the people who receive an organ first. This would be a "first come, first served" principle. Alternatively, a lottery might seem fair, so that everyone diagnosed as needing an organ would have the same chance of receiving one. Questions could be raised, however, about the fairness of this type of lottery. Some might suggest, for example, that someone whose lifestyle choices put her at risk for illness, such as when alcoholism results in liver failure, is less deserving of a transplant. It might alternatively be thought that people who have better prognoses should receive some sort of priority. A weighted lottery could incorporate these considerations, giving smaller or larger chances to members of particular populations. In practice, the U.S. United Network for Organ Sharing (UNOS) uses a complex point system that is different for each organ, where matching, urgency, time on waiting list, expected health outcome, and patient age are typically taken into account.[41] Other countries have similar systems.

Some ways to allocate scarce resources are obviously unfair. Prioritizing certain people's health needs over others because they are of a particular ethnic group or sexual orientation is unethical. The "first come, first served" system, for example, might accidentally favor the well-connected or people who already have access to good-quality medical care and so are likely to get an early diagnosis.[42]

There are various alternative ways to allocate resources that may seem fairer. The justification underlying most plausible allocation proposals is one or more of four basic ethical principles:

- Health maximization
- Equity
- Extra priority to the worse off
- Personal responsibility

Most ethical frameworks, as well as countries that have developed guidelines for priority setting, include some variants of the first three principles.[43-45] Personal responsibility for health is more controversial.

In addition, there is agreement among ethical theories that priority setting should be impartial and treat people as equals. In global health, there is growing consensus that priority setting should aim to promote health maximization and fair distribution.[45,46] Both level and distribution matter.

The principle of **health maximization** tells us that we should allocate healthcare resources in such a way that the total beneficial impact on health is as large as possible. For example, if someone proposed allocating kidneys based on the criterion of best prognosis for the recipient, this would be a form of health maximization. If health maximization were the only principle used, then people making health investments might simply look at the DALYs averted by different allocations of interventions and choose the most cost-effective way to avert DALYs.

Health maximization has obvious appeal: it means producing the greatest benefit that we can. In addition, choosing to prioritize services based on their cost-effectiveness is important, considering that improving the length and quality of life has both direct and indirect value for people. Even if the principle of health maximization cannot stand alone, there are very few ethicists who would argue that it is not relevant—to *not* improve health as much as possible would have substantial opportunity costs in terms of healthy life years forgone.[47] However, the principle of health maximization also has drawbacks. One important drawback is illustrated by one of the vignettes at the beginning of this chapter. Sometimes a given amount of money could do the greatest good if it is spent helping people who are already well off. For example, if a government wants a new clinic to vaccinate the greatest number of children possible, it should locate the clinic in a city, not in the countryside. But people living in cities are usually already better off than people living in the country—they are likely to make more money, have

better education, and have improved water supplies and sanitation. So, just focusing on helping people in cities looks unfair. The principles of equity and priority to the worse off may weigh in favor of locating the clinic in a rural area.

There are several ways to interpret the principle of **equity**. One interpretation is that we should try to ensure that everyone has an equal chance at receiving a scarce resource or having access to health care. In this case, people are treated equally by being treated the same. Another interpretation of equity is concerned with equal access to health services or equal health outcomes regardless of socioeconomic status, neighborhood, or other types of disadvantages. Most egalitarians recognize that health maximization is also important, so the two principles must sometimes be balanced.

Giving extra **"priority to the worse off"** is different from the principle of equity and should be seen together with the principle of health maximization. When we adopt this principle, we make decisions about providing health care on the basis of who is already disadvantaged, rather than only on the basis of who would benefit the most (as maximization would dictate). Priority to the worse off is important because benefiting them matters more than benefiting those who are better off.[48] Put differently, we should give priority to those we can help the most and who are in greatest need. The worse off can be defined as those with the most severe disease (largest individual disease burden), or those who are the poorest or otherwise most disadvantaged.[45] Because the most cost-effective services do not always benefit the worse off, services targeting the worse off should be assigned extra value. The relative priority to be given to maximizing health compared to giving priority to the worse off is, in the end, a choice that the decision maker must make.

This principle works well when the worse off can be helped relatively easily. It works less well when helping the worse off would be a severe drain on resources, such as when terminally ill patients require continuous expensive therapies. There is also the question of how to identify the worse off. Are they the people who are sickest now or those who will be sickest in the future? Those who have the worst health over a lifetime? Those who are poorest, even if their health is not the worst? A careful definition of the "worse off" is therefore necessary. For example, some have argued that priority to the worse off, defined as those with least health over a lifetime, implies that low-income countries should continue to prioritize reductions in communicable diseases, neonatal conditions, and maternal health, despite the shift toward a burden of noncommunicable diseases that typically affect those that have longer lives.[49]

Each of these three principles has some plausibility. In general, if each is taken to an extreme, it would justify allocations of resources that seem unfair. Most people therefore think that some balance of maximizing benefits, giving equal chances, securing equal outcomes, and prioritizing the worse off is the best way to decide how to invest resources in health. Exactly how to balance these principles in any particular case is difficult, although new methods are now being developed.[50]

Finally, some people cite **personal responsibility** as a principle that can be used in combination with other principles to make decisions about health investments.[51] Those who think that personal responsibility can be a basis for allocation decisions argue that when spending society's resources, lower priority should be given to people whose health problems may relate to their own health behaviors. Why, they may ask, should the tax money of responsible citizens be spent treating lung cancer in smokers, providing methadone and clean needles to people addicted to heroin, or providing ICU beds to motorcycle riders who refuse to wear helmets? Alternatively, it may be proposed that people who contribute to society should be rewarded by giving them greater priority. For example, organ donors might be given greater priority to be organ recipients.

Doctors' decisions about whether to treat are traditionally based only on need and not on actions that have led to that need. Generally, those analyzing these decisions believe that it would only be fair to give a lower priority to the care of people whose behaviors appear to have caused the need for care under the following conditions:

> The needs must have been caused by the behavior; the behavior must have been voluntary; the persons must have known that the behavior would cause the health needs and that if they engaged in it their health needs would receive lower priority.[52]

At present, these conditions are rarely, if ever, met.

Others have argued that the principle of responsibility simply states that individuals should be held responsible for their choices, not for the consequences of their choices. It is only in the special case where the outcome only depends on the individual's choices and not on any other factors that this principle implies that individuals should be held responsible for the consequences of their actions. To hold people responsible for the actual consequences of their choice would therefore be to *hold them responsible for too much*. Some people are lucky and some are unlucky when they engage in risky behavior. It would be unfair to hold people responsible for differences in luck. We could therefore reward or tax the behavior as such, rather than the consequences of the behavior. This means that the correct way to introduce responsibility is not at the sick bed or beside the road accident victim, but through taxation. Levying taxes on certain types of behavior, such as smoking, is one way of holding individuals responsible that avoids most of the objections presented here.[53]

Fair Processes

Whatever the content of a decision about health investments, there are better and worse ways to make the decision. If an unelected civil servant in a ministry of health were to unilaterally decide which medicines would be provided in the public healthcare system, this would be troubling. Justice is not just a matter of the result, but of the process, too. The idea of fair process is accorded great importance in contemporary democracies. For example, people accused of crimes are supposed to get a fair trial, and political leaders are supposed to be fairly elected. The proper processes for making health investment decisions have not been completely worked out. However, it seems clear that a fair process will involve at least transparency about how decisions are made and representation from stakeholders affected by the results of the process. The National Institute for Health and Clinical Excellence (NICE) in the United Kingdom, which makes recommendations for how the National Health Service should provide treatments and procedures, is one example of an institution that has attempted to combine fair processes for making recommendations about health spending with an appropriate use of scientific data and medical expertise.[54-56]

In cases where disagreement about principles of distribution seems intractable, the introduction of a fair process has been proposed as a way to resolve the disagreement.[57] Even reasonable people may disagree about the right principles and what weight they should have in concrete situations. This procedural framework suggests that governments or other providers should make explicit their priorities and that reasons for inclusion or exclusion are made transparent and provided to all affected parties. A fair process is inclusive and has broad stakeholder involvement and mechanisms for critical assessment and revision. The process itself should be institutionalized. If satisfied, these conditions can connect decisions about priority setting to broader democratic processes. Most countries that have implemented procedures for priority setting, such as through institutions for health technology assessment, combine them with substantive principles such as health maximization and fair distribution.[44]

The idea here is that even if people cannot agree, for example, on how their state should spend its tax revenue on health and welfare, they may still be able to agree on a process for making such decisions. By analogy, a divorcing couple might not be able to agree on how to divide up their possessions; however, they might be able to agree on a process of mediation by a third party, which would lead to a division that they would both accept. This may be one solution to disagreements. However, it has its own potential problems. First, there may be similarly intractable disagreement about what counts as a fair process. Second, the fact that people agree on a process does not guarantee that either the process or its results are fair.

This overview has only scratched the surface of the ethical problems involved in deciding how to allocate resources for health. Many other questions arise when considering investment choices in health and the use of cost-effectiveness analysis. One concerns the way that cost-effectiveness analyses are conducted; for example, measuring health benefits in DALYs may seem to discriminate against disabled people, because the methodology for DALYs inherently values a condition of disability less highly than a condition of good health. Another important question is how to balance present benefits with future benefits. Should governments give greater priority to giving people vital medications now, or should they equally focus on training doctors, building infrastructure, and conducting medical research to help future patients? One could consider these and other related issues at great length. The important point of this section, however, is that, when considering investment choices and the tools one will use to make decisions about them, it is necessary to critically assess the value judgments that are implicit in them.

▶ Case Studies

Ethical Priority Setting in Norway

Norway is one of the richest countries in the world and, in principle, can afford to spend more per capita on health than almost any other country. Nonetheless, Norway has a long tradition of trying to achieve the most health for its people, in fair ways, through systematic priority setting at the national level.[58,59]

As a reflection of this, a third Norwegian Committee on Priority Setting in the Health Sector laid out a new, comprehensive framework for setting priorities in 2014.[60,61] This framework comprises four general principles:

Priority setting should

1. pursue the goal of "the greatest number of healthy life years for all, fairly distributed";
2. be based on clear criteria;
3. be open, systematic, and involve user participation; and
4. be supported by a coherent set of effective instruments.

The framework, with some minor adjustments, was approved by the parliament.

The first principle of the framework underscores that the goal of Norway's investment in health is not only to maximize population health but also to ensure that healthy life years are fairly distributed. From this followed three new criteria, as adopted by the parliament:

- *The health-benefit criterion:* The priority of an intervention increases with the expected health benefit and other relevant welfare benefits from the intervention.
- *The resource criterion:* The more the priority of an intervention increases, the fewer the resources it requires.
- *The severity of disease criterion:* The priority of an intervention increases with the expected future health loss of the beneficiary in the absence of such an intervention.

The first two criteria are well known in the priority setting literature, while the third is not. The severity criterion is intended to capture a key aspect of fairness: the concern for the worse off. The worse off are defined, at the individual level, as those with the highest risk of death, loss of physical and mental functioning, pain, and other discomfort. At the group level, the worse off are defined as those who have a larger future health loss as a result of their condition. The loss of future health is defined as the difference between normal healthy life expectancy, at the time of treatment or onset of disease, and the length and quality of life a person would have without the new intervention being considered. At the group level, this is called the **prognostic loss** and can be measured as loss of **quality-adjusted life years (QALYs)**.

Related to this, conditions are put into three severity (or health loss) classes: low, medium, and high. The severity criterion addresses the core problem with

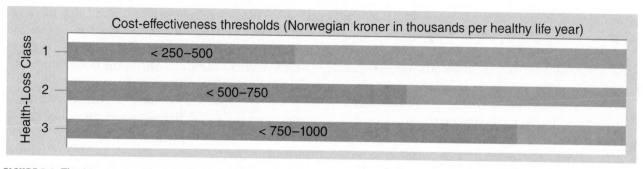

FIGURE 5-1 The Norwegian "Staircase Model" for Cost-Effectiveness Thresholds, with Illustrative Threshold Values

Note: 1 million Norwegian kroner (NOK) equals about US $125,000 as of 2018.

Ottersen, Trygve. (2016). *A new proposal for priority setting in Norway: Open and fair.* Amsterdam, The Netherlands: Elsevier.

setting priorities solely on the basis of magnitude of benefits or cost-effectiveness, namely the problem that it ignores the distribution of benefits and is unconcerned with how disadvantaged people are, as long as the total benefits are the same. The introduction of a severity criterion can thus make cost-effectiveness information more relevant and useful.

The committee further suggested how the three criteria could be balanced with each other. A key feature of the proposal is assigning weights to health benefits according to the health loss of the beneficiary. As a starting point, a simple rule—the "1–2–3 rule"—was proposed, which could be easily understood and used by multiple decision makers. According to this rule, the weight assigned to health benefits increases gradually with health loss.

The three criteria can be used either to directly rank competing interventions or used together with predefined cost-effectiveness thresholds. The committee recommended that such thresholds be based on the opportunity cost of implementing the intervention being considered. This refers to what else could be "purchased" with the same amount of money to be spent on the proposed intervention. Rather than one single threshold value, the committee recommended multiple thresholds, differentiated according to the average health loss of the target group (**FIGURE 5-1**). Thus, a higher cost-effectiveness threshold is accepted if the condition is very severe.

This framework is now used in Norway and has an impact on reimbursement decisions for new costly medications. For example, the drug kabazitaxel (Jevtana) for metastatic prostate cancer was rejected because it was not cost-effective enough, while the drug pertuzumab (Perjeta) for metastatic breast cancer was approved because the condition was considered more severe and price negotiations made it cost-effective.

WHO: Helping Countries Make Fair Choices on the Path to Universal Health Coverage

In 2014, WHO published a report with the findings of its Consultative Group on Equity and Universal Health Coverage. This report recommended the following strategy for countries seeking to implement universal coverage in a progressive manner over time and in a way that would be fair:

Categorize services into priority classes. Relevant criteria for this categorization include factors related to:

a. cost-effectiveness
b. priority to the worse off
c. financial risk protection.

Expand coverage for high-priority services to everyone, as a first step in service expansion. As countries take this step, they should eliminate out-of-pocket payments while increasing mandatory, progressive prepayment with pooling of funds.

While implementing the above, they should also ensure that disadvantaged groups are not left behind. These will often include low-income groups and rural populations.[62]

A key concept in WHO's important report on priority setting was the concept of "fair priority setting." Fairness is fundamentally concerned with the overall distribution of benefits and burdens in society. Equity in health has traditionally been most concerned with equitable access to services regardless of socioeconomic status. Fairness is a broader concept. We all react to unfairness: it is unfair if someone with a very severe disease is denied coverage for a high-priority service simply because he or she is poor and unable to pay. In more technical language, we may say that a fair system will expand service coverage with financial risk protection by giving priority to policies benefiting the worse off, where the worse off are defined both in terms of health itself and in terms of socioeconomic status.[63,64]

Fair health systems are concerned with the worse off in terms of health, socioeconomic status, or overall well-being. One motivation can be that those defined as worse off typically have a greater need for the benefits that come with improved coverage.[65,66] Another, related motivation can be the promotion of equality.[67,68] Priority to the worse off can also be motivated by the right to health.[69] When considering the worse off in terms of health or well-being, there are good reasons to adopt a population perspective and focus not merely on those *currently* worse off but also on the people who are expected to be worse off over their lifetime.[68,70]

This framework for priority setting is now used in Ethiopia, where the government is in the process of revising its essential health services package. *The Disease Control Priorities Project, 3rd Edition*,[71] also used this framework when recommending highest priority packages for low- and middle-income countries.[72] Several other countries, including Iran and Afghanistan, have also decided to implement these recommendations.

▶ Challenges for the Future

Efforts to incorporate ethical and human rights concerns into global health work face a number of challenges. Some of these are briefly explained here.

First, many students of public health and global health get insufficient exposure in their training to ethical and human rights issues. Normally, they do have to understand the core concepts of research on human subjects and how an institutional review board functions. However, they may have few opportunities to take courses that cover broader issues of human rights and health or give them the tools to think systematically through the ethical aspects of research and policymaking. This chapter is a small attempt to correct that gap.

Second, there are deficits in implementation of human rights concerns. As noted earlier, compliance with human rights norms is self-reported by countries. There are few indicators for measuring such compliance and no mechanisms for enforcement. Some also argue that the right to health and health care remains an unrealistic ideal in a world with scarce resources. On the other hand, some human rights advocates and ethicists concerned about fair priority setting in global

health have come together and argued that there are a number of ways in which the right to health and rights-talk can aid priority setters, as well as ways in which priority setting can help in the realization of the right to health.[73]

The governance of human subjects research has been more successful. In most countries there are systems for ethics review. However, these remain patchy in some settings. There is still a shortage of trained personnel for reviewing research; research ethics committees are understaffed, underfunded, and often undervalued; and it is not known how effective even established review systems are at protecting research participants.

There is a lack of explicit review of the fairness of many of the investment choices that are made, both by countries and by the development assistance agencies with which they work. In addition, students of global health are not given enough exposure to the concept of and tools for fair priority setting. If one reviews the documents that relate to investments in health in low- and middle-income countries, attention is generally paid to ensuring that project benefits go to disadvantaged people. However, it is rare that there are explicit reviews or articulation of how investment choices are made and the ethical choices that are a part of them. With respect to HIV/AIDS, for example, what criteria will be used to allocate drugs if there are more people clinically eligible for drugs than the amount of drugs available? Will it be access to the health center, so that there is a greater likelihood that the person will comply with treatment? Will it be pregnancy, so that one can reduce mother-to-child transmission?[74] If there were greater pressure to articulate these choices openly, then these decisions might be made more fairly.

Third, there are many unsolved ethical problems for people working in global health. For example, if human rights are going to guide decisions about global health interventions, we need to know exactly what those rights include. How do we work out what is included in the right to health and what is not? The discussion of the ethics of research in low- and middle-income countries indicated a number of unanswered questions about what is owed to research participants and poor communities in which researchers work.

Those studying global health or working in the global health field are encouraged to think carefully about their answers to the ethical questions that this chapter has left open and to articulate the reasons that justify their answers.

Study Questions

1. The chapter begins with four vignettes. Briefly explain what ethical or human rights issue each vignette reveals.

2. What do the human rights documents mentioned in this chapter say about health?

3. Consider a disease other than HIV/AIDS, such as tuberculosis. How might public health efforts with respect to this disease raise human rights concerns?

4. Explain the three ethical principles stated in the Belmont Report. Give an example of a research study and show how the three principles apply to it.

5. What are the most important ethical concerns that arise when research is conducted with people in low- and middle-income countries?

6. Do you think the short-course AZT trials were ethical? Give reasons why or why not.

7. What principles might be used to justify a decision about how to allocate scarce resources for health care?

8. Why should we pay attention to the process by which health investment decisions are made?

9. How do you think cost-effectiveness analysis should be used by a government making an ethical decision about allocating a scarce health care resource, such as antiretroviral therapy for HIV/AIDS?

References

1. Rudy Van Puymbroeck, then of Georgetown University, co-authored the original version of this chapter. Joseph Millum, a bioethicist who serves as a staff scientist at the Clinical Center Department of Bioethics and the Fogarty International Center, U.S. National Institutes of Health, co-authored in his personal capacity the version of this chapter that appeared in the second and third editions. Ole Norheim, of the University of Bergen, co-authored the version of the chapter that appears in the fourth edition. The opinions expressed are the authors' own. They do not reflect any position or policy of the National Institutes of Health, U.S. Public Health Service, or Department of Health and Human Services.

2. Mann, J., Gostin, L., Gruskin, S., Brennan, T., Lazzarini, Z., & Fineberg, H. (1994). Health and human rights. *Health and Human Rights, 1*(1), 6–23.

3. Hannum, H. (1998). The UDHR in national and international law. *Health and Human Rights, 3*(2), 144–158.

4. United Nations General Assembly. (1948). *Universal declaration of human rights.* Reprinted with the permission of the United Nations. Retrieved from http://www.un.org/en/universal-declaration-human-rights/index.html

5. Office of the United Nations High Commissioner for Human Rights. (1966). *International covenant on economic, social and cultural rights.* Retrieved from http://www.ohchr.org/en/professionalinterest/pages/cescr.aspx

6. Office of the United Nations High Commissioner for Human Rights. (1966). *International covenant on civil and political rights.* Retrieved from http://www.ohchr.org/en/professionalinterest/pages/ccpr.aspx

7. United Nations Human Rights, Office of the High Commissioner. (n.d.). *Status of ratification interactive dashboard.* Retrieved from http://indicators.ohchr.org/

8. Gruskin, S., & Tarantola, D. (2004). Health and human rights. In S. Gruskin, M. A. Grodin, G. J. Annas, & S. P. Marks (Eds.), *Perspectives on health and human rights* (pp. 3–58). New York, NY: Routledge.

9. Mokhiber, C. G. (2005). Toward a measure of dignity: indicators for rights-based development. In S. Gruskin, M. A. Grodin, G. J. Annas, & S. P. Marks (Eds.), *Perspectives on health and human rights* (pp. 383–392). New York, NY: Routledge.

10. Office of the United Nations High Commissioner for Human Rights, World Health Organization. (2008, June). *The right to health: Fact sheet no. 31.* Retrieved from http://www.ohchr.org/documents/publications/factsheet31.pdf

11. Yamin, A. E., & Gloppen, S. (Eds.). (2011). *Litigating health rights: Can courts bring more justice to health?* Cambridge, MA: Harvard University Press.

12. Biehl, J., Petryna, A., Gertner, A., Amon, J. J., & Picon, P. D. (2009). Judicialisation of the right to health in Brazil. *The Lancet, 373*(9682), 2182–2184.

13. Annas, G. J. (2003). The right to health and the nevirapine case in South Africa. *New England Journal of Medicine, 348*(24), 2470–2471.

14. Torres, M. A. (2005). The human right to health, national courts, and access to HIV/AIDS treatment: A case study from Venezuela. In S. Gruskin, M. A. Grodin, G. J. Annas, & S. P. Marks (Eds.), *Perspectives on health and human rights* (pp. 507–516). New York, NY: Routledge.

15. Ely Yamin, A. E., & Parra-Vera, O. (2009). How do courts set health policy? The case of the Colombian constitutional court. *PLoS Med, 6*(2), e1000032.

16. Norheim, O. F., & Wilson, B. M. (2014). Health rights litigation and access to medicines: Priority classification of successful cases from Costa Rica's constitutional chamber of the Supreme Court. *Health and Human Rights, 16*(2), E47–61.

17. United Nations. (1979). *Convention on the elimination of all forms of discrimination against women.* Retrieved from http://www.un.org/womenwatch/daw/cedaw/cedaw.htm

18. Office of the United Nations High Commissioner for Human Rights. (1989). *Convention on the rights of the child.* Reprinted with the permission of the United Nations. Retrieved from http://www.ohchr.org/en/professionalinterest/pages/crc.aspx

19. Gostin, L. O. (2014). *Global health law.* Cambridge, MA: Harvard University Press.

20. Yamin, A. E. (2016). *Power, suffering, and the struggle for dignity: Human rights for health and why they matter.* Philadelphia, PA: University of Pennsylvania Press.

21. Wilkinson, R., & Marmot, M. (2003). *Social determinants of health: The solid facts.* Geneva, Switzerland: World Health Organization. Retrieved from http://www.euro.who.int/__data/assets/pdf_file/0005/98438/e81384.pdf

22. Easley, C. E., Marks, S. P., & Morgan, R. E., Jr. (2005). The challenge and place of international human rights in public health. In S. Gruskin, M. A. Grodin, G. J. Annas, & S. P. Marks (Eds.), *Perspectives on health and human rights* (pp. 519–526). New York, NY: Routledge.

23. Weindling, P. J. (2008). The Nazi medical experiments. In E. Emanuel, C. Grady, R. A. Crouch, et al. (Eds.), *The Oxford textbook of clinical research ethics* (pp. 18–30). Oxford, UK: Oxford University Press.

24. Moe, K. (1984). Should the Nazi research data be cited? *Hastings Center Report, 14*(6), 5–7.

25. Jones, J. H. (2008). The Tuskegee syphilis experiment. In E. Emanuel, C. Grady, R. A. Crouch, et al. (Eds.), *The Oxford textbook of clinical research ethics* (pp. 86–96). Oxford, UK: Oxford University Press.

26. Centers for Disease Control and Prevention. (n.d.). The Tuskegee timeline. Retrieved from http://www.cdc.gov/tuskegee/timeline.htm

27. Connor, E. M., Sperling, R. S., Gelber, R., Kiselev, P., Scott, G., O'Sullican, M. J., . . . Balsley, J. (1994). Reduction of maternal-infant transmission of human immunodeficiency virus type 1 with zidovudine treatment. *New England Journal of Medicine, 331,* 1173–1180.

28. Angell, M. (1997). The ethics of clinical research in the third world. *New England Journal of Medicine, 337,* 847–849.

29. Lurie, P., & Wolfe, S. M. (1997). Unethical trials of interventions to reduce perinatal transmission of the human immunodeficiency virus in developing countries. *New England Journal of Medicine, 337*(12), 853–856.

30. Wendler, D., Emanuel, E., & Lie, R. (2004). The standard of care debate: Can research in developing countries be both ethical and responsive to those countries' health needs? *American Journal of Public Health, 94*(6), 923–928.

31. World Medical Association. (2013). *WMA declaration of Helsinki: Ethical principles for medical research involving human subjects.* Retrieved from https://www.wma.net/policies-post/wma-declaration-of-helsinki-ethical-principles-for-medical-research-involving-human-subjects/

32. U.S. National Institutes of Health. (1947). *The Nuremberg code.* Retrieved from http://history.nih.gov/about/timelines/nuremberg.html

33. Office for Human Research Protections. (1976). *The Belmont report.* Retrieved from https://www.hhs.gov/ohrp/regulations-and-policy/belmont-report/index.html

34. Emanuel, E. J., Wendler, D., & Grady, C. (2000). What makes clinical research ethical? *JAMA, 283*(20), 2701–2711.

35. Millum, J. (2011). Post-trial access to antiretrovirals: Who owes what to whom? *Bioethics, 25*(3), 145–154.

36. Slack, C., Stobie, M., Milford, C., Lindegger, G., Wassenaar, D., Strode, A., & Ijsselmuiden, C. (2005). Provision of HIV treatment in HIV preventive vaccine trials: A developing country perspective. *Social Science & Medicine, 60,* 1197–1208.

37. Glantz, L. H., Annas, G. J., Grodin, M. A., & Mariner, W. K. (1998). Research in developing countries: Taking "benefit" seriously. *Hastings Center Report, 28*(6), 38–42.

38. Council for International Organizations of Medical Sciences. (2002). *International ethical guidelines for biomedical research involving human subjects* (2nd ed.). Geneva, Switzerland: CIOMS.

39. Participants in the 2001 Conference on Ethical Aspects of Research in Developing Countries. (2004). Moral standards for research in developing countries: From "reasonable availability" to "fair benefits." *Hastings Center Report, 34*(3), 17–27.

40. Richardson, H. S., & Belsky, L. (2004). The ancillary-care responsibilities of medical researchers: An ethical framework for thinking about the clinical care that researchers owe their subjects. *Hastings Center Report, 34*(1), 25–33.

41. UNOS. (n.d.). *How we match organs.* Retrieved from https://unos.org/transplant/how-we-match-organs

42. Persad, G., Wertheimer, A., & Emanuel, E. J. (2009). Principles for allocation of scarce medical interventions. *The Lancet, 373*(9661), 423–431.

43. Norheim, O. F. (2016). Ethical priority setting for universal health coverage: Challenges in deciding upon fair distribution of health services. *BMC Medicine, 14,* 75.

44. Sabik, L. S, & Lie, R. (2008). Priority setting in health care: Lessons from the experiences of eight countries. *International Journal for Equity in Health, 7*(4). doi: 10.1186/1475-9276-7-4

45. World Health Organization. (2014). *Making fair choices on the path to universal health coverage.* Geneva, Switzerland: Author.

46. Norheim, O. F., Baltussen, R., Johri, M., Chisholm, D., Nord, E., Brock, D. W., . . . Wikler, D. (2014). Guidance on priority setting in health care (GPS-Health): The inclusion of equity criteria not captured by cost-effectiveness analysis. *Cost Effectiveness and Resource Allocation, 12*(1), 18.

47. Ord, T. (2013). *The moral imperative toward cost-effectiveness in global health.* Retrieved from www.cgdev.org/content/publications/detail/1427016

48. Ottersen, T. (2013). Lifetime QALY prioritarianism in priority setting. *Journal of Medical Ethics, 39,* 175–180.

49. Sharp, D., & Millum, J. (2015). The post-2015 development agenda: Keeping our focus on the worst off. *American Journal of Tropical Medicine and Hygiene, 92*(6), 1087–1089.

50. Asaria, M., Griffin, S., & Cookson, R. (2016). Distributional cost-effectiveness analysis: A tutorial. *Medical Decision Making, 36*(1), 8–19.

51. Segall, S. (2010). *Luck, health, and justice.* Princeton, NJ: Princeton University Press.

52. Brock, D., & Wikler, D. (2006). Ethical issues in research allocation, research and new product development. In D. T. Jamison, J. G. Breman, A. R. Measham, et al. (Eds.), *Disease control priorities in developing countries* (2nd ed., pp. 259–270). New York, NY: Oxford University Press.

53. Cappelen, A. W., & Norheim, O. F. (2005). Responsibility in health care: A liberal egalitarian approach. *Journal of Medial Ethics, 31*(8), 476–480.

54. Rawlins, M. D. (2005). Pharmacopolitics and deliberative democracy. *Clinical Medicine, 5*(5), 471–475.

55. Rawlins, M. D., & Culyer, A. J. (2004). National Institute for Clinical Excellence and its value judgements. *BMJ, 329,* 224–226.

56. National Institute for Health and Clinical Excellence. (n.d.). *What we do.* Retrieved from http://www.nice.org.uk/about/what-we-do

57. Daniels, N., & Sabin, J. E. (2002). *Setting limits fairly: Can we learn to share medical resources?* New York, NY: Oxford University Press.

58. Norges Offentlige Utredninger. (1997). *Priority setting revisited* [Norwegian]. Oslo, Norway: Statens forvaltningstjeneste. Statens trykking.

59. Norheim, O. F. (2005). Rights to specialized health care in Norway: A normative perspective. *Journal of Law, Medicine, & Ethics, 33*(4), 641–649.

60. Norges Offentlige Utredninger. (2014). *Åpent og rettferdig—prioriteringer i helsetjenesten. NOU 2014: 12* [Norwegian]. Oslo, Norway, Author.

61. Ottersen, T., Førde, R., Kakad, M., Kjellevold, A., Melberg, H. O., Moen, A., . . . Norheim, O. F. (2016). A new proposal for priority setting in Norway: Open and fair. *Health Policy, 120*(3), 246–251.

62. World Health Organization. (2014). *Making fair choices on the path to universal health coverage: Final report of the WHO Consultative Group on Equity and Universal Health Coverage.* Geneva, Switzerland: Author.

63. Eyal, N., Hurst, S. A., Norheim, O. F., & Wikler, D. (2013). Inequalities and inequities in health. In N. Eyal, S. A. Hurst, O. F. Norheim, & D. Wikler (Eds.), *Inequalities in health: Concepts, measures, and ethics* (pp. 1–10). New York, NY: Oxford University Press.

64. Lippert-Rasmussen, K., & Eyal, N. (2012). Equality and egalitarianism. In R. Chadwick (Ed.), *Encyclopedia of applied ethics* (pp. 141–148). San Diego, CA: Academic Press.

65. Parfit, D. (1995). *Equality or priority?* Lawrence, KS: University of Kansas.

66. Brock, D.W. (2002). Priority to the worse off in health-care resource prioritization. In R. Rhodes & A. Silvers (Eds.), *Medicine and social justice: Essays on the distribution of health care* (pp. 362–372). New York, NY: Oxford University Press.

67. Daniels, N. (2008). *Just health: Meeting health needs fairly.* Cambridge, UK: Cambridge University Press.

68. Williams, A. (1997). Intergenerational equity: An exploration of the "fair innings" argument. *Health Economics, 6*(2), 117–132.

69. Wolff, J. (2012). *The human right to health.* New York, NY: W. W. Norton & Co., p. 192.

70. Ottersen, T. (2013). Lifetime QALY prioritarianism in priority setting. *Journal of Medical Ethics, 39*, 175–180.

71. The World Bank. (2015). *Disease control priorities.* Washington, DC: Author. Retrieved from http://dcp-3.org/

72. Jamison, D. T., Alwan, A., Mock, C. N., Nugent, R., Watkins, D., Adeyi, O., . . . Zhao, K. (2017). Universal health coverage and intersectoral action for health: Key messages from *Disease control priorities* (3rd Ed.). *The Lancet, 394*(10125), 1108–1120.

73. Rumbold, B., Baker, R., Ferraz, O., Hawkes, S., Krubiner, C., Littlejohns, P., . . . Hunt, P. (2017). Universal health coverage, priority setting, and the human right to health. *The Lancet, 390*(10095), 712–714.

74. Macklin, R. (2004). *Ethics and equity in access to HIV treatment—3 by 5 initiative.* Geneva, Switzerland: World Health Organization.

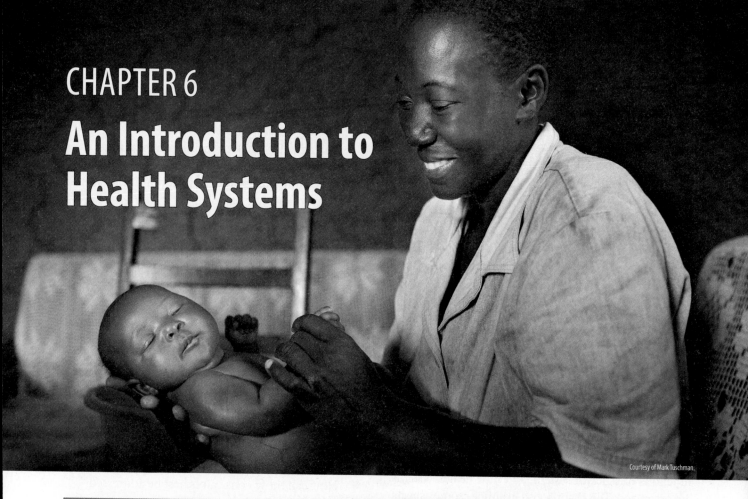

Courtesy of Mark Tuschman.

CHAPTER 6
An Introduction to Health Systems

LEARNING OBJECTIVES

By the end of this chapter, the reader will be able to do the following:

- Describe the main functions of a health system
- Review how health systems are organized
- Discuss selected examples of health systems
- Outline key health system issues and how they might be addressed
- Note the main features of universal health coverage (UHC) and measures that low- and lower middle-income countries can take to achieve UHC over time

▶ Vignettes

Uchenna lived in Nigeria. She had a high fever and suspected she had malaria. Her family took her to the local health clinic. When they arrived at 11:00 in the morning, the clinic was not open. In addition, the community health worker who staffed the clinic was nowhere to be found. Uchenna's family knew that the clinic rarely operated as it was supposed to, so they took her instead to the district hospital. She waited 6 hours to be seen, but was finally examined by a doctor and given medicine for malaria. Happily, she had a full recovery.

Sajitha lived in a small village in northern India. She woke up with a rash that covered the upper half of her body. Her family lived quite far from the government health center and had little faith in the quality of the staff there. Thus, they took Sajitha to a local medical practitioner. He came from the village, was always polite to people, could be paid in cash or in kind, and seemed to have a good record in curing people of their ills. He examined Sajitha, gave her an injection of vitamin B_{12}, and told her she would be fine. In due course, Sajitha did recover, as she would almost certainly have done anyway and without the cost or risk of the medically unnecessary injection.

Melissa lived in the state of Virginia in the United States. She had been unemployed for some time, had little money, and had no health insurance. She also had cancer. She was thousands of dollars in debt to doctors and hospitals for the tests and treatment she had received so far. However, she needed more treatment, more drugs, and additional surgery. Several physicians would not take her as a patient because she had no health insurance. Eventually, after she became sicker, she found a physician who would do the surgery for very low cost. Unfortunately, she was so ill by the time she got the operation that she died a few months later from the cancer.

Cesar lived in San José, the capital of Costa Rica, and had been ill for some time. He visited his local health center, where he was referred to the national hospital because it appeared that he might have cancer. The hospital confirmed the diagnosis of cancer and then treated him with drugs and surgery. He stayed several weeks in the hospital during his recovery. The national health insurance program of Costa Rica covered the cost of Cesar's care. His cancer was detected early and treated appropriately, and 10 years later Cesar remains cancer free.

▶ Introduction

This chapter is about health systems and the aim of attaining **universal health coverage (UHC)**. The chapter introduces the definition of a health system, the functions of a health system, and how health systems are organized. The chapter also examines some aspects of how health systems are financed. The chapter briefly reviews some examples of health systems in different countries before turning to critical issues that health systems face, especially in low- and middle-income countries, and how they might be addressed. The chapter then examines the quest for universal health coverage and how countries might achieve it as rapidly as possible, at least cost, and in the fairest possible ways. The chapter concludes with a series of case studies that are meant to illustrate the key themes of the chapter.

It is especially important to learn about health systems early in one's study of global health for several reasons:

- Health systems are the vehicle through which health services are delivered.
- The health of individuals has an important relationship with the effectiveness of health systems.
- Most countries spend a substantial share of national income on their health system, often with major gaps in effectiveness and efficiency.
- Individuals in many countries spend an important share of their family income on health, and the costs of health care can be immiserating.
- Global forces such as population aging are exerting pressure on health systems.
- Achieving the best population health at the lowest possible cost, in fairly distributed ways, is an important goal for all countries.

- Developing and sustaining an effective and efficient system of universal health coverage can be challenging for resource-poor countries to achieve.

This chapter focuses mainly on health services, which is only one important aspect of a health system. When reading this chapter, it is important to keep in mind the following questions:

- To what extent do different health systems value the "right to health"?
- What is the extent to which universal health coverage has been achieved?
- What is the role in various health systems of individuals, and of the public, private, and nongovernmental organization (NGO) sectors?
- What is the extent to which different actors in the system are engaged in the financing and provision of health services?
- How are different health systems organized and managed?
- What are key issues constraining the effectiveness and efficiency of health systems in different settings?
- How can those constraints best be addressed?

Before reading this chapter, it will be valuable to review some key terms that will be used, which are shown in **TABLE 6-1**.

▶ What Is a Health System?

The World Health Organization (WHO) defines a **health system** as "the sum total of all the organizations, institutions and resources whose primary purpose is to improve health."[1] A related definition of a health system is "the combination of resources, organization, and management that culminate in the delivery of health services to the population."[2]

Another way to put this would be to see the health system as composed of the following[3]:

- Agencies that plan, fund, and regulate health care
- The money that finances health care
- Those who provide preventive health services
- Those who provide clinical services
- Those who provide rehabilitative services
- Those who provide specialized inputs into health care, such as the education of healthcare professionals and the production of drugs and medical devices

It is important to remember when considering health systems that they are composed of a set of interdependent parts. The organizations, money, and

TABLE 6-1 Key Terms

Term	Definition
Health System Organization and Management	
Brain Drain	The migration of health personnel in search of a better standard of living and quality of life, higher salaries, access to advanced technology, and more stable political conditions in different places worldwide.
Governance	The actions and means adopted by a society to organize itself in the promotion and protection of the health of its population.
Health System	The sum of organizations, institutions, and resources whose primary purpose is to improve health.
Primary Care	The provision of first contact, person-focused, ongoing care over time that meets the health-related needs of people, refers (to a hospital) only those problems too uncommon to maintain competence, and coordinates care when people receive services at other levels of care.
Responsiveness to the Expectations of the Population	How the system performs relative to nonhealth aspects, meeting or not meeting a population's expectations of how it should be treated by providers of prevention, care, or nonpersonal services.
Secondary Care	Medical care provided by a specialist or facility upon referral by a primary care physician.
Stewardship	The wide range of functions carried out by governments as they seek to achieve national health policy objectives.
Task Shifting	The rational redistribution of tasks among health workforce teams. Specific tasks are moved, where appropriate, from highly qualified health workers to health workers with shorter training and fewer qualifications in order to make more efficient use of the available human resources for health.
Tertiary Care	Specialized consultative care, usually on referral from primary or secondary medical care personnel, by specialists working in a center that has personnel and facilities for special investigation and treatment.
Financing Health Systems	
Conditional Cash Transfers	Programs that provide cash payments to poor households that meet certain behavioral requirements, generally related to children's health care and education.
Contracting In (Health Services)	One level of government or a public institution contracts with a lower level of government facility, such as a district, a province, or another facility, to deliver services.
Contracting Out (Health Services)	A financing agency (government, insurance entity, or development partner), also known as a "purchaser," provides resources to a nonstate provider (NSP, such as an NGO or private sector firm), also known as a "contractor," to provide a specified set of services, in a specified location, with specified objectives.

(continues)

TABLE 6-1 Key Terms   (continued)

Term	Definition
Financing Health Systems	
Fairness of Financial Contribution	The risks each household faces due to the costs of the health system are distributed according to ability to pay rather than to the risk of illness.
Financial Protection	Financing health care in a way that does not cause people to be denied access to health care or to become impoverished because of their inability to pay for health services.
Out-of-Pocket Health Expenditure	Any direct outlay by households, including gratuities and in-kind payments, to health practitioners and suppliers of pharmaceuticals, therapeutic appliances, and other goods and services whose primary intent is to contribute to the restoration or enhancement of the health status of individuals or population groups. It is a part of private health expenditure.
Private Health Expenditure	The sum of total expenditure on health by private entities, notably commercial insurance, nonprofit institutions, and households, including out-of-pocket health expenditures, patient copayments, private health insurance premiums, and health expenditures by nongovernmental organizations.
Public Health Expenditure	The sum of outlays by government entities to purchase healthcare services and goods, notably by ministries of health and social security agencies. The revenue base may comprise multiple sources, including external funds.
Results-Based Financing	Any program that rewards the delivery of one or more outputs or outcomes by one or more incentives, financial or otherwise, after the principal has verified that the agent has delivered the agreed-upon results.
Right to Health	The highest attainable standard of health is a fundamental right of every human being, including access to timely, acceptable, and affordable health care of appropriate quality.
Risk Pooling	Those who are healthy subsidize those who are sick, and those who are rich subsidize those who are poor.
Total Expenditure on Health	The sum of general government expenditure on health (commonly called public expenditure on health) and private expenditure on health.
Universal Health Coverage	Ensuring that all people can use the promotive, preventive, curative, rehabilitative, and palliative health services they need, of sufficient quality to be effective, while also ensuring that the use of these services does not expose the user to financial hardship.
User Fees	Charges levied at the point of use for any aspect of health services. For example, registration fees, consultation fees, fees for drugs and medical supplies, or charges for any health service rendered, such as outpatient or inpatient care.

people that make up health systems may be public; private, for-profit; or private, not-for-profit.

TABLE 6-2 lists several examples of how health systems relate to achieving key targets of the Sustainable Development Goal (SDG) targets.

▶ The Functions of a Health System

The *World Health Report 2000*, produced by WHO, was about making health systems more effective and

TABLE 6-2 Health Systems and Selected SDG Targets

Goal 3: Ensure healthy lives and promote well-being for all at all ages.

Target 3.1

By 2030, reduce the global maternal mortality ratio to less than 70 per 100,000 live births.

Health systems will have to play a central role in the provision of family planning services, prenatal care, and emergency obstetric care if this goal is to be met.

Target 3.2

By 2030, end preventable deaths of newborns and children under 5 years of age, with all countries aiming to reduce neonatal mortality to at least as low as 12 per 1,000 live births and under-5 mortality to at least as low as 25 per 1,000 live births.

One critical step in reducing neonatal and young child death is to ensure that all births are attended by skilled personnel. Health system efforts to reduce maternal mortality will also reduce neonatal and young child mortality.

Target 3.3

By 2030, end the epidemics of AIDS, tuberculosis, malaria, and neglected tropical diseases and combat hepatitis, waterborne diseases, and other communicable diseases.

To meet this target, health systems will need to play central roles in immunization for TB and hepatitis; early diagnosis and appropriate treatment of malaria; and preventive treatment against neglected tropical diseases. Health promotion, testing, and treatment will also be central to reducing the burden of HIV/AIDS.

Target 3.4

By 2030, reduce by one-third premature mortality from noncommunicable diseases through prevention and treatment and promote mental health and well-being.

Meeting this target will require that health systems play an expanded role in promoting healthy diets and exercise; the diagnosis of high blood pressure and high fasting plasma glucose; and treatment for noncommunicable diseases. Much greater attention will also need to be paid to creating more systemic and community-based approaches to diagnosing and addressing mental health.

Target 3.5

Strengthen the prevention and treatment of substance abuse, including narcotic drug abuse and harmful use of alcohol.

Health systems will need to work closely with others to help governments implement an intersectoral package of efforts to try to deal with these issues. This will have to include, for example, health promotion, taxation, laws on sales to minors, and the measures to treat narcotic drug abuse as a public health problem.

Target 3.6

By 2020, halve the number of global deaths and injuries from road traffic accidents.

Here, too, health systems will need to work with other agencies. These efforts will need to encourage better driver training, safer vehicles and appropriate helmet use, better traffic enforcement, improved road engineering, and better emergency health services for accident victims.

(continues)

TABLE 6-2 Health Systems and Selected SDG Targets	*(continued)*
Goal 3: Ensure healthy lives and promote well-being for all at all ages.	
Target 3.7	
By 2030, ensure universal access to sexual and reproductive healthcare services, including for family planning, information and education, and the integration of reproductive health into national strategies and programs.	
Health systems will need to take the leading role in meeting these aims.	
Target 3.8	
Achieve universal health coverage, including financial risk protection, access to quality essential healthcare services, and access to safe, effective, quality, and affordable essential medicines and vaccines for all.	
This goal represents the essence of the goals of an effective, efficient, and fair health system.	
Target 3.9	
By 2030, substantially reduce the number of deaths and illnesses from hazardous chemicals and air, water, and soil pollution and contamination.	
Achieving this goal will also require that health systems work with others to take the policy measures needed to achieve these targets.	

United Nations Sustainable Development Goals Knowledge Platform. (n.d.). Sustainable Development Goals. © United Nations. Reprinted with the permission of the United Nations.

efficient.[4] That report has been widely read and has been the basis for considerable analysis of the goals of health systems, their functions, how they are organized, and how well they perform.

The *World Health Report 2000* suggests that there are three goals for every health system[5]:

- Good health
- Responsiveness to the expectations of the population
- Fairness of financial contribution

The report further suggests that if these are the goals of health systems, then each health system has four functions to play[5]:

- Provide health services
- Raise money that can be spent on health, referred to as "resource generation"
- Pay for health services, referred to as "financing"
- Govern and regulate the health system, referred to as "stewardship"

Elaborating somewhat on those ideas, one could say that all health systems should do the following[6]:

- Provide access to a comprehensive range of health services, including prevention, diagnosis, treatment, and rehabilitation

- Protect the sick and their families against the financial costs of ill health and disability through the establishment and operation of some type of insurance scheme
- Improve the health of populations through appropriate governance of the health system, regulation of that system, promotion of good health, and the carrying out of key public health functions, such as surveillance, the operation of public health laboratories, and food and drug regulation

WHO has also developed a framework for considering the different parts of health systems and the roles they play in health system performance.[7] This framework includes the six building blocks of a health system, depicted in **FIGURE 6-1**.

WHO defines the health system building blocks in the following ways:

- *Good health services* deliver safe and effective health interventions to people where and when they need them, in an efficient manner.
- A *health workforce* performs well when it has an appropriate number of trained staff, in the right fields, in the places they are needed, and they perform their work as effectively and efficiently as possible.

The WHO health system framework

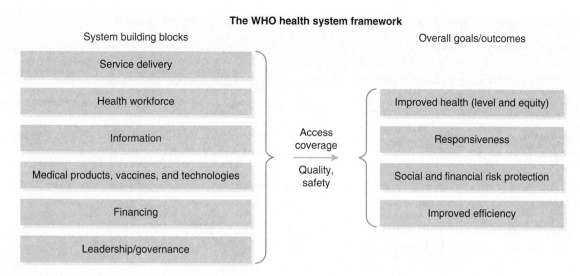

FIGURE 6-1 Health System Building Blocks

Used with permission from World Health Organization (WHO). (2007). *Everybody's business: Strengthening health systems to improve health outcomes: WHO's framework for action.* Geneva, Switzerland: Author.

- A *health information system* functions well when it delivers the information needed for monitoring health status and health system performance in a reliable and timely manner.
- A health system should ideally provide equitable access to *medical products, vaccines,* and *technologies* that are safe, of appropriate quality, have been procured at the best available prices, and can be used in cost-effective ways.
- An effective *health financing system* is one that raises enough money to fund an agreed-upon health program and protect individuals from financial harm due to the costs of health services.
- *Leadership* and *governance* concern the management, oversight, and regulation of health systems in open, participatory, and accountable ways, that seek to maximize health for the money spent.

The WHO framework suggests that if countries combine these building blocks with attention to ensuring quality, safety, and universality of coverage, then the services are most likely to improve health in equitable ways that are responsive to the needs of individuals, protect them from financial risk, and get as much health for the money spent as possible.

▶ How Are Health Services Organized?

Categorizing Health Services

The manner in which health systems are organized is related to the history, politics, and values of individual countries. Countries generally spend more money per capita on health as their incomes rise. At the same

time, as countries become better-off, they usually focus greater attention on trying to ensure universal access to a basic package of health services and universal coverage of health insurance. As they develop economically, they normally pay increasing attention to improving the quality, effectiveness, efficiency, and fairness of their health systems. Of course, one goal of low- and middle-income countries must be to address these aims, to the greatest extent possible, even before their incomes have risen to substantially higher levels.

There is no ideal way of categorizing healthcare systems because they are so varied and so complex. However, **TABLE 6-3** reflects one way of thinking about how health systems are organized.[8] Nonetheless, keep in mind that the table represents a dramatic oversimplification of a very complicated subject.

In Table 6-3, health systems are organized into three types:

- Some systems are organized around a national health service. In this approach, outside of a relatively small private health sector, the government is the sole payer for health care and owns most of the healthcare facilities. This is the case, for example, in the constituent parts of the United Kingdom. In this case, some, but not all, healthcare providers are essentially state employees. It is also worth noting that in Cuba essentially all health services, facilities, and personnel are part of a government-operated healthcare system. Such systems were the case in the former Soviet Union.
- Other systems operate through a national health insurance scheme, such as in Canada, France, Germany, and Japan. These systems, in

TABLE 6-3 Simplified Categorization of Approaches to Selected Health System Issues

	National Health Service	**National Health Insurance**	**Pluralistic**
Health as a Right	Fundamental	Fundamental	Health as a personal good
Ownership of Facilities	Overwhelmingly public	Vast majority public and private, not-for-profit	Public; private, for-profit; and private, not-for-profit
Employment of Providers	The health service and private	Largely private	Largely private
Form of Insurance	Overwhelmingly public insurance linked to the health service	Largely government single payers and firms working with government schemes	Public insurance; private, for-profit insurance, and private, not-for-profit insurance, with substantial numbers lacking insurance
Financing of Insurance	Overwhelmingly tax based	Some based on individual premiums, others based on employee and employer payroll taxes, some are tax based	Taxes, employer and employee insurance contributions, individual purchase of insurance, and out of pocket
Country Examples	United Kingdom, Cuba	France, Canada, Japan, Germany, Brazil, Mexico, Thailand	India, Nigeria, United States

Data from Birn, A.-E., Pillay, Y., & Holtz, T. H. (2009). *Textbook of international health*. New York, NY: Oxford University Press.

principle, offer health insurance to all people for an agreed package of services. People often refer to such systems as having "social health insurance." Some systems include a number of different insurance providers who cover similar or identical service packages. In other systems, insurance is generally provided through a government entity or entities, as in Canada. Many countries in Latin America have health systems that can also best be described as a "social health insurance" model. An increasing number of low- and middle-income countries also have or are developing systems that best fit this description.

■ Pluralistic systems, such as those in the United States, India, and Nigeria, are those systems in which the public sector; private, for-profit sector; and private, not-for-profit sectors all play important roles. In some of these systems, the private sector dominates the system. In all of them it plays a large role.

Table 6-3 first examines the approach of each type of health system to providing universal coverage

of an insured basic package of health services as a "right." Most high-income countries do have such an approach, except the United States. Most middle-income countries have accepted the principle of universal health care as a right, but not all of them have attained it. A number of low-income countries, such as Ghana and Rwanda, are also striving to implement universal health care as a right. However, most low-income countries have not yet moved very far toward implementing such an approach, even if it is sometimes enshrined in their laws.

The table also examines who owns health facilities. In the health systems of most high-income countries, facilities are generally owned by the public sector or by private, not-for-profit organizations. In more pluralistic systems, however, including both the United States and a number of low- and middle-income countries, facilities could be owned by the public sector; private, for-profit sector; or private, not-for-profit sector.

Table 6-3 also examines the manner in which insurance is operated in different healthcare systems. In the United Kingdom model, the public insurance scheme is inherent to and linked with the National

Health Service. In social health insurance models like those in some high-income countries, a number of organizations, which could be for-profit or non-profit, provide insurance for a package of services that is agreed upon with the government. The price of the insurance is generally the same across all insurers. In pluralistic systems, insurance can come in many forms, and many people may lack insurance. The public sector may operate some insurance schemes. In addition, people may purchase insurance from private, for-profit insurers and from private, not-for-profit insurers.

Another dimension for examining health systems is the manner in which they finance their insurance schemes. The constituent parts of the National Health Service of the United Kingdom raise their funds through general taxes. The Canadian government and provincial governments also raise money for their health insurance schemes through general taxes. In some of the other countries with national insurance schemes, such as Germany, however, most of the funding for health insurance comes from payroll tax contributions from employers and employees. In social health insurance schemes, governments usually use funds from general taxes to purchase insurance for those who are not able to make contributions to the insurance scheme, such as the unemployed. In more pluralistic settings, the government may finance health insurance for special groups, such as the disabled, poor, and aged, through general and earmarked taxes. In addition, individuals and employers often jointly contribute to the purchase of insurance. In these systems, significant numbers of people may be without insurance, and such systems usually feature substantial out-of-pocket expenditures.

Most low-income countries have very fragmented and pluralistic health systems that include both public and private providers. Many of these countries have a publicly supported and provided health system and a range of private providers and facilities. They often have publicly organized insurance programs for government employees and relatively small private insurance markets. They may also have a number of community-based insurance schemes. As noted above, an increasing number of low- and lower middle-income countries are also implementing social health insurance schemes. Private out-of-pocket payments represent a substantial share of the costs of health in countries that lack widespread insurance programs.

Many of the middle-income countries, particularly in Latin America, have organized a substantial part of their health system around a social health insurance scheme or schemes. Many of them are also working to better coordinate and expand the schemes

to be universal in coverage, as noted later in this chapter. Private out-of-pocket expenditures are generally lower in these countries than in many other low- and middle-income countries and are concentrated in those individuals who are not covered by the insurance schemes.

It is very important to keep the concepts of *financing* and *provision* of healthcare services conceptually separate and then to examine whether the public or private sector delivers healthcare services in settings with varying financing arrangements. These comments are a very simplified summary of some of these arrangements:

- Cuba is the only country today in which the public sector essentially finances and delivers all healthcare services.
- In many countries in which the private healthcare sector is not well developed, a large share of formal healthcare services will be provided by the public sector. They will generally be financed through a combination of public funds and private payments for some services.
- The National Health Service (or its related entities) finances most healthcare services in the United Kingdom. It owns most healthcare facilities. The National Health Service can purchase services from providers it does not employ.
- There are many countries, such as Canada, Thailand, and New Zealand, in which the private sector delivers services, but the public sector is largely responsible for healthcare financing.
- There are also countries in which most healthcare services are in the private sector, with some of those services being paid for through public financing schemes and some through privately financed schemes. Such countries usually also contain a substantial establishment of government-owned healthcare services, which are generally financed through the public sector and through private payments for services. Such countries would include, for example, the United States and a number of low- and middle-income countries, such as India and Nigeria.

Levels of Care

Health systems are generally organized into three levels of care that are referred to as primary, secondary, and tertiary. In most high-income countries, primary care is provided by a physician who is the first point of contact with the patient. In many systems, nonemergency patients must see a primary care provider before they can be treated by a specialist, and such providers are often referred to as "gatekeepers." Secondary care

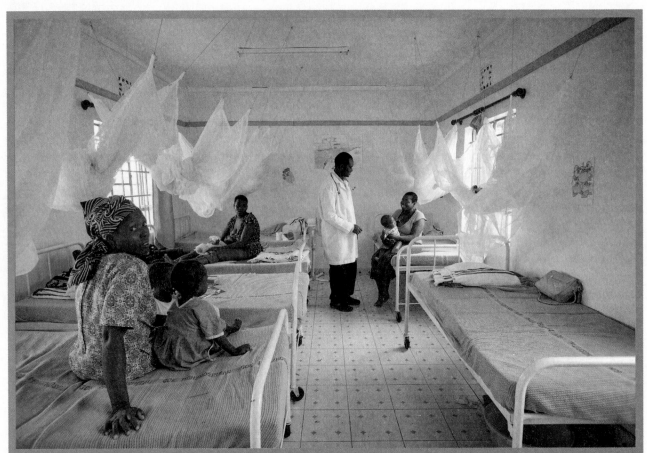

PHOTO 6-1 This is a view of a hospital ward in Uganda. Although the ward seems rudimentary compared to a hospital in high-income countries, this ward appears to be cleaner, better organized, and better equipped than hospital wards in small hospitals in many low- and middle-income countries. How can health systems in these countries raise the money they need to improve facilities such as this one?
Courtesy of Mark Tuschman.

is usually provided by physicians and general hospitals, which are often located in towns and cities. At these physician services and hospitals, one would get treatment for certain illnesses and conditions, including some emergency procedures and other medical procedures and surgery that primary-level providers cannot do. Tertiary care is provided in specialized hospitals that are generally located only in cities. In principle, these specialized hospitals are staffed with a wide range of physicians and can address a diverse array of illnesses with higher-level diagnostics, treatments, and surgeries.

Many low- and middle-income countries have established primary, secondary, and tertiary level facilities by geographic area, depending on the size of the population. These countries, for example, might have a center for primary care for every 5,000 to 10,000 people, a secondary hospital in each district, and a tertiary hospital in large cities. In many low-income countries, medical assistants, nurses, or nurse–midwives would staff the lowest level of the system. The first level at which there might be a trained physician would be in

large primary healthcare centers or district hospitals. **TABLE 6-4** shows the types of services that one might typically expect to find at the different service levels in a low-income country.

Primary Health Care, from Alma-Ata to the Present

One of the historic and core ideas about health systems is the notion of "primary health care," which springs partly from a historic conference in 1978 in Alma-Ata (now called Almaty) in Kazakhstan in the former Soviet Union. This was one of the most important meetings in the history of global health, and it produced the Declaration of Alma-Ata.[9]

To a large extent, the declaration discusses two matters. First, it speaks of health as a human right. These parts of the declaration note the right to health, the unacceptable levels of health disparities, and the need for social and economic development to enable better health, as better health would promote social and economic development. It also speaks about

TABLE 6-4 Selected Examples of Health Services by Level in a Low-Income Country

Primary Level
- Family planning
- Maternal health care
- Well-baby care
- Diagnosis and treatment of simple childhood ailments
- Diagnosis and treatment of simple adult ailments and injuries
- Diagnosis and treatment of malaria and TB

Secondary Level
As above, plus:
- Emergency obstetric care
- Diagnosis and treatment of sick children
- Diagnosis and treatment of adult illness
- Basic surgical services
- Some emergency care

Tertiary Level
As above, plus:
- Treatment of complicated pediatric cases
- Treatment of complicated adult cases
- Specialist surgical services
- Advanced emergency care

people's right to participate in the planning and implementation of health care. In addition, it set a goal of ensuring that there would be "health for all" by the year 2000, such that people would enjoy the health needed to fulfill their capabilities.

The document also outlines the concept of primary health care, which is distinct from primary care. Primary health care is care that is essential and socially acceptable. It must also be based on evidence and made universally available. It addresses the needs of the community and is affordable. It provides preventive, promotive, curative, and rehabilitative services. Personnel who are sensitive to the needs of the community would staff primary healthcare services. The base of such an approach to health would be linked to other levels of health services through a referral system. It would also be linked to action on the key determinants of health, including health education, water supply and sanitation, and nutrition. The implementation of primary health care would promote self-reliance in the community. It would pay particular attention to infectious diseases and other common causes of morbidity and mortality, family planning, immunization, and the provision of essential drugs.

This notion of primary health care that was articulated at Alma-Ata remains an important one. Many countries, at all income levels, continue to work toward a model of primary health care that is effective and efficient and grounded in the community.

In October 2018, in fact, a global conference on primary health care was held in Astana, Kazakhstan, to celebrate the 40th anniversary of the Declaration of Alma-Ata and examine steps in furthering the agenda for primary health care globally. The Astana conference also produced an important declaration.[10] This document reaffirmed the commitment of the global community to the following:

- Health as a human right
- The importance of primary health care as the foundation for achieving better health
- The imperative to take more integrated approaches to enhancing health and to preventive, promotive, and rehabilitative services of appropriate quality
- The need to make greater progress in reducing inequities in health
- The need to focus greater attention on the growing burden of noncommunicable diseases

The declaration further states that efforts to achieve these goals will have to focus on enhancing knowledge and building capacity; strengthening human resources for health; broadening the use of technologies; improving the financing of health, including financial protection; and empowering individuals and communities. The declaration also includes recommendations for periodically reviewing progress toward the achievement of its aims.

It is important to be familiar with the concept of primary health care, its place in history, and efforts underway to achieve it. It is also important not to confuse this concept with primary care, which is the first level of health services.

▶ The Roles of the Public, Private, and NGO Sectors

It is important to distinguish among the different actors that participate in health systems and the different functions they play. The public sector is the first actor in most health systems. The involvement of the public sector could be at the national, state, or municipal level, depending on the country. The public sector is responsible for the stewardship of the system, meaning its governance, policy setting, rule making, and enforcement of rules. The public sector is also responsible for raising the funds for the health system, making decisions about allocating those funds, and establishing approaches to health insurance—often referred to as "financial protection" from health costs. In addition, the public sector is responsible for managing and financing key public health functions, such as setting public health policies, enforcing laws related to health, disease surveillance, and food and drug regulations. In some countries, as noted later, the public sector provides health services through facilities that it owns and operates. However, the public sector can also purchase health services from the private, for-profit or private, not-for-profit sectors.

Although some people believe that health is a right that should not be "for sale," the private, for-profit sector is involved in the provision and financing of health systems in all countries. There are many types of private health service providers that go beyond those involved in formal health services. Especially in low- and middle-income countries, people often buy health services from medicine men, shamans, healers, and bonesetters. There is also a range of nonlicensed medical practitioners who operate in many roles, including as traditional birth attendants. In addition, many people get medical advice from drug vendors that operate small kiosks or mobile drug stores, or from pharmacies and pharmacists. Many people also seek care from practitioners of traditional forms of medicine, such as those in China and India. In high-income countries, too, people make use of a wide range of health practitioners. When considering the ways in which health systems function and how they can be made more effective and efficient, it is essential to keep in mind where people get their health services, the role those providers play in the health system, and how people pay for these different kinds of services.[11]

In some countries, physicians operate in the private, for-profit sector. In some countries, the private sector may also operate health clinics, hospitals, and health services. Private sector health insurers are also involved in health in many countries. The private sector might also operate laboratories. The private, for-profit sector can operate on its own financing, sell selected services to the government, or operate under contract to the government for a range of services. The private, for-profit sector can play a very important role for those people who are willing and able to pay for it, or whose care is paid for by others, such as employers or by insurance.

When one thinks about the private, not-for-profit sector, particularly in low- and middle-income countries, one is often thinking about **nongovernmental organizations (NGOs)**. Broadly defined, an NGO is

A not for-profit, voluntary citizens' group, which is organized on a local, national or international level to address issues in support

TABLE 6-5 Examples of NGOs Involved in Health in Selected Countries

BRAC—Bangladesh
Christian Health Association—Kenya
PHILCAT—Philippines
Profamilia—Dominican Republic
Tilganga Eye Center—Nepal
Treatment Action Campaign—South Africa
Voluntary Health Services—India

of the public good. Some are organized around specific issues, such as human rights.[12]

NGOs may be large or small; may be local, national, or international; and may work in one or many areas of activity. Some examples of NGOs that play important roles in health are given in **TABLE 6-5**.

NGOs are actively involved in many areas of health in a large number of countries. Typical examples would be in community-based efforts to promote better health through health education and improved water supply and sanitation. NGOs are also very involved in carrying out various health services. Like the private, for-profit sector, NGOs can operate with their own financing or they can work under contract to the government, the private sector, or the philanthropic sector.

A critical issue in designing and operating health systems is the roles that ought to be assigned to the public; private, for-profit; private, not-for-profit; and NGO sectors and how those roles should be paid for. It is particularly important to carefully consider the extent to which the public sector should provide services, compared to the extent to which it would be more cost-efficient for the public sector to buy certain services from the private, for-profit; and private, not-for-profit sectors. It could be the case that public sector health services at the primary level are not as effective and efficient as similar services operated by the NGO sector. As Afghanistan engaged in reconstruction after its civil war, for example, it contracted out a package of primary healthcare services to the NGO sector.[13] In Bangladesh, BRAC, a large NGO with a significant presence throughout the country, has carried out a number of nutrition programs under contract to the government of Bangladesh.[14]

▶ Health Sector Expenditure

The health sector is an important part of the economy in all countries and a matter on which governments and private individuals spend a substantial amount of resources. **TABLE 6-6** shows the total current expenditure on health as a share of gross domestic product (GDP) for selected countries. The table also shows

TABLE 6-6 Total Health Expenditure as a Percentage of GDP and Private Expenditure on Health as a Percentage of Total Health Expenditure, Selected Countries, 2015

	Total Health Expenditure as Percentage of GDP	Private Health Expenditure as Percentage of Total Health Expenditure
South Sudan	2.5	64.7
Pakistan	2.7	68.8
Indonesia	3.6	61.2
Nigeria	3.6	73.7
Thailand	3.8	21.1
India	3.9	73.5
Peru	5.3	37.8
China	5.3	40.2
Vietnam	5.7	47.5
Ghana	5.9	39.5
Nepal	6.2	71.4
Dominican Republic	6.2	52.4
Jordan	6.3	36.1
Haiti	6.9	40.5
Costa Rica	8.2	24.0
South Africa	8.2	44.0
Brazil	8.9	56.5
Afghanistan	10.3	78.4
Denmark	10.3	15.9
France	11.1	21.1
United States	16.8	49.6

Data from The World Bank. (n.d.). Data: Current health expenditure (% of GDP). Retrieved from https://data.worldbank.org/indicator/SH.XPD.CHEX.GD.ZS; The World Bank. (n.d.). Data: Domestic private health expenditure (% of current health expenditure). Retrieved from https://data.worldbank.org/indicator/SH.XPD.CHEX.GD.ZS

the share of total expenditure that is from the private sector—including private, for-profit; private, not-for-profit; and out-of-pocket expenditures.

Table 6-6 highlights a number of important points. First, total health expenditure as a share of GDP varies substantially across countries. It is around 2 percent to 4 percent in a number of countries, such as Indonesia, Pakistan, and Nigeria. Several low- and middle-income countries spend about 4 percent to 7 percent of their GDP on health. Most of the higher-income countries spend between 8 percent and 12 percent of their GDP on health. However, the United States spends almost 17 percent of its GDP on health. In addition, there are some countries that spend a substantially higher share of GDP on health than one might anticipate given their income level, including Afghanistan, Costa Rica, Cuba, and Brazil.

We can also see a very wide range in the share of total expenditure on health that is attributable to the private sector. Only about 15 percent to 25 percent of total expenditure on health is private sector expenditure in a number of high-income countries that have substantial health insurance programs, such as Denmark and France. In some other high-income countries, such as Ireland and Israel, private sector expenditure as a share of total expenditure on health is between 35 percent and 40 percent. On the other hand, in a number of low- and lower middle-income countries such as India, Nepal, Nigeria, and Pakistan, which lack widespread coverage with formal insurance, private sector expenditure on health as a share of total expenditure on health is around 60 percent to 75 percent.

In some respects, these data are contrary to what one might expect—or wish: poorer countries, in which people can least afford to spend for health out-of-pocket, have the highest private expenditure. Better-off countries, in which people can most afford out-of-pocket expenditure, spend relatively less out-of-pocket, because their insurance schemes are generally well-developed. Among high-income countries, the United States has the highest proportion of private expenditure as a share of total expenditure.

It is valuable when examining data on health expenditure to compare it to health outcomes. As you will see later in this chapter, Thailand has managed to achieve relatively good health with a relatively low level of expenditures and low out-of-pocket costs. This raises important questions about how other countries might do the same.

TABLE 6-7 shows health expenditure per capita for a sample of countries from across the range of country income groups.

TABLE 6-7 Current Health Expenditure per Capita, Selected Countries, 2015

	Health Expenditure per Capita (US$)
South Sudan	28
Haiti	54
Afghanistan	60
India	63
Ghana	80
Nigeria	97
Indonesia	112
Thailand	217
Jordan	257
Dominican Republic	397
South Africa	471
Brazil	780
Costa Rica	929
France	4,026
United States	9,536

Data from The World Bank. (n.d.). Data: Current health expenditure per capita (current US$). Retrieved from https://data.worldbank.org/indicator/SH.XPD.CHEX.PC.CD

As one can surmise from Table 6-7, countries spend more per capita on health as their incomes rise. This is in part because they have more to spend, they face a burden of noncommunicable diseases, and the popular demands on their systems are significant. In fact, the average per capita spending on health annually is as follows:[15]

Low-income: $37
Lower middle-income: $82
Upper middle-income: $457
High-income: $4,875

Levels of expenditure, both as a share of GDP and per capita, however, need to be considered for their effectiveness and efficiency. What outcomes does a country achieve for its expenditure on health? The goal of a country is not to spend high sums on health; rather, it is to enable the best health of its people at least cost, in doable, sustainable, and fairly distributed ways.

▶ The Quest for Universal Health Coverage

As noted earlier, the goal of a health system should be the attainment of universal health coverage, in as cost-efficient a manner as possible, in fairly distributed ways, with particular attention to the marginalized members of society. According to WHO, the aim of universal health coverage is to ensure "that people get the health services they need, without suffering financial hardship when paying for them."[16] WHO also suggests that this aim reflects three fundamental concerns[16]:

- Fairness of access to services, regardless of people's ability to pay for them
- Appropriate quality of services
- Financial arrangements for services that protect people from suffering financial hardship

In the simplest terms, as noted earlier, universal health coverage can be seen as ensuring that all people have access to an agreed set of at least basic healthcare services either for free or at such low cost that it does not constrain access or cause hardship.

The importance of universal health coverage should be clear, in light of the comments earlier in the text on equity and on the financing of health care. The costs of care are an important barrier to many people seeking health services. In addition, in general, the poorer the country, the larger the share of health costs that are met by out-of-pocket costs—and these costs often lead to temporary or even permanent impoverishment. Moreover, as the Nobel Laureate Amartya Sen has written, universal health coverage is a foundation for better health, and better health is a foundation for social well-being and economic prosperity at the level of individuals, families, and societies.[17]

In principle, the achievement of universal health coverage requires, first of all, a health system that works. Building on the WHO health systems framework described earlier in the chapter, this would ideally mean a system that has the following components[18]:

- Offers an integrated package of basic services for maternal and child health, noncommunicable diseases, and the control of key communicable diseases, such as HIV, TB, malaria, and neglected tropical diseases (NTDs)
- Is affordable
- Offers fair access to essential medicine and medical technologies
- Has a well-trained and highly motivated workforce

Of course, these inputs must also be managed effectively if a health system is to function properly and achieve desired outcomes at a reasonable cost.

Although countries can provide financial protection in a number of ways, most have chosen to do so by pooling risks across part or all of the population through insurance. As countries seek to develop an insurance scheme, they face a number of key questions. The following are among the most fundamental, of course[19]:

- Who should be covered?
- What services should be covered?
- What share of the costs should the insurance scheme pay?

Countries, especially low-income ones, must also wrestle with how they will finance the provision of insurance. Generally, countries may finance insurance through some combination of payroll taxes on employers and employees, general taxes, and contributions from the insured in the form of premiums. The options for financing, however, are constrained in countries that have only a small formal sector of the economy and a large informal sector. In these countries, the people who pay taxes are a relatively small share of the population. In addition, trying to collect contributions from participants who are largely rural and poor can be challenging and costly.[19]

As countries establish programs for UHC, they must also assess the most efficient and effective ways to pay the healthcare providers from whom the insurance system will buy services. Should this be on a fee-for-service basis, a fixed fee per person covered per year (capitation), paying for the achievement of certain health goals, or the successful completion of certain procedures?[19]

It will also be important for some countries, as they seek to achieve universal health care, to increase the financial resources available to the health sector. Although this will not happen quickly, many countries do have the capacity to increase the efficiency of tax collection, orient more public resources toward health, and improve the effectiveness and efficiency of existing healthcare expenditure.[19]

Countries must also wrestle with questions concerning how they will organize their risk-pooling—

insurance—arrangements. Should they have a single national insurance scheme, many schemes operated by different groups, or many schemes based on different kinds of beneficiaries?[19]

The operation of insurance schemes also requires careful attention to deciding how those schemes will finance the purchase of services. Should insurance cover the costs of public sector services, private sector services, or both? Will it be fair, effective, or efficient if the public sector continues to offer free or nearly free but often low-quality services to mostly poor people, whereas other people are able to purchase insurance and buy services that are often of higher quality in the private sector?[19,20]

For many years, there was enormous skepticism about the possibility that some countries, especially low-income ones, could achieve universal health coverage. Today, however, there is a global movement around ensuring that all countries achieve UHC as rapidly as possible. In fact, there have been a number of countries that have made important progress toward achieving UHC, including some countries that continue to have very low per capita income. In the last decade or so, Mexico has made important progress toward achieving universal health coverage through a health reform effort that has been the subject of substantial study. Ghana, Nigeria, and Rwanda have also moved in important ways toward UHC. South Korea, Singapore, and Taiwan have had universal health coverage for some time. In addition, Thailand and the Philippines have made important progress toward UHC over the last decade, and other countries, such as China, Indonesia, and Vietnam, are now also moving toward UHC. Countries in South Asia are also making progress toward UHC, such as India's implementation of an insurance program for the poor.[20-24]

TABLE 6-8 shows one framework for considering where countries are on the path toward UHC.

Moving toward UHC is a highly political matter, and achieving it will not come quickly or easily in most settings. This suggests that many countries may

TABLE 6-8 Framework for Progress Toward Universal Health Coverage

	Group 1	Group 2	Group 3	Group 4
Status of UHC policies and programs	Agenda setting: piloting new programs and developing new systems	Initial programs and systems in place, implementation in progress; need for further systems development and capacity building to address remaining uncovered population	Strong political leadership and citizen demand lead to new investments and UHC policy reforms; systems and programs develop to meet new demands	Mature systems and programs: adaptive systems enable continuous adjustments to meet changing demands
Status of health coverage	Low population coverage at the early stage of UHC	Significant share of population gains access to services with financial protection but population coverage is not yet universal and coverage gaps in access to services and financial protection remain	Universal population coverage achieved but countries are focusing on improving financial protection and quality of services	Universal coverage sustained with comprehensive access to health services and effective financial protection
Countries	Bangladesh Ethiopia	Ghana Indonesia Peru Vietnam	Brazil Thailand Turkey	France Japan

wish to take a phased approach, such as Mexico did, by incrementally increasing the coverage of both more people and more services.[23] At the same time, as countries move forward, they will want to take account of the accumulating body of evidence about what works in efforts to achieve UHC. It will also be essential to focus on the achievement of the goals of UHC through research and rigorous data collection on the impacts and outcomes of UHC. It appears that the establishment of UHC does increase the use of health services. However, in the absence of other measures to improve the quality of services, it is clear that access alone will not lead to better health at a reasonable cost.[20] Additional comments on the importance of the quality of services are offered later in the chapter.

▶ Selected Examples of Health Systems

The section that follows provides very brief comments on the main features of a small number of health systems. It is important to note the common approaches of some of the countries to selected issues. However, it is also important to remember that each country has its own health system, built from its unique historical experience.

High-Income Countries

Germany

Germany was the first country in the world to have a universal program of health insurance, which started in the 1880s.[25] The federal and state governments have established a legal environment for health services but are not engaged in the direct provision of medical services. The German system is based on achieving universal health coverage on the basis of four principles[26]:

- Compulsory insurance: Anyone earning under a certain amount must have statutory health insurance (SHI). Others can get private health insurance (PHI).
- Funding through insurance premiums: Most of the funding for health insurance is raised through premiums paid by employers and employees. Tax funding is generally used as a supplement to these funds to help pay for those unable to contribute.
- Solidarity: In Germany, the health system is based, in principle, on the idea that the system must cover all people and cross-subsidize as

appropriate—for example, from the young and healthy to the older and less healthy.
- Self-governance: The German health system is founded on the idea that it is primarily governed by "sickness funds" and organizations of doctors and hospitals. This is to be done under the policy direction of a national body, The Joint Committee, that represents all of the key actors in the system.

The Joint Committee sets the regulations on the minimum package of services that all insurance firms must offer. The Joint Committee is supported by foundations that oversee the cost-effectiveness of drugs and the quality of care. The states own most university hospitals. About half of the hospitals are public, a third are private and not-for-profit, and the remainder are for-profit. States determine hospital capacity. Regulations on ambulatory care are set by The Joint Committee.[27]

There are two main insurance schemes: SHI and PHI. About 85 percent of the population is covered by SHI, and about 11 percent is covered by PHI. The remainder, such as the military, are covered by their own health plans. Those people earning less than 4,800 Euros per month are required to be covered by statutory health insurance. Others, including the self-employed and those earning more than this amount, may opt for a voluntary private health insurance scheme. These schemes also cover the dependents of the enrolled person.[28]

The insurance carriers for the mandatory insurance in Germany are 110 "sickness funds." These are not-for-profit insurance funds that are financed by contributions from employers and employees. In 2017, employees and pensioners paid 14.7 percent of their wages or pension up to an agreed limit, which was shared equally with the employer.[28] Various arrangements are made to pay for the health insurance contributions for people who are disabled or unemployed. Those participating in the statutory health insurance scheme have small copayments for certain medicines, inpatient hospital stays, and medical aides. The private health insurance schemes are underwritten by 42 companies, of which most are for-profit companies. Employers also make a contribution to these schemes.[27]

The statutory health insurance package of benefits covers a wide range of medical, dental, and eye care services. It also covers prescription medicines, medical aids, and physical therapy. The package includes a range of preventive services, such as well-baby checkups, immunizations, some cancer screenings, and dental checkups.[29] The package of services offered by the private insurance scheme is broader than that offered by the statutory health insurance scheme.[28,29]

In the German healthcare system, sickness funds contract physician associations to provide care to people who do not require hospitalization. Most physicians work in their own private practices. The sickness funds also make arrangements for hospital services for the people they insure by entering into agreements with hospitals about how many services they will be able to render at a certain price that the sickness fund will pay. Generally, individuals can choose the general practitioner, specialist, or hospital that they want to use.[29]

In 2015, Germany spent about 11 percent of its GDP on health. This was at the high end of expenditure for European countries, surpassed only by Switzerland.[15] About 13 percent of total health expenditure in Germany is private.[27] Overall, the German healthcare system is one that has a relatively expansive package of benefits, with relatively low out-of-pocket costs. Given an aging population and the split of the insurance schemes, Germany will wrestle in the coming years with trying to keep the costs of the system under control while also ensuring the insurance schemes do not create unacceptable disparities in access to services or health outcomes.[27]

England

The United Kingdom established a system of universal healthcare coverage in 1946, following World War II.[25] It aims to provide a comprehensive set of health services to all people in the United Kingdom, without regard to their ability to pay for such services, and is meant to be free at the point of care. The National Health Service (NHS) England is that part of the health system that is responsible for health services in England.

NHS England has a constitution that lays out the rights and responsibilities of the different actors involved in the health system. The Department of Health and the Secretary of State oversee the NHS, which is responsible for the day-to-day operation of the healthcare system. The NHS works closely with institutions responsible for encouraging the system to be cost-effective and for providing high-quality care, such as the Care Quality Commission, NHS Improvement, and the National Institute of Clinical Effectiveness. NHS England oversees the NHS budget. The overwhelming majority of hospital beds are public. Publicly owned hospitals are established as either "NHS trusts" or "foundation trusts." These hospitals are supported by the Care Quality Commission and NHS Improvement.[30,31]

The system includes 195 Clinical Commissioning Groups. They are clinically led bodies established by statute under the NHS. They are responsible for planning and purchasing healthcare services in their local areas.[32] Most general practitioners work as private independent contractors to the NHS. Specialist physicians overwhelmingly work in hospitals for the NHS. In principle, people can choose their general practitioners, who play a gatekeeping role in the NHS system.[33] Increasingly, the NHS has created an internal market for services, and NHS funds can be used to purchase funds from NHS or private providers.[32]

The NHS is universal in coverage. The NHS covers a wide range of preventive and therapeutic services, mental health care, physical therapy, some palliative care, and dental and eye care. People can buy supplementary voluntary private insurance if they would like, which they mostly use to reduce waiting times for services that are not urgent or to seek what they believe to be higher quality care. About 11 percent of the population has such insurance.[31,33]

Three-quarters of NHS funding comes from general taxes, and the rest mostly from a payroll tax. The system requires minimal copayments for drugs prescribed outside a hospital and for dental services. The system offers a safety net of exemptions from copayments for certain groups who may be financially unable to make the required payments.[33]

The United Kingdom as a whole spent close to 10 percent of its GDP on health in 2015. This is below what France, Germany, Sweden, and Switzerland spend on health, but is similar to expenditure on health as a share of GDP in Denmark and The Netherlands.[15] About 83 percent of all expenditure on health in the United Kingdom is public, which is higher than the average for high-income countries.[34]

The United States

The United States has a complex and very fragmented healthcare system. It is the only high-income country whose health system is not based on the premise that health is a human right. It is also the only high-income country that does not have universal health coverage. In addition, the United States spends a higher percentage of GDP on health than any other high-income country, almost 17 percent in 2015. In fact, this was almost 50 percent higher than the country with the next highest expenditure, Switzerland.[15] The United States also spends more on health per capita than any other country.[35] Yet life expectancy in the United States is ranked near the bottom of all high-income countries.[36]

The federal government oversees and operates health programs for some special groups, such as the military medical services, the health services under the Department of Veterans Affairs, and the Indian Health Service for Native Americans. The federal government also oversees, works with state governments on, and helps to fund a number of other programs such as Medicaid, which provides insurance to the indigent; Medicare, which provides insurance to the elderly; and the Children's Health Insurance Program, for uninsured children whose modest family incomes are too high to be eligible for Medicaid.[37]

The majority of care in the United States is provided in the private sector. The overwhelming majority of U.S. physicians work as private practitioners, either on their own or in group practices. Patients are usually free to choose the doctor or hospital they wish to use, unless they are part of an insurance plan that limits providers to those who are preferred. In most cases, primary care physicians in the United States are not formally charged with being gatekeepers, although some insurance plans do require referral from a primary care physician. Most payments to physicians are on a fee-for-service basis. There are some public hospitals, but most hospitals are private. Private hospitals can be not-for-profit or for-profit. About 70 percent of all hospital beds in the United States are not-for-profit, about 15 percent are public, and about 15 percent are for-profit.[37]

In 2015, about 67 percent of the population was covered by private voluntary insurance, which could be from a not-for-profit or a for-profit organization. Public programs, such as the those noted earlier, covered about 37 percent of the population. In early 2016, almost 9 percent of the population did not have health insurance.[37]

There is no standard package of insurance benefits in the United States, although the health reform of 2010, if fully implemented, would move the United States closer to ensuring that those who have health insurance are covered for at least a minimum package of services. However, political issues have constrained the implementation of that reform. Thus, today, different insurers continue to offer different insurance packages, with substantial variation in what is covered and what copayments and deductibles apply. The typical policy, however, covers selected physicians' services and hospitalization. Many policies and Medicare also cover prescription drugs, and some cover dental and eye care, which some people can also purchase separately.[38]

Almost half of all healthcare expenditure in the United States is public. Slightly more than half of all expenditure is private. Those who get insurance through their employer generally share the cost of the insurance with their employer, through tax-exempt premiums.[37] It was estimated in 2016 that about 13 percent of all healthcare expenditure, or almost $1,400 per capita, was out-of-pocket payments.[39]

Upper Middle-Income Countries
Costa Rica[40–42]

Costa Rica has had a commitment to universal health coverage for many years. Costa Rica is also a country that is well-known for having achieved high levels of health outcomes even before it had achieved a relatively high national income per capita.

The health system of Costa Rica resembles the health systems of many Latin American countries in some ways; it also resembles the National Health Service of the United Kingdom. The most important part of the health system is the Costa Rican Social Security Administration (Caja Costaricense de Seguro Social—CCSS). The CCSS is both a financier and a provider of health services.

The CCSS has three main parts: illness and maternal health; disability, old age, and death; and the noncontributive regime. People who work in the formal sector of the economy are obliged to participate in the CCSS. Informal sector workers may also join the CCSS, with fees that depend on their income. More than 90 percent of the financing of the CCSS comes from employer and employee taxes, with the remainder coming from government. The government has a mechanism, related to the noncontributive regime, to cover the costs of insurance of those unable to pay into the system. Participants in the CCSS receive most services for free, but do have copayments for some services.

Costa Rica has established a national system of primary care that is community oriented. The government has divided the country into health regions and 103 health areas, each of which has 30,000 to 60,000 people. The basic unit of health coverage is 1,094 "health teams for integrated primary care" (EBAIS), which each serve 3,500 to 4,000 people.[40]

The CCSS insures 95 percent of the people in Costa Rica. It also guarantees emergency services for all people, even if they are not insured. About 15 percent of all services are provided in the private sector under CCSS financing. Less than 1 percent of the population participates in voluntary private insurance. The CCSS has a standard benefits package for primary care and a national drug list. In 2015, Costa Rica spent about 8 percent of its GDP on health, which is lower than most high-income countries.[15] Private expenditure as a share of total health expenditure in 2015 was about 24 percent. This would be among the lowest in Latin America but toward the higher end of private expenditure compared to high-income countries.[43]

Compared to many countries, Costa Rica achieves quite good outcomes from its health system for relatively low costs and low out-of-pocket expenditures. However, Costa Rica will face a number of health system challenges in the future. Among the most important will be how to sustain financing that is largely employer-based when the population is aging and a smaller share of the population will be engaged in formal sector employment.

Lower Middle-Income Countries

India[44,45]

The health system in India bears many resemblances to the health system in the United States. India's health system is highly fragmented, with a range of public and private financiers and providers. In addition, India is a federal system; health is largely under state jurisdiction, but the federal government nevertheless plays an important role in many aspects of the system. This federal role focuses in principle on public goods such as family planning and the control of communicable diseases. India has only recently made a commitment to moving toward universal health coverage.

One part of the Indian healthcare system is a publicly financed and provided set of healthcare services. For this, India has a tiered network of health services in the public sector. At the lowest level is a health subcenter, which serves 3,000 to 5,000 people, depending on whether it is in a difficult geographic area or serves tribal people. Subcenters are staffed by at least one auxiliary nurse–midwife or female health worker and one male multipurpose worker. India has almost 150,000 subcenters. Primary health centers (PHCs) serve 20,000 to 30,000 people. The primary healthcare centers are the referral point for 6 subcenters and have 6 patient beds. The PHCs are staffed with a physician, a nurse, a female multipurpose worker, a health educator, a laboratory technician, and assistant-level staff. India has almost 25,000 primary healthcare centers. Community health centers (CHC) serve 80,000 to 120,000 people and are staffed with a physician, a pediatrician, a gynecologist, and a surgeon, as well as a number of paramedical staff. Each operates as a small hospital with 30 beds and a laboratory and x-ray facilities. India has about 4,500 CHCs.

At the top of the Indian publicly provided healthcare system are hospitals of varying sizes and complexities. These hospitals are at the district, regional, and national levels, with the latter able to treat very complicated cases with a full range of staff.

In addition to having an extensive array of public facilities, India also has a very large private healthcare sector. This ranges from unlicensed medical practitioners, to practitioners of Indian systems of medicine, to very well-trained practitioners of allopathic medicine. In addition, there is an equally wide variety of private healthcare facilities, from simple nursing homes to the most sophisticated hospitals. The private sector treats almost 80 percent of outpatients and 60 percent of inpatients. Estimates suggest that about 40 percent of all care in the private sector is provided by unqualified practitioners.

In principle, services provided by the public sector are free or have small copayments. In practice, however, there are major issues of accessing public sector services of appropriate quality. Many facilities, especially hospitals and their outpatient clinics, are overwhelmed with patients; have inadequate budgets, materials, supplies, and equipment; and offer services of varied quality. These issues encourage people to seek care in the private sector. Private hospitals, for example, provide about 6 percent of outpatient care and 80 percent of inpatient care. The costs of health care are among the leading causes of falling into poverty in India.

India is just beginning to develop more extensive approaches to insurance. It previously had schemes for the military and government workers. In addition, many people in formal private employment bought private insurance. India, however, more recently developed a scheme, Rashtriya Swasthya Bima Yojana (RSBY), which means "National Health Insurance Program" in Hindi and is intended to insure people living below the poverty line. In 2015–2016, more than 40 million families enrolled in this program. India also established a National Health Mission, which recruited almost 1 million community-based health promoters. Most recently, India has announced a larger initiative for insuring more of its poorer people, with higher levels of insurance coverage, for a wide range of services.[46]

India has historically spent very small amounts of public funds on health, compared even to low-income countries. In 2015, for example, India's total expenditure on health was just under 4 percent of GDP. However, private expenditure on health was almost 75 percent of total expenditure. Thus, one challenge for India to achieve universal health coverage of appropriate quality will be to substantially raise public expenditure on health. Other key challenges will be to reduce the fragmentation of the health system, enhance the quality of care, improve the distribution of qualified healthcare providers, and expand insurance coverage.

Ghana

The health system in Ghana is moving from one that was overwhelmingly dependent on public funding and publicly provided services to a system based on everyone having access to insurance that allows them to purchase services from a variety of providers. Ghana is among the first African countries to commit to universal coverage, and, as a result, it is important to learn from Ghana's experience.[47]

Until recently Ghana's health system was largely publicly financed and provided. Like the foundation of the Indian system and the systems in many other low- and middle-income countries, Ghana has had a public system that is a pyramid of services at different levels, following population-based norms. In addition to the public system, Ghana has had services provided by NGOs, other nonprofits, and the for-profit private sector.[48]

Although the government largely financed the public system, it also required that those using the system pay user fees for the services they received. In Ghana, this became known as the "cash and carry system," which has been shown to be an important constraint to the demand for and use of health services by the poor.[48]

The health system was a major issue in the 2000 presidential elections in Ghana, and the winning candidate pledged to eliminate the "cash and carry" system. Therefore, Ghana established the National Health Insurance System (NHIS) in 2003, which was financed by a value-added tax. The NHIS is meant to be universal in coverage. Prior to the launching of the NHIS, less than 1 percent of the population was insured.[48]

The NHIS is financed largely by government, which raises most of the money for the scheme through a value-added tax. In addition, those in formal employment have a mandatory contribution to the scheme. Those who are not formally employed pay premiums to the scheme, in accordance with their ability to pay. The latest estimates suggest that the NHIS covers about 40 percent of all of the eligible families in Ghana.[49]

In 2015, Ghana devoted almost 6 percent of its GDP to health.[15] That same year, about 40 percent of total expenditure on health was private expenditure. This is a dramatic change from the 70 percent of total expenditure on health that was private in 2000.[43]

Despite important progress in improving access to health services of appropriate quality, the financing of health services, and financial protection, Ghana faces a number of critical issues as it further seeks to achieve universal health coverage. First, Ghana needs to ensure that a larger share of the population enrolls in NHIS, especially the more marginalized members of society. There are still large gaps in enrollment across different segments of Ghana's population. Second, while Ghana has some centers of excellence in the health sector, it also faces substantial problems of quality. Some of these relate to continuing shortages of competent healthcare workers at all levels. Third, universalizing the NHIS will require improvements in the effectiveness, efficiency, and management of the NHIS itself, as well as more public funding.[49,50] It will also require substantial amounts of additional financing, which it will almost certainly have to raise through taxation, because a large share of the population will not be able to bear the cost of premiums for some time.

▶ Key Health Sector Issues

When we consider the extent to which various health systems meet the criteria WHO has set for measuring health system performance, it is clear that some health systems produce better outcomes than others. Health systems in high-income countries, for example, produce better results than the systems in low-income countries. The systems in high-income countries will be better organized and managed, have greater financial resources, and have better trained and more abundant human resources for health. Almost all high-income countries have also had universal health coverage for many years, with substantial amounts of financial protection linked to it. By contrast, the health systems of the poorest countries will lack universal coverage and have limited financial protection. They will also be severely lacking in financial and human resources and will tend to be not very well organized and managed. They will also suffer substantial issues of the quality of care.

Nonetheless, even countries that are resource poor can achieve good health outcomes if they are committed to the health of their people, make cost-efficient and fair choices about the policies that should lead the health sector, manage that sector with rigor, and also invest in addressing the determinants of health in effective and efficient ways. A number of countries, such as Costa Rica, as noted earlier, Cuba, and China, for example, were able to substantially enhance the health of their people, even when they had relatively low levels of income. Indeed, the goal of all resource-poor countries, in principle, is to achieve greater gains in health than would be expected for a country at their income level.

As we explore health systems in greater detail, it is clear that all systems wrestle with a variety of challenges and constraints. Some of the most important challenges are related to changing epidemiologic and demographic patterns, governance of the health sector, having an appropriate number and placement of healthcare personnel, the financing of health care, and the role of the private sector in the overall health system. Other important issues include the quality of care, how to finance services so that people are protected from their costs, and the extent to which people have access to and get covered by the most appropriate health services for their needs. As discussed earlier, the health systems in many countries also face critical issues of equity and financial protection. Finally, health systems face a number of problems concerning their design and the overall achievement of health outcomes, some of which have been the subject of health sector reform efforts and some of which will relate to the growing need to address noncommunicable diseases. These themes are explored briefly here.

Demographic and Epidemiologic Change

Demographic and epidemiologic changes raise critical challenges for the health systems of most countries. Except in countries in conflict, people are living longer. As they do so, societies face higher burdens of noncommunicable diseases. Many of these conditions are chronic, and the cost of treating them is high compared to acute bouts of communicable diseases or conditions that occur at younger ages. As a result, relatively poor countries, with few resources to spend on health and weak institutions to address health issues, face a triple burden of disease simultaneously—the burdens of noncommunicable disease, communicable disease, and injuries.[51]

Stewardship

The quality of governance is an important determinant of outcomes in the health sector, as well as in many other sectors. In high-income countries, the health sector will tend to be governed in relatively open and transparent ways. These countries will usually have clear rules and regulations for the management and operation of the health sector, and high-income countries can enforce those regulations. There is usually relatively little corruption in the health sectors of high-income countries.

Unfortunately, however, there are major problems of governance in many low- and middle-income countries. These problems often affect the performance of the healthcare system and penalize poor people more than other people, because the poor have fewer choices about where they can go for their health care and have less power in dealing with healthcare personnel. Governance in these settings will tend to be weak across most sectors, and governments in low- and middle-income countries are often unable to enforce health sector rules and regulations. This may be especially

true with respect to the inability of the health sector to oversee the work of the private healthcare sector.[52]

The management of human resource matters is often especially weak, with staff sometimes being recruited by virtue of their connections, rather than their merit or fit with existing hiring rules. In addition, some staff that are recruited have to pay off the people who are recruiting them by giving them an upfront payment for their post or a percentage of their salary each month. Healthcare personnel are often absent from their jobs without sanction. When health services procure goods or construct facilities, they sometimes do not get the best prices available, often because they engage in corrupt practices with the providers of those goods or because they do not have the capacity to engage in sound procurement practices. In many countries, healthcare personnel arrange to get payments from patients for services that are intended to be free.[52]

Human Resource Issues

The most severe human resource issues in better-off countries will tend to be imbalances in the number of certain types of healthcare personnel. Some countries do not produce enough physicians. Others do not produce enough nurses, and they tend to make up these shortages through the recruitment of healthcare personnel from other countries, particularly low- and middle-income countries. This contributes to the problem of "brain drain" in the healthcare sector of low- and middle-income countries.[53]

The human resource issues in many low-income countries are considerable. The very poorest countries, especially in sub-Saharan Africa, will not have enough healthcare personnel to operate a health system effectively. They will face shortages of physicians, midwives, nurses, and laboratory and other technicians. Despite their needs for better stewardship, they will also face important gaps in qualified health service managers, both clinical and nonclinical. In addition, the quality of training, knowledge, and skills of many of their healthcare staff will be deficient. Those staff who are well-trained will usually be clustered in major cities, and there are often important shortages of appropriately trained healthcare personnel everywhere else in the country, especially in rural and poor areas. Public sector salaries of staff may be very low compared to salaries in the private sector, and they will almost certainly be very low compared to comparable positions overseas. As a result, many staff lack the incentive to perform their jobs properly, often practice in both the private and public sectors even if this is not allowed, and are

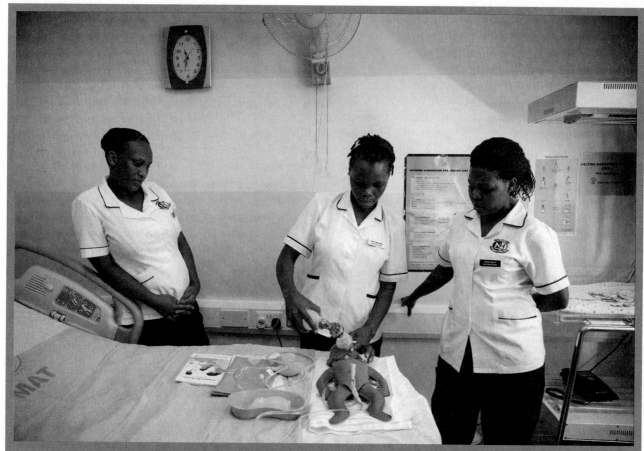

PHOTO 6-2 This photo shows the training of nurses in Uganda in a simulation exercise. There is a critical shortage of key healthcare personnel in many low- and middle-income countries. In addition, they are often trained in substandard ways and lack the knowledge they need to do their job to an appropriate level of quality. What measures can resource-scarce nations take to increase the number of healthcare workers being trained and the quality of their training?
Courtesy of Mark Tuschman.

frequently absent from work. In the face of poor salaries and working conditions in which they often lack the facilities, equipment, and materials needed to perform their work well, many healthcare personnel move to other countries, particularly higher-income countries, in which salaries and working conditions are much better.[53,54]

Quality of Care

The United States Institute of Medicine (IOM) defines quality as "the degree to which health services for individuals and populations increase the likelihood of desired health outcomes and are consistent with current professional knowledge."[55(p3)] According to the IOM approach, the following are qualities health services need to have[55]:

- Safe
- Effective
- Patient centered
- Timely
- Efficient
- Equitable

There is good evidence from low-, middle-, and high-income countries that many health systems suffer from important problems of quality, and that quality varies considerably within health systems. Studies in the United States, for example, showed that "physicians complied with evidence based guidelines for at least 80 percent of patients in only 8 of 306 U.S. hospital regions."[56(p1295)] In a study in Papua New Guinea, a low-income country with rampant malaria, only 24 percent of health workers could indicate the correct treatment for malaria.[57] In a similar study in Pakistan, only 35 percent of the health workers could indicate the proper treatment for a certain type of diarrhea.[58] In another study of clinical practices in seven low- and middle-income countries, 76 percent of medical cases were not adequately diagnosed, treated, or monitored, and inappropriate treatment with antibiotics, fluids, feeding, or oxygen occurred for 61 percent of the patients.[59]

A study that further reflects the depth of quality issues was published in 2015. This examined how health practitioners in rural India treat childhood diarrhea and pneumonia. This was assessed by seeing how the practitioners responded both to descriptive scenarios and to standardized patients. Only 3.5 percent of those given a diarrhea scenario offered oral rehydration for diarrhea, despite this being the standard of care and it being available locally. None of those given a standard patient offered the correct care for diarrhea, but 13 percent of them offered the correct treatment for pneumonia. Seventy-two percent of those given the standard patient prescribed potentially harmful treatments for diarrhea.[60]

In fact, the global health community is now examining and acting on quality issues in health with much greater attention and rigor than ever before. One very important recent study suggested, for example, that almost 10 percent of all deaths worldwide could have been prevented with appropriate quality health care.[61] A recent survey of facilities for primary health care suggested major gaps in the quality of care.[62] Moreover, WHO suggests that the quality of care in most countries, but especially in low- and middle-income countries, is suboptimal. In a recent report on quality of care, WHO noted the following[63]:

- Practitioners followed clinical practice guidelines less than 50 percent of the time in eight low- and middle-income countries, resulting in low-quality antenatal and child care and deficient family planning.
- The Service Delivery Indicators initiative in seven low- and middle-income countries showed very low scores and significant variation in provider absenteeism, daily productivity, diagnostic accuracy, and adherence to clinical guidelines.
- A systematic review of 80 studies showed that suboptimal clinical practice is common in both private and public primary healthcare facilities in several low- and middle-income countries.
- Organization for Economic Cooperation and Development (OECD) data showed that even in the high- and middle-income countries, 19 percent to 53 percent of women ages 50 to 69 years did not receive mammography screening, and that 27 percent to 73 percent of older adults did not receive influenza vaccination.

There are many causes of poor-quality health services in low- and middle-income countries, including poor management, a lack of financial resources, poorly trained and inappropriately deployed staff, a failure of staff to do their work as intended, and unempowered patients, as discussed throughout this chapter. Many

health systems also provide very little supervision of healthcare personnel and have only weak systems for monitoring the performance of their health system.[56]

It is important to remember that in the health sector, poor-quality services are not just a waste of money. Rather, in this sector, as in some others, there is a direct link between the poor quality of services and people's health and well being. Thus, it is essential that all health systems seek to achieve high-quality health services.

The Financing of Health Systems

The health systems in many countries battle continuously for sufficient financing to meet their highest priorities in effective and efficient ways. Many countries, especially better-off ones, face issues of rising costs because of aging populations and the ever-increasing demands for the use of new technologies and new drugs. In addition, all health systems ration health services to some extent. In many high-income countries, a critical issue is how to find the funding that is needed, even with increased efficiency, to reduce the waiting times for certain medical procedures that are financed through the national insurance program. This has been a highlight of the healthcare debates in the United Kingdom and Canada, for example. A few of the high-income countries, such as Switzerland and the United States, also face important questions about the share of their total GDP that they are devoting to health and the implications of this for the rest of the economy.

As one might expect, the financing issue in most low- and middle-income countries often revolves around the absolute lack of public sector financial resources for health. It is true that many countries do not spend effectively or efficiently the financial resources that they do have for health. However, it is also true that many countries do not provide the health sector with the public funds needed to ensure that an appropriate basic package of health services is available to all people regardless of their ability to pay.

Financial Protection

The capacity of people to pay for health services *is* a barrier to their access to health care, and catastrophic health costs impoverish people in many settings. In most high-income countries, this is not a significant problem because they have social health insurance schemes and essentially offer health insurance to all of their people. However, the lack of financial protection is a common problem in poorer countries. Studies in India have shown, for example, that expenditure on health is a leading cause of families falling below the poverty line and a major cause of families selling assets to pay their bills for health care.[64] Although the evidence is of poor quality and mixed, some studies have shown a decline in the use of tuberculosis medicines and hospital deliveries of babies when charges were levied on these services.[65]

Access and Equity

Health disparities are an important feature of many health systems. It is always important to assess health status, the provision of health services, and health outcomes by sex, age, ethnicity, income, education, and location. In low- and middle-income countries, disparities in access to services and in equity are often reflected in the following ways, among others:

- A lack of coverage of basic health services in areas where poor, rural, and minority people live
- Service coverage with a lower level of inputs in the areas previously noted, compared to other areas, such as fewer trained personnel and less equipment and drugs
- Service coverage that varies, such as already illustrated for immunization programs, with income and education levels, as well as by location, with urban dwellers getting preference
- Better-off people getting access to relatively expensive services that are generally less available to lower-income and socially marginalized groups

It is very important as we assess the performance of health systems that we examine the coverage of health programs for different groups of people. It is also important that we examine how accessible services are to lower-income and other disadvantaged groups compared to the services available to higher-income and other advantaged groups.

▶ Addressing Key Health Sector Concerns

There are few easy answers to effectively addressing the most critical health sector issues, particularly in low-income countries. Nevertheless, there is an increasing body of evidence about measures that can be taken to deal with some of the specific problems noted previously and to design and manage health systems more effectively and efficiently. These are discussed briefly here.

Demographic and Epidemiologic Change

The very poorest countries can take only a limited number of steps at once to deal with the multiple burdens of communicable and noncommunicable diseases and injuries. Yet, all of these countries will face an increasing burden from noncommunicable disease, particularly cardiovascular disease and road traffic accidents.

Perhaps the single most important step that low- and middle-income countries can take today to reduce the future burden of cardiovascular disease is to reduce the disease burden that is related to tobacco use. There is very good evidence that even in low-income settings, measures to make it harder and more expensive to buy cigarettes can reduce tobacco smoking.[66] Even with their limited financial resources and management capacity, low-income countries need to start taking these steps now. They can also take other measures to begin to reduce road traffic accidents, including better engineering of roads, safer cars, and more traffic enforcement.[67]

The way in which health systems are organized and operated in many low- and middle-income countries will need to be strengthened to address the growing burden of noncommunicable diseases. These countries will need to pay increasing attention to these problems, even as they continue to confront the problems of communicable diseases and undernutrition. To an important extent, countries will need to assess the six building blocks of health systems from the perspective of managing prevention, treatment, and care related to noncommunicable diseases. Addressing chronic noncommunicable diseases requires prolonged and frequent contacts with patients, unlike care for most communicable diseases, with the exception of HIV/AIDS treatment. Countries will need to develop or adopt models of care that can sustain more frequent contacts with patients over a longer period of time than they have had to do thus far.[68]

Stewardship

It will also be difficult to improve health system governance in countries in which overall governance is weak and corruption is high. Nonetheless, a number of measures are proving to be useful in addressing key governance issues in health. Corruption has been reduced, for example, in countries like Poland that have launched national anticorruption programs with strong political backing. In addition, reforming procurement systems and making them more open and transparent has been associated with reducing corruption in contracting in countries such as Chile and Argentina. Increasing audits of the health system and enforcing penalties to deal with adverse findings have assisted Madagascar in reducing corruption. There is an increasing number of efforts at reducing corruption and enhancing management through oversight by communities. In a number of cases, such as in Uganda, the Philippines, and Bolivia, community boards were provided more information about the money and services that the community should have received and the authority to provide oversight of these resources in a way that could lead to the firing of corrupt officials. Contracting out some services, carrying out customer satisfaction surveys among the users of the health system, and letting communities provide services with "citizen report cards" are also proving to be helpful to enhancing governance in some settings.[52]

Human Resources

The problems of human resources for health relate largely to a lack of staff, a maldistribution of staff, the inadequate training and quality of personnel, and the poor environment in which many of them have to carry out their work. An international group examining human resources for health has suggested that there needs to be more shared global responsibility for these resources, given the extent to which health workers migrate in search of better pay and working conditions. In addition, they suggested that countries need to have much more explicit strategies for workforce development that would focus on coverage, motivation, and competence. They also highlighted the need for countries and their development partners to provide greater support for education and training of health personnel and to develop better policies and programs for retaining personnel.[69]

Even as they seek to address these problems in more comprehensive ways, some countries have taken steps to deal with human resource issues. Countries might be able to reduce the share of their health workers who are migrating, for example, by training them so they gain needed skills but do not get credentials for those skills that would be recognized by other countries.[54] Moreover, lower-level health personnel can be trained to carry out a number of functions often reserved for higher-level staff, a strategy known as **task shifting**. In Malawi, where there is an acute shortage of doctors, nurses were trained to perform caesarean sections.[54] As antiretroviral therapy is being scaled up for HIV/AIDS, community-based workers are being taught how to dispense drugs for patients who have been doing well on treatment and to recognize when the patients are having problems and need to be referred for more specialized care. These are tasks reserved for doctors in some HIV/AIDS treatment programs. A number of mental health programs in places where there are very few mental health professionals are training healthcare workers at the primary

level or community health workers to be the front line in the diagnosis and treatment of mental health issues.

A number of countries also use financial incentives to encourage better performance of healthcare personnel. These might include better salaries, additional payments for serving in hard-to-reach areas, bonus payments for meeting certain health service or health outcome objectives, providing housing for people who work in those areas, or special allowances for training. The design of incentives and provider payment mechanisms, of course, has to take account of what one is trying to achieve and of the local culture. Incentives might be different, for example, if one were trying to reduce migration, trying to get staff to serve in rural areas, or just trying to get staff to come to work in a timely way.[54]

Financing Health Services

The scope for very low-income countries to raise additional resources for health is limited, given the overall scarcity of resources. Nevertheless, there is some scope for shifting resources from other areas of the economy in some countries, given the potentially high returns to investments in health. Some of the low-income countries, however, will require development assistance for health for some time in order to boost expenditure on health and more effectively address some of their key health concerns, such as HIV/AIDS.[70]

There is, however, some scope for enhancing health outcomes by shifting expenditure within the health sector. By focusing expenditure on a selected group of low-cost investments that are known to be effective if managed properly, even very poor countries may be able to improve health outcomes of their poorest people.[4,71] To assist in raising and managing resources for health more effectively, many countries will need to enhance the data they have on health expenditure and also monitor health investments and expenditures more carefully.

Many countries also have substantial room for improving the efficiency of the resources they spend on health. WHO has estimated that between 20 percent and 40 percent of the expenditures on health in low-income countries are wasted by spending that is not effective or efficient. Improvements in the efficiency of expenditures could help to free resources for high-priority expenditures. In addition, the better management of financial resources by ministries of health will strengthen any arguments they make to ministries of finance about the need for additional financing for health and their ability to use it wisely.[7]

Financial Protection and Universal Coverage

WHO has suggested that countries need to take a number of steps to enhance people's protection from the burden of health expenditure and to achieve universal coverage with a basic package of health services. These measures would include raising additional revenue for health, improving the efficiency of health sector expenditure, reducing dependence on out-of-pocket expenditures, and enhancing equity. Although efforts to achieve universal coverage were once generally considered possible only in middle- and high-income countries, a number of low- and middle-income countries in the last decade have made substantial progress toward providing universal coverage, including Brazil, Ghana, Mexico, Rwanda, and Thailand.[7] Ghana was discussed briefly earlier. The case studies later in this chapter include additional comments on efforts to achieve universal coverage.

Over the longer term, today's low- and middle-income countries aspire to having a health system that provides universal health coverage, coupled with a high degree of financial protection. We can think of this, for example, as their wanting to move as rapidly as possible toward having a system like that of France or the Netherlands—a system that covers all of the population for many health conditions with a generous insurance package and limited out-of-pocket payments.

A recent study defined a package of the highest priority investments that could be a starting point for the further development of UHC in low- and lower middle-income countries. This package would include key efforts to address outstanding Group I causes and the highest priority investments for noncommunicable diseases and injuries. The package was estimated to cost about $42 per person in low-income countries and $58 in lower middle-income countries. As countries make progress in implementing this "highest-priority package," they could expand services that are part of their UHC scheme to an even broader package. The study estimated that this expanded package would cost $76 in low-income countries and $110 in lower middle-income countries.[72]

This progressive movement toward a broad package of services under a universal health coverage scheme is depicted in **FIGURE 6-2**. One can think of everything inside the outer circle as a "full coverage UHC package" to which a low- or lower middle-income country could aspire in the longer term. Given their present health system and resources, however, these countries might start their move toward full universal

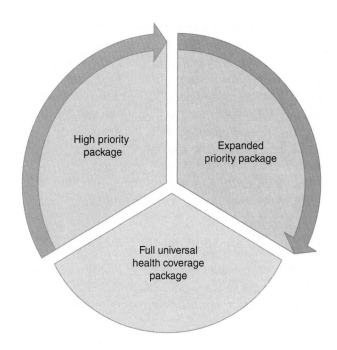

FIGURE 6-2 Essential Universal Health Coverage and Highest Priority Packages

Modified from Jamison, D. T., Gelband, H., Horton, S., Jha, P., Laxminarayan, R., Mock, C. N., & Nugent, R. (Eds.). (2018). Disease control priorities: Improving health and reducing poverty. In *Disease control priorities* (3rd ed., Vol. 9). Washington, DC: The World Bank. doi: 10.1596/978-1-4648-0527-1

health coverage, with the "highest-priority package." As they further develop their health system, they would add services to implement the "expanded priority package." Ultimately, they would move to include all services in the circle, as they put in place a package for "full universal health coverage." WHO suggests that countries move in these directions by first expanding coverage for high-priority services to everyone. WHO also highlights the importance of ensuring while doing so that marginalized groups are not left behind.[72]

As the quest for universal health coverage has become more global, considerable attention has been paid to the criteria and principles that countries should use to define their package of services. WHO has recommended that countries "make fair choices" as they do this by including such criteria as "cost-effectiveness, priority to the worse off, and financial risk protection."[73]

Additional Comments on Access and Equity

Improving access to and equity of services is largely a question of political will and health systems planning. Many countries have not focused sufficient attention on the health of their disadvantaged people and have not been sufficiently aware of the kinds of gaps in health coverage and health status that these people face. There is much evidence, however, like that cited earlier, that the coverage of health services is inequitable in many countries and often leaves out those living in difficult regions and those with less income, less education, and less empowerment. Countries need to use the data they get from national surveys, such as the Demographic and Health Surveys,[74] to identify gaps in health status and health coverage. They then need to specifically target health resources to the places and people most in need. Very substantial gains could be made in health status within many countries, for example, if the coverage of effective programs for at least childhood vaccination, TB, and malaria were increased among the poor. The enhancements in health would be even greater if carried out in conjunction with improvements in water supply, sanitation, nutrition, and overall hygiene and health-caring behaviors. This can be partly accomplished through improvements in knowledge that also need to be at the core of efforts to improve the health of the poor.

Quality

As noted earlier, low-quality health services waste money and are dangerous to people's health. Although most of us probably believe that low quality is primarily a reflection of inadequate financial resources, this issue has many sources. In addition, there is good evidence that quality can be enhanced in a number of ways even in the absence of substantial additional resources.

The recent global commission on the quality of care suggested a number of broad measures that are essential to quality improvement[75]:

- Governments must make quality the foundation of their systems and part of "system DNA" and govern for quality in partnership with other institutions.
- Governments and their citizens must ignite a demand for quality services.
- Services need to be redesigned to focus on quality outcomes rather than access alone.
- Countries should revise the training of providers to focus on competency-based training and providing better support to those workers.
- Health systems should measure and report on what matters most—outcomes, competent care, user experience, and confidence in the system.

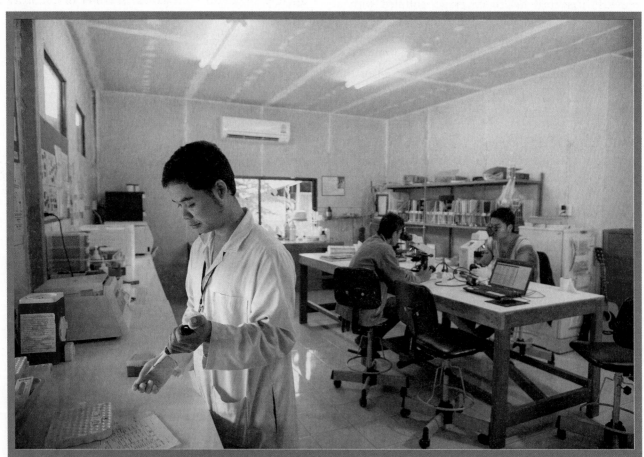

PHOTO 6-3 This is a scene from a laboratory in a health center in Singapore, which has a well-developed healthcare system. Although laboratories are central to the proper functioning of a healthcare system, many low-income countries face serious shortages of laboratories of acceptable quality and the people to manage and operate them. What steps might be taken to enhance the numbers, distribution, and quality of laboratories in such countries?

Courtesy of Mark Tuschman.

As countries move in these directions, it is very important, first, that health systems carry out assessments that will help them understand the quality gaps in their programs. Second, there is evidence that better professional oversight, supervision, and continuing training can enhance the quality of care provided by health service providers. Third, the use of clear guidelines, protocols, and algorithms for services can also improve quality, particularly where health workers are not well-educated or trained. Fourth, when contracting services to the private and NGO sectors, governments can link their payments with performance against specific goals and can independently verify that they have been achieved. This can also be done through results-based financing schemes in the public sector, as discussed in the case studies later in this chapter. Finally, focusing some health staff on becoming very proficient at a small number of services is consistently associated with better quality of care.[76]

There is also evidence that total quality management approaches can enhance the quality of care, even in low-income countries. In this approach, groups of health providers define goals, measure how the system is doing in achieving them, together decide how they might best address the gaps in their program, and then evaluate whether their proposed improvements are working. Even in the poorest areas of North India, this kind of effort, coupled with standard guidelines for managing certain services, has produced improvements in the quality of care. The safety of anesthesia has been enhanced in Malaysia in similar ways.[76]

Delivering Primary Health Care

In the end, of course, trying to enhance health outcomes for the poor through better health services in low- and middle-income countries is not just a question of addressing the specific issues discussed previously. Rather, it is also a question of the overall orientation of the health system and how it will carry out the services that can potentially have the biggest impact on improving health outcomes for disadvantaged groups.

There is a broad consensus that a number of measures are needed to achieve this aim. First, services should be focused on the most important burdens of disease. Second, health outcomes can only be achieved if the health system is strengthened to deliver those services effectively, efficiently, and at an appropriate level of quality. Third, the core of activities to meet these goals should be through primary health care and the district hospital.[77]

There have been a number of very important declarations, studies, and reports that have suggested what the basic healthcare package should contain at the primary healthcare level. The most important elements such a package might contain are noted in **TABLE 6-9**.

Although there are differences in the exact content of the suggested package, there is consensus around most of the elements it might contain. To a large extent, it is recommended that countries deliver the services listed in **TABLE 6-10** as close to where people live as possible, through close collaboration between primary healthcare services and the district hospital. The hospital would help to supervise the work in primary health care as well as serve as the referral service for activities that cannot be handled adequately at the primary level, such as complications of pregnancy. The components of the package are outlined in Table 6-10.[77] It is important to note that services like those outlined in Table 6-10 need to be provided regardless of whether countries organize their health system along public or private provision of services.

Ideally, these services would be delivered in an integrated manner. However, because of weaknesses in the health systems of many countries, especially low-income ones, a substantial number of countries have established "vertical" programs to address some of these health problems. These have historically been used to deal with diseases such as smallpox, malaria, neglected tropical diseases, and tuberculosis, for example, for which governments set up separate management, financing, procurement, staffing, and reporting in parallel with the regular health programs of the government.

Although in principle this vertical approach may not be the most efficient and effective manner in which to operate health services, in practice it has sometimes been seen as the only way to accomplish urgent goals in weak health systems. There is an increasing consensus, however, that if such approaches are going to be taken, then they should be linked with efforts to improve related aspects of the health system. The polio eradication program, for example, can be used to strengthen laboratories, surveillance, and the management of the cold chain for some medicines and vaccines. In any case, there is now a growing effort globally to focus on health systems strengthening and to try to ensure that countries increasingly take more integrated approaches to their health systems, centered around the quest for UHC.[78]

▶ Case Studies

Four case studies follow to illustrate some of the concepts that were discussed in this chapter. The first discusses key issues in the management of

TABLE 6-9 Model Primary Care Package of Essential Health Service Interventions

Maternity-related interventions
Prenatal care
Tetanus vaccine
Skilled attendant at delivery
Treatment of complications during pregnancy
Emergency obstetric care
Postpartum care
Family planning

Childhood disease–related interventions (prevention)
Bacillus Calmette-Guérin vaccination for tuberculosis
Polio vaccination
Diphtheria-pertussis-tetanus vaccination
Measles vaccination
Hepatitis B vaccination
Haemophilus influenza type B vaccination
Rotavirus vaccination
Pneumococcal vaccination
Vitamin A supplementation
Anthelmintic treatment
School health program (incorporating micronutrient supplementation, school meals, anthelmintic treatment, and health education)

Childhood disease–related interventions (treatment)
Acute respiratory infections early diagnosis and treatment
Diarrhea—oral rehydration with zinc
Causes of fever—early diagnosis and treatment
Undernutrition—measures to enhance protein, energy, and needed micronutrients, including iron, iodine, vitamin A, and zinc
Feeding and breastfeeding counseling

Malaria prevention
Insecticide-treated nets
Residual indoor spraying
Intermittent treatment of pregnant women

Malaria treatment
Early diagnosis and treatment with artemisinin-based combination therapy

Tuberculosis treatment
Patient-centered TB care

HIV prevention
Youth-focused interventions
Interventions with sex workers and clients and interventions for other most at risk populations, such as men who have sex with men
Condom social marketing and distribution
Workplace interventions
Strengthening of blood transfusion systems
Voluntary counseling and testing
Prevention of mother-to-child transmission
Treatment for sexually transmitted infections

HIV care
Palliative care
Clinical management of opportunistic illnesses
Prevention of opportunistic illnesses
Home-based care
Provision of antiretroviral therapy (ART) for HIV

Tobacco control program
Taxes
Ban smoking in public places, advertising, sales to minors
Health education
Nicotine replacement

Alcohol control program
Taxes
Ban advertising, sales to minors
Laws against drunk driving
Short counseling sessions

Modified from Tollman, S., Doherty, J., & Mulligan, J. A. (2006). General primary care. In D. T. Jamison, J. G. Breman, A. R. Measham, et al. (Eds.), *Disease control priorities in developing countries* (2nd ed., pp. 1193–1209). New York, NY: Oxford University Press.

pharmaceuticals. The second examines "essential surgery." Two additional country cases then follow, concerning efforts to enhance health services and move toward UHC.

Pharmaceuticals

The Importance of Pharmaceuticals

Pharmaceuticals play an essential role in the health systems of all countries. They are essential for the care of many health conditions, and people can spend a significant part of their income on medicines. Additionally, many countries spend an important part of

their health budgets on pharmaceuticals. It has been estimated, for example, that expenditure on pharmaceuticals as a share of total health expenditure ranges from approximately 20 percent in high-income countries to 30 percent in low-income countries.[79]

In the simplest terms, countries should ensure that they can procure in a timely manner drugs of appropriate quality for key health conditions their people face. They must also ensure that the drugs are affordable for those who need them. In addition, of course, they need to be able to transport the drugs so they can get where they are needed and be able to safely store them. They must also ensure that they are prescribed,

TABLE 6-10 Selected Essential Healthcare Interventions by Level of Service in a Close-to-the-Client System

Level of Care	Tuberculosis	Malaria	HIV	Childhood Diseases	Maternal/Perinatal	Smoking
Outreach services		Epidemic planning and response Indoor residual spraying	Peer education for vulnerable groups Needle exchange	Specific immunization campaign Outreach for integrated management of childhood illness (IMCI) Home management of fever Outreach for micronutrients and deworming		
Health center/ health post	Patient-centered TB care	Treatment of uncomplicated malaria Intermittent treatment of pregnant women for malaria	Antiretrovirals Prevention of opportunistic infections (OIs) and treatment of uncomplicated OIs Voluntary counseling and testing (VCT) Treatment of sexually transmitted infections (STIs)	IMCI Immunization Treatment of severe anemia	Skilled birth attendants Antenatal and postnatal care Family planning postpartum	Cessation advice Pharmacological therapies for smoking
Hospital	Treatment for complicated tuberculosis cases	Treatment of complicated malaria	Treatment of severe OI for AIDS Palliative care	IMCI (severe cases)	Emergency obstetric care	

Modified from Jha, P., & Mills, A. (2002). *Improving health outcomes for the poor: Report of Working Group 5 of the Commission on Macroeconomics and Health* (p. 5). Geneva, Switzerland: World Health Organization.

dispensed, and used properly for the appropriate health conditions.

This section briefly explores some of the key questions concerning the role of pharmaceuticals in health systems, critical issues in procuring appropriate medicines at reasonable prices, and selective issues in the appropriate management and use of those medicines. This section does not deal with prescribing practices and antimicrobial resistance, which is dealt with in the chapter on communicable diseases.

Procuring the Right Drugs

Countries need to manage their drug supplies effectively and efficiently. Historically, many countries have purchased a wide array of drugs, not always consistent with clinical needs. In addition, many countries have failed to procure those drugs at the lowest cost.

To assist in getting more appropriate medicines at better prices, WHO has helped countries improve the effectiveness and efficiency of their procurement of medicines by producing lists of essential medicines. The broader focus of this effort has been to help countries and their public health systems procure the medicines that are most needed, in the most effective and efficient ways, in order to get better prices than would otherwise be possible. This effort began in 1977, and many countries have been able to achieve better outcomes at lower cost through the use of the essential medicines approach.[80] WHO has published an updated model list of essential medicines every 2 years since 1977, the most recent of which was issued in 2017.[81]

Medications that are procured, of course, need to have certain quality standards. Low-quality medicines cannot provide the intended therapeutic benefit; they can also cause harm. In addition, the purchase of low-quality medicines is a waste of money by individuals and by health systems.

To ensure that medicines sold in their country are safe and effective, countries need to have a competent regulatory authority. The U.S. Food and Drug Administration (FDA) is one such regulatory body, and there are similar bodies in Australia, the European Union, India, and Japan. However, many low- and middle-income countries do not have the resources necessary to establish competent organizations for ensuring the quality of medicines.

Partly related to these institutional gaps in some countries, a widespread problem in pharmaceutical quality is counterfeit or fake medicines. These "falsified or substandard" medicines often look, taste, and are packaged exactly like real medications. However, they have none, too little, or too much of the active ingredients. Internet pharmacies have been a major source of falsified and substandard pharmaceuticals. Over 50 percent of medicines sold on internet pharmacies are counterfeit. The main driver for these counterfeit medicines is financial gain, as global sales of counterfeit medications were estimated even by 2010 at $75 billion worldwide.[82] This is despite the fact that the distribution of counterfeit or falsely labeled medicines is universally considered a crime.[80]

In 2010, WHO established a working group on spurious, falsely labeled, fake, or counterfeit medicines (SFFC). This group collected data and information about SFFCs around the world. Some of their findings, for example, showed surprising amounts of counterfeit medicines in major global markets[83]:

- In 2009, two deaths and nine hospitalizations occurred in China from a traditional medicine for diabetes containing six times the normal dosage.
- In 2011, 3,000 Kenyan HIV patients received a false batch of the antiretroviral Zidolam-N.
- In 2012, 19 U.S. medical facilities found that they were using a counterfeit version of Avastin, a widely used cancer therapy.

In fact, the U.S. FDA earlier estimated that around 10 percent to 15 percent of all medicines on the global market are fake medicines. In some low- and middle-income countries, this number is estimated to exceed 50 percent.[84] A major recent study of falsified and substandard medicines in Africa and Asia suggested that almost 20 percent of antimalarials and 12 percent of antibiotics were substandard or falsified.[85]

A recent WHO report on substandard and falsified medical products suggests that these products have enormous health and economic consequences[86]:

- Endangering health, prolonging illness, and even killing
- Promoting antimicrobial resistance and the spread of drug-resistant infections
- Undermining confidence in health professionals and health systems
- Creating distrust about the effectiveness of vaccines and medicines
- Eating into the limited budgets of families and health systems
- Providing income to criminal networks

In 2013, WHO launched a Global Surveillance and Monitoring System for Substandard and Falsified Medical Products. It works with member states to improve the quantity, quality, and analysis of accurate data concerning these medical products. It then seeks to protect public health by using the data to better prevent, detect, and respond to those products. WHO also developed a global reporting system on substandard and falsified medical products. This system shares information across countries about these products and can issue medical alerts about a product that is found to be harmful to public health. Under this program, WHO also assists in training people from its member countries on this issue.[87]

A collaboration of nongovernmental organizations, pharmaceutical companies, healthcare providers, legitimate internet pharmacy organizations, and patient advocacy organizations have also worked together in a campaign called Fight the Fakes.[88] This group works across borders to raise public awareness about the dangers of shopping outside of regulated markets, as well to educate governmental and other leaders about the issue of counterfeit medicines.[89] The partnership is working with new mobile technologies to increase reporting of counterfeit medicines. The campaign has noted that antibiotics are some of the most counterfeited medications, which has serious implications for the issue of antimicrobial resistance.

Procuring Drugs at the Right Price

Pharmaceutical companies are mostly for-profit businesses that design, produce, and market medications. These medications can incur high investment costs, from discovery of basic molecules to clinical trials for safety and efficacy. The cost to bring a single medicine through this process can be between $500 million and $2 billion.[90] The costs for research and development can be a large barrier for new medicines to make it to market, as well as a contributor to high prices for medicines.

Moreover, because pharmaceutical companies are businesses, they have to make a profit to continue to exist. In order to incentivize the development and sale of new medicines, governments grant temporary monopolies on them called patents. A patented medicine is under the sole ownership and control of the patent holder.[91] While patents may inspire innovation, they also contribute to medicine prices that may be unaffordable for low- and middle-income countries.

Beyond the essential medicines approach, a number of measures have also been taken to make these medicines more affordable in low- and middle-income countries. Many pharmaceutical companies, for example, sell medicines at reduced prices in some resource-poor settings. Pharmaceutical companies also donate drugs to countries and to global health campaigns, and a number of companies have made long-term commitments to donate drugs to address the neglected tropical diseases.

Companies also engage in **tiered pricing**. Under this mechanism, companies sell medicines at different prices, depending on the income level of the country involved. However, tiered pricing is often criticized as providing only a temporary solution to a permanent problem, as well as not lowering the cost of the medicine to an affordable price for individuals.[92]

Low- and middle-income countries can also gain access to quality medicines at affordable prices through procurement programs set up in partnership with a range of organizations. The Global Drug Facility,[93] the Global Fund,[94] and the Supply Chain Management System that works with PEPFAR,[95] UNITAID,[96] and the Clinton Foundation,[97] among others, have helped negotiate reduced prices for some medicines, such as HIV drugs needed by low- and middle-income countries.

Some international trade agreements, including the Trade-Related Aspects of Intellectual Property Rights (TRIPS) Agreement, have been criticized as being significant constraints to access to affordable medicines by low- and middle-income countries. However, under these arrangements, countries *can* issue a "compulsory license" that allows outside parties, such as generic manufacturers, to produce and distribute patented drugs without the drug company's consent in order to meet public health needs or help deal with a public health emergency.[98] For example, in 2007 Thailand used compulsory licenses for the heart disease drug Plavix. With this approach, the government predicted a decrease in costs for Plavix from $2 to $0.20 per pill.[99] Compulsory licensing has also been used for HIV/AIDS drugs in Brazil, South Africa, and Malaysia, among others.[100]

The "patent pool" funded by UNITAID is another approach that is now used to enable the production of generic medicines. The patent pool is a collection of HIV drug patents for which the patent holders voluntarily allow the manufacture of generics for low- and middle-income countries.

Procuring Drugs at the Right Time

A country must have an effective supply chain in order to ensure that medicines reach the patients who need them, in a timely manner and at an affordable price. An interruption in the supply chain can have serious or even disastrous effects. For example, interruption in treatment for TB, among other diseases, can breed drug-resistant strains and cause the death of patients who are lacking necessary medications.

A supply chain for medicines includes multiple actors[101]:

- Manufacturers who produce the raw materials and medicines required
- Procurement agents such as ministries of health; government procurement offices; public organizations that assist countries with procurement of medicines, such as UNICEF; or private organizations that also do this, such as IDA or Crown Agents
- Distributors to transport medicines at national, regional, and district levels
- Warehouses at each level of the system to safely store medicines
- Service providers who order and dispense medicines

Unfortunately, many low- and middle-income countries lack the capacity to manage an effective supply chain for essential medicines. They may lack staff trained in logistics or an appropriate logistical management system that can keep inventory, track the medicines given out, and ensure that orders for new medicines are placed in a timely manner. Many countries also lack appropriate storage facilities for medicines or vaccines, some of which have to be kept cold. Vaccines for polio, influenza, and hepatitis, for example, require storage temperatures between 2°C and 8°C.[102]

Many low- and middle-income countries, however, have taken steps to improve supply chain management for pharmaceuticals. They have established supply chain organizations, trained staff, and improved the legal environment for procurement. Some countries have also sought innovative approaches to enhancing their supply chain management.

The Tanzanian Medical Supplies Department and the Coca-Cola Company, for example, began working with the Global Fund in 2010[103] to strengthen the supply chain for essential medicines in Tanzania. In 2011, staff of Yale University joined this effort, which has been called Project Last Mile. This effort seeks to build on the strong supply chain of Coca-Cola and the company's knowledge of supply chain management to ensure that the Tanzanian government can get pharmaceuticals to the right place at the right time and at affordable prices. Based on the successes of the Tanzania collaboration, Project Last Mile was to be expanded to 10 African countries by 2019.[104]

Procuring Drugs for the Right People

Even if countries can get the right drugs to the right place, at the right time, and at the right price, countries still have to ensure that the right people take them in the appropriate manner. In fact, it has been estimated that around half of all prescribed medicines are dispensed incorrectly. Moreover, even when distributed adequately, only half of all patients take them correctly.[105]

Another global effort, therefore, has focused on the rational use of medicines. WHO has emphasized several measures to promote rational use[105]:

- Establishing regulatory bodies to set rules for medicine use
- Following clinical guidelines from WHO and other authorities
- Developing national lists of essential medicines
- Creating local committees in hospitals and districts to monitor medicine use and distribution
- Improving medical training to include problem-based curricula
- Requiring continued medical education on medicines for healthcare providers
- Ensuring supervision of medicine use, audits of facilities, and feedback reviews
- Using information about medicines from sources outside the company creating them
- Rolling out public education on medicine use
- Avoiding the use of financial incentives for drug usage
- Enforcing appropriate regulations on medication use
- Ensuring adequate numbers of human resources and medicines needed for the system

There are significant challenges to rational use in all countries, but achieving more rational use of medicines can be especially challenging in low- and middle-income countries. This is due to the poor quality of some care, including misdiagnosis, prescribing the wrong medicines, and overprescribing; medical and financial reasons; patient demands for medicines even if they are not needed; and the failure of patients to adhere to treatment regimens, some of which can be long and have unpleasant side effects.

Measures to improve the use of medicines can yield high returns. Correct diagnostic tests and rational use of antimalarial artemisinin combination therapy (ACT), for example, were vital to successfully reducing malaria in Senegal.[105] In 2007, Senegal moved from primarily clinical assessment for malaria to rapid diagnostic tests, which are low-cost and accurate.[105] As a result, ACT has been used only for confirmed cases, curbing the overuse of ACT and reducing unnecessary costs of malaria control.

The Antibiotics Smart Use program in Thailand decreased the use of antibiotics while maintaining high treatment success rates between 2007 and

2012.[105] The Thailand Food and Drug Administration trained medical staff on rational antibiotic use and educating patients through easy-to-read brochures.[105] As a result, there was an 18 percent to 23 percent decrease in antibiotic use in community hospitals, with a decrease in primary hospitals as high as 46 percent.[105,106]

Essential Surgery

The Relative Neglect of Essential Surgery

A number of health conditions, including injuries, malignancies, congenital anomalies, obstetrical complications, cataracts, glaucoma, and perinatal conditions, require surgery to be addressed. However, these surgeries are often not available in a timely or appropriate way in low- and lower middle-income countries. Moreover, until recently, relatively little attention was paid to surgical needs in these settings, as countries and their partners focused most of their attention on women and children's health and the control of communicable diseases.

In the last decade or so, however, increasing attention has been paid to the role that surgery can play in low- and lower middle-income settings in averting deaths and disability in cost-effective ways. An important work published in 2006, *Disease Control Priorities in Developing Countries, Second Edition* (DCP2), included a chapter on essential surgery. The third edition of that work, *Disease Control Priorities in Developing Countries, Third Edition* (DCP3), builds upon the earlier work and further examines the needs for essential surgery, the cost-effectiveness of such surgeries, and measures that low- and lower middle-income countries can take to improve access to, the quality of, and outcomes from such surgery.[107] In addition, *The Lancet* has recently established a commission on global surgery.

This case study outlines the findings of the essential surgery volume of DCP3, as they were summarized in an article in *The Lancet*.[108]

What Is Essential Surgery?

The term essential surgery is not commonly used, and it is important to define it:

> Essential surgical disorders can be defined as those that are mainly or extensively treated by surgery (procedures and other surgical care), have a large health burden, and can be successfully treated by a surgical procedure (and other surgical care) that is cost-effective and feasible to promote globally.[108(p2210)]

It is especially important to note that the term *surgical care* includes preoperative care, including assessment of whether or not to perform surgery; safe anesthesia; and postsurgical care.

TABLE 6-11 indicates a proposed package of essential surgical interventions and the level of the health system at which low- and lower middle-income countries should aim to carry out such surgeries.

The Burden of Disease

It has been estimated that about 6.5 percent of all deaths in low- and lower middle-income countries could be averted if the package of essential surgery noted previously could be made universally available in those countries.

It should also be noted, however, that there are substantial gaps in the data on this point. In addition, the proportion of deaths that are avertable through the application of this package will be very sensitive to the share of the population that lacks access to such services.

Gaps in Access to Essential Surgery of Good Quality

In fact, only about 3.5 percent of all surgeries take place in low- and lower middle-income countries, which are home to about 35 percent of the world's population. This discrepancy should not be a surprise and reflects, among other things, the lack of skilled human resources in such countries, the lack of facilities, and the lack of equipment and supplies. The United States, for example, has more than 60 times the number of general surgeons per 100,000 population and more than 100 times the number of anesthesiologists per 100,000 population than some of the lowest-income countries. The United States has about 6 times more general surgeons per 100,000 population and more than 2 times the number of anesthesiologists per 100,000 population than even the better-off of the lower middle-income countries. In addition, the United States has more than 10 times more operating rooms (theaters) per 100,000 people than the countries of sub-Saharan Africa and South Asia.

There are also major gaps in the quality of surgical care in many countries. The risk of a complication or death from caesarean section is 6 to 10 times greater in South Asia than in Sweden and 100 times higher in sub-Saharan Africa than in Sweden. The deaths related to complications from anesthesia are more than 5 times higher in low- and middle-income countries than in high-income countries.

TABLE 6-11 An Essential Surgery Package

DELIVERY PLATFORM

	Community Facility and Primary Health Centers	First-Level Hospitals	Referral and Specialized Hospitals
Dental procedures	Extraction Drainage of dental abscess Treatment for caries		
Obstetric, gynecological, and family planning	Normal delivery	Caesarean birth Vacuum extraction or forceps delivery Ectopic pregnancy Manual vacuum aspiration and dilation and curettage Tubal ligation Vasectomy Hysterectomy for uterine rupture or intractable postpartum hemorrhage Visual inspection with acetic acid and cryotherapy for precancerous cervical lesions	Repair obstetric fistula
General surgical	Drainage of superficial abscess Male circumcision	Repair of perforations (perforated peptic ulcer, typhoid ileal perforation, etc.) Appendectomy Bowel obstruction Colostomy Gallbladder disease (including emergency surgery for acute cholecystitis) Hernia (including incarceration) Hydrocelectomy Relief of urinary obstruction; catheterization or suprapubic cystostomy (tube into bladder through skin)	
Injury	Resuscitation with basic life support measures Suturing laceration Management of non-displaced fractures	Resuscitation with advanced life support measures, including surgical airway Tube thoracostomy (chest drain) Trauma laparotomy Fracture reduction Irrigation and debridement of open fractures Placement of external fixator, use of traction Escharotomy or fasciotomy (cutting of constricting tissue to relieve pressure from swelling) Trauma-related amputations Skin grafting Burr hole	

Congenital		Cleft lip and palate repair Club foot repair Shunt for hydrocephalus Repair of anorectal malformations and Hirschsprung's disease
Visual impairment		Cataract extraction and insertion of intraocular lens Eyelid surgery for trachoma
Nontrauma orthopedic	Drainage of septic arthritis Debridement of osteomyelitis	

Closing the Gaps in Access and Quality

In the long run, it would be valuable if low- and lower middle-income countries could train the highly skilled surgeons needed to effectively and universally implement a package of essential surgery. Indeed, some countries, such as Ghana, have made important strides in increasing the number of trained surgeons.

Nonetheless, it is clear that it will be many years before the poorest countries will have the number of licensed surgeons they need to implement a package of essential surgical interventions. Thus, they will for some time need to engage in task shifting for an important part of that work. This would include training general practitioners and nonphysician clinical personnel to carry out such work. There is good evidence from a number of countries, including Burkina Faso, Mozambique, and Tanzania, that these staff can be more cost-effective than surgeons in doing procedures such as cataract surgeries and caesarean surgeries.

Some countries, such as Vietnam, have also made progress in improving their equipment and supplies for essential surgery, often following guidelines produced by WHO on the infrastructure needed for surgical care at first-level hospitals and for emergency and essential surgery care.

More and more countries are moving toward programs of universal health coverage. Access to a package of essential surgery would be enhanced if countries include such a package in their programs for universal health coverage.

Addressing issues of the quality of care will not be easy in countries that lack many of the inputs needed to implement a package of essential surgical interventions and that have such large gaps in quality compared to the standard of care in better-off countries. However, a number of models for quality improvement have shown excellent and sustainable results. These approaches are also uncomplicated and inexpensive. Such measures could include, for example, implementing the WHO 19-point checklist on surgical safety, the use of which has improved outcomes in low-, middle-, and high-income countries for both elective and emergency surgery.

Many higher-income countries have made substantial progress in reducing complications from anesthesia by adopting standards of care and careful monitoring of patients' breathing, level of oxygen saturation, and flow of blood to the capillaries. This has been helped in these countries by the use of certain medical equipment, such as the pulse oximeter, which monitors the patient's level of oxygen saturation. As countries begin to make progress in improving the quality and safety of anesthesia, it would be helpful if lower-cost versions of key equipment, like the pulse oximeter, could be developed and made available to them. Work is ongoing in this direction.

Essential Surgery Is Cost-Effective

The evidence suggests that essential surgery is a cost-effective investment. In fact, some of the procedures that are part of the essential surgery package are as cost-effective, in terms of dollars per DALY averted, as almost any other of the best buys in global health. Surgical repair of a cleft lip or inguinal hernia, cataract surgery, and caesarean section, for example, appear to be as cost-effective or almost as cost-effective as vitamin A supplementation and more cost-effective than oral rehydration therapy or antiretroviral therapy for HIV/AIDS.

Studies have also shown that these basic and essential surgeries are cost-effective at first-, second-, or third-level hospitals. However, the studies also show that these surgeries are more cost-effective when done at first-level hospitals.

Conclusion

Low- and lower middle-income countries should implement a package of essential surgery. In the long run, they should aim to have such surgeries performed by fully trained personnel. For now, however, countries can engage in task shifting coupled with the use of WHO guidelines on equipment and materials and the quality and safety of care, to produce good outcomes in highly cost-efficient ways. As countries increase the coverage of such programs, they can avert a substantial burden of deaths and DALYs at reasonable costs. Like the tropical diseases that had previously been neglected but now get more attention, it is important that countries increasingly understand the burden of surgical needs and act to address it.

Improving Health Outcomes in Rwanda Through Pay-for-Performance Schemes[109]

This case study, adapted from *Millions Saved: New Cases of Proven Success in Global Health*, explores an initiative in Rwanda to align health worker incentives with delivering high-quality care.

Introduction

In 1994, genocide took the lives of one-tenth of the Rwandan population and left the country reeling in its wake. Between 1993 and 1995, infant mortality rose by 15 percent and child mortality by 41 percent. The effects of the genocide lingered: the infant and under-5 mortality rates were still higher in 2000 than before the genocide.

These poor health outcomes were partially attributable to the deterioration of healthcare infrastructure after the genocide. During the genocide, a staggering 75 percent of health workers fled Rwanda or lost their lives to the conflict, and nearly all health facilities were demolished. The acute lack of human resources and health infrastructure exacerbated problems of low motivation and poor performance among remaining workers. Furthermore, instability in the years after the conflict prevented the Rwandan government from investing in health infrastructure.

The Intervention

The political climate stabilized in Rwanda in the late 1990s, allowing the government to turn its attention toward rebuilding its health system. It was essential for the government to find ways to motivate workers to deliver high-quality services even in underresourced settings.

Around this time, NGOs in selected regions of Rwanda were piloting a new method for reimbursing healthcare providers called pay-for-performance (P4P). Instead of receiving payment solely based on a salary, part of the compensation for health providers would depend on the performance of their health center, including quality and appropriateness of services, number of services provided, and health outcomes for patients.

Initial evaluations of these pilot P4P projects showed that they seemed to be improving family planning coverage, facility-based childbirth, and service quality in several regions of Rwanda. Although it was difficult to determine if these results were attributable directly to P4P schemes, improvements coinciding with the P4P approach made policymakers optimistic.

In light of these initial promising results, the Rwandan Ministry of Health sought to scale up the P4P scheme to the rest of the country beginning in 2006. With support from the World Bank, the Rwandan government launched a plan to expand P4P schemes to the 17 districts not covered by the early P4P initiatives. The Rwandan government rolled out the scheme in two phases in order to facilitate an impact evaluation of the program. The first group of districts would introduce the P4P in 2006, while the second group would delay implementation until 2008. To ensure fairness between the districts that participated and did not participate in the first phase of the scheme, the second group of districts received payments equal to the average P4P scheme payment in the years between the first and second phases of the program. However, these payments were not linked to performance.

The national P4P was set up to work in the following manner. Health facilities received incentive payments linked to the provision of a package of 14 different maternal, child, and general health services. Each health facility tracked the number of times healthcare workers performed each service, and submitted their records to a district committee. These committees calculated a baseline payment based on the quantity of services delivered, then factored in quality-of-care measures before disbursing the final incentive payment. Health facilities were free to allocate incentive funds at their own discretion, and most used the additional payments to raise staff salaries. On average, salaries were 38 percent higher than before the P4P scheme.

Impact

An evaluation of the P4P scheme found that districts that implemented the program saw improvements in quality of care, service utilization, and health outcomes compared to those that did not implement the scheme. The quality of prenatal care, for example, improved under the P4P scheme. As compared to control regions, in P4P districts, the number of preventive visits for children under age 2 increased by 27 percent, the proportion of births taking place in a hospital by 14 percent, and the proportion of mothers receiving a tetanus vaccine by 8 percent.

Districts implementing the P4P program also made substantial gains in infant and child nutrition. Infants in P4P districts had greater gains in weight for age than infants in control districts. The rate of stunting in children ages 2 to 4 was also significantly lower in P4P districts than in control districts.

It is important to note that several health systems strengthening initiatives in Rwanda coincided with the P4P scheme scale-up. Thus, the improvements in health indicators may not be entirely attributable to the P4P alone, but to the confluence of multiple factors that helped improve health status. Still, it is estimated that the scheme contributed to the 35 percent to 40 percent decrease in maternal, child, and infant mortality observed over the course of the scale-up of the P4P approach.

Despite these gains, some healthcare providers and administrators reported that the P4P scheme had adverse effects on their work. Some facilities noted that the scheme incentivized workers to "cheat the system" by falsifying patient records, or by refusing to dispense remaining medications to prevent stock-outs, which

were penalized under the P4P scheme. Others complained that the scheme placed an excessive administrative burden on health workers trying to both document their work and care for patients in settings with strained resources.

Costs

Implementing P4P required substantial investment. The P4P scheme contributed to a 500 percent increase in per capita health spending in Rwanda—from US$8 in 2002 to US$47 in 2008. Beyond the incentive payments, P4P required additional administrative costs to document and verify performance measures. These administrative costs amounted to approximately US$0.30 per person per year, or 1.2 percent of combined donor and government spending.

Lessons Learned

The Rwandan P4P program was the first program of its kind to undergo an evaluation based on a comprehensive, randomized controlled trial. The scheme demonstrated that giving providers financial incentives to provide better care can improve healthcare quality, service utilization, and health outcomes. Nonetheless, the Rwandan P4P still faces several challenges moving forward, including how to address attempts to "cheat" by misreporting information, as well as how to reduce the administrative burden on health facilities. Questions also remain as to whether the costing of each service is appropriate, what the most objective method is for measuring quality, and how to best design provider incentives.

It is important to note that several additional factors facilitated the success of the P4P. In 2001, Rwanda undertook a major effort to decentralize its health system and delegate control over finances and human resources to local health facilities. This meant that local health centers had the flexibility to adequately adapt to the new structure of the P4P. Implementation of community insurance schemes, or *mutuelles*, also coincided with scale-up of the P4P scheme, reaching 85 percent coverage by 2008. These programs helped Rwandans access the care they needed with a small copay, improving service utilization. Donor support and increased government spending on health also made the P4P possible.

The P4P program in Rwanda has inspired similar initiatives around the globe with support from a wide range of donors. Many questions remain, however, about how to best implement this type of program.

Health for All in Thailand Through the Universal Coverage Scheme[110]

The following case study describes how Thailand, a middle-income country, was able to achieve universal health coverage for its citizens. The following is a summary of the case study that appears in *Millions Saved: New Cases of Proven Success in Global Health*.

Background

Before universal health coverage was implemented in Thailand, nearly one out of every four individuals did not have health insurance, and many only had partial insurance coverage. Uninsured individuals often spent a large proportion of their household income on health care when illness struck. This was impoverishing for many families. In fact, as a result of the large proportion of uninsured people in Thailand, out-of-pocket spending on health care pushed one in every five of the poorest Thai households below the poverty line.

Thailand made several attempts to improve health equity and affordability before introducing universal health coverage. The Thai government made free health services available to people living in poverty in 1975. Between 1982 and 1986, the government redirected investments from urban hospitals to strengthen rural hospitals and health centers in order to address the lack of health services in rural areas. Despite these efforts, however, inequities in healthcare coverage were intensified when the Asian financial crisis hit in 1997. Unemployment rates increased, as did the number of people living under the poverty line. The cost of medical supplies and drugs rose, too, while the Ministry of Public Health lost much of its funding. Thus, 25 percent of the Thai population was still uninsured in 2001.

The Intervention

By 1999, Thai public health experts and other reformers produced convincing evidence that implementing a universal health coverage program would be a feasible endeavor. In the past, however, advocates in the Ministry of Public Health had been unable to convince politicians and lawmakers to prioritize a universal health coverage scheme.

The legislative election of 2001 offered a chance for universal health coverage advocates to garner political support for their healthcare reform plan. The populist Thai Rak Thai party, led by Thaksin Shinawatra, made universal health coverage central to its platform. With the slogan "30 baht treats all diseases" (BHT30

is approximately US$0.70), the Thai Rak Thai party promised insurance for all.

Other activists and members of civil society also played a role in mobilizing organizations in support of the "30 baht" scheme. Jon Ungphakorn, a senator in the Thai parliament, brought together 11 nongovernmental organizations to campaign for equity in healthcare coverage and financial protection for all. Five members of civil society also held seats on the parliamentary commission to review drafts of the universal health coverage bill, giving them influence over policy design.

When the Thai Rak Thai party won the 2001 general election, they immediately began to roll out their proposed healthcare plan, formally called the Universal Coverage Scheme (UCS). Senior advisers at WHO and the World Bank recommended implementing the plan gradually. However, Thai leaders believed that rapid implementation would bolster confidence in their leadership. Thus, despite the Thai leaders' caution—especially regarding budget execution—they began a rapid course of action to implement the UCS.

Thai government leaders initially planned to combine resources from four different health coverage schemes in order to fund the UCS: the Medical Welfare Scheme (MWS), Health Card Scheme (HCS), Social Security Scheme (SSS), and Civil Servants Medical Benefits Scheme (CSMBS). However, the departments responsible for these schemes resisted the merger—particularly the civil servants and trade unionists who benefited from the employment-based CSMBS and SSS. The implementers were able to circumvent this resistance by pooling resources from only the MWS and HCS schemes, which provide financial support for the poor and near-poor. With funding secured, the National Health Security Act passed in 2002, and the UCS was ready to be set in motion.

The Thai government began piloting the UCS in six districts in mid-2001, and by mid-2002, almost all districts in Thailand had introduced the scheme. Every citizen was eligible to participate in the program. The UCS covered approximately 18 million additional individuals less than a year after its rollout. By 2011, the program covered 48 million Thais and their families, and the uninsured rate dropped to 2 percent.

People enrolled in the UCS by registering at a district health center. Upon registration, they received a gold card that covered free care at local health centers and referrals to tertiary-care hospitals in cities. In its initial stages, the UCS covered a comprehensive set of benefits, including outpatient and inpatient care, accident and emergency services, dental care, diagnostics, medicines, and medical supplies. The UCS has also supported preventive services at clinics and health promotion programs at health centers. The UCS has since expanded its package of benefits by using an ethical decision-making process that considers equity and cost-effectiveness in determining which additional services should be covered.

In order to maintain accountability with healthcare providers, the government separated oversight of the provider and purchaser responsibilities between two distinct departments. The Ministry of Public Health provided health services, while the National Health Scrutiny Office (NHSO)—a new, independent government agency—managed purchasing of health services through the UCS.

Impact

The UCS successfully reduced financial risk, increased access to care, and even contributed to improvements in infant mortality and the health of young women. The proportion of households that fall into poverty due to expenditure on medicine and health care annually decreased from 2.7 percent in 2000 to below 0.5 percent in 2009.

Although it is difficult to measure the impact of the UCS on health outcomes, several studies suggest a correlation between the UCS implementation and improvements across various health indicators. One study found that UCS reduced infant mortality to a greater extent among poor UCS beneficiaries than among wealthier individuals already insured through their employer. Another found that exposure to the UCS was correlated with minimized risk of missing work due to illness.

Costs

Thailand has achieved universal health coverage at a slightly lower expenditure relative to GDP than similar upper middle-income countries. From 2001 to 2008, the government expenditure on health increased from the equivalent of $3.6 billion to $7.6 billion. The UCS budget itself increased from the equivalent of $35 per person to $80 per person between 2002 and 2012.

The UCS was funded mostly through general income taxes, although users were initially expected to pay a BHT30 copay for each visit to health services. The BHT30 copayment was eventually eliminated because the costs of collecting the copayments exceeded the revenue these payments generated.

Lessons Learned

Strong and committed leadership was a key factor in the success of the UCS. The Thai Rak Thai held their 2001 election promise to deliver universal health coverage to their constituents, and leaders who pushed for the scheme remained in key leadership positions post-election. These leaders continued to work with the same dedication to get politicians and citizens to support the UCS. The benefits of the UCS helped the Thai Rak Thai remain popular and sustain power for several years.

Also essential to the success of the UCS was the ethical, evidence-based decision-making mechanism the Thai government used to determine which services and technologies the scheme would cover. Partly in response to the large increase in public health spending, the Thai government established the Health Intervention and Technology Assessment Program (HITAP). The agency uses cost-effectiveness, equity, and other feasibility considerations to determine which items should be covered under the UCS. HITAP allowed the Thai government to transparently evaluate which additional benefits it would include as the UCS package expanded.

The UCS benefited from many other factors that created the conditions necessary for its swift rollout. For example, Thai reformers incorporated lessons learned from previous public schemes in creating the UCS structure. Investments in the health system infrastructure prior to UCS rollout also helped pave the way for the scheme's success. Thailand's experience demonstrates that with careful decision making, low- and middle-income countries can achieve universal health coverage.

▶ Main Messages

A health system is "the combination of resources, organization, and management that culminate in the delivery of health services to the population."[2(p31)] The goal of every health system, in principle, should be universal health coverage. This means that every person in a country should have access to a package of healthcare services that is coupled with an insurance program that protects them from suffering financial hardship as a result of the costs of those services. An increasing number of countries, including low-income countries, are making progress toward UHC.

WHO recommends that countries seek to achieve UHC in a progressive manner. Countries with the least developed health systems, for example, could start by covering as much of their population as possible with a package of essential services. Over time, the country could implement an expanded package of services. Ultimately, each country, of course, aspires to offer all of its people an extensive package of services like that in today's high-income countries, such as France and Norway, and to link it with an insurance scheme that protects people from financial hardship and minimizes out-of-pocket costs. As countries expand toward UHC, they should pay particular attention to the needs of their poor and marginalized populations.

The main functions of a health system are to raise money for health services, provide health services, pay for health services, and engage in governance and regulation of health activities. In line with this, health systems provide prevention, diagnosis, treatment, and rehabilitative services; protect the sick and their families against the cost of ill health; and carry out key public health functions, such as surveillance, the operation of public health laboratories, and food and drug regulation. Health systems are important parts of all economies.

Health systems have three levels of health care: primary, secondary, and tertiary. Depending on the country, the public, private, and nongovernmental sectors participate in different parts of the health system. A critical issue in the design of health systems is the roles that each of these sectors should play. There is agreement that governments must regulate and provide oversight of the health system. However, there is also a growing view that the government does not need to provide all services but should instead consider how they might most effectively be provided, which could mean government contracting the private or NGO sectors for some services.

The notion of primary health care, as developed at the Alma-Ata Conference in 1978, and confirmed at a global conference in 2018, remains very important. Many countries continue to try to provide essential and socially acceptable health services close to the people who need them most. They also seek to embody preventive, promotive, curative, and rehabilitative services in their primary healthcare programs and to link them with higher levels of the health system. Achieving such programs, however, has remained a challenge for many countries, especially low-income countries.

Health systems reflect the unique history and culture of each country. They are also diverse, complex, and very difficult to categorize. One very simplified approach to thinking about health systems, however, considers those that are based on a national health service model, like the United Kingdom; those that have social health insurance programs, such as Canada,

Japan, and Germany; and those that have pluralistic systems, like the United States, India, or Nigeria. When thinking about different approaches to health systems, it is valuable to consider the roles different actors play in the regulation, financing, and provision of services. It is also important to consider the extent to which these systems offer financial protection through insurance, how such insurance is organized, and how insurance is financed.

Countries spend a wide range of their GDP on health, from about 3 percent in South Sudan to about 17 percent in the United States. Most of the high-income countries have health systems that provide a universal package of insured health benefits. In low-income countries that lack national health insurance, most expenditure on health is private and out of pocket. In general, the health systems of high-income countries are more effective at meeting health system aims than are the systems in low- and middle-income countries.

The health systems of all countries, but especially those in low- and middle-income countries, face a number of important challenges:

- How to cope with an aging population and increasing prevalence of noncommunicable disease
- Quality of governance
- Number, quality, and distribution of healthcare personnel
- Mobilization of sufficient financial resources for the health sector
- How to provide health care at an appropriate level of quality
- How to ensure access to and equitable provision of services
- Creation of mechanisms to provide the poor with protection from the costs of health services

Governance is a difficult issue to address because governance issues are generally problems across all sectors, not just the health sector. Nonetheless, by giving communities more control over health sector resources, having them openly monitor their use, enhancing the capacity of the health sector to engage in procurement functions, and contracting out services that can most effectively and efficiently be delivered by the private or NGO sectors, governance can be improved.

Ensuring that countries have the right number of trained health personnel in the right places will continue to be difficult. However, there is evidence that different kinds of incentives, such as housing, additional pay, and greater access to training, can encourage health personnel to serve in underserved areas. The productivity of health providers can also be encouraged through appropriate incentives.

It will continue to be difficult for low-income countries to raise the resources they need to finance a cost-effective package of health services. However, given the potential returns on investments in health, even very poor countries must consider allocating a larger share of their overall resources to health. In addition, existing expenditure on health is very inefficient in many countries, and some financial savings can be generated from improving the efficiency of existing expenditure and by allocating a higher share of resources to areas that will yield the highest returns.

The quality of services can and must be improved, even in low-income settings, and countries must make this a central concern. The lack of quality is both a waste of resources and a danger to people's health and well-being. Accreditation of services is potentially promising, but not yet a proven way of improving health outcomes. Oversight by senior health staff in structured ways has improved outcomes in some settings. Providing health personnel with clear guidelines, protocols, and algorithms for treatment of patients can also improve the quality of care. There is also increasing evidence that total quality management activities can improve health outcomes, even in very low-income settings. Efforts at improving quality through results-based financing are also becoming more prominent.

Greater attention needs to be paid in most countries to enhancing health system coverage of poor and marginalized populations. One way to do this is to engage these communities in the planning and design of health system interventions. Improving services for the poor and ensuring that these services do not hurt families financially will also require that greater attention be paid to various insurance schemes.

In addition, low- and middle-income countries can help enhance the health of their poor by moving in the previously noted directions, achieving universal health coverage, and then focusing expenditure on a package of services that at relatively low cost will have the highest impact on preventing illness among the poor and on treating the illnesses that most affect them:

- Promoting access to safe water and enhanced sanitation and encouraging improved hygiene
- Enhancing people's eating habits and providing selective nutrition supplementation
- Providing a basic package of reproductive health services, including emergency obstetric care
- Providing a basic package of neonatal health services
- Vaccinating and deworming young children, providing oral rehydration for diarrhea, and treating pneumonia and malaria in a timely and appropriate way
- Preventing and treating, as appropriate, HIV/AIDS, TB, and malaria
- Preventing tobacco use and reducing salt consumption
- Treating hypertension and high cholesterol, aspirin for heart attacks, and community-based mental health services

Study Questions

1. What is the meaning of universal health coverage?
2. What are the primary functions of a health system?
3. What are primary, secondary, and tertiary health care, and what services are generally rendered at each level?
4. How might one compare and contrast the organization of the healthcare systems of the United Kingdom, Germany, and the United States?
5. What proportion of their GDP do countries generally spend on health? Why is there such a wide range?
6. Which types of countries tend to have a larger share of private expenditure on health than public expenditure on health? Why is this so, compared to countries that have health systems that are mostly publicly funded?
7. What are some of the significant issues that arise in trying to govern health systems in low- and middle-income countries?
8. What are some of the key human resource challenges that low- and middle-income countries face in staffing and operating their health systems?
9. What are the most important epidemiologic and demographic issues that face health systems, and what are the implications of these issues for healthcare costs?
10. What are some of the most important steps that can be taken to improve the effectiveness and efficiency of weaker health systems in low- and middle-income countries?

References

1. WHO. (n.d.). *Q&As: Health systems.* Retrieved from https://www.who.int/topics/health_systems/qa/en/.

2. Roemer, M. (1991). *National health systems of the world* (Vol. 1: The Countries). Oxford, UK: Oxford University Press.

3. Roberts, M. J., Hsiao, W., Berman, P., & Reich, M. R. (2004). *Getting health reform right: A guide to improving performance and equity.* New York, NY: Oxford University Press.

4. World Health Organization (WHO). (2000). *The world health report 2000.* Geneva, Switzerland: Author.

5. World Health Organization (WHO). (2000). *Overview: The world health report 2000.* Geneva, Switzerland: Author.

6. Southby, R. (2004). *Health system organization.* Presented at George Washington University, Washington, DC.

7. World Health Organization (WHO). (2007). *Everybody's business: Strengthening health systems to improve health outcomes: WHO's framework for action.* Geneva, Switzerland: Author.

8. Birn, A.-E., Pillay, Y., & Holtz, T. H. (2009). *Textbook of international health.* New York, NY: Oxford University Press.

9. World Health Organization (WHO). (1978). *Declaration of Alma-Ata.* International Conference on Primary Health Care, September 6–12, 1978, Alma-Ata, USSR. Geneva, Switzerland: Author.

10. Global Conference on Primary Health Care. (2018). *Declaration of Astana.* Retrieved from https://www.who.int/docs/default-source/primary-health/declaration/gcphc-declaration.pdf

11. Bloom, G., Champion, C., Lucas, H., Rahman, M. H., Bhuiya, A., Oladepo, O., & Peters, D. (2008). Health markets and future health systems: innovation for equity. *Global forum update on research for health, 5,* 30–33.

12. United Nations Civil Society Unit (n.d.). *United Nations: Definitions and terms.* Retrieved from https://www.apa.org/international/united-nations/acronyms.pdf

13. The World Bank. (2003). *Afghanistan health sector and emergency reconstruction and development project.* Washington, DC: Author.

14. The World Bank. (1995). *Bangladesh integrated nutrition project.* Washington, DC: Author.

15. The World Bank. (n.d.). *Data: Current health expenditure (% of GDP).* Retrieved from https://data.worldbank.org/indicator/SH.XPD.CHEX.GD.ZS

16. World Health Organization (WHO). (2014). *Health financing for universal coverage.* Retrieved from http://www.who.int/health_financing/universal_coverage_definition/en/

17. Sen, A. (2015, January 6). Universal healthcare: The affordable dream. *The Guardian.* Retrieved from http://www.theguardian.com/society/2015/jan/06/-sp-universal-healthcare-the-affordable-dream-amartya-sen

18. World Health Organization (WHO). (2014). *What is universal health coverage?* Retrieved from http://www.who.int/features/qa/universal_health_coverage/en/

19. World Health Organization (WHO). (2010). *World health report 2010.* Geneva, Switzerland: Author.

20. Langomarsino, G., Gabarant, A., Adyas, A., Muga, R., & Otoo, N. (2012, September 8). Moving towards universal health coverage: Health insurance reforms in nine developing countries in Africa and Asia. *The Lancet, 380,* 933–943.

21. Tangcharoensathien, V., Patcharanarumol, W., Ir, P., Aljunid, S. M., Mukti, A. G., Akkhavong, K., . . . Mills, A. (2011, January 25). Health-financing reforms in southeast Asia: Challenges in achieving universal coverage. *The Lancet, 377,* 863–873.

22. Kumar, A. K. S., Chen, L. C., Choudhury, M., Ganju, S., Mahajan, V., Sinha, A., & Sen, A. (2011, January 12). India: Towards universal health coverage 6—Financing health care for all: Challenges and opportunities. *The Lancet, 377,* 668–679.

23. Atun, R., de Andrade, L. O., Almeida, G., Cotlear, D., Dmytraczenko, T., Frenz, P., . . . Wagstaff, A. (2014, October 16). Universal health coverage in Latin America 1—Health-system reform and universal coverage in Latin America. *The Lancet.* doi: 10.1016/S0140-6736(14)61646-9

24. Reich, M. R., Harris, J., Ikegami, N., Maeda, A., Cashin, C., Araujo, E. C., . . . Evans, T. G. (2016). Moving towards universal health coverage: Lessons from 11 country studies. *The Lancet, 387,* 811–816.

25. Basch, P. (2001). *Textbook of international health* (2nd ed.). New York, NY: Oxford University Press.

26. Health Care Online. (2015). *Health care in Germany: The German health care system.* Retrieved from https://www.ncbi.nlm.nih.gov/pubmedhealth/PMH0078019/

27. Blumel, M., & Busse, R. (2016). International health care system profiles. The German health care system. *The Commonwealth Fund.* Retrieved from https://international.commonwealthfund.org/countries/germany/

28. Expatica. (2019). *The German health care system: A guide to healthcare in Germany.* Retrieved from https://www.expatica.com/de/healthcare/Your-guide-to-the-German-healthcare-system_103359.html

29. Blumel, M. (2013). The German health care system, 2013. In S. Thomson, R. Osborn, D. Squires, & M. Jun (Eds.), *International profiles of health care systems, 2013* (pp. 57–66). New York, NY: The Commonwealth Fund.

30. NHS Improvement. (n.d.). *Who we are.* Retrieved from https://improvement.nhs.uk/about-us/who-we-are/

31. Tunstall, L. (n.d.). The UK health care system. *Evidence-Network.* Retrieved from https://evidencenetwork.ca/the-uk-health-care-system/

32. NHS Clinical Commissioners. (n.d.). About CCGs. Retrieved from https://www.nhscc.org/ccgs/

33. Harrison, A. (2013). The English health care system, 2013. In S. Thomson, R. Osborn, D. Squires, & M. Jun (Eds.), *International profiles of health care systems, 2013* (pp. 37–45). New York, NY: The Commonwealth Fund.

34. Smith, P. C. (2018). Advancing universal health coverage: What countries can learn from the English experience. *Universal Health Coverage Series, 40,* 10. Washington, DC: The World Bank.

35. Index Mundi. (n.d.). *Health expenditure per capita (current US$).* Retrieved from https://www.indexmundi.com/facts/indicators/SH.XPD.PCAP

36. The World Bank. (n.d.). *Data: Life expectancy at birth, total (years).* Retrieved from https://data.worldbank.org/indicator/sp.dyn.le00.in

37. The Commonwealth Fund. (n.d.). *The U.S. healthcare system.* Retrieved from https://international.commonwealthfund.org/countries/united_states/

38. The Commonwealth Fund. (2013). The U.S. health care system, 2013. In S. Thomson, R. Osborn, D. Squires, & M. Jun (Eds.), *International profiles of health care systems, 2013* (pp. 128–135). New York, NY: Author.

39. Kalorama Information. (2017). *Out of pocket health care expenditures in the United States.* Retrieved from https://www.kaloramainformation.com/Pocket-Healthcare-Expenditures-10781903/

40. Torres, F. M. (2013). *Costa Rica case study: Primary health care achievements and challenges in the framework of social health insurance.* Washington, DC: The World Bank.

41. Saenz, M. dR., Bermudez, J. L., & Acosta, M. (2010). *Universal coverage in a middle-income country: Costa Rica.* Geneva, Switzerland: World Health Organization.

42. Organization for Economic Cooperation and Development (OECD). (2017). *OECD reviews of health systems: Costa Rica 2017.* Paris, France: Author.

43. The World Bank. (n.d.). *Data: Domestic private health expenditure (% of current health expenditure).* Retrieved from https://data.worldbank.org/indicator/SH.XPD.PVTD.CH.ZS

44. Swedish Agency for Growth Policy Analysis. (2013). *India's healthcare system—Overview and quality improvement.* Stockholm, Sweden: Author.

45. Gupta, I., & Bhatia, M. (2017). The India healthcare system. In E. Mossialos, A. Djordjevic, R. Osborn, & D. Sarnak (Eds.), *International profiles of health care systems* (pp. 77-84). New York, NY: The Commonwealth Fund.

46. Abraham, R. (2018, February 2). What is "Modicare" and how will it affect you? *The Hindu.* Retrieved from https://www.thehindu.com/business/budget/what-is-modicare-and-how-will-it-affect-you/article22635372.ece

47. Saleh, K. (2013). *The health sector in Ghana.* Washington, DC: The World Bank.

48. Gajate-Garrido, G., & Owusua, R. (2013). *The national health insurance scheme in Ghana.* Washington, DC: IFPRI.

49. Wang, H. H., Otoo, N., & Dsane-Selby, L. (2017). *Ghana national health insurance scheme: Improving financial sustainability based on expenditure review.* Washington, DC: The World Bank.

50. Haruna, U., & Sugiri, M. A. (2018). Ghana. In J. Johnson, C. Stoskopf, & L. Shi (Eds.), *Comparative health Systems: A global perspective* (2nd ed., pp. 335–352). Burlington, MA: Jones & Bartlett.

51. Mathers, C. D., Lopez, A. D., & Murray, C. J. L. (2006). The burden of disease and mortality by condition: Data, methods, and results for 2001. In A. D. Lopez, C. D. Mathers, M. Ezzati, D. T. Jamison, & C. J. L. Murray (Eds.), *Global burden of disease and risk factors* (pp. 45–93). New York, NY: Oxford University Press.

52. Lewis, M. (2006). *Tackling healthcare corruption and governance woes in developing countries* (Working Paper 78). Washington, DC: Center for Global Development.

53. Physicians for Human Rights. (2004). *An action plan to prevent brain drain: Building equitable health systems in Africa.* Retrieved from http://physiciansforhumanrights.org/library/reports/action-plan-to-prevent-brain-drain-africa-2004.html

54. Hongoro, C., & Normand, C. (2006). Health workers: Building and motivating the workforce. In D. T. Jamison, J. G. Breman, A. R. Measham, et al. (Eds.), *Disease control priorities in developing countries* (2nd ed., pp. 1309–1322). New York, NY: Oxford University Press.

55. Institute of Medicine (IOM). (1999). *Measuring the quality of health care.* Washington, DC: Author.

56. Peabody, J. W., Taguiwalo, M. M., Robalino, D. A., & Frenk, J. (2006). Improving the quality of care in developing countries. In D. T. Jamison, J. G. Breman, A. R. Measham, et al. (Eds.), *Disease control priorities in developing countries* (2nd ed., pp. 1293–1307). New York, NY: Oxford University Press.

57. Beracochea, E., Dickenson, R., Freemand, P., & Thomason, J. (1995). Case management quality assessment in rural areas of Papua New Guinea. *Tropical Doctor, 25*(2), 69–74.

58. Thaver, I. H., Harpham, T., McPake, B., & Garner, P. (1998). Private practitioners in the slums of Karachi: What quality of care do they offer? *Social Science & Medicine, 46*(11), 1441–1449.

59. Nolan, T., Angos, P., Cunha, A. J., Muhe, L., Qazi, S., Simoes, E. A., . . . Pierce, N. F. (2001). Quality of hospital care for seriously ill children in less-developed countries. *The Lancet, 357*(9250), 106–110.

60. Mohanan, M., Vera-Hernandez, M., Das, V., Giardili, S., Goldhaber-Fiebert, J. D., Rabin, T., Raj, S. S., . . . Seth, A. (2015). The know-do gap in quality of health care for childhood diarrhea and pneumonia in rural India. *JAMA Pediatrics, 169*(4), 349–357.

61. Kruk, M. A., Gage, A. D., Joseph, N. T., Danaei, G., García-Saisó, S., & Salomon, J. A. (2018). Mortality due to low-quality health systems in the universal health coverage era: A systematic analysis of amenable deaths in 137 countries. *The Lancet, 392*(10160), 2203–2212. doi: 10.1016/S0140-6736(18)31668-4

62. Macarayan, E. K., Gage, A. D., Doubova, S. V., Guanais, F., Lemango, E. T., Ndiaye, Y., . . . Kruk, M. E. (2018). Assessment of quality of primary care with facility surveys: A descriptive analysis in ten low-income and middle-income countries. *The Lancet Global Health, 6*(11), e1176–e1185.

63. Kieny, M.-P., Evans, T. G., Scarpetta, S., Kelley, E. T., Klazinga, N., Firde, I., . . . Donaldson, L. (2018). *Delivering quality health services: A global imperative for universal health coverage.* Washington, DC: World Bank Group.

64. Peters, D. H., Preker, A. S., Yazbek, A. S., Sharma, R. R., Ramana, G. N. V., Pritchett, L. H., Wagstaff, A. (2002). *Better health systems for India's poor.* Washington, DC: The World Bank.

65. Lagarde, M., & Palmer, N. (2011). *The impact of user fees on access to health services in low- and middle-income countries* (Review). Hoboken, NJ: The Cochrane Collaboration.

66. Jha, P., Chaloupka, F. J., Moore, J., Gajalakshmi, V., Gupta, P. C., Peck, R., . . . Zatonski, W. (2006). Tobacco addiction. In D. T. Jamison, J. G. Breman, A. R. Measham, et al. (Eds.), *Disease control priorities in developing countries* (2nd ed., pp. 869–885). New York, NY: Oxford University Press.

67. Norton, R., Hyder, A. A., Bishai, D., & Peden, M. (2006). Unintentional injuries. In D. T. Jamison, J. G. Breman, A. R. Measham, et al. (Eds.), *Disease control priorities in developing countries* (2nd ed., pp. 737–753). New York, NY: Oxford University Press.

68. Samb, B., Desai, N., Nishtar, S., Mendis, S., Bekedam, H., Wright, A., . . . Etienne, C. (2010). Prevention and management of chronic disease: A litmus test for health-systems strengthening in low-income and middle-income countries. *The Lancet, 376,* 1785–1797.

69. Joint Learning Initiative. (2004). *Human resources for health: Overcoming the crisis.* Cambridge, MA: Author.

70. Resch, S., Ryckman, T., & Hecht, R. (2015). Funding AIDS programmes in the era of shared responsibility: An analysis of domestic spending in 12 low-income and middle-income countries. *The Lancet Global Health, 3,* e52–e61.

71. Jamison, D. T., Breman, J. G., Measham, A. R., Alleyne, G., Claeson, M., Evans, D. B., . . . Musgrove, P. (Eds.). (2006). *Priorities in health*. Washington, DC: The World Bank.

72. Jamison, D.T., Gelband, H., Horton, S., Jha, P., Laxminarayan, R., Mock, C. N., & Nugent, R. (Eds.). (2018). *Disease control priorities: Improving health and reducing poverty* (3rd ed., Vol. 9). Washington, DC: The World Bank.

73. World Health Organization (WHO). (2014). *Making fair choices on the path to universal health coverage*. Geneva, Switzerland: Author.

74. USAID. (n.d.). *Demographic and health surveys*. Retrieved from http://dhsprogram.com/

75. Kruk, M. E, Gage, A. D., Arsenault, C., Jordan, K., Leslier, H. H., Roder-DeWan, S., . . . Pate, M. (2018). High-quality health systems in the Sustainable Development Goals era: Time for a revolution. *The Lancet Global Health*, 6(11), e1196–e1252. doi: 10.1016/S2214-109X(18)30386-3

76. Peabody, J. W., Taguiwalo, M. M., Robalino, D. A., & Frenk, J. (2006). Improving the quality of care in developing countries. In D. T. Jamison, J. G. Breman, A. R. Measham, et al. (Eds.), *Disease control priorities in developing countries* (2nd ed., pp. 1293–1307). New York, NY: Oxford University Press.

77. Tollman, S., Doherty, J., & Mulligan, J.-A. (2006). General primary care. In D. T. Jamison, J. G. Breman, A. R. Measham, et al. (Eds.), *Disease control priorities in developing countries* (2nd ed., pp. 1193–1210). New York, NY: Oxford University Press.

78. Sepulveda, J., Bustreo, F., Tapia, R., Rivera, J., Lozano, R., Oláiz, G., . . . Valdespino, J. L. (2006). The improvement of child survival in Mexico: The diagonal approach. *The Lancet*, 368(9551), 2017–2027.

79. Lu, Y., Hernandez, P., Abegunde, D., & Edejer, T. (2011). *The world medicines situation 2011*. Geneva, Switzerland: World Health Organization. Retrieved from http://www.who.int/health-accounts/documentation/world_medicine_situation.pdf

80. World Health Organization (WHO). (2012). *The pursuit of responsible use medicines: Sharing and learning from country experiences*. Retrieved from http://apps.who.int/iris/bitstream/10665/75828/1/WHO_EMP_MAR_2012.3_eng.pdf?ua=1

81. World Health Organization (WHO). (2017). *The selection and use of essential medicines: Report of the WHO Expert Committee, 2017 (including the 20th WHO model list of essential medicines and the 6th WHO model list of essential medicines for children)* (WHO Technical Report Series no. 1006). Geneva, Switzerland: Author. Retrieved from http://apps.who.int/iris/bitstream/handle/10665/259481/9789241210157-eng.pdf?sequence=1

82. World Health Organization (WHO). (2010). *Growing threat from counterfeit medications*. Retrieved from http://www.who.int/bulletin/volumes/88/4/10-020410/en/

83. World Health Organization (WHO). (2018). *Substandard and falsified medical products*. Retrieved from http://www.who.int/mediacentre/factsheets/fs275/en/

84. Cockburn, R., Newton, P. N., Agyarko, E. K., Akunyili, D., & White, N. J. (2005). The global threat of counterfeit drugs: Why industry and governments must communicate the dangers. *PLOS Medicine*. Retrieved from http://journals.plos.org/plosmedicine/article?id=10.1371/journal.pmed.0020100

85. Ozawa, S., Evans, D. R., Bessias, S., Haynie, D. G., Yemeke, T. T., Laing, S. K., & Herrington, J. E. (2018). Prevalence and estimated economic burden of substandard and falsified medicines in low- and middle-income countries: A systematic review and meta-analysis. *JAMA Network Open*, 1(4), e181662. doi: 10.1001/jamanetworkopen.2018.1662

86. World Health Organization (WHO). (2017). *WHO global surveillance and monitoring system for substandard and falsified medical products*. Geneva, Switzerland: Author.

87. World Health Organization (WHO). (n.d.). *WHO global surveillance and monitoring system*. Retrieved from http://www.who.int/medicines/regulation/ssffc/surveillance/en/

88. Fight the Fakes. (n.d.). Homepage. Retrieved from http://fightthefakes.org/

89. Fight the Fakes Campaign. (2014). *Fight the Fakes Campaign joint statement*. Retrieved from http://fightthefakes.org/wp-content/uploads/2014/06/Joint-statement-_Fight-the-Fakes-Campaign-06022014.pdf

90. Adams, C.P., & Brantner, V.V. (2006). Estimating The Cost Of New Drug Development: Is It Really $802 Million? *Health Affairs*. Retrieved from https://www.healthaffairs.org/doi/full/10.1377/hlthaff.25.2.420

91. Hoen, E. (2009). *The global politics of pharmaceutical monopoly power: Drug patents, access, innovation, and the application of the WTO Doha Declaration on TRIPS and public health*. Diemen, The Netherlands: AMB.

92. Moon, S., Jambert, E., Childs, M., & von Schoen-Angerer, T. (2011). A win-win solution? A critical analysis of tiered pricing to improve access to medicines in developing countries. *Globalization and Health*, 7, 39.

93. STOP TB Partnership. (2015). *What is the GDF?* Retrieved from http://www.stoptb.org/gdf/whatis/default.asp

94. The Global Fund. (2015). *Updated guide to global fund policies on procurement and supply management of health products*. Retrieved from https://www.theglobalfund.org/en/sourcing-management/updates/2019-02-05-updated-guide-to-global-fund-policies-on-procurement-and-supply-management/

95. Management Sciences for Health. (n.d.). *Supply chain management system*. Retrieved from https://www.msh.org/our-work/projects/supply-chain-management-system

96. Unitaid. (n.d.). *About us*. Retrieved from http://www.unitaid.eu/en/who/about-unitaid

97. Clinton Health Access Initiative. (2015). *About CHAI*. Retrieved from http://www.clintonhealthaccess.org/about

98. Doha WTO Ministerial. (2001). *Declaration on the TRIPS agreement and public health*. Retrieved from https://www.wto.org/english/thewto_e/minist_e/min01_e/mindecl_trips_e.htm

99. Savoie, B. (2007). Thailand's test: Compulsory licensing in an era of epidemiologic transition. *Virginia Journal of International Law*, 48, 212–246.

100. Beall, R., & Kuhn, R. (2012). Trends in compulsory licensing of pharmaceuticals since the Doha declaration: A database analysis. *PLOS Medicine*, 9(1), e1001154. Retrieved from http://journals.plos.org/plosmedicine/article?id=10.1371/journal.pmed.1001154

101. Raja, S., & Mohammad, N. (2005). *National HIV/AIDS programs: A handbook on supply chain management for HIV/AIDS medical commodities*. Washington, DC: The World Bank.

102. Centers for Disease Control and Prevention (CDC). (2012). *Appendix C: Vaccine storage & handling.* Retrieved from http://www.cdc.gov/vaccines/pubs/pinkbook/downloads /appendices/appdx-full-c.pdf

103. Coca-Cola Company. (2012). *coca-cola and the global fund announce partnership to help bring critical medicines to remote regions.* Retrieved from https://www .coca-colacompany.com/press-center/press-releases/coca -cola-and-the-global-fund-announce-partnership-to-help -bring-critical-medicines-to-remote-regions

104. Coca-Cola Company. (2014). *"Project Last Mile" expands to improve availability of life-saving medications in additional regions of Africa.* Retrieved from http://www.coca -colacompany.com/press-center/press-releases/% 20project-last-mile-expands-in-africa

105. World Health Organization (WHO). (2012). *The pursuit of responsible use medicines: Sharing and learning from country experiences.* Retrieved from http://apps.who.int /iris/bitstream/10665/75828/1/WHO_EMP_MAR_2012.3 _eng.pdf?ua=1

106. So, A., & Woodhouse, W. (2014). Thailand's antibiotic smart use initiative. In *Alliance for Health Policy and Systems Research Flagship Report 2014: Medicines in health systems: Advancing access, affordability and appropriate use.* Retrieved from http://www.who.int/alliance-hpsr/resources/FR_Ch5 _Annex3a.pdf

107. Jamison, D.T., Gelband, H., Horton, S., Jha, P., Laxminarayan, R., Mock, C. N., & Nugent, R. (Eds.). (2018). *Disease control priorities* (3rd ed., Vol. 9). Washington, DC: The World Bank.

108. Mock, C. N., Donkor, P., Gawande, A., Jamison, D. T., Kruk, M. E., & Debas, H. T. for the DCP3 Essential Surgery Author Group. (2015). Essential surgery: Key messages from *Disease Control Priorities (3rd ed.). The Lancet, 385,* 2209–2219.

109. This case is based on Glassman, A., Temin, M., & the Millions Saved Team and Advisory Group. (2016). Motivating health workers, motivating better health: Rwanda's pay-for-performance scheme for health services. In *Millions saved* (pp. 13–22). Washington, DC: Center for Global Development. Those interested in a more complete account of the case and additional references will want to read the case in *Millions Saved.*

110. This case is based on Glassman, A., Temin, M., & the Millions Saved Team and Advisory Group. (2016). Health access for all: Thailand's universal health coverage scheme. In *Millions saved* (pp. 89–96). Washington, DC: Center for Global Development. Those interested in a more complete account of the case and additional references will want to read the case in *Millions Saved.*

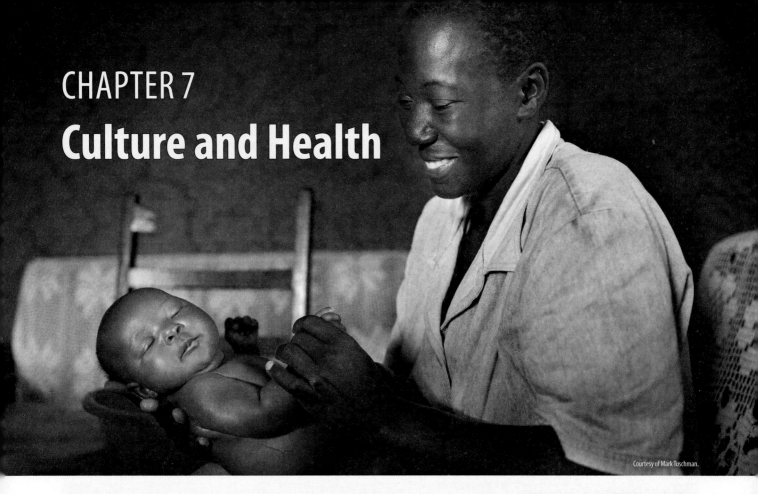

CHAPTER 7
Culture and Health

Courtesy of Mark Tuschman.

▶ Vignettes

Joshua was 1 year old and lived in eastern Zimbabwe. His mother could tell that he had a fever. She wondered what caused it. Was it the food that he ate? Was it the mixing of the "hot" foods and the "cold" foods? Or, did they do something to offend local custom? If the fever did not get better by the next day, then she would take Joshua to the local healer.

Siu-Hong was 80 years old and lived in Hong Kong. He had a severe toothache for more than a week. His children repeatedly encouraged him to go to the dentist, but he would not go. He did not like dentists or "Western medicine." In addition, he would

have to wait in line to be seen at the dentist's office and would miss work at the clothes market. His children finally convinced him to go to the dentist by giving him a present of $25 and offering to take him to "dim sum," the traditional South Chinese brunch.

Dorji lived in Bhutan, just outside the capital city of Thimpu. He felt tired, weak, and dizzy for some time but had no fever. After another week of feeling this way, Dorji went to visit his local health clinic. Each clinic in Bhutan had two medical practitioners, one who practiced the indigenous system of medicine and the other who practiced "Western biomedical medicine."[1] In light of Dorji's symptoms, he visited the indigenous practitioner inside the clinic. The "doctor" gave him some herbs that he thought would help his condition. However, he also thought Dorji had an underlying infection and took him across the hall to the "other doctor," who prescribed antibiotics for him.

Arathi was a young mother in southeast India. She and the other women in her village were participating in the Tamil Nadu Nutrition Project. They were all young mothers, many of whose babies were underweight for their age. Arathi nursed her baby as she had learned to do from her mother and grandmother. She also gave the baby some other foods as she had learned from them. Despite this, her baby was quite small for her age. As part of the project, the community nutrition workers taught all the women and children in the village songs about proper feeding and about the vitamins the children needed. They also sponsored weekly "weighing parties," in which all of the babies of the village were weighed and the mothers together decided if the baby was growing properly and what could be done to make the baby healthier. They also helped the mothers make a food supplement for the babies who were "too small."

▶ The Importance of Culture to Health

Culture is an important determinant of health in a number of ways. First, culture is related to health behaviors. People's attitudes toward foods and what they eat, for example, are closely related to culture. The food that pregnant women eat, birthing practices, and how long women breastfeed their children are also linked to their cultural backgrounds. Hygiene practices are closely tied to culture as well. Second, culture is an important determinant of people's perceptions of illness. Different cultural groups may have different beliefs about what constitutes good health and what constitutes illness. Third, the extent to which people use health services is also very closely linked with culture. Some groups may use health services as soon as they feel ill. Others, however, may visit health practitioners only when they feel very sick. Fourth, different cultures have different practices concerning health and medical treatment. Chinese and Indian cultures

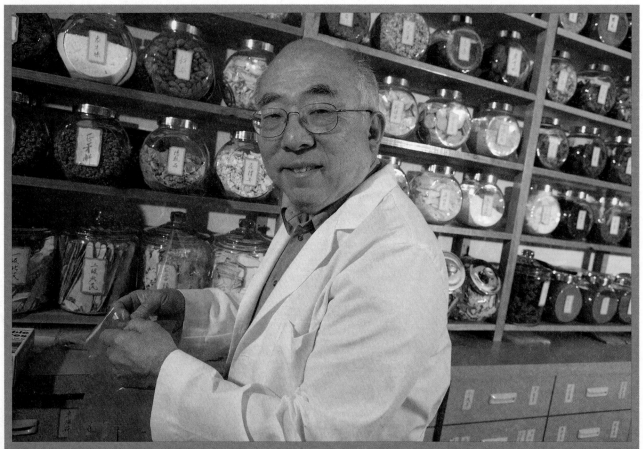

PHOTO 7-1 China has a well-articulated system of "traditional medicine," reflected in this Chinese medicine shop. What is the extent to which people use traditional medicines in cultures with which you are familiar? From whom do they get them?
© Barry Austin/Photodisc/Getty Images.

have well-defined indigenous systems of medicine. There is a long history of local systems of medicine that include notions of illness, various types of practitioners, and different kinds of medicines in many other societies as well.

The purpose of this chapter is to introduce you to the most important links between health and culture, particularly as they relate to global health and people in low- and middle-income countries. The chapter begins by introducing you to the concept of culture. It then examines how views of health, illness, the use of health services, and the role of different health providers vary by culture. The chapter also reviews some of the theories of behavior change that relate to enhancing people's health. The chapter concludes with three case studies that reflect some of the critical relationships between culture and health and how they need to be taken into account in efforts to improve health. This chapter is based on the premise that understanding and addressing health issues requires an understanding of the deep relationship between culture and health in different settings and among different culture groups.

As you review this chapter, it is also important to note that some cultural values enhance health and others do not enhance health. A culture, for example, that puts a strong emphasis on monogamy in marriage should have lower rates of HIV/AIDS than cultures in which having concurrent sexual partners is more tolerated. However, a cultural preference for heaviness in people as a sign of prosperity or wealth, for example, may be harmful to health because it would increase the risk of cardiovascular disease and diabetes. Some cultures have taboos against pregnant women eating certain foods, therefore preventing them from getting all of the nutrients they need. This chapter aims to help you understand the relationship between culture and health, identify practices that are helpful or hurtful to good health, and learn about approaches to promoting healthier behaviors.

▶ The Concept of Culture

Anthropologists developed the concept of culture at the end of the 19th century. There have been many definitions of culture. An early definition suggested that culture was "that complex whole which includes knowledge, beliefs, art, law, morals, custom and any other capabilities and habits acquired by man [sic] as a member of society."[2(p43)] A relatively modern definition states that culture is "a set of rules or standards shared by members of a society, which when acted upon by the members, produce behavior that falls within a range of variation the members consider proper and acceptable."[3(p30)] In the simplest terms, one

may call culture "behavior and beliefs that are learned and shared."[4]

Cultures operate in a variety of domains, including the following[4]:

- The family
- Social groups beyond the family
- Individual growth and development
- Communication
- Religion
- Art
- Music
- Politics and law
- The economy

As one thinks about the links between culture and health, it is also important to understand the term society, which refers to "a group of people who occupy a specific locality and share the same cultural traditions."[3] Societies have social structures that are the "relationships of groups within society that hold it together."[3(p31)] In addition, we must note that there is heterogeneity within all cultures. Sometimes this is reflected in what people call subcultures. There are many shared aspects, for example, of Chinese culture. However, China is a very large country, and even among the Han Chinese—the largest ethnic group—there are important variations as one moves across China in language, food, wedding customs, and music, among other things. The same would be true of North India. People across North India have much in common. Yet, there are variations of North Indian culture in different places, such as in the state of West Bengal as compared to the state of Rajasthan. This can be seen, again, in language, music, art, and food.

When thinking about the links between culture and health, one also needs to consider that some cultural practices may be well adapted to some settings but poorly adapted to others. Alternatively, they may be well adapted to the way people have been living, but less well adapted to the way people live after important changes or developments in their communities.[3(p46)] The culture of nomadic people, for example, may be well suited to their nomadic lifestyle. However, their culture may be ill equipped to deal with a lifestyle after societal change that would cause them to be more sedentary.

As we consider the relationship between culture and health, we should be aware of the ways in which a culture is viewed by people from outside that culture group. This helps us to understand the difference between looking at another culture from our perspective and looking at it from the perspective of those who live within that culture.

Especially in the early days of anthropology, those who studied cultures other than their own often viewed them solely through the prism of their own society and judged much of what they saw to be lacking. This view is called **ethnocentrism**. Contrary to this view is **cultural relativism**, or the idea that "because cultures are unique, they can be evaluated only according to their own standards and values."[3(p51)]

The approach that will guide the rest of this chapter and, indeed, the text as a whole, is the question: "How well does a given culture satisfy the physical and psychological needs of those whose behavior it guides?"[3(p51)] For example, is female circumcision, also called female genital mutilation, a health-enhancing procedure or a harmful procedure? Is it good or bad for the health of a newborn to be given sugar water? How should one see cultural practices that discriminate against women and cause them to eat less well than men, as in India and China? How should one see cultural practices that discriminate against sexual minorities, that drive them underground, and that therefore may contribute to less healthy sexual practices? On the other hand, what about cultures that encourage exclusive breastfeeding for 6 months? What about male circumcision, which is associated with reduced transmission of HIV?

You will realize as you make your way through the text that those responsible for guiding health policies and programs in different countries must have a good understanding of the cultures with which they are working if they are to be helpful in enhancing health for the members of those societies. This is also true of outsiders, including development assistance agencies. They must be very sensitive to local cultures, while simultaneously considering with their government partners and with insiders to the culture what behavior changes may be needed to enhance individual and population health in a particular setting.[1(p56)]

▶ Other Key Concepts and Definitions

A number of other key concepts and definitions are central to understanding the relationship between culture and health. They also relate in important ways to work in global health. These are summarized here.

Cultural competence: "Cultural competence is the ability to interact effectively with people of different cultures. In practice, both individuals and organizations can be culturally competent. . . . Cultural competence means to be respectful and responsive to the health beliefs and practices—and cultural and linguistic needs—of diverse population groups. Developing cultural competence is also an evolving, dynamic process that takes time and occurs along a continuum."[5] To work effectively in public health and global health, one needs to be culturally competent.

Cultural humility: This concept builds on cultural competence and takes it further. Cultural humility can be described as "a lifelong process of self-reflection and self-critique whereby the individual not only learns about another's culture, but one starts with an examination of her/his own beliefs and cultural identities. This critical consciousness is more than just self-awareness, but requires one to step back to understand one's own assumptions, biases and values."[6] Understanding another culture and its attitudes toward health and health practices is essential to effective work in public and global health. However, it is not sufficient unless one brings to this understanding an appreciation for one's own assumptions. The difference between cultural competence and cultural humility may seem subtle to those new to the global health field. However, it is fundamental and substantial.

Health literacy: "Health literacy is the degree to which individuals have the capacity to obtain, process, and understand basic health information and services needed to make appropriate health decisions."[7] Clearly, the more literate a group is in health matters, the more we expect that group to engage in healthy behaviors. We would also expect groups that are more health literate to be able to respond more quickly to messages and measures meant to promote better health.

Traditional medicine: The World Health Organization (WHO) defines traditional medicine as "the sum total of the knowledge, skill, and practices based on the theories, beliefs, and experiences indigenous to different cultures, whether explicable or not, used in the maintenance of health as well as in the prevention, diagnosis, improvement or treatment of physical and mental illness."[8] This text does not discuss traditional medicine at length. However, readers should understand that this is an important topic on which there is an extensive literature. Traditional medicines are also of great importance in a number of settings, and there is a substantial literature on them, as well. The National Center for Complementary and Integrative Medicine at the U.S. National Institutes of Health also has a research program on medicine that is not "conventional"—meaning not Western biomedicine.[9]

Western biomedicine: This refers to "a system in which medical doctors and other healthcare professionals (such as nurses, pharmacists, and therapists) treat symptoms and diseases using drugs, radiation, or surgery. Also called allopathic medicine, biomedicine, conventional medicine, mainstream medicine, and orthodox medicine."[10] One could also say that it is "the sum total of knowledge, skills and practices of the modern Western scientific tradition, used for the diagnosis and treatment of illness."[11] The overwhelming majority of the literature on global health will refer to the approaches of Western biomedicine.

▶ Health Beliefs and Practices

Different cultures vary in their perceptions of the body and their views of what is illness, what causes illness, and what should be done about it. They have different views on how to prevent health problems, what health care they should seek, and the types of remedies that health providers might offer.[4] This section highlights selected aspects of belief systems about health that one would see most in low- and middle-income countries, in immigrant populations in high-income countries, and in what some might call "traditional societies."

Perceptions of Illness

Perceptions of illness vary considerably across culture groups. What one culture may view as entirely normal, for example, another culture may see as an affliction. Worms are so common among children in some cultures that people do not see infection with worms as an illness. Malaria is so common in much of sub-Saharan Africa that many families see it as normal. In much of South Asia, back pain among women is very common and is also seen as just a part of being a woman.[12] Schistosomiasis is very common in Egypt. It causes blood in the urine, which is referred to in Egypt as "male menstruation," and it is often considered normal because it is so widespread.[1(p57)]

Perceptions of Disease

Medical anthropologists, among others, define **disease** as the "malfunctioning or maladaptation of biologic and psychophysiologic processes in the individual."[13(p252)] Pneumonia is a disease. HIV is a disease. Polio is a disease. **Illness**, however, is different from disease. "Illness represents personal, interpersonal, and cultural reactions to disease or discomfort."[13] People may feel like they have an illness. They can describe it and its symptoms. They may have a name in their culture for this problem. However, they may not have a "disease," which is a physiological condition. This is a very important point, because different cultures may have very different perceptions of the causes of illness.

Most people in high-income countries follow the "Western medical paradigm" in explaining the causes of disease. This will be familiar to you. You get influenza and colds from viruses. You get diabetes as an adult from an inability to control your blood sugar, although there may be a genetic component to it. You raise the risk of heart disease from smoking, from having obesity, or from having cholesterol that is too high.

On the other hand, many people, especially those in or from low- and middle-income countries and more traditional societies, often see illness as being caused by factors other than disease as defined in the Western biomedical model. There are many cultures, for example, that believe the body being "out of balance" brings on illness. Among the most common of these concepts is the notion of "hot" and "cold." In this case, the body may get out of balance if one engages in certain unhealthy practices. In certain cultures, some foods are regarded as "hot" and some foods are regarded as "cold," and people are supposed to achieve a balance between these foods to avoid illness.

Many people also believe that illness has supernatural origins. A study done among people of Caribbean and African descent in the United States showed that many people believed that the symptoms of illness stem from supernatural causes.[14] There are many cultures in which people believe that illness comes from being affected by "the evil eye," being bewitched or possessed, losing their soul, or offending gods.[1] Some First Nations people in Canada have a belief that "illness is not necessarily a bad thing, but instead a sign sent by the Creator to help people re-evaluate their lives."[15(p81)] A study of the cultural perceptions of illness among Yoruba people in Nigeria found that illness could be

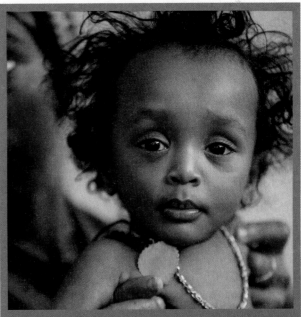

PHOTO 7-2 People in many cultures believe that amulets, like the one shown on this child, can protect the child from falling ill. In your culture, are there beliefs not based on Western biomedicine about the reasons people get sick?
Courtesy of Mark Tuschman.

"traced to enemies, including witchcraft, sorcery, gods, ancestors, natural illnesses, or hereditary illness."[16(p328)]

Emotional stresses are also seen in different cultures as direct causes of illness. This could come about as a result of being stressed or extremely frightened. Being too envious is also viewed as a cause of illness in some cultures.[1] Sexual matters are seen as causes of illness in some cultures as well. In several cultures, for example, frequent sexual relations are believed to weaken men by taking away their blood.[1] These beliefs are quite common in parts of India.

Folk Illnesses

Many cultures also have what are called folk illnesses. These are local, cultural interpretations of physical states that people perceive to be illnesses without a physiological cause. *Empacho* is an illness that is commonly described in a number of Latin American cultures. This is often described as a condition caused by food that "gets stuck to the walls of the stomach or intestines, causing an obstruction."[17(p693)] *Empacho* is said to be caused by any of a variety of inappropriate food practices, and in children it is said to produce a number of gastrointestinal symptoms, including bloating, diarrhea, and a stomachache.

To cure *empacho*, families may, for example, limit some foods or give abdominal massages with warm oil. They will also often consult a local healer, such as the *santiguadora* in the Puerto Rican community and *sobadora* in the Mexican community. Some Mexican communities in both the United States and Mexico also treat this "illness" with medicinal powders.

To understand health problems in low- and middle-income countries and in traditional societies, it is very important to understand the existence of folk illnesses such as *empacho*. It may be that the condition described by communities as *empacho* has no known or real biomedical basis. However, even if this condition

has no biomedical basis, if people believe it is an important illness, any efforts to improve the health of the community will have to consider such beliefs.[17] **TABLE 7-1** lists some of the culturally defined causes of illness.

The Prevention of Illness

Given the wide range of views on what causes illness, it is not surprising that there are many different cultural practices that concern avoiding illness. Many cultures, for example, have taboos, or behaviors and practices that they forbid people from engaging in if they are to stay healthy. A large number of taboos concern what not to eat during pregnancy, as was suggested in a study of traditional beliefs in western Malaysia, including avoiding certain important sources of protein.[18] A study in southern Nigeria about traditional beliefs concerning eating in pregnancy found widespread belief that pregnant women must avoid foods such as the following[19]:

- Sweet foods, so the baby would not be weak
- Eggs, so the baby would not grow up to be a thief
- Snails, so the baby would not be dull, would not salivate excessively, or would develop speech properly

A study in Brazil found that many people believed that women should not eat game meat and fish during pregnancy, although both could be good sources of protein.[20] A study of poor women in South India showed that the intake of fruits and legumes was affected by taboos, and legumes are among the most important sources of protein for many Indian women.[21]

There is also a wide array of ritual practices that people undergo to avoid illness. Related to this, there are traditions in some cultures to get rid of bad spirits or evil forces to ensure that one does not fall ill. There are beliefs among the Yoruba people in Nigeria, for example, that charms, amulets, scarification, or some oral potions can prevent illness that is caused by one's

TABLE 7-1 Selected Cultural Explanations of Illness and Disease

Body Balances	Emotional	Supernatural	Sexual
Temperature	Fright	Bewitching	Sex with forbidden person
Energy	Sorrow	Demons	Overindulgence in sex
Blood	Envy	Spirit possession	
Dislocation	Stress	Evil eye	
Problems with organs		Offending God or gods	
Incompatibility of horoscopes		Soul loss	

Modified from Scrimshaw, S. C. (2006). Culture, behavior, and health. In M. H. Merson, R. E. Black, & A. Mills (Eds.), *International public health: Diseases, programs, systems, and policies* (pp. 53–78). Sudbury, MA: Jones and Bartlett.

enemies.[16] Some tribal groups in Rajasthan, India, put charms at certain crossings to inflict harm on others, to avoid harm to themselves, to appease an evil spirit, or to leave their affliction there with the spirit.[22] In rural Senegal, a special ritual is performed for women who have lost two children, had two miscarriages, or appear to be infertile. The ritual is intended to prevent the causes of child death and infertility.[23]

The Diagnosis and Treatment of Illness and the Use of Health Services

In many cultures, when people are ill, they first try to care for the illness themselves or with the help of family members, using home remedies. This is often followed by a visit to some type of local healer and the use of indigenous medicines from that healer. Only if the illness does not resolve after that will families seek the help of a "Western doctor." Even then, it is quite common for people to use modern medicines and indigenous medicines at the same time.

The manner in which people and families care for illnesses is called patterns of resort. People seek help from different healthcare providers at different times for a number of reasons.[1] One important concern is the cost of services, both direct, such as fees, and indirect, such as the cost of transportation, time en route, or waiting. Another concern is the means of payment. People with little cash may prefer to visit a healer or doctor who takes payment in kind, rather than in cash. This could be in small gifts or payment in farm products such as fruits, vegetables, or poultry. People are also driven by the reputation of the provider. They will go to a provider who is reputed in their community to have good results over a provider who does not enjoy this type of reputation.

The manner in which the provider treats them socially is also an important determinant of the use of services. People generally prefer to go to a provider who is from their community, speaks their language, is known to them, and treats them with respect, rather than an outsider who may be disrespectful. It is interesting to note that many people around the world tend to treat illnesses at home and then go to a local healer. As a last resort, they may go to a licensed physician who practices Western biomedicine.[17]

It is very important to understand the extent to which a large share of the treatment of illness in most cultures takes place first at home. People in high-income countries may take some aspirin, drink plenty of water, eat a certain soup, and try to rest when they first develop symptoms. They may also take a variety of different types of herbal products or vitamins. Only if people do not feel better by a certain time will many people try to see a health provider. People in more traditional societies have analogous patterns of behavior when they believe themselves to be ill. Understanding these patterns, of course, is central to any efforts to enhance health.

Health Providers

There are also many different types of health service providers. Some of these are shown in **TABLE 7-2**. As you can see in the table, some of the providers are practitioners of indigenous systems of medicine, such as ayurvedic practitioners in India and practitioners of Chinese systems of medicine like herbalists and acupuncturists. Other practitioners will be part of a wide array of local health providers. These include, for example, traditional birth attendants, priests, herbalists, and bonesetters. The types of practitioners of Western biomedicine will depend on the size and

TABLE 7-2 Selected Examples of Health Service Providers

Indigenous	Western Biomedical	Other Medical Systems
Midwives Shamans Curers Spiritualists Witches Sorcerers Priests Diviners Herbalists Bonesetters	Pharmacists Nurse–midwives Nurses Nurse practitioners Physicians Dentists	Chinese medical system practitioners Chemists/herbalists Acupuncturists Ayurvedic practitioners

Modified from Scrimshaw, S. C. (2006). Culture, behavior, and health. In M. H. Merson, R. E. Black, & A. Mills (Eds.), *International public health: Diseases, programs, systems, and policies* (pp. 53–78). Sudbury, MA: Jones and Bartlett.

location of the place in which they work, and could include, for example, community health workers, nurses, midwives, nurse–midwives, physicians, and dentists. You should also be aware that in many low- and middle-income countries, pharmacists or stores that sell drugs also frequently dispense both drugs and medical advice. Although prescriptions for drugs may be legally required, many low- and middle-income countries are unable or unwilling to enforce this requirement. It is also important to note that many healthcare providers will combine indigenous health practices with Western biomedicine.[1]

▶ Health Behaviors and Behavior Change

When one considers the burden of disease, one quickly realizes that many of the leading causes of disability and death are related to health behaviors, which, in turn, are often related to culture. The leading causes of death globally for all age groups and both sexes in 2016 were ischemic heart disease, stroke, chronic obstructive pulmonary disease, Alzheimer's disease, and lower respiratory infections. Lung cancer, diarrhea, diabetes, road injuries, and tuberculosis (TB) were also among the top 10 causes of death globally in 2016.[24] The most important risk factors for deaths globally for all ages and both sexes in 2016 were high blood pressure, smoking, high fasting plasma glucose, high body mass index, high total cholesterol, ambient particulate matter, alcohol use, household air pollution, impaired kidney function, and low whole grains. There are many behaviors that *are* conducive to good health. However, it is important to ask the question: what are the behaviors that contribute to the leading risk factors for illness and premature death? A number of examples are discussed next.

An infant being underweight for age is among the most important risk factors for premature death in low-income countries. Although income and education are closely linked with nutritional status of both mother and child, cultural variables are also important determinants of their nutrition. As noted earlier, many cultures have food taboos for pregnant women that are not helpful to birth outcomes; other cultures encourage pregnant women to eat less rather than more. In addition, how much women breastfeed their babies is closely linked with culture, as is the timing for the introduction of complementary foods and the types of foods that are offered. Undernutrition also stems from other eating practices that are also closely tied to culture. Can behaviors be changed so that pregnant women will eat the most nutritious foods they can, given their level of income, and exclusively breastfeed their babies for 6 months?

Unsafe sex is the major risk factor for HIV in low-, middle-, and high-income countries. Some people, such as commercial sex workers, may not have the bargaining power with their clients to negotiate sex with a condom. The same will often be true of women who are forced into unsafe sex by their husbands and boyfriends or because of their own economic position. However, many people who engage in unsafe sex do have control over whether or not to use a condom. What would it take to ensure that people use protection?

Hygiene is another area that closely relates to health behaviors, and the lack of safe water and sanitation is a major risk factor for diarrheal disease. In many low- and middle-income countries, hygiene practices may be poor, and families need to learn to use water safely, dispose of human waste in sanitary ways, and wash their hands with soap and water after defecating. Behaviors regarding hygiene, of course, are intimately linked with culture. How can they be changed?

Household air pollution is another major risk factor for respiratory infections. This relates largely to the fact that families in many cultures cook indoors with biomass fuels without appropriate ventilation. Some families may not be able to afford an improved stove. However, other families cook as they do because of tradition and the lack of knowledge of the health impacts of indoor air pollution. How could the way people cook be changed?

Tobacco smoking is a leading risk factor for cardiovascular disease and cancer. Most people who smoke cigarettes start smoking as adolescents. Are there measures that can be taken to change these behaviors? How would the efforts to change behavior differ if one tried to stop adolescents from taking up smoking, compared to if one helped adult smokers quit?

Of course, behaviors are closely linked with culture and health not only in low- and middle-income countries but also in high-income countries. Moreover, in high-income countries, as well as in low- and middle-income countries, there is a wide array of behaviors that do not promote good health. In high-income countries, for example, an increasing number of people are physically inactive and consume poor diets, leading to obesity and diabetes. Many people also continue to smoke, even though smoking is a major risk factor for both cardiovascular disease and cancer. Despite the widespread availability of seat belts in cars, some people still do not use them. What needs to be done to get people to change these behaviors to ones that are healthier?

Improving Health Behaviors

There are a number of models or theories that explain why people engage in certain health behaviors and what can be done to encourage changes in those behaviors. Those interested in learning more about health behaviors can review *The Essentials of Health Behavior, Second Edition*, another book in this series.[25] Some of the most important concepts about health behavior and models about behavior change, however, are examined very briefly here.

The Ecological Perspective

As one considers the factors that influence behaviors that relate to health, it is important to take what is called an ecological perspective. This is a concept that suggests that the factors influencing health behaviors occur at several levels. These are noted in **TABLE 7-3**.

The basic precepts concerning the ecological approach are the following:

- "Health related behaviors are affected by, and affect, multiple levels of influence: intrapersonal or individual factors, interpersonal factors, institutional factors, community factors, and public policy factors."[26(p4)]
- "Behavior both influences and is influenced by the social environments in which it occurs."[26(p5)]

You can try to imagine, for example, whether or not an adolescent male will take up smoking. This will depend on how he feels about smoking, what he thinks others think of his smoking, the setting in which he operates, how expensive it is to buy cigarettes, and how easy it is to buy them. Of course, if he does start smoking, some of his own peer group may follow.

The Health Belief Model

The Health Belief model was the first effort to articulate a coherent understanding of the factors that enter into health behaviors. It was developed by the U.S. Public Health Service as it tried to understand why people did or did not avail themselves of the opportunity to get chest x-rays for TB.[27] The premises of this model are that people's health behaviors depend on their perceptions of the following:

- Their likelihood of getting the illness
- The severity of the illness if they get it
- The benefits of engaging in behavior that will prevent the illness
- The barriers to engaging in preventive behavior

In this model, people's health behavior also depends on whether or not people feel that they could actually carry out the appropriate behavior if they tried, which is called **self-efficacy**.[26]

One could think about how this model pertains to HIV and engaging in safe sex. The extent to which a young man uses a condom will be influenced by how easy he thinks it is to become infected with HIV, how serious a disease he believes it to be, the extent to which a condom can prevent HIV, and how easy it is to buy a condom and get a partner to agree to use it. The young man must also feel that he is capable of buying the condom and using it.

TABLE 7-3 The Ecological Perspective

Factors	Definition
Individual	Individual characteristics that influence behavior, such as knowledge, attitudes, beliefs, and personality traits
Interpersonal	Interpersonal processes, and primary groups including family, friends, and peers
Institutional	Rules, regulations, policies, and informal structures
Community	Social networks and norms or standards that exist formally or informally among individuals, groups, and organizations
Public policy	Local, state, and federal policies and laws that regulate or support healthy actions and practices for disease prevention, early detection, control, and management

Modified with permission from Murphy, E. (2005). *Promoting healthy behavior. Health bulletin 2.* Washington, DC: Population Reference Bureau.

The Stages of Change Model

The Stages of Change model was developed in the 1990s in the United States in conjunction with work on alcohol and drug abuse.[26] The premise behind this model is that change in behavior is a process and that different people are at different stages of readiness for change. The stages of change are outlined in **TABLE 7-4**.

It is easy to see how this model might apply to alcohol and drug abuse. You can imagine an excessive drinker who is not aware of his problem or who will not face it and needs help doing so. This individual would be in the "precontemplation" stage of change. Other people who are aware of their problem and willing to do something about it may need help to stop. Still others, who have already broken their addictions, need positive reinforcement to maintain their health.[26]

The Diffusion of Innovations Model

The Diffusion of Innovations model originates from work that was done on promoting agricultural change in the United States. In this model, "an innovation is an idea, practice, service, or other object that is perceived as new by the individual or group."[1(p66)] This model is based on the notion that communication is needed to promote social change and that "diffusion" is the process by which innovations are communicated over time among members of different groups and societies.[28] This model focuses on how people adopt and can be encouraged to adopt innovations, but does not discuss how they might maintain what they have adopted.

TABLE 7-5 outlines the stages that have to be undertaken to try to diffuse a health innovation.

This model also suggests that as the innovation begins to be diffused, people will fall into six groups[1,28]:

- Innovators
- Early adopters
- Early majority
- Late majority
- Late adopters
- Laggards

TABLE 7-4 The Stages of Change Model

Stages
- Precontemplation
- Contemplation
- Decision/Determination
- Action
- Maintenance

Reprinted with permission from Murphy, E. (2005). *Promoting healthy behavior. Health bulletin 2*. Washington, DC: Population Reference Bureau.

TABLE 7-5 The Diffusion of Health Innovations Model

Stages of Diffusion
- Recognition of a problem or need
- Conduct of basic and applied research to address the specific problem
- Development of strategies and materials that will put the innovative concept into a form that will meet the needs of the target population
- Commercialization of the innovation, which will involve production, marketing, and distribution efforts
- Diffusion and adoption of the innovation
- Consequences associated with adoption of the innovation

Modified from Scrimshaw, S. C. (2006). Culture, behavior, and health. In M. H. Merson, R. E. Black, & A. Mills (Eds.), *International public health: Diseases, programs, systems, and policies* (pp. 53–78). Sudbury, MA: Jones and Bartlett.

In addition, the model also indicates that the pace of adoption will be influenced by several factors[1,28]:

- The gains people think they will get by adopting the innovation
- How much the innovation fits in with their existing culture and values
- How easy it is to try the innovation
- Whether or not there are role models who are already trying the innovation
- The extent to which potential adopters see the innovation as cost-efficient and not taking too much of their time, energy, or money

One can imagine how the Diffusion of Innovations model may apply to efforts to change diets in high-income countries away from certain fats and toward more fruits and vegetables, fewer processed foods, and more whole grains. Some people change their diets relatively quickly. Others in the community make these shifts only as they can overcome some of their long-held dietary patterns. Some people shift as they learn more from their friends, some of whom become role models for change. The relatively high costs of some organic and other healthy foods may be a constraint to the adoption of change by some people. Others may simply not be willing or able to change the way they and their families have always eaten.

▶ Understanding and Engendering Behavior Change

As you can clearly see, in many instances, improving health requires that the behaviors of individuals, families, and communities be changed. You also see, however, that behaviors are intimately connected to culture, which is inherently difficult to change. Under these circumstances, what can be done, first to understand what behaviors need to be changed and, second, to change them? These questions are answered briefly here.

Understanding Behaviors

A first step in trying to promote behavior change must be to gain a good understanding of the behaviors that are taking place. This requires a careful assessment of several factors:

- The behaviors that are taking place
- The extent to which they are helpful or harmful to health
- The underlying motivation for these behaviors
- The likely responses to different approaches to changing the unhealthy behaviors

By taking a look at breastfeeding, for example, we can get a sense of how one would carry out such an assessment. One can consider how infant deaths might be reduced. As part of this effort, it is important to get a better sense of the extent to which any nutritional issues are harmful to infant health and how they might be improved. One important part of this effort would be to examine breastfeeding practices. In doing so, we would try to answer the following questions, among others:

- When do women start breastfeeding?
- Do they feed on schedule or on demand?
- Do they feed male and female children the same way?
- For how long do they breastfeed exclusively?
- At what age do they introduce complementary foods?
- Until what age do they continue to breastfeed, even while the children are getting complementary foods?
- Why do they engage in these practices?
- Why do some women not breastfeed?
- Who breastfeeds and who does not?
- Who has influence over their breastfeeding practices?

The answers to these questions, of course, will vary by culture group; however, once we get answers to them, we can begin to formulate a plan for behavior change that is built on the cultural values and approaches of the people. Without understanding current practices, the rationale for them, and who has influence over them, it will be impossible to promote behavior change. When we do have a sense of the existing practices and why they take place, what can be done to change behaviors?

Changing Health Behaviors

There are many different approaches to changing health behaviors. Some operate at the level of the individual, some at the level of the community, and some at the level of society as a whole. Generally, they include some combination of communication through the mass media and more personal communication. Several approaches to behavior change are discussed briefly here.

Community Mobilization

One very important way to encourage change in health behaviors is to engage in community mobilization. In this case, the effort focuses on getting an entire community to engage in the effort of promoting more healthy behaviors. This requires considerable efforts aimed at helping people across the community identify the problems they face, find potential solutions to the problems, and then work together to implement those solutions. Generally, it also requires that the leaders within the community are mobilized, willing to be champions for the needed change, and then willing to promote that change.[26] One example comes from the Tamil Nadu Nutrition Project, which was noted in one of the vignettes at the opening of this chapter. Communities which participated in this project were involved in promoting a variety of innovations, including weighing babies together, identifying together the babies who were not thriving, and working together to make supplementary food for their children. In addition, all of the community was involved in learning about appropriate foods and needed micronutrients. You will read later about this program and a variety of other community-based activities, including a campaign to address polio in India.

Mass Media

The mass media is often used to promote change in health behaviors. Most people in low- and middle-income countries have access to radio, which is often used for this purpose. Many of those engaged in promoting better health use a tool referred to as "entertainment-education." Some of these efforts have focused on soap opera series in which the characters bring out the main messages about healthy behaviors. The British Broadcasting Company has a group, for example, that works with low- and middle-income countries to produce soap operas on health topics of importance such as HIV/AIDS. Such a series was done on HIV/AIDS in India and Nigeria. The government of Myanmar had a soap opera about leprosy that featured Myanmar's best-known actress. The aims of the soap opera were to help destigmatize leprosy, let people know how to diagnose leprosy, inform them that it could be treated completely if treated early, and get people to come forward for treatment at an early stage. The Population Media Center's radio serial drama *Yeken Kignit* in Ethiopia reached nearly half of the population and addressed reproductive health and gender equality. After 2.5 years of the show being broadcast, demand for contraceptives increased by 157 percent and listeners were five times more likely than those who did not listen to the show to know three or more family planning methods. Additionally, male listeners requested HIV tests at four times the rate of male nonlisteners.[29]

Social Media

Social media is defined as "activities, practices, and behaviours among communities of people who gather online to share information, knowledge, and opinions using conversational media . . . that make it possible to create and easily transmit content in the form of words, pictures, videos, and audios."[30] One might notice that there is some overlap between social media and mass media. A helpful distinction between social media and mass media is that social media allows people to engage with content rather than passively receive it.

Efforts to promote behavior change through social media are fairly new. Thus, there are a limited number of studies that have examined the impact of social media interventions on health behavior change. A meta-analysis of 12 such studies found that health interventions on social networking sites resulted in a modest beneficial impact on health behavior change.[31] However, all the studies included in the analysis were taken from high-income countries.

To date, no studies in low- or middle-income countries have measured the effect of a social media intervention on health behavior change.[32] However, there are a number of promising areas in which social media may be deployed for health behavior change in low- and middle-income countries. For example, in Turkey, a social marketing enterprise company called DKT International recently implemented a social media campaign to promote condom use.[33] The company created a condom company called "Fiesta" and promoted the brand on several digital platforms.

By creating a Facebook page with interactive questions about condoms and sexual health, as well as targeted advertisements on Facebook's platform, Fiesta attracted 7,000 Facebook members to join its page and generated 141,000 total "clicks" through advertising. Combined with other initiatives, including an e-newsletter, Google Adwords, banner advertisements, and creation of viral videos, Fiesta sold 4.3 million condoms in its first 18 months.[33]

An important consideration in any effort to use social media to influence health is the fact that social media use may not be uniform across different sectors of society. For example, if only people in the higher-wealth quintiles of a country can purchase the smartphones and internet to engage with social media, those who belong to lower-wealth quintiles will not be reached by a social media intervention. In a similar vein, those who are elderly and are less accustomed to social media may be more difficult to reach through behavior change initiatives on social networking platforms.

It is also important to consider the fact that messages on social media platforms may spread misinformation about health, or may be used by other parties to promote unhealthy behaviors. For example, the alcohol companies in Australia that sponsor sports teams have been found to use the interactive nature of social media in their advertising strategies to normalize alcohol consumption during sports victory celebrations.[34] Due to the rapid transmission of information through social networking sites, it can be difficult to control or prevent the dispersal of misinformation on these platforms.

Information technologies, such as social media networks, are becoming increasingly accessible in low- and middle-income countries. A recent report by the Pew Research Center found that approximately two-thirds of adults in "emerging and developing economies" use the internet or own a smartphone, and approximately half use online social networking sites.[35] One should expect that as internet access increases in these settings, the use of social networking sites such as Facebook and Twitter, among others, may become important tools for promoting healthy behaviors.

Social Marketing

Social marketing is the application of the tools of commercial marketing to try to promote behavior change and the uptake of important health actions or products. This has been used widely in family planning work. It is also being used in other fields, such as in selling bednets for malaria control. In social marketing, a local brand of a product is often created, such as a condom, a contraceptive pill, or an insecticide-treated bednet. Mass media, social media, and other forms of communication are then used to promote the brand and the behaviors related to the product. You might recall that DKT International used a social marketing approach to promote condom use in Turkey. Of course, successful marketing depends on very careful market research and a good understanding of the local culture, values, and behaviors. It also depends on what is called "the four Ps" in social marketing[26]:

- Attractive product
- Affordable price
- Convenient places to buy the product
- Persuasive promotion

Often the products being marketed through social marketing are sold through commercial channels but the government subsidizes their price.

Health Education

Health education is something with which every reader of this text will be familiar. It comes in many forms, such as in the classroom, in the news media, on the radio and television, and on the internet. Successful health education programs that are aimed at sex education have several features in common that hold lessons for other efforts at making health education effective[26]:

- They focus on risky behaviors and are clear about abstinence and consistent condom use
- They provide accurate information
- They address how to deal with social pressures
- They select teachers and peer educators who believe in the program
- They gear the content of the program to the age, sexual experience, and culture of the students

Cash Transfers

A number of countries have turned to the use of economic incentives to encourage behavior change in health and help reduce poverty. These incentives are called **cash transfers**, some of which are conditional. In the case of a **conditional cash transfer**, a government program offers a payment to families on an agreed-upon time frame, provided that the family engages in agreed-upon nutrition, health, or education behaviors. The desired behaviors could include activities such as giving birth in a hospital; engaging in regular well-baby care like immunizations; participating in a nutrition program that checks on the nutritional status of a child and offers food supplements,

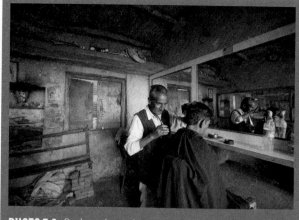

PHOTO 7-3 Barber shops in many countries are "community centers" in which men often congregate for discussion, as well as for a haircut. Several countries, including the United States, have created programs in which barbershops and barbers provide health education messages, such as on HIV. What are other places in which people congregate and how could they be used for health promotion?
Courtesy of Mark Tuschman.

as needed; or sending female children to school on a regular basis.

Some cash transfers are not conditional. Rather, they are given more like income support, without being directly tied to behavior change. Considerable study has been done on cash transfers and the extent to which they need to be conditional to be effective or cost-effective. The evidence suggests that conditionality may encourage better impact under some circumstances, but this is not always the case.[36]

Achieving Success in Health Promotion

The previous sections refer to specific types of health promotion that can be used to encourage a change in health behaviors or the adoption of healthy behaviors. There are a number of lessons that have emerged both about these approaches and about what constitutes an effective health promotion effort. These are noted in **TABLE 7-6**.

▶ Social Assessment

Concerning the links between health and culture, **social assessment** or **social impact assessment** must also be addressed. A social impact assessment is "a process for assessing the social impacts of planned interventions or events and for developing strategies for the ongoing monitoring and management of those impacts."[37(p2)] In more expansive terms,

Social impact assessment includes the processes of analyzing, monitoring, and managing the intended and unintended social consequences, both positive and negative, of planned interventions (policies, programs, plans, projects) and any social change processes invoked by those interventions. Its primary purpose is to bring about a more sustainable and equitable biophysical and human environment.[37(p2)]

The social impact assessment looks at a variety of domains that go beyond health. These include impact on historical artifacts and buildings, communities, demography, gender, minority groups, culture, and

health. The assessment should be carried out in a way that builds on local processes, engages the community fully, and proactively tries to maximize the potential good that can come from the proposed investment. It "promotes community development and empowerment, builds capacity, and develops social capital."[37(p2)] The detailed approach of a social impact assessment is outlined in **TABLE 7-7**.

Many readers will be familiar with environmental assessment of proposed investment schemes, and many countries require such assessments be done before any major physical investment. In some respects, a social assessment is the social analogue to an environmental assessment. In this case, let us suppose that a development agency and a government are going to

---

TABLE 7-6 Selected Factors for Success in Health Promotion

Identify specific health problems, related behaviors, and key stakeholders.
Know and use sound behavioral theories.
Research motivations and constraints to change, considering biological, environmental, cultural, and other contextual factors.
Use participatory assessment tools and include relevant stakeholders in the design, implementation, and evaluation of the intervention.
Plan and budget carefully.
Identify people who exhibit healthy behaviors that differ from the social norm.
Create an environment that enables behavior change through policy dialogue, advocacy, and capacity building.
Organize an intervention that addresses both specific behaviors and contextual factors.
Work to ensure sustainability.
Evaluate from the beginning.
Form partnerships to scale up and/or adapt the most successful interventions for implementation in other settings.

Modified with permission from Murphy, E. (2005). *Promoting healthy behavior. Health bulletin 2.* Washington, DC: Population Reference Bureau.

TABLE 7-7 Selected Focuses of Social Impact Assessment

Identifies interested and affected peoples
Facilitates and coordinates the participation of stakeholders
Analyzes the local setting of the planned intervention to assess likely impacts to it
Collects baseline data to allow for evaluation of the impact of the intervention
Gives a picture of the local cultural context, and develops an understanding of local community values, particularly how they relate to the planned intervention
Identifies and describes the activities that are likely to cause impacts
Predicts likely impacts and how different stakeholders are likely to respond
Assists in evaluating and selecting alternatives
Recommends measures to mitigate any likely negative impacts
Assists in the evaluation process and provides suggestions about compensation for affected peoples
Describes potential conflicts between stakeholders and advises on resolution processes
Develops coping strategies for dealing with residual and nonmitigatable impacts
Contributes to skill development and capacity building in the community
Assists in devising and implementing monitoring and management programs

Modified from Vanclay, F. (2003). International principles for social impact assessment. *Impact Assessment and Project Appraisal, 21*(1), 5–11.

collaborate to develop a series of health centers in a particular region of a country. First, the country would carry out a social assessment to set the foundation for the project design. The affected communities should participate in this assessment. The country would also ensure that the design took account of the needs of various groups in the community and was based on their culture and values, and it would keep in mind how programs need to be tailored to address them. The assessment would seek to identify any negative consequences that might emerge from the investment and how those consequences might be mitigated. The plan emerging from the assessment would also include a scheme for monitoring and evaluating the social impacts of the project and determining if the program design is consistent with local values and the underlying needs of the community.

Some years ago, very little attention was paid in some development assistance agencies and in some governments to social assessment. Little effort was spent on examining the social and cultural issues involved in designing appropriate interventions in health. In addition, little attention was paid to the potential impact on health or on other social areas of investments in sectors outside of health. Although the quality of the social assessment may vary both within and across some agencies and governments, they are now done more frequently for major development projects.

▸ Case Studies

Three case studies follow. They are meant to illustrate some of the key issues concerning the relationship between culture and health and how better health can be engendered through behavior change.

The first examines breastfeeding practices in Burundi and the barriers to exclusive breastfeeding for 6 months, as WHO recommends. The second case reviews some of the cultural issues related to efforts to eradicate polio in India and how communications programs have been enhanced to address them. The last case examines some of the key linkages between cultural practices and the spread of the Ebola virus.

Breastfeeding in Burundi[38]

There is substantial evidence that giving only breast-milk to an infant for the first 6 months of life is a critical health-promoting practice. This is called **exclusive breastfeeding (EBF)**. Nonetheless, WHO estimates that only about one-third of all of the infants in the

world are exclusively breastfed.[39] In order to promote exclusive breastfeeding and enhance the health of young children, it is critical to understand why many women do not engage in EBF at higher rates.

An examination of the factors that motivate the duration of EBF was carried out in December 2009 in Burundi, a low-income country in Africa. Although the study was done some time ago, its approach and findings remain highly relevant today. The study focused on breastfeeding practices in families in two provinces, Cancuzo and Ruyigi. In Burundi, the rate of EBF for the first 4 months was then about 74 percent. However, many women stopped exclusive breastfeeding after the fourth month, and the rate of EBF for 6 months was only 45 percent.

Given the importance of cultural beliefs to health behaviors, the study aimed at understanding how certain beliefs affected whether a woman chose to breastfeed exclusively for 6 months. The goal of the study was to understand barriers to EBF in order to develop an effective EBF promotion program.

The study was based on an approach called **barrier analysis**, which focuses on trying to understand barriers to the adoption of positive health behaviors so that more effective behavior change communication messages and support activities can be developed.[40] This methodology has been used for work not only on breastfeeding but also on other nutrition practices, the use of latrines, and the use of bednets. With respect to exclusive breastfeeding, the study set out to gain a better understanding of the extent to which a mother believes the following:

- People important to her would approve of EBF
- God would approve of EBF
- She has sufficient knowledge, capacities, and resources to successfully perform EBF
- Malnutrition is a serious problem
- Her child could become malnourished
- EBF is effective in preventing malnutrition
- She can remember to practice EBF
- In certain negative or positive attributes of practicing EBF

Following barrier analysis methods, 45 women with children under 1 year of age who had exclusively breastfed their children were interviewed. Forty-nine women who had not exclusively breastfed their children under 1 year of age were also interviewed. The questions they were asked included the following:

- Do you think that exclusive breastfeeding until the age of 6 months could help your child avoid becoming malnourished?

- Do you think that God approves of mothers exclusively breastfeeding their children until the age of 6 months?
- In your opinion, would most of the people you know approve of your exclusively breastfeeding your child?
- Who are the people who would approve of your breastfeeding your child?
- With your current knowledge and abilities, do you think you would be able to exclusively breastfeed your next child until the age of 6 months?
- What are the disadvantages of exclusively breastfeeding your child?
- If you wanted to exclusively breastfeed your child until the age of 6 months, would it be difficult to remember not to give your child foods or liquids other than breastmilk?

A number of statistically significant findings emerged from the research:

- Those who exclusively breastfed were 21 times more likely than those who did not to say that a child who does not exclusively breastfeed will become malnourished.
- Those who did not exclusively breastfeed were 17.6 times more likely than those who did to say that God does not approve of exclusive breastfeeding.
- Those who exclusively breastfed were many times more likely than those who did not to say that mothers-in-law, husbands, cousins, and mothers, respectively, approved of exclusive breastfeeding (10.4, 6.5, 5.9, 3.8 times, respectively).
- Those who exclusively breastfed were 8 times more likely than those who did not to say that they had the knowledge and abilities to practice exclusive breastfeeding.
- Those who did not exclusively breastfeed were 7 times more likely than those who did to believe that exclusive breastfeeding would lead to babies always being hungry.
- Those who exclusively breastfed were 6.3 times more likely to say that it is not difficult at all to remember to practice EBF.

Among these findings, three stood out as especially significant in terms of designing a breastfeeding promotion program. These included the extent to which women believed (1) that a child who is not exclusively breastfed can become malnourished, (2) God approved of exclusive breastfeeding, and (3) persons important to them approved of exclusive breastfeeding.

With these findings in mind, the study authors and local staff made a number of recommendations for strengthening the promotion of breastfeeding in these two provinces:

- Track and expose to the communities positive deviants who faithfully practice EBF and who also have healthy, well-nourished babies.
- Provide peer-based lactation counseling to help women understand the importance of EBF in combating malnutrition.
- Educate health promotion trainers on how to effectively demonstrate the link between EBF and good nutrition.
- Mobilize spiritual leaders to show support for EBF.
- Give pastors and priests sermon guidelines related to breastfeeding practices and good nutrition.
- Use radio broadcasts featuring mothers-in-law, husbands, cousins, and mothers who support EBF.
- Train some of these mothers-in-law, female cousins, and mothers to be "Leader Mothers," the community-level cadre of health promoters in the project.

Polio Vaccination in India

In early 2014, India was declared polio free, having gone three consecutive years without a single case of polio. India had become a success story, from once having the highest burden of polio in the world to celebrating zero cases.[41]

In 1988, India launched its Polio Eradication Initiative. India's polio eradication program is a part of the Global Polio Eradication Initiative and includes a social mobilization and communication component.[42] This is meant to encourage universal immunization by providing accurate information about the vaccine, mobilizing demand for vaccination, and countering popular beliefs and behaviors that might constrain vaccination against polio.

India's polio program is a collaborative effort of national and international partners. These include India's national and local governments, via the Ministries of Health and Family Welfare, UNICEF, the World Health Organization National Polio Surveillance Project, Rotary International, the U.S. Centers for Disease Control and Prevention, and numerous nongovernmental organizations.[43,44]

India has the second largest population of any country in the world and has over 1.3 billion people.[45] The country is divided into 29 states and 7 union territories and has a very diverse population.[46] As would be expected, health beliefs vary across India and among different social groups.

Until recently, India was one of the last four countries in the world with endemic polio.[47] In addition, there were periodic outbreaks of polio in India, with the annual number of cases jumping to 1,600 in 2002 and 874 in 2007, from considerably lower levels in most other years.[47] The more recent polio outbreaks occurred primarily in the states of Uttar Pradesh and Bihar.[48]

These outbreaks were attributed to a variety of biological, social, political, and programmatic factors. Biological factors contributing to persistent polio outbreaks included high population density, poor sanitation, and pervasive poverty in certain regions. The primary social forces that contributed to the outbreaks were resistance to immunization among minority communities, as well as difficulty in vaccinating the children of the great numbers of people who migrate for work. Political forces that inhibited the polio program were rooted in tensions between Muslim minorities and the Hindu-dominated government. Programmatic challenges, such as low coverage of immunization activities and falsification of data, also affected some regions of India.[48]

Certain communities and social groups, primarily marginalized Muslim minority groups, had been resistant to giving oral polio vaccine to their children. This was attributed partly to a failure on the part of parents to understand the need for repeated vaccinations. It was also due to misinformation that circulated in some communities that the vaccine is ineffective, causes illness in children, causes infertility, or is part of a plot to curb the population growth of Muslims.[49] The strength of these rumors was likely exacerbated by the fact that most health professionals and community health workers tend to be Hindu.

In the face of these difficulties, public health leaders in India and from key international organizations collaborated to enhance the health communication and social mobilization aspects of India's polio program. Greater focus was put on reaching those resistant to vaccination and convincing them both to immunize their children and to continue vaccinating them with the appropriate number of doses.[49] In addition, efforts at communication and social mobilization were decentralized to the district, block, and village level, which allowed them to be more closely tailored to local mores. The program also enlisted community members in communication efforts to a greater extent than earlier.[43,50] These measures were intended to ensure that families receive information about the program from respected community members whom they trusted and with whom they already had a relationship.[50]

Some of the major steps that were taken to support this approach included the following:

- The establishment of a social mobilization network that extended to the village level.
- The linking of the social mobilization network, including community mobilization coordinators, with vaccination teams. These teams worked in booths on immunization days and then went house to house to immunize children who were missed on those days.
- Greater involvement of community and religious leaders in mobilizing members of their communities to be vaccinated.
- More use of intensive, house-to-house, interpersonal communications to ensure families would vaccinate their children.
- Greater engagement of well-known celebrities for mass media advertisements to support the polio program.
- Greater involvement in the program of professional associations, such as the Pediatric Association.

The evidence suggests that communities in which these social mobilization and communications activities took place had higher rates of immunization coverage than other communities.[49] These measures have also been associated with a decrease in the number of new polio cases. In the first 9 months of 2010, for example, as these measures were implemented, India had 37 new cases of polio, compared to 367 during the same period in 2009.[47]

The implementation of the Polio Eradication Initiative in India suggests that health communication efforts must pay particular attention to cultural context as well as epidemiologic factors and the political environment. The polio program in India also highlights these important factors[48]:

- The importance of engaging effectively with marginalized communities
- The importance of ensuring messages reach the village level
- The need in some settings for intensive interpersonal communications from respected people with influence who are seen as members of the community
- The power of involving religious leaders in programs

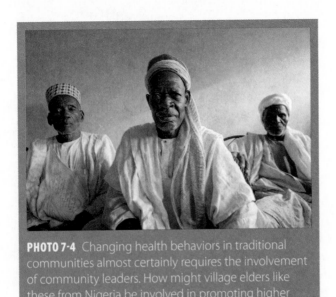

PHOTO 7-4 Changing health behaviors in traditional communities almost certainly requires the involvement of community leaders. How might village elders like these from Nigeria be involved in promoting higher uptake of vaccination in their community?
Courtesy of Mark Tuschman.

Ebola and Culture

Introduction

Culture affects how individuals think and feel about many aspects of life, including illness and disease. Cultural practices, beliefs, customs, and rituals can often increase or mitigate the risk of individuals being exposed to pathogens, which can then affect the transmission patterns of diseases. With this in mind, in order to be successful, disease control efforts must take into account the unique beliefs and actions of different groups.

Sensitivity to cultural factors associated with the control of infectious and parasitic disease has increased in the past 20 years. However, until recently, relatively little attention was given to cultural factors associated with emerging infectious diseases, especially diseases with high case fatality rates such as Ebola.[51] The challenges of the 2014 Ebola epidemic have brought to light the importance of paying much more attention to cultural issues when designing and implementing programs for the control of emerging and re-emerging infectious diseases.

What Is Ebola?

Ebola virus disease (EVD) is an acute, serious illness that is transmitted to people from wild animals. It spreads in the human population through human-to-human transmission via direct contact with bodily fluids of infected people or surfaces contaminated with these fluids. People remain infectious as long as their blood and body fluids, including semen and breast milk, contain the virus. The average EVD case fatality rate is around 50 percent, but case fatality rates have varied from 25 percent to 90 percent in past outbreaks.[52]

The first Ebola outbreak occurred in Yamuku, Democratic Republic of the Congo (DRC), in 1976.[53] Major outbreaks have also occurred in the DRC in 1995, northern Uganda from 2000 to 2001, the DRC and Uganda in 2008, and the DRC and Uganda in 2018/19. However, the 2014 outbreak in West Africa was the most complex to date and led to more cases and deaths than all previous outbreaks combined.[52,54]

Impact of Culture on Ebola Transmission

Culture is related to Ebola outbreaks in several unique ways, including through burial practices, caregiving practices, and societal stigma. A greater understanding of the relationship between these cultural elements and EVD has shed light on how Ebola is transmitted and has allowed for more effective disease control interventions. The following illustrations are examples of how knowledge of local culture can help us understand the dynamics of disease transmission and disease control in certain settings.[55]

Burial practices are the most notable and discussed cultural factor related to Ebola. It is estimated that 60 percent of the cases in the 2014 outbreak in Guinea were associated with burial practices.[55] There is a risk of transmission of Ebola after a patient is deceased because the bodies and bodily fluids of the deceased patient remain contagious many days after death.[56] Nonetheless, many local customs call on a family member, often a paternal aunt, to wash and prepare the body for burial, potentially exposing this individual to a high viral load.[51]

Ebola infections can also occur during burials when family and community members perform religious rites that require directly touching the body.[57] Moreover, the potential exists for transmission to distant areas when visiting funeral attendants are exposed to the body itself and when family members distribute personal property of the loved one, which may have been infected with the virus.[57,58] In Liberia, for example, among Muslims, Christians, and followers of indigenous Liberian religious customs, it is common for family and friends of the deceased to hold a wake in the home before the burial, both to console each other and to celebrate the life of the deceased. At this occasion, family members usually handle the corpse themselves and funeral attendees pay their respects by touching or kissing the body of the deceased.[59] In November 2014, the WHO released a safe burial protocol that acknowledges the necessity of religious washing before burial and other sacred rituals such as praying over the body and describes how these rituals can be maintained in a safe way. It also discusses safe alternatives to these practices.[57]

Interestingly, evidence exists that gender roles can explain why it has been observed that men are more likely to be infected early in an Ebola outbreak, whereas the number of female cases greatly exceeds the number of male cases over the course of the outbreak. Men are likely to be the ones hunting in rural areas. This puts them at greater risk for coming into contact with forest animals, which often triggers the initial animal-to-human transmission of the virus.[60] However, as an outbreak continues, women are increasingly affected by Ebola. This relates to the fact that women are usually the ones to feed and clean up after sick relatives, which heightens their exposure to the Ebola virus. In addition, women traditionally are also more likely to perform the funeral rituals.[59] Despite the evidence that women are also severely affected, men still seem to dominate meetings and remain the main participants in discussions of control strategies at the community level.[62] This imbalance suggests that women need to play a greater role in future campaigns.

Stigma on the local and international levels can also complicate the Ebola response. In local areas, the stigma carried by Ebola survivors and family members of Ebola victims could exacerbate disease spread. In particular, misinformation can result in families hiding relatives and friends infected with Ebola to avoid being shunned by their own communities. Individuals remaining in their homes can undermine the need for treatment in hospitals. This can also pose threats to household members who are then put at risk for Ebola infection.[59,63]

On an international level, stigma can result from paranoia and fear of the disease, which can interfere with response efforts and humanitarian aid. Some countries have imposed harsh travel restrictions, travel bans, or compulsory quarantines for individuals upon return. These efforts to reduce risk limit the exchange of physical and human resources that disease-afflicted areas need.[63] In November 2014, the UN called on the global community to work to understand the roots of this stigma and to address these roots in order to promote solidarity,[64] or unity in action.[65] Many parallels have been drawn between the 2014 Ebola epidemic and the early HIV/AIDS epidemic, and, as a result, local education interventions for Ebola have been built off of the grassroots, community-based stigma reduction initiatives developed to combat stigma associated with HIV/AIDS.[65]

In addition to the factors discussed here, there are many other important cultural factors related to Ebola transmission and control dynamics. For example, the use of bushmeat has been identified as the primary mechanism of spillover of the Ebola virus from wildlife reservoirs to humans. In Liberia, it was estimated at the time of the outbreak that about 75 percent of meat consumption was bushmeat.[56] In addition, traditional healers in the informal healthcare system can also influence disease parameters. Traditional healers can be used as important mechanisms to spread correct public health information. During the 2014 outbreak, for example, traditional healers in one district of Sierra Leone decided to stop treating patients until they received appropriate training on the Ebola virus.[55] On the other hand, traditional healers sometimes advocate for prevention or treatment efforts that differ from those suggested by the biomedical or foreign aid communities. They might also spread misinformation, such as in northern Uganda, when traditional healers shared that drinking bleach would cure Ebola.

Lessons Learned

Cultural practices are often referred to as barriers to controlling an epidemic. Overall, a limited number of studies have investigated the influence of cultural factors on disease transmission and control of emerging and re-emerging diseases. The few studies that have been conducted, however, have made clear that if cultural knowledge is embraced, it can be used as a tool to effectively craft a response that engages afflicted communities and resources in order to save lives as quickly as possible.

The first sociocultural study of Ebola, conducted in 2003, determined that although some cultural elements such as burial practices can amplify an outbreak at first, many in-place cultural belief systems or practices can be used to control outbreaks. This is because many of these belief systems have had to evolve to survive diseases with high fatality rates for many years.[51] For example, this first study conducted outside Gulu, Uganda, identified that residents, mostly of the Acholi ethnic group, came to identify Ebola as a *gemo*, a traditional explanation for the disease outside of a biomedical context. After this, the Acholi people modified their practices in a way that matched suggested WHO epidemic control measures, including isolation of patients and suspension of public events such as funerals. These adaptions were not achieved by promoting a biomedical explanation for disease, but rather by promoting one that reflects a more holistic understanding of illness common in many parts of the world. Local and international health workers could then work with the Acholi people more effectively to help combat the outbreak.[51]

Ebola outbreaks and outbreaks of other similar diseases are rare events. Nonetheless, the 2014 Ebola epidemic heightened awareness of the relevance of cultural factors to understanding transmission. It also raised attention to the need for sensitivity to culture in designing control campaigns.

▶ Main Messages

Culture is a set of beliefs and behaviors that are learned and shared. Culture operates, among other areas, in the domains of the family, social groups beyond the family, religion, art, music, and law. Culture is an important determinant of health in many ways. It relates to people's health behaviors, their perceptions of illness, the extent to which they use health services, and forms of medicine that they have practiced traditionally. This chapter examines the links between culture and health from the perspective of the extent to which a culture satisfies the physical and psychological needs of those who follow it.

Perceptions of illness vary considerably across cultures. What is seen as normal in some societies may be seen as illness in others. Different societies also have differing perceptions of the causes of illness and disease. In addition to perceptions related to "Western biomedicine," diseases may be viewed, for example, as a result of the body "being out of balance," supernatural causes, offending the gods, emotional stress, or witchcraft. Different cultures also take an array of steps, beyond the Western biomedical paradigm, to prevent illness. Some of these include rituals, the wearing of charms, and the observance of certain food taboos.

When people believe themselves to be ill, they usually resort to trying home remedies first. Following that, people in traditional societies often visit some type of traditional healer. It may be some time before they consult a physician practicing "modern medicine"—often only when they are certain that they are ill and when other forms of treatment have not brought relief.

Many forms of traditional behavior *are* conducive to good health. This might include, for example, traditional practices that allow the mother to spend some time with her baby before she returns to her normal work and household chores. Male circumcision, as practiced in many cultures, reduces the transmission of HIV. Other traditional practices, however, are not health promoting. Feeding sugar water to infants, for example, is not good for the health of the infants, who should be exclusively breastfed for 6 months. It is important to consider how healthy behaviors can be promoted.

There are a number of models of how behaviors can be changed, including the Health Belief model, the Diffusion of Innovations model, and the Stages of Change model. To encourage behavior change, of course, requires a good understanding of the behaviors that are taking place, how they relate to health, the underlying motivation for them, and the likely response to various approaches aimed at changing them.

When thinking about trying to change behavior on a large scale, such as promoting an immunization program, the use of seat belts, or the willingness to seek treatment for leprosy, several approaches are important. One way to engender change is to engage in community mobilization. Promoting messages about desirable and undesirable health behaviors can also be done effectively using mass media, and, increasingly, social media. Social marketing and health education efforts are also important. Cash transfers are also being used to promote behavior change. An effective tool for setting the foundation for any efforts at investing in health or trying to change behaviors is to carry out a social assessment, which will identify the social basis of the health issues one is trying to influence, as well as the likely social impacts of the proposed activities.

Study Questions

1. What is culture? Give some examples of aspects of culture that vary across different societies.
2. Why is it important to assess the relationship between culture and health in specific societies by the extent to which cultural practices promote or discourage good physical and mental health?
3. Name three cultural practices that are health promoting. Name three cultural practices that are harmful to health.
4. How does culture relate to people's perceptions of illness? Why would some cultures regard some illnesses as normal?
5. What might low-income people in traditional societies see as possible causes of illness?
6. What is the difference between illness and disease?
7. When an infant is ill in a traditional society in a low-income country, from whom and in what order are the parents likely to seek help?

8. Why would members of a community seek treatment for illness from traditional healers?

9. If you wanted to encourage the large-scale adoption of a healthy behavior, such as giving up cigarette smoking, what information would you want to know as you plan your effort?

10. Why are social assessments important? If they are done well, what gains would they produce that might not come if there were no such assessment?

References

1. Scrimshaw, S. C. (2001). Culture, behavior, and health. In M. H. Merson, R. E. Black, & A. Mills (Eds.), *International public health: Diseases, programs, systems, and policies* (pp. 53–78). Gaithersburg, MD: Aspen.

2. Tylor, E. (1871). *Primitive culture*. London, UK: J. Murray.

3. Haviland, W. A. (1990). The nature of culture. In *Cultural anthropology* (6th ed.). Fort Worth, TX: Holt, Rinehart & Winston, Inc.

4. Miller, B. (2004). *Culture and health*. Presentation given at George Washington University, Washington, DC.

5. Substance Abuse and Mental Health Service Administration (SAMSHA). (2016). *Cultural competence*. Retrieved from https://www.samhsa.gov/capt/applying-strategic-prevention/cultural-competence

6. Yeager, K. A., & Bauer-Wu, S. (2013). Cultural humility: Essential foundation for clinical researchers. *Applied Nursing Research, 26*(4), 251–256. doi: 10.1016/j.apnr.2013.06.008.

7. Health.gov. (n.d.). *A quick guide to health literacy*. Retrieved from https://health.gov/communication/literacy/quickguide/factsbasic.htm

8. World Health Organization. (n.d.). *Traditional, complementary, and integrative medicine*. Retrieved from http://www.who.int/traditional-complementary-integrative-medicine/about/en/

9. National Center for Complimentary and Integrative Medicine. (2017). *About NCCIH*. Retrieved from https://nccih.nih.gov/about

10. National Cancer Institute. (n.d.). Western medicine. In *Dictionary of cancer terms*. Retrieved from https://www.cancer.gov/publications/dictionaries/cancer-terms/def/western-medicine

11. IGI Global. (n.d.). *What is Western biomedicine*. Retrieved from https://www.igi-global.com/dictionary/multiple-voices-multiple-paths/56656

12. Murphy, E. M. (2003). Being born female is dangerous for your health. *American Psychologist, 58*(3), 205–210.

13. Kleinman, A., Eisenberg, L., & Good, B. (1978). Culture, illness, and care: Clinical lessons from anthropologic and cross-cultural research. *Annals of Internal Medicine, 88*(2), 251–258.

14. Hopper, S. (1993). The influence of ethnicity on the health of older women. *Clinics in Geriatric Medicine, 9*, 231–259.

15. Letendre, A. D. (2002). Aboriginal traditional medicine: Where does it fit? *Crossing Boundaries, 1*(2), 78–87.

16. Jegede, A. S. (2002). The Yoruba cultural construction of health and illness. *Nordic Journal of African Studies, 11*(3), 322–335.

17. Pachter, L. M. (1994). Culture and clinical care. Folk illness beliefs and behaviors and their implications for health care delivery. *JAMA, 271*(9), 690–694.

18. Bolton, J. M. (1972). Food taboos among the Orang Asli in West Malaysia: A potential nutritional hazard. *American Journal of Clinical Nutrition, 25*(8), 788–799.

19. Chiwuzie, J., & Okolocha, C. (2001). Traditional belief systems and maternal mortality in a semi-urban community in southern Nigeria. *African Journal of Reproductive Health, 5*(1), 75–82.

20. Trigo, M., Roncada, M. J., Stewien, G. T., & Pereira, I. M. (1989). [Food taboos in the northern region of Brazil]. *Revista de Saúde Pública, 23*(6), 455–464.

21. Sundararaj, R., & Pereira, S. M. (1975). Dietary intakes and food taboos of lactating women in a South Indian community. *Tropical and Geographical Medicine, 27*(2), 189–193.

22. Bhasin, V. (2003). Sickness and therapy among tribals of Rajasthan. *Studies of Tribes and Tribals, 1*(1), 77–83.

23. Fassin, D., & Badji, I. (1986). Ritual buffoonery: A social preventive measure against childhood mortality in Senegal. *The Lancet, 18*(1), 142–143.

24. Institute of Health Metrics and Evaluation. (n.d.). GBD Compare: Viz Hub. Retrieved from https://vizhub.healthdata.org/gbd-compare/

25. Edberg, M. (2013). *The essentials of health behavior* (2nd ed.). Burlington, MA: Jones & Bartlett Learning.

26. Murphy, E. (2005). *Promoting healthy behavior. Health bulletin 2*. Washington, DC: Population Reference Bureau.

27. Rosenstock, I. M., Strecher, V. J., & Becker, M. H. (1988). Social learning theory and the Health Belief Model. *Health Education Quarterly, 15*(2), 175–183.

28. Rogers, E. (1983). *Diffusion of innovations* (3rd ed.). New York, NY: Free Press.

29. Population Institute. (n.d.). *Soap operas: Making a difference in developing nations*. Retrieved from https://www.populationinstitute.org/resources/populationonline/issue/1/7/

30. Safko, L., & Brake, D. (2012). *The social media bible: Tactics, tools, and strategies for business success* (3rd ed.). Hoboken, NJ: Wiley.

31. Laranjo, L., Arguel, A., Neves, A. L., Gallagher, A. M., Kaplan, R., Mortimer, N., . . . Lau, A. Y. S. (2015). The influence of social networking sites on health behavior change: A systematic review and meta-analysis. *Journal of the American Medical Informatics Association, 22*(1), (243–256). doi: 10.1136/amiajnl-2014-002841

32. Hagg, E., Dahinten, V. S., & Currie, L. M. (2018). The emerging use of social media for health-related purposes in low and middle-income countries: A scoping review. *International Journal of Medical Informatics, 115*, 92–105. doi: 10.1016/j.ijmedinf.2018.04.010

33. Purdy, C. H. (2011). Using the Internet and social media to promote condom use in Turkey. *Reproductive Health Matters, 19*(37), 157–165.

34. Westberg, K., Stavros, C., Smith, A. C. T., Munro, G., & Argus, K. (2018). An examination of how alcohol brands use sport to engage consumers on social media. *Drug and Alcohol Review, 37*(1), 28–35. doi: 10.1111/dar.12493

35. Poushter, J., Bishop, C., & Chwe, H. (2018). Social media use continues to rise in developing countries but plateaus across developed ones. *Pew Research Center.* Retrieved from http://www.pewglobal.org/2018/06/19/social-media-use-continues-to-rise-in-developing-countries-but-plateaus-across-developed-ones/

36. Hagen-Zanker, J., Bastagli, F., Harman, L., Barca, V., Sturge, G., & Schmidt, T. (2016). Understanding the impact of cash transfers: The evidence. *ODI.* Retrieved from https://www.odi.org/sites/odi.org.uk/files/resource-documents/11465.pdf

37. Vanclay, F. (2003). *Social impact assessment: International principles.* Special Publication Series No. 2. Fargo, ND: International Association for Impact Assessment. Retrieved from https://www.iaia.org/uploads/pdf/IAIA-SIA-International-Principles.pdf

38. This policy and program brief is adapted with permission from a paper prepared in May 2010 by Josephine E.V. Francisco, titled *Barrier Analysis of Exclusive Breastfeeding Practices in Ruyigi and Cancuzo Provinces, Burundi.* This paper was part of a culminating experience to meet the requirements for the master of public health degree at The George Washington University.

39. World Health Organization. (n.d.). *Increasing breastfeeding could save 800,000 children and US$ 300 billion every year.* Retrieved from http://www.who.int/maternal_child_adolescent/news_events/news/2016/exclusive-breastfeeding/en/

40. Food for the Hungry. (n.d.). *Barrier analysis.* Retrieved from http://barrieranalysis.fhi.net

41. Chan, M. (2014, February 11). *WHO director-general celebrates polio-free India.* Retrieved from http://www.who.int/dg/speeches/2014/india-polio-free/en/

42. Centers for Disease Control and Prevention. (1998). *Progress toward poliomyelitis eradication—India, 1998. MMWR, 47*(37), 771–781.

43. The Communication Initiative Network. (2004). *Social mobilisation-communication polio eradication partnership—India.* Retrieved from http://www.comminit.com/en/node/127845/292

44. UNICEF. (n.d.). India polio eradication. Retrieved from http://unicef.in/Whatwedo/5/Polio

45. PopulationPyramid.net. (n.d.). India 2017. Retrieved from https://www.populationpyramid.net/india/2017/

46. Know India. (n.d.). *States and union territories.* Retrieved from http://knowindia.gov.in/states-uts/

47. Global Polio Eradication Initiative. (2010). *Annual Report 2010.* Retrieved from http://polioeradication.org/wp-content/uploads/2016/07/GPEI_AR2010_EN.pdf

48. Chaturvedi, S., Dasgupta, R., Adhish, V., Ganguly, K. K., Rai, S., Sushant, L., . . . Arora, N. K. (2009). Deconstructing social resistance to pulse polio campaign in two north Indian districts. *Indian Pediatrics, 46*(11), 963–974.

49. Obregón, R., Chitnis, K., Morry, C., Feek, W., Bates, J., Galway, M., & Ogden, E. (2009, August). Achieving polio eradication: A review of health communication evidence and lessons learned in India and Pakistan. *Bulletin of the World Health Organization, 87*(8), 624–630.

50. Bhagat, P. (2005). *Vaccination campaign focuses on tackling social resistance to vaccine.* Retrieved from http:www.unicef.org/infobycountry/india_25290.html

51. Hewlett, B. S., & Amola, R. P. (2003, October). Cultural contexts of Ebola in northern Uganda. *Emerging Infectious Diseases, 9*(10). Retrieved from http://wwwnc.cdc.gov/eid/article/9/10/02-0493

52. World Health Organization. (2014, September). *Ebola fact sheet.* Retrieved from http://www.who.int/mediacentre/factsheets/fs103/en/

53. Hewlett, B. S., & Hewlett, B. L. (2008). *Ebola, culture, and politics: The anthropology of an emerging disease.* Belmont, CA: Thomson Wadsworth.

54. Centers for Disease Control and Prevention. (n.d.). *Outbreaks chronology: Ebola virus disease.* Retrieved from http://www.cdc.gov/vhf/ebola/outbreaks/history/chronology.html

55. Alexander, K. A., Sanderson, C. E., Marathe, M., Lewis, B. L., Rivers, C. M., Shaman, J. M., . . . Eubank, S. (2014). What factors might have led to the emergence of Ebola in West Africa? *PLoS Neglected Tropical Diseases.* Retrieved from http://blogs.plos.org/speakingofmedicine/2014/11/11/factors-might-led-emergence-ebola-west-africa/

56. Centers for Disease Control and Prevention & World Health Organization. (1998). *Control for viral haemorrhagic fevers in the African health care setting.* Atlanta, GA: Centers for Disease Control and Prevention.

57. World Health Organization. (2014, November 7). *New WHO safe and dignified burial protocol—Key to reducing Ebola transmission.* Retrieved from http://www.who.int/mediacentre/news/notes/2014/ebola-burial-protocol/en/

58. Chowell, G., & Nishiura, H. (2014). Transmission dynamics and control of Ebola virus disease (EVD): A review. *BMC Medicine, 120.* Retrieved from http://www.biomedcentral.com/1741-7015/12/196

59. Ravi, S., & Gauldin, E. (2014). Sociocultural dimensions of the Ebola virus disease outbreak in Liberia. *Biosecurity and Bioterrorism: Biodefense, Strategy, Practice, and Science, 12*(6). doi: 10.1089/bsp.2014.1002

60. World Health Organization. (2007). *Addressing sex and gender in epidemic-prone infectious diseases.* Geneva, Switzerland: Author. Retrieved from http://www.who.int/csr/resources/publications/SexGenderInfectDis.pdf?ua=1

61. Wolfe, L. (2014, August 20). Why are so many women dying from Ebola? *Foreign Policy.* Retrieved from http://www.foreignpolicy.com/articles/2014/08/20/why_are_so_many_women_dying_from_ebola

62. Hitchen, J. (2014, November 5). *Ebola in Sierra Leone: Stigmatization.* Africa Research Institute. Retrieved from http://www.africaresearchinstitute.org/blog/ebola-stigma/

63. UN News Center. (2014, November 12). *Ebola: UN special envoy says combating stigma integral to overall crisis response.* Retrieved from https://news.un.org/en/story/2014/11/483462-ebola-un-special-envoy-says-combating-stigma-integral-overall-crisis-response

64. Solidarity. (n.d.). *Oxford Dictionary.* Retrieved from http://www.oxforddictionaries.com/us/definition/american_english/solidarity

65. Davtyan, M., Brown, B., & Oluwatoyin Folayan, M. (2014). Addressing Ebola-related stigma: Lessons learned from HIV/AIDS. *Global Health Action, 7,* 26058. doi: 10.3402/gha.v7.26058

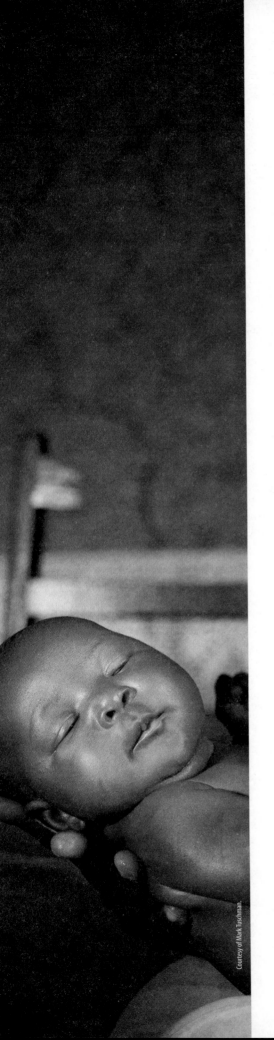

PART III

The Burden of Disease

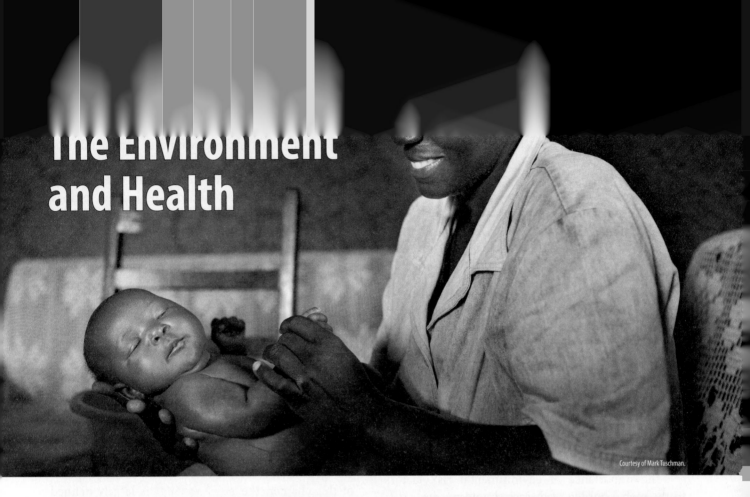

The Environment and Health

Courtesy of Mark Tuschman.

LEARNING OBJECTIVES

By the end of this chapter, the reader will be able to do the following:

- Discuss the most important environmental threats to health, especially for low- and middle-income countries
- Review the burden of disease related to environmental risks
- Comment on the costs and consequences of key environmental health burdens
- Describe some of the most cost-effective ways of reducing the global burden of environmental health problems

▶ Vignettes

Rashmi lived in the eastern part of Nepal in a modest home. She often had difficulty breathing. This was linked to the way Rashmi cooked, with an unvented household stove that was fueled by cow dung or wood. She cooked two meals a day on the stove, and she often held her new baby on her back as she did so. She heard about different stoves and about using kerosene or gas for fuel. However, she lacked the money to buy a new stove or to use kerosene or gas for cooking.

Sunisa was a young mother in a rural area in northern Laos. She had two children, a 1-year-old and a 3-year-old. Sunisa was not wealthy. Her house had no water connection. Thus, she collected water daily from the stream about half a mile from her house in containers she carried on her head. She stored the containers at the edge of her house, covered by cloth. Sunisa had only a little formal education and did nothing to purify the water. Her two daughters regularly had bouts of diarrhea, partly the result of drinking unsafe water.

Juan had lived in Mexico City his whole life and was now 70 years old. He remembered a time when the city was not so crowded, had few cars, and when the views from the city were magnificent. He lamented the fact that today the city was too crowded to enjoy, the traffic was overwhelming, and the air was often unbreathable. It was so polluted that on many days there was no view at all. Juan had a very hard time breathing because he suffered from chronic obstructive pulmonary disease (COPD). Juan suspected that outdoor air pollution contributed to his illness.

Raj and his family lived in a slum at the edge of Patna, India. The slum was the size of a small city. Most of the houses were made of scrap wood with scrap metal roofing. The houses had no water connection and people had to walk to the edge of the slum to get their water from a standpipe or buy it from a tanker truck if the standpipe did not work. There were no private toilets either. There were a few toilets that were shared, but they were always dirty. For this reason, many people in the slum, especially the women, waited until dark and then went to defecate in fields near the slum.

▶ The Importance of Environmental Health

Environmental health issues are major risk factors for the global burden of disease. One important study, which took a broad view of environmental risk factors, concluded that 22 percent of global deaths and 23 percent of the global burden of disease are attributable to environmental risk factors. A study of the burden of ambient particulate matter pollution suggested that this pollution alone causes 7.6 percent of total global deaths and 4.2 percent of global DALYs.[1]

The importance of environmental risk factors to the global burden of disease should not be a surprise. The third-leading cause of death in low- and middle-income countries is COPD, the fifth-leading cause of death is lower respiratory infections, and the seventh is diarrheal diseases. Each of these is closely linked with environmental factors. In addition, environmental risk factors are even more important when considering the causes of death of children in low- and middle-income countries. Lower respiratory conditions are the leading cause of death for children 0–5 years of age in these countries, and diarrheal diseases are fifth. For children 5–14 years old, lower respiratory conditions are the fourth leading cause of death, and diarrhea is the fifth leading cause of death.[2]

Environmental health matters are also of special importance because addressing them effectively is central to the achievement of the Sustainable Development Goals (SDGs), as shown in **TABLE 8-1**.

This chapter aims to introduce some of the most important links between health and the environment. Environmental health is a very broad topic. Given the introductory nature of this text, this chapter focuses largely on only three of the most important risk factors in terms of the burden of environmentally related diseases in low- and middle-income countries. These include unsafe water, sanitation, and hygiene; ambient particulate air pollution; and household air pollution that comes from the use of solid fuels.[3]

The chapter begins by covering some of the most important terms and concepts that relate to environmental health. It then explores the burden of disease related to the risk factors noted previously. After that, it briefly reviews some of the costs and consequences of the selected environmental risk factors.

The chapter concludes with case studies that discuss some of the most challenging environmental health issues and some of the most cost-effective ways to address them in low- and middle-income settings. Much has been written about environmental health. Readers who wish to explore environmental health in greater detail are encouraged to examine those writings, possibly starting with an introductory text on environmental health.[4,5]

▶ Key Concepts

It is important to understand how the word *environment* is used in this chapter. In some cases, the word *environment* in a health context is defined very broadly, meaning everything that is not genetic. In other cases, when considering health, the word *environment* includes only physical, chemical, or biological agents that directly affect health. For the purposes of this chapter, the **environment** is largely defined as "external physical, chemical, and microbiological exposures and processes that impinge upon individuals and groups and are beyond the immediate control of individuals."[6(p379)]

It is also valuable to understand the meaning of **environmental health**. This generally refers to a set of public health efforts that "is concerned with preventing disease, death, and disability by reducing exposure to adverse environmental conditions and promoting behavior change. It focuses on the direct and indirect causes of disease and injuries and taps resources inside and outside the healthcare system to help improve health outcomes."[7]

The World Health Organization (WHO) takes a broad view of environmental health and says:

> Environmental health comprises those aspects of human health, including quality of life, that are determined by physical, chemical, biological, social, and psychosocial factors in the environment. It also refers to the theory and practice of assessing, correcting, controlling, and preventing those factors in the environment that can potentially affect adversely the health of present and future generations.[8]

It is important to note that in discussing the burden of disease and other topics, this chapter will use a number of terms taken from the Global Burden of Disease Study 2016 (GBD 2016). That study refers

TABLE 8-1 Selected Links Between Environmental Health, Human Health, and the SDGs

Goal 1: End poverty in all its forms everywhere

Degradation of the environment reduces economic prosperity and generally takes its heaviest toll among the poor. The lack of access to safe water and sanitation are major causes of ill health. This leads to lower human productivity, greater expenditure on health, and greater risks of living in poverty.

Goal 3: Ensure healthy lives and promote well-being for all at all ages

About a quarter of all DALYs in 2016 were attributed to environmental health risks, including lack of safe water and sanitation, poor hygiene, and indoor and outdoor air pollution.

Goal 5: Achieve gender equality and empower all women and girls

The lack of safe water imposes a substantial economic burden on women, who are generally responsible for getting water for families in places in which access is lacking. This reduces the time they can spend at school and doing other work, both of which have a negative impact on their health.

Goal 6: Ensure access to water and sanitation for all

The lack of access to safe water and sanitation is a major risk factor for morbidity and mortality, especially in lower-income countries and among lower-income people.

Goal 7: Ensure access to affordable, reliable, sustainable and modern energy

Cooking with biofuels in unventilated settings is a major risk to health, especially in lower-income countries.

Goal 10: Reduce inequality within and among countries

Environmental health issues are a substantial barrier to good health and human productivity in many settings and disproportionately affect the poor. Thus, they pose a major barrier to reducing disparities.

Goal 13: Take urgent action to combat climate change and its impacts

Climate change poses a range of risks to health globally by its possible links, for example, to coastal flooding, migration, a loss of livelihoods, and the spread to new settings of some vector-borne diseases.

Modified from United Nations Sustainable Development Goals Knowledge Platform. (n.d.). Sustainable Development Goals. © United Nations. Reprinted with the permission of the United Nations.

to what we commonly call "outdoor air pollution" as "ambient particular matter pollution." This chapter will use that term as well. GBD 2016 refers to what we commonly call "indoor air pollution" as "household air pollution from solid fuels." This chapter will use the GBD 2016 term for that as well.

Another term that is commonly used when speaking about environmental health is WASH. This refers to "water, sanitation, and hygiene." This chapter will speak specifically about water, sanitation, and hygiene, and it is important to be familiar with the term *WASH*.

In thinking about the environment and health, it is important to consider the key types of environmental risk, the setting and scale at which one is exposed to such risks, and how one might be exposed to them.

TABLE 8-2 highlights some types of environmental exposures that occur at various levels:

- The household
- The workplace
- The community
- Regionally
- Globally

We are generally exposed to such risks through air, water, or food.

TABLE 8-3 further highlights some examples of environmental health issues, their determinants, and their consequences. It organizes these examples by their level of impact: the household, the community, or globally.

TABLE 8-2 Selected Examples of Unhealthy Environmental Exposures

Types of Exposure	Household	Workplace	Community	Regional	Global
Microbiological	Contaminated drinking water	Needlestick injuries in health services	Fecal contamination of lakes and rivers	Spread of pathogenic bacteria through major waterways	Global spread of infectious disease associated with climate change
Chemical	Lead exposure from paint	Exposure to solvents in manufacturing	Urban air pollution from vehicles	Spread of air pollution to larger areas	Greenhouse gas emissions
Physical	Indoor temperatures too hot or too cold	Noisy workplace machinery	Traffic noise	Radiation from nuclear accidents	Increased ultraviolet radiation related to ozone depletion

Modified from McMillan, A, Kjellstrom, Smith, KR, Pillarisetti, A, Woodward, A. Environmental and Occupational Health. Merson, M. Mills, A, Black, R. , eds. (2018). In Merson, M, Black, R, Mills, A., eds. *Global Health Diseases, Systems, Programs, and Policies*. (Fourth Edition). Burlington, Ma., p. 479.

TABLE 8-3 Typical Environmental Health Issues: Determinants and Health Consequences

Underlying Determinants	Selected Adverse Health Consequences
Household	
Unsafe water, inadequate sanitation and solid waste disposal, improper hygiene	Diarrhea and vector-related diseases, such as malaria, schistosomiasis, and dengue
Crowded housing and poor ventilation of smoke	Respiratory diseases and lung cancer
Exposure to naturally occurring toxic substances	Poisoning from arsenic, manganese, and fluorides
Community	
Improper water resource management, including poor drainage	Vector-related diseases, such as malaria and schistosomiasis
Exposure to vehicle emissions and industrial air pollution	Respiratory diseases, some cancers, and reduced IQ in children
Global	
Climate change Ozone depletion	Injury/death from extreme heat/cold, storms, floods, and fires Aggravation of respiratory diseases, population dislocation, water pollution from sea level rise, etc. Skin cancer, cataracts Indirect effects: spread of vector-borne diseases and compromised food production

Adapted from The World Bank. (n.d.). Environmental health. Retrieved from http://siteresources.worldbank.org/INTPHAAG/Resources/AAGEHEng.pdf

Key Environmental Health Burdens

This section very briefly examines the most important health conditions that relate to the environmental issues that are discussed in this chapter. The section then examines the burden of disease from those conditions.

As you read the next section, it is important to keep in mind how families cook, get water, and dispose of human waste and how these change as family income grows. **FIGURE 8-1** indicates what are often called "service ladders" for access to improved water and sanitation services and facilities for handwashing.

Household Air Pollution from Solid Fuels

WHO estimates that about 3 billion people in the world depend on solid fuel for their cooking and heating. Such fuels include the fossil fuel coal and the biomass fuels of animal dung, wood, logging wastes, and crop waste.[9] In the cases that most concern us, cooking and heating are done on open stoves that are not vented to the outside. These are generally used by lower-income groups, because people usually move to kerosene or gas for cooking and switch to improved stoves and better ventilation as their family income grows.

Biomass fuels and coal do not completely combust when they are burned. Instead, they leave behind

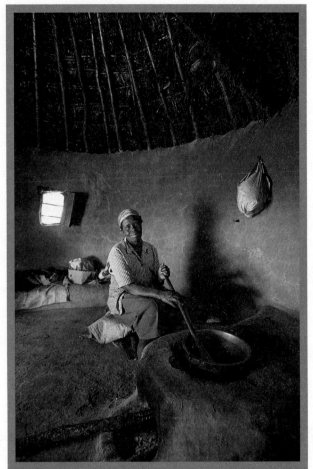

PHOTO 8-1 Indoor air pollution is a major health risk. This stems from cooking indoors with a biofuel without sufficient ventilation. This woman is cooking according to traditional methods, but these methods are not health-enabling for her and her family. What is the state of the art for developing and using more efficient cookstoves?
Courtesy of Mark Tuschman.

breathable particles of a variety of gases and chemical products. The amount of these substances in a poorly ventilated home can exceed WHO norms by more than 20 times.[10] Smoke from burning biomass inside the home can produce conjunctivitis, upper respiratory irritation, and acute respiratory infection. The carbon monoxide produced can lead to acute poisoning. Other gases and smoke are associated over the long term with cardiovascular disease, chronic obstructive pulmonary disease, adverse reproductive outcomes, and cancer.[10] Women and children are especially vulnerable to the effects of household air pollution.

Ambient Particulate Matter Pollution

Many pollutants can be found in the ambient air. The most common effects of ambient air pollution are respiratory symptoms, including cough, irritation of the nose and throat, and shortness of breath.[11] **TABLE 8-4** indicates

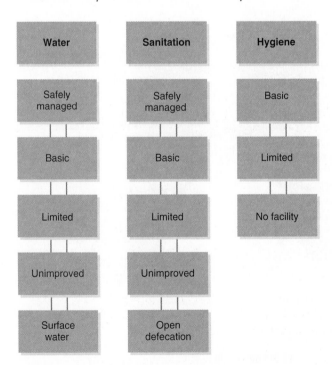

FIGURE 8-1 Ladders of Progress in Access to Water, Sanitation, and Hygiene

Modified from World Health Organization & UNICEF. (2017). *Progress on drinking water, sanitation and hygiene: 2017* (p. 2). Retrieved from http://www.who.int/mediacentre/news/releases/2017/launch-version-report-jmp-water-sanitation-hygiene.pdf

TABLE 8-4 Common Air Pollutants and Their Health Effects

Name of Pollutant	Example of Source	Health Effects
Carbon monoxide	Combustion of gasoline and fossil fuels; cars	Reduction in oxygen-carrying capacity of the blood
Lead	Leaded gasoline, paint, batteries	Brain/central nervous system damage; digestive problems
Nitrogen dioxide, nitrogen oxides	Combustion of gasoline and fossil fuels; cars	Damage to lungs and respiratory system
Ozone	Variety of oxygen formed by chemical reaction of pollutants	Breathing impairment; eye irritation
Particulate matter	Burning of wood and diesel fuels	Respiratory irritation; lung damage
Smog	Mixture of pollutants, esp. ozone; originates from petroleum-based fuels	Irritation of respiratory system and eyes
Sulfur dioxide	Burning of coal and oil	Breathing problems; lung damage
Volatile organic compounds (VOCs)	Burning fuels; released from certain chemicals (e.g., solvents)	Acute effects similar to those of smog; possible carcinogen

Data from U.S. Environmental Protection Agency. (2007). The plain English guide to the Clean Air Act: The common air pollutants. Retrieved from https://www.epa.gov/sites/production/files/2015-08/documents/peg.pdf; U.S. Environmental Protection Agency. (n.d.). Air & radiation: Six common air pollutants. Retrieved from http://www.epa.gov/air/urbanair/

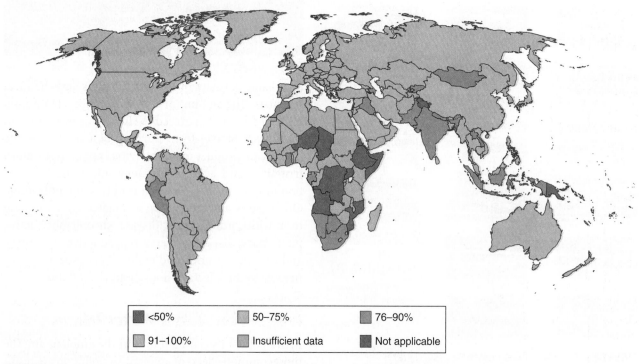

■ <50%	■ 50–75%	■ 76–90%
■ 91–100%	■ Insufficient data	■ Not applicable

FIGURE 8-2 Percentage of Population with Access to Improved Water Supplies, 2015

World Health Organization & UNICEF. (2017). *Progress on drinking water and sanitation, 2017.* Retrieved from http://www.who.int/mediacentre/news/releases/2017/launch-version-report-jmp-water-sanitation-hygiene.pdf some of the most common pollutants in the ambient air, examples of their sources, and the most important health effects. Certain preexisting health factors make some people susceptible to being harmed by ambient particulate matter pollution. In addition, older and younger people are generally most susceptible to the health effects of ambient particulate matter pollution.

There have been a number of instances in which severe ambient particulate matter pollution has been associated with considerable excess mortality in a very short time. Among the most famous cases was in London, England, in 1952. Because of what is called a temperature inversion, a dense fog, full of pollutants, hung over the city center for several days. The value of certain particulates in the air was 3 to 10 times the normal level. On December 13, 1952, the city administration reported a death rate per 100,000 people that was more than four times the normal daily death rate for that period.[11]

Water, Sanitation, and Hygiene

WHO estimated that in 2015 about 71 percent of the global population, or about 5.2 billion people, had access to "a safely managed drinking water service." This is defined as "one located on premises, available when needed, and free from contamination." WHO also estimated that about 1.3 billion people had access to only "basic service" for water. This is defined as "an improved drinking-water source within a round trip of 30 minutes to collect water." Another 263 million people were estimated to have had only "limited service," requiring more than 30 minutes to collect water. Unfortunately, about 160 million people still depend on surface water sources. Moreover, it is estimated that almost 2 million people in the world depend on water sources that are contaminated with human waste.[12] In addition, access to safe water generally varies with country income level and the income levels of different regions within countries. Access to an improved water source is depicted graphically in **FIGURE 8-2**.

In fact, water-related infections are among the most important in terms of the burden of disease, and they are numerous in low- and middle-income countries. **TABLE 8-5** indicates how water-related infections may be classified. Some of the most important waterborne pathogens are shown in **TABLE 8-6**.

These pathogens are associated with diarrhea and many other gastrointestinal problems. They can be deadly when they lead to severe diarrhea and dehydration. Such diseases are especially risky for the very young, the very old, and people who have compromised immune systems, such as people living with HIV/AIDS.

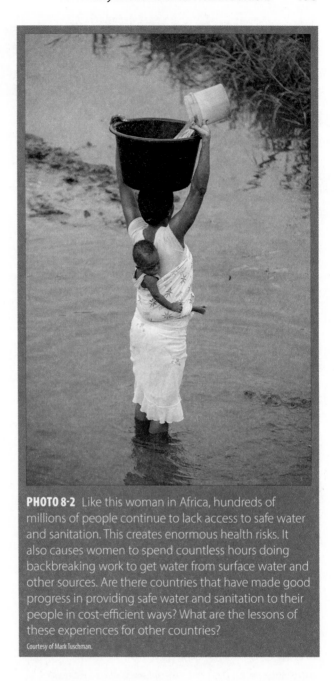

PHOTO 8-2 Like this woman in Africa, hundreds of millions of people continue to lack access to safe water and sanitation. This creates enormous health risks. It also causes women to spend countless hours doing backbreaking work to get water from surface water and other sources. Are there countries that have made good progress in providing safe water and sanitation to their people in cost-efficient ways? What are the lessons of these experiences for other countries?

Courtesy of Mark Tuschman.

WHO estimated that in 2015 about 68 percent of the world's population, or about 5 billion people, had access to at least a basic sanitation service. Only about 60 percent of the people in the world had access to improved sanitation. Almost 3 billion used a "safely managed sanitation service," which is defined as "use of a toilet or improved latrine, not shared with other households, with a system in place to ensure that excreta are treated or disposed of safely." Almost 2 billion people used sanitation facilities that were connected to sewers from which wastewater was treated. Another almost 1 billion people used sanitation facilities in which waste was treated on site. Unfortunately, about 2.3 billion people have no sanitation facilities and almost 900 million people are still defecating in

TABLE 8-5 Classification of Water-Related Infections

Transmission	Water-Related Infections
Waterborne	The pathogen is in water that is ingested.
Water-washed (or water-scarce)	Person-to-person transmission because of a lack of water for hygiene.
Water-based	Transmission via an aquatic intermediate host.
Water-related insect vector	Transmission by insects that breed in water or bite near water.

Data from Cairncross, S., & Valdmanis, V. (2006). Water supply, sanitation, and hygiene promotion. In D. T. Jamison, J. G. Breman, A. R. Measham, et al. (Eds.), *Disease control priorities in developing countries* (2nd ed., p. 775). Washington, DC, and New York, NY: The World Bank and Oxford University Press.

TABLE 8-6 Selected Waterborne Pathogens

Enteric protozoal parasites
- *Entamoeba histolytica*
- *Giardia intestinalis*
- *Cryptosporidium parvum*
- *Cryptosporidium cayetanensis*

Bacterial enteropathogens
- *Salmonella*
- *Shigella*
- *Escherichia coli*
- *Vibrio cholerae*
- *Campylobacter*

Viral pathogens
- Enteroviruses
- Adenoviruses
- Noroviruses

Modified from Friis, R. H. (2007). Water quality. In *Essentials of environmental health* (p. 211). Sudbury, MA: Jones and Bartlett.

the open.[13] Access to improved sanitation also generally varies by country and regional income level. **FIGURE 8-3** shows access to improved sanitation facilities in 2015.

There is good evidence that improved disposal of human waste is associated with reductions in diarrheal disease, intestinal parasites, and trachoma. Failure to dispose properly of human waste contaminates water and food sources and leads to an increase in transmission of pathogens through the oral–fecal route. Failure to improve sanitation is also associated with the spread of parasitic worms, such as ascaris and hookworm.[14] Improved sanitation reduces the burden of trachoma, because the flies that are significantly

involved in the spread of that disease often breed in human waste.[14]

One area of hygiene, handwashing with soap, is especially important for good health. Unfortunately, however, there is little data about the rates of handwashing with soap, or even on the availability of soap and water at designated places, which is used as a proxy for handwashing. The best available data in 2015 was from a sample of 70 countries throughout the world. North America and Europe showed consistently high rates of basic handwashing facilities. The five countries surveyed in East and Southeast Asia also showed rates between 65 and 90 percent. In Latin America, the rates varied from about 25 to over 90 percent, similar to the rates for western Asia and northern Africa. The rates in central Asia and southern Asia varied from only about 5 percent to almost universal facilities. In sub-Saharan Africa the rates varied from about 0 percent to about 50 percent. Clearly, much of the world, especially low- and lower middle-income countries, is very far from having universal access to handwashing facilities so that people might wash their hands with soap and water when, for example, preparing food, feeding their children, or after defecating.[15]

▶ The Burden of Environmentally Related Diseases

The sections that follow explore further the burden of disease related to household air pollution, ambient particulate matter pollution, and unimproved water and sanitation. One section also comments on hygiene.

To assist in reviewing the sections that follow, **TABLE 8-7** shows the leading risk factors for deaths in 2016

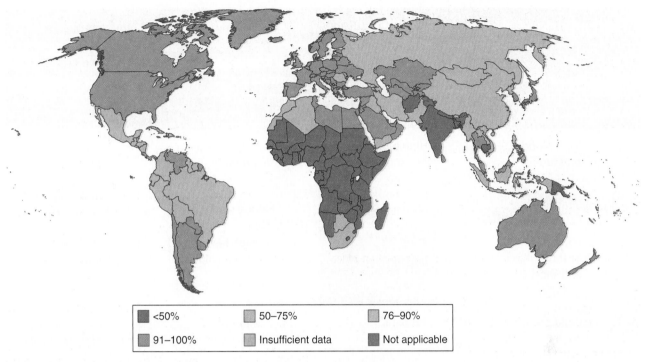

FIGURE 8-3 Percentage of the Population with Access to Improved Sanitation Facilities, 2015

World Health Organization & UNICEF. (2017). *Progress on drinking water and sanitation, 2017* (p. 4). Retrieved from http://www.who.int/mediacentre/news/releases/2017/launch-version-report-jmp-water-sanitation-hygiene.pdf

by country income group. **TABLE 8-8** shows the same data for disability-adjusted life years (DALYs). Both tables highlight the key environmentally related risk factors.

Household Air Pollution

Household air pollution was the eighth most important risk factor in 2016 for deaths globally, for both sexes and all ages. However, it was the second most important risk factor in low-income countries and the sixth most important risk factor for lower middle-income countries.[2]

In fact, household air pollution is almost 20 times greater a risk for death in low-income than in upper middle-income countries and about 2.5 times the risk in low-income countries as in lower middle-income countries.[2] Almost all of the deaths associated with household air pollution from the use of solid fuels occur in low- and lower middle-income countries.

WHO estimates that about 3.8 million people die yearly from exposure to household air pollution. WHO has further estimated that such deaths are distributed in the following way[9]:

- 27 percent are due to pneumonia
- 18 percent from stroke
- 27 percent from ischemic heart disease
- 20 percent from COPD
- 8 percent from lung cancer

When looking at this another way, we see that household air pollution is a major attributable risk for

all of the above conditions. WHO further estimates that household air pollution is responsible for the following deaths[9]:

- 45 percent of deaths from pneumonia in children under 5 years of age
- 25 percent of deaths from COPD in adults in low- and middle-income countries
- 12 percent of deaths from stroke
- 11 percent of deaths from ischemic heart disease
- 17 percent of premature deaths from lung cancer in adults

These figures include only those diseases for which there is solid evidence of a link to household air pollution from the use of solid fuels. However, this may be an underestimate of the real burden of disease from household air pollution because there is some evidence that household air pollution of this type is also associated with cataracts and tuberculosis. There is also tentative evidence of links with adverse pregnancy outcomes, especially low birthweight, and two types of cancer other than lung cancer.[9]

Ambient Particulate Matter Pollution

In 2016, ambient particulate matter pollution was the sixth leading attributable risk factor for death globally. It was also sixth in low-income and upper middle-income countries. It was the third leading attributable risk factor for death in lower middle-income countries.[2]

TABLE 8-7 Leading Environmental Risk Factors for Deaths by World Bank Country Income Group, 2016

Low-Income Countries		Lower Middle-Income Countries		Upper Middle-Income Countries		High-Income Countries	
Rank	Risk Factor	Rank	Risk Factor	Rank	Risk Factor	Rank	Risk Factor
1	High blood pressure	1	High blood pressure	1	High blood pressure	1	High blood pressure
2	Household air pollution	2	High fasting plasma glucose	2	Smoking	2	Smoking
3	Low birthweight and short gestation	3	Ambient particulate matter	3	High fasting plasma glucose	3	High body mass index
4	Child growth failure	4	Smoking	4	High body mass index	4	High fasting plasma glucose
5	Unsafe sex	5	High total cholesterol	5	High total cholesterol	5	High total cholesterol
6	Ambient particulate matter	6	Household air pollution	6	Ambient particulate matter	6	Alcohol use
7	High fasting plasma glucose	7	High body mass index	7	Alcohol use	7	Impaired kidney function
8	Unsafe water	8	Low birthweight and short gestation	8	High sodium	8	Low whole grains
9	Smoking	9	Impaired kidney function	9	Low whole grains	9	Ambient particulate matter
10	Unsafe sanitation	10	Low fruit	10	Impaired kidney function	10	High sodium

Note: Highlighted risk factors represent environmental risks.

Data from: Institute of Health Metrics and Evaluation (IHME). (n.d.). GBD Compare: Viz Hub. Retrieved from https://vizhub.healthdata.org/gbd-compare/

WHO estimates that ambient particulate matter pollution contributes to about 4.2 million deaths a year globally. WHO also estimates that more than 90 percent of those deaths occur in low- and middle-income countries. A commission from *The Lancet* on pollution and health made similar estimates.[16] The WHO regions of South-East Asia, which includes India, and the Western Pacific, which includes China, suffer a disproportionate share of such deaths.[17]

Globally, ambient particulate matter pollution is responsible for the following[9]:

- 25 percent of all deaths and disease from lung cancer
- 17 percent of all deaths and disease from acute lower respiratory infection
- 16 percent of all deaths from stroke
- 15 percent of all deaths and disease from ischemic heart disease
- 8 percent of all deaths and disease from COPD

Children are especially susceptible to the effects of ambient particulate matter pollution, particularly

TABLE 8-8 Leading Environmental Risk Factors for DALYs by World Bank Country Income Group, 2016

Low-Income Countries		Lower Middle-Income Countries		Upper Middle-Income Countries		High-Income Countries	
Rank	*Risk Factor*	*Rank*	*Risk Factor*	*Rank*	*Risk Factor*	*Rank*	*Risk Factor*
1	Low birthweight and short gestation	1	Low birthweight and short gestation	1	High blood pressure	1	Smoking
2	Child growth failure	2	High blood pressure	2	Smoking	2	High blood pressure
3	Household air pollution	3	High fasting plasma glucose	3	High body mass index	3	High body mass index
4	Unsafe water	4	Ambient particulate matter	4	High fasting plasma glucose	4	High fasting plasma glucose
5	Unsafe sex	5	Smoking	5	Alcohol use	5	Alcohol use
6	Unsafe sanitation	6	Child growth failure	6	High total cholesterol	6	High total cholesterol
7	Handwashing	7	High body mass index	7	Ambient particulate matter	7	Low whole grains
8	High blood pressure	8	Household air pollution	8	High sodium	8	Drug use
9	Ambient particulate matter	9	High total cholesterol	9	Low whole grains	9	Impaired kidney function
10	High fasting plasma glucose	10	Unsafe water	10	Low fruit	10	Low fruit

Note: Highlighted risk factors represent environmental risks.

Data from: Institute of Health Metrics and Evaluation (IHME). (n.d.). GBD Compare: Viz Hub. Retrieved from https://vizhub.healthdata.org/gbd-compare/

at critical times in their early development. Cities are also disproportionately affected.[16] The data given here may underestimate the health effects of ambient air pollution because there is evidence it is also associated with pre-term birth, low birthweight, and small gestational age births; poor neurological development in children; and diabetes.[9]

Water, Sanitation, and Hygiene

The *Global Burden of Disease Study 2016* estimated that unsafe water was the 18th leading risk factor for deaths

globally, but the 8th leading risk factor in low-income countries and the 12th leading risk factor in lower middle-income countries. The same study estimated that unsafe sanitation was the 21st leading risk factor for deaths globally, but the 10th leading risk factor for low-income countries and the 17th for lower middle-income countries. No access to a handwashing facility was the 24th leading risk factor globally, but the 11th leading risk factor in low-income countries and the 20th leading risk factor in lower middle-income countries.[2]

We should expect that the burden of disease related to these risk factors will fall disproportionately on children, who suffer a large share of the burden of disease from diarrhea. In fact, the *Global Burden of Disease Study 2016* estimated that unsafe water was the third leading risk factor for deaths of children under 5 years of age, unsafe sanitation was the fourth leading risk factor, and no access to handwashing was the sixth leading risk factor.[2] The burden of these risk factors will also fall overwhelmingly on poor and less educated people in the lower-income countries. They have less access than others to improved water supply and sanitation and to the knowledge of good hygiene they need in order to avoid illness in the face of unsafe water and sanitation.

It is very complicated to try to assess individually the relative contribution of unsafe sanitation, unsafe water, and poor hygienic practices to the burden of diarrheal disease, partly because they are all so closely linked with each other. Nonetheless, both historical experiences in what are now the high-income countries and a number of studies in low- and middle-income countries suggest that improving water supply alone will not reduce diarrheal disease as needed. This seems to stem from the large share of diarrhea that is associated with food that is unsafe and with poor personal hygiene. More will be said about these later.

Separate from any impact on the reduction of diarrheal disease, improvements in water supply are associated with important reductions in the burden of disease from dracunculiasis, schistosomiasis, and trachoma.[14]

▶ The Costs and Consequences of Key Environmental Health Problems

For a number of reasons, the social and economic consequences of the key environmental health issues that have been discussed are enormous. First, the fact that more than 20 percent of the total global burden of disease is due to environmental risk factors suggests substantial social and economic costs related to these issues.[18]

Second, as indicated earlier, the burden of these risk factors and their related causes of disease fall disproportionately on relatively poorer people. It is poorer people who cook with biomass fuels and coal, not better-off people. These burdens also fall on low- and middle-income countries more than on high-income countries. People in high-income countries do not customarily cook with biomass fuel or coal, and they do not have to contend with the problems of

unsafe water and sanitation to the extent that people in lower- and middle-income countries do. Their knowledge of good hygiene practices is also often greater than the level of knowledge of most people in low- and middle-income countries.

Third, these environmental health burdens have very negative consequences on productivity. The consequences of household air pollution, for example, are very costly to women in terms of morbidity, disability, and days of reduced productivity from both acute and chronic illnesses. In addition, the economic and social consequences of ill health for women in many low- and middle-income countries go considerably beyond just women's health. Rather, they spill over into the health of the rest of the family, especially young children, whose own health and survival depend in important ways on the health of the mother.

Young children are especially at risk from all three environmental issues discussed in this chapter. They are especially vulnerable to unsafe water, and diarrheal disease can put them into a cycle of infection and malnutrition that may ultimately stunt their growth and development or be deadly. Household air pollution can also lead to a cycle of illness and respiratory infection, death from pneumonia, or disability from asthma. Ambient particulate matter pollution can do the same. The elderly face particular risks from this pollution, which can exacerbate chronic health problems they already have, leading to additional disability and its attendant reduction in productivity.

▶ Reducing the Burden of Disease

Important progress has been made in some settings in addressing the environmental health issues discussed here. **TABLE 8-9** summarizes some of the key measures that can be taken to address environmental health issues related to these matters. The next section examines some of those measures further.

Ambient Particulate Matter Pollution

Ambient particulate matter pollution is a very broad topic, and there is relatively little published data on the cost-effectiveness of approaches to addressing it in low- and middle-income countries. The studies that have been done on high-income countries, however, suggest that low- and middle-income countries could take a number of cost-effective steps to reduce the health burden of ambient air pollution.[19] These can be in the domains of law, policy, regulation, and

TABLE 8-9 Essential Environmental Policies

Domain of action	Fiscal and Intersectoral Policies		Regulation	Information, education, and communication
	Taxes and subsidies	**Infrastructure and built environment**	**Regulation**	**Information, education, and communication**
Water and sanitation	Targeted subsidies to poor and vulnerable groups Incentives for private sector to become more involved with WASH for supply chain and service provision	Quality WASH facilities in schools, workplaces, public spaces, and healthcare facilities	Defined WASH standards per setting (household, outside household)	National awareness campaigns (for example, on handwashing) WASH behavior-change interventions, such as community-led total sanitation
Outdoor air pollution	Fuel taxes Fines for residential trash burning Fines for not controlling construction dust Tax polluters Cap and trade policies for specific pollutants (for example, SO_2) No more subsidies for coal	Relocation of industrial sources, such as brick kilns Municipal trash collection Diesel to CNG transition for fleets Movement toward banning solid fuels in cities Regular street cleaning to control dust	Diesel retrofits Coal to natural gas transition Brick kiln retrofits for emissions control PM, SO_2, and NO_2 emissions control Acceleration of European Union standards for vehicles National regulation to reduce household emissions to outdoors Construction and road dust controls Adoption of European Union fuel standards	Updated health information systems to include vulnerability, adaptation, and capacity assessment
Household air pollution	Advanced biomass stove subsidies Targeted and expanded LPG and other clean fuel subsidies to the poor Subsidies for clean alternatives to kerosene Campaigns for middle class to give up subsidies intended for poor	Improved ventilation as part of building codes and norms Enhanced clean fuel distribution networks Electrification as a health measure Application of modern digital technology to enhance access to household clean fuel	Lower barriers and expanded licensure requirements for clean fuel distribution Kerosene ban National regulation on clean household fuels to match UN SE4ALL goals Smoke-free communities	Ventilation HAP health effects education Promotion of kitchen retrofits to encourage HAP-reducing interventions and behaviors

(continues)

TABLE 8-9 Essential Environmental Policies

(continued)

Domain of action	Fiscal and Intersectoral Policies			
	Taxes and subsidies	Infrastructure and built environment	Regulation	Information, education, and communication
Chemical contamination		Regulations on hazardous waste disposal covering land, air, and water	Arsenic: monitoring of groundwater supplies and provision of alternatives if needed Asbestos: banning of import, export, mining, manufacture, and sale Mercury: monitoring and reduction or elimination of use in artisanal mining, large-scale smelting, and cosmetics Established and enforced toxic element emissions limits for air and water Restricted access to contaminated sites Strict control and movement to selective bans of highly hazardous pesticides	Notification of public of locations of contaminated sites
Lead exposure	Concessionary financing for remediation of worst conditions	Minimization of occupational and environmental exposures in maintaining, renovating, and demolishing buildings and other structures with lead paint	Ban on lead paint and leaded fuels Ban on lead in water pipes, cookware, drugs, food supplements, and cosmetics Reduction in corrosiveness of drinking water National take-back requirements for collecting used lead batteries Regulations governing land-based waste disposal Risk-based limits for lead in air, water, soil, and dust	Lead poisoning training for healthcare providers

TABLE 8-9 Essential Environmental Policies

Domain of action	Fiscal and Intersectoral Policies			Information, education, and communication
	Taxes and subsidies	Infrastructure and built environment	Regulation	
Global climate change	Carbon tax or cap and trade (mitigation) Subsidies to renewable energy	Mitigation policies and incentives, including land use plans, building design, and transportation, to reduce GHGs Resilient design in buildings and infrastructure (adaptation) Consideration of climate change in public health infrastructure (mitigation and adaptation)	Energy efficiency and fuel-efficient vehicles (mitigation) Mainstreaming of climate change into public health planning and programs, and into health system policies and plans Methane control regulations	Early warning and emergency response systems

(continued)

Note: CNG = compressed natural gas; GHG = greenhouse gas; HAP = household air pollution; LPG = liquefied petroleum gas; NO_2 = nitrogen dioxide; PM = particulate matter; SO_2 = sulfur dioxide; UN SE4ALL = United Nations Sustainable Energy for All program; WASH = water, sanitation, and hygiene.

Reproduced from Mock, C.N., R. Nugent, O. Kobusingye, and K.R. Smith, editors. 2017. *Injury Prevention and Environmental Health.* Volume 7, *Disease Control Priorities* (third edition). Washington, DC: World Bank.

technology. Estimates suggest that such measures are a "good buy," with a $30 return on average for every dollar spent on pollution control.[16]

A number of cities, for example, including Jakarta, Manila, Kathmandu, and Mumbai, participated in a World Bank–assisted effort to assess their ambient particulate matter pollution and take measures to reduce it. They examined the following[19]:

- The amount and type of pollution
- How it was being dispersed
- The health impacts of reductions in particulate matter
- Time and cost to implement reductions
- Health benefits
- The value of those health benefits
- How the benefits compared to the costs of the intervention

The following are some of the first measures that these cities and some other large cities in low- and middle-income countries have taken to reduce ambient particulate matter pollution[19]:

- The introduction of unleaded gasoline
- Low-smoke lubricant for two-stroke engines
- The banning of two-stroke engines
- Shifting to natural gas to fuel public vehicles
- Tightening emissions inspections on vehicles
- Reducing the burning of garbage

It would also be reasonable to ensure that governments in low- and middle-income countries use their regulatory authority to incorporate information about ambient particulate matter pollution in their policies on transportation and industrial development.[19] In line with this, many of the lowest-income countries do not yet have a significant problem of ambient particulate matter pollution. It will be much more effective for those countries to put in place cost-effective approaches now to minimize ambient particulate matter pollution and its health effects than it will be to try later to mitigate those effects. In doing so, they should take account of vehicular and industrial pollution.

Household Air Pollution from Solid Fuels

There are a number of areas in which actions could be taken to reduce household air pollution from the burning of solid fuels for cooking and heating. In terms of the source of pollution, cooking devices can be improved, less polluting fuels can be used, and families can reduce their need for these fuels by using solar cooking and heating. Some changes can also be made to the living environment. Mechanisms for venting smoke can be built into the house, for example, or

the kitchen can be moved away from the main part of the house. People can also change their behaviors to reduce pollution or exposure to it by using dried fuels, properly maintaining their stoves and chimneys, and keeping children away from the cooking area.[20]

Public policy can also play a helpful role in trying to reduce household air pollution. The public sector, for example, can promote information and education about such pollution and how to reduce it in schools, in the media, and in communities. The government can also use tax policy to reduce the cost of cooking appliances and fuels that will reduce this pollution. If necessary, it could subsidize the cost of improved fuels and appliances for those below a certain income level. Governments could also undertake surveillance of the problem and, if possible, set and enforce standards for household air pollution, although this will certainly be beyond the capacity of most low-income countries.[20]

Calculating the cost-effectiveness of different approaches to reducing the health effects of household air pollution is a very complicated matter and requires many assumptions. Nonetheless, the conclusions of the analyses that have been done are instructive. The main finding is that the most cost-effective approach to reducing household air pollution in sub-Saharan Africa and South Asia, where the needs are greatest, would be to promote the use of improved stoves. The most cost-effective approach in East Asia would be to promote the use of better fuels, such as kerosene and gas. Of course, this conclusion presumes that the stoves are maintained and the fuels are of good quality, which may not always be the case and the failure of which would detract from the effectiveness of these approaches.[20]

In addition, a number of lessons have been learned about how to encourage the uptake of better stoves and better fuels, some drawn from extensive experiences in China and India. These include the following[20]:

- Involve end users, especially women, in helping to assess needs and design approaches.
- Promote demand for better stoves and fuels to encourage the development of competitive suppliers and market choice.
- Consider subsidies and microcredit for selected interventions to help defray the cost of improvements for the poor.
- Establish national and local policies that encourage the needed changes in stoves and fuels.

Sanitation

There are a number of different levels of technology associated with excreta disposal, many different forms

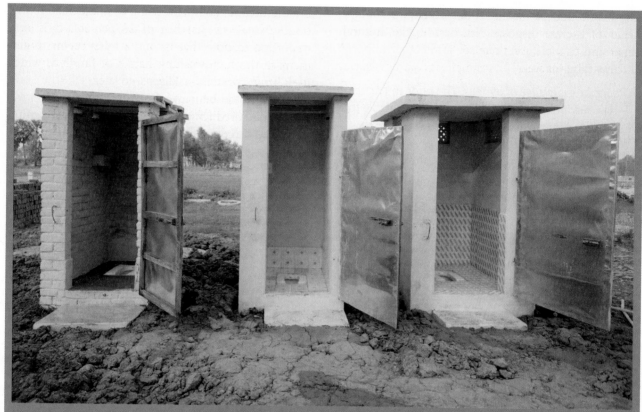

PHOTO 8-3 Here is a photo of pit latrines in India. They were constructed under the 3SI Project, funded by the Bill & Melinda Gates Foundation in partnership with Unilever. The project is implemented by Population Services International (PSI), a U.S.-based nongovernmental organization working in global health. 3SI facilitates the sanitation market by enabling both demand and supply of toilets in remote districts of the Indian state of Bihar, where in 2013 only 20 percent of households had toilets. Now, 68 percent of homes in Bihar have a toilet.
© Kiran Thejaswi/Population Services International.

TABLE 8-10 Selected Sanitation Technologies

- Simple pit latrine
- Small-bore sewer
- Ventilation-improved latrine
- Pour-flush
- Septic tank
- Sewer connection

Data from Cairncross, S., & Valdmanis, V. (2006). Water supply, sanitation, and hygiene promotion. In D. T. Jamison, J. G. Breman, A. R. Measham, et al. (Eds.), *Disease control priorities in developing countries* (2nd ed., p. 780). Washington, DC, and New York, NY: The World Bank and Oxford University Press.

of toilets, and a wide array of costs associated with them. Sanitation could range from the simple technology of bucket latrines to modern urban sewage systems. **TABLE 8-10** lists the different approaches to excreta disposal. Although we usually think of toilets as owned by individuals, they can also be public and shared by many individuals and families.

The cost per person for methods of sanitary removal of human waste varies considerably. At the bottom levels of service, it appears that pour-flush latrines, ventilation-improved latrines, and simple pit latrines can be constructed in low- and middle-income settings for about $60. Assuming that these last approximately 5 years, the annual cost per capita would be about $12. The construction cost of conventional sewage systems in some countries is more than 10 times that amount. In addition, they need water to function properly, and water is often in short supply.[14] Work is ongoing to develop more cost-effective toilets, and in Bangladesh a simple pour-flush pan has been developed that costs only about $0.27 per household to construct.[14]

Contrary to what we might believe, all of these systems can be operated in a hygienic manner that addresses health concerns. A very important review that was conducted in the early 1980s, for example, concluded that from the point of view of health, pit latrines would be just as hygienic as modern sewage systems, even if they were considerably less convenient.[21]

Given the relatively low cost of simple methods of sanitation and their relative effectiveness, it might be surprising that such a small share of households in low- and middle-income countries have a sanitary means of excreta disposal. Yet, besides the cultural constraints to their use, there are some other important constraints as well[14]:

- *Lack of knowledge of options*: The poor in particular may not understand the options available to them and may believe that toilets cost more to install than they do.
- *Cost*: Even at relatively low prices, the poor may not have the money to pay for the up-front costs of a toilet.
- *Construction*: There may be a lack of skills to help install the toilets.
- *Local laws*: Particularly in urban areas, local laws may forbid low-cost sanitation, even if the area has no modern sewage system.

In some countries the public sector leads the effort to build low-cost sanitation systems. The public sector may also subsidize the cost of toilets for the poorest families, given that these sanitation improvements provide benefits to society as a whole. In addition, the public sector can try to enforce regulations to require the use of toilets. Although such regulatory authority is weak in most low-income and many middle-income countries, one of the main cities in Burkina Faso was able to promote toilet construction by taking away the title of homes if their owners did not install a toilet within a specific period of time.[14]

It is also possible, if the private sector believes that there is a market for low-cost sanitation, for such efforts to be handled in the private sector. In this case, the public sector may confine its role to areas needed to encourage private sector involvement and public demand for the toilets. This would include, for example, promoting the use of toilets, encouraging private sector involvement, setting technical standards, and helping to train people in installation and maintenance techniques.[14]

Promotion of improved sanitation can also be done with a public–private partnership and led by nongovernmental organizations (NGOs). Two of the most successful cases of improving low-cost sanitation were led by NGOs in Zimbabwe and Bangladesh. In Zimbabwe, an NGO was able to help communities construct 3,400 latrines for about $13 per unit, or only about $2.25 per person served.[22] In Bangladesh, an NGO has helped to make 100 villages free of open defecation for a cost of only about $1.50 per person served.[23] In both of these cases, the families in these communities paid for the latrines themselves.

The largest impact of improved sanitation is in the reduction of diarrhea. Some studies[24] suggest that improved sanitation facilities in low- and middle-income countries result in an average reduction in cases of diarrhea of 28 percent. It is very important to note that having a toilet seems to also increase the handwashing habits of families, which itself brings benefits, as discussed later.

Finally, the benefits of sanitary excreta removal go beyond reducing diarrhea. Improving sanitation should reduce the prevalence of several worms, including ascaris, trichuris, and hookworm.[14] Given the low cost of some forms of latrines, they would be cost-effective approaches to reducing the prevalence of these worms. As noted earlier, the same would be true in terms of the positive impact and low costs of reducing trachoma through improved sanitation.[25]

Water Supply

There are many analogies between water supply and sanitation. For water, as well as for sanitation, there are many different levels of technology, and costs vary considerably according to the level of technology employed. One could get water, for example, from the following types of improved water sources:

- House connection
- Standpost
- Borehole
- Dug well
- Rainwater collection

This section offers brief comments on different approaches to achieving health benefits from improved water supply. In considering the costs and benefits to these approaches, reasonable access to water was considered to be access to at least 20 liters per day per person from one of these sources from not more than 1-kilometer distance. (It is now considered 50 to 100 liters per day). Although some of the data are not very recent, they are still valuable.[14,26]

Improving water supply can lead to a variety of health benefits. The most important studies that have been done have shown that providing a continuous supply of water with good bacteriological quality can reduce the morbidity of a number of diseases, as shown in **TABLE 8-11**. Studies showed a median reduction in trachoma, for example, of 27 percent, schistosomiasis of 77 percent, and dracunculiasis of 78 percent.[14]

Other studies have looked at the health benefits from different combinations of investments in water quantity, water quality, sanitation, and the promotion of hygiene. The results of these studies are somewhat surprising to those not involved in the environmental health field. They suggest that the largest reductions in diarrhea morbidity—approximately 30 percent—come from investing in sanitation only, water and

TABLE 8-11 Potential Morbidity Reduction from Excellent Water Supply

Condition	Percentage Reduction
Scabies	80
Typhoid fever	80
Trachoma	60
Most diarrheas and dysentery	50
Skin and subcutaneous infections	50
Paratyphoid, other *Salmonella*	40

Modified with permission from Cairncross, S., & Valdmanis, V. (2006). Water supply, sanitation, and hygiene promotion. In D. T. Jamison, J. G. Breman, A. R. Measham, et al. (Eds.), *Disease control priorities in developing countries* (2nd ed., p. 776). Washington, DC, and New York, NY: The World Bank and Oxford University Press.

sanitation, or hygiene only. The lowest reductions, between 15 and 20 percent, came from investing in water quantity only, or a combination of water quality and quantity, all without complementary investments in hygiene or in sanitation.

As noted earlier, many of the pathogens that are waterborne are also carried on food. Thus, sanitation has a large potential impact on reducing those pathogens. By contrast, investing in water interventions alone may not yield the results that sanitation would. For this, among other reasons, complementary investments for the promotion of hygiene are critical to realizing gains from water and sanitation.[14]

Another important lesson is that the greatest effect of investments in water is realized when people have water connections in their homes. Unfortunately, community standpipes, for example, do not produce the same level of health gains as individual household water connections.[14] A review in New Guinea, for example, showed that there was 56 percent less diarrhea in homes with an individual connection than in homes that got their water from standpipes.[14] This may partly be the case because people with individual connections use considerably more water than those without such connections and much of the additional water may be used to engage in better hygiene.

Nonetheless, it is also important to realize that it is estimated that over 1 billion people engage in home treatment of water to improve its safety. In surveys of countries representing about 40 percent of the global population, about 36 percent of urban dwellers and 30

percent of rural dwellers engaged in home water treatment. On average, about 21 percent of households boiled water, almost 6 percent added chlorine to the water, about 4 percent used filtration, and a very small percentage engaged in solar disinfection. The range of these practices across countries was wide, with almost universal boiling in Indonesia, for example. About 10 percent of households surveyed engaged in home water treatment using methods that will not make their water safe.[27]

Hygiene

Unfortunately, there have been relatively few studies of the impact of hygiene promotion on actual health behaviors and on related reductions in the burden of disease. The studies that have been done showed that investing in hygiene promotion led to a 33 percent reduction in diarrhea. They also found that hygiene promotion efforts need to focus on simple messages about handwashing and avoid trying to promote too many messages at once, if they are to be successful and sustainable. It appears that the messages that families acquire through hygiene promotion do stay with them and that retraining is necessary only once every 5 years.[14] Studies have also been done on the impact of handwashing on respiratory infections. Handwashing was associated in these studies with a significant reduction in acute respiratory infections.[14]

Integrating Investment Choices About Water, Sanitation, and Hygiene

When the information from the studies previously discussed is reviewed together, it appears that the promotion of hygiene, the promotion of sanitation, and the construction of standposts are all likely to be cost-effective in low- and middle-income countries. However, using public funds to provide individual household connections to water supply systems is likely to be above the cutoff for cost-effective investments. This is shown in **TABLE 8-12**. Although the data are not recent, they still shed important light on the relative cost-effectiveness of a range of investments in water, sanitation, and hygiene.

The costs of hygiene and sanitation promotion compare favorably, for example, with the costs per DALY averted of oral rehydration. In addition, such investments might help to reduce the burden of diarrhea and decrease the need for oral rehydration.

On that basis, what would be a sensible approach to improving health through investments in water supply, sanitation, and hygiene in low- and middle-income countries? First would be to promote hygiene. This is necessary both for its own sake and to maximize

TABLE 8-12 Cost per DALY Averted of Selected Investments in Water, Sanitation, and Hygiene

Investment	$/DALY Averted
Hygiene promotion	3.35
Sanitation promotion only	11.15
Water sector regulation and advocacy	47.00
Hand pump or standpost	94.00
House connection	223.00
Construction and promotion	270.00

Modified with permission from Cairncross, S., & Valdmanis, V. (2006). Water supply, sanitation, and hygiene promotion. In D. T. Jamison, J. G. Breman, A. R. Measham, et al. (Eds.), *Disease control priorities in developing countries* (2nd ed., p. 791). Washington, DC, and New York, NY: The World Bank and Oxford University Press.

the value that will accrue from investments in water supply and sanitation. Second, governments should promote low-cost sanitation schemes. In doing this, they should encourage the private sector to invest in this business, encourage demand from consumers, try to ensure that there are skills to install the latrines, and try to set and enforce standards to which they have to be built. Third, low-cost water supply schemes should also be developed. This can often be done best in conjunction with communities and with community-based approaches. Finally, the government should use its regulatory and other authority to be sure that it helps consumers meet the costs of these schemes and also encourages investment in water supply schemes with household connections that families pay for.

Much has been written about approaches to water and sanitation. Those interested in how such schemes are designed, built, operated, and financed are encouraged to review some of the literature on those topics, which is beyond the scope of this text.

▶ Case Studies

Four case studies follow. The first discusses a program for handwashing with soap in Senegal. The second concerns a campaign for "total sanitation" in East Java, Indonesia. Both cases were largely successful in meeting their goals and have valuable lessons for other countries trying to improve hygiene and sanitation. The third case speaks of the health gains from putting concrete floors into the homes of lower-income people

in Mexico. The last case summarizes the findings of some of the most important studies completed to date on possible links between climate change and health.

Handwashing with Soap in Senegal[28]

Handwashing with soap is key to preventing the spread of disease because it kills various agents, such as harmful bacteria, that can cause infection. Nonetheless, the rate of handwashing with soap in Senegal has been relatively low, as it is in many low- and middle-income countries. According to a study conducted in Senegal in 2004, for example, the rate of handwashing with soap was 18 percent after cleaning a child, 18 percent before handling food, and 23 percent after going to the toilet. Distance between soap and a source of water, soap being controlled by people who do not want to share it, and the lack of a designated place for handwashing have all been barriers to handwashing with soap in Senegal.

The Public-Private Partnership for Handwashing with Soap (PPPHW) was created in Senegal in 2003 with the mission to promote handwashing with soap. With technical assistance from an international partnership housed at the World Bank, the Water and Sanitation Program (WSP), PPPHW was originally housed within the Senegalese government unit that oversees sanitation within the Ministry of Health.

The PPPHW launched a communications campaign in 2004 with the goal of educating people about the importance of using soap when washing hands, in addition to the most critical times for handwashing. "Water rinses but soap cleans" was the main message of this first phase of communications efforts.

The campaign made use of a number of communications methods to send its message. Television and radio spots were aired nationally, especially during times when mothers were preparing meals. At the time, more than 87 percent of Senegalese owned radios and 40 percent owned televisions, explaining why mass media can be an effective tool for exposing the campaign's slogan and visual aspects. Billboards, which are prevalent in Senegal, were also used.

The campaign also hosted interactive local community events to extend its messages directly to the population. Local marketplaces and schools hosted live entertainment and demonstrations to educate women and children about the importance of handwashing with soap. In addition, small-group discussions were held at women's associations and waiting rooms of local health centers to facilitate communication about the importance of using soap.

The PPPHW project introduced a second phase of activities to promote handwashing with soap in 2008 after being incorporated into the WSP's Global Scaling Up Handwashing Project, which sought to "apply innovative promotional approaches to behavior change to generate widespread and sustained improvements in handwashing with soap."[28(p1)] The project expanded in this phase to reach 8 of the 11 regions in Senegal with a more defined target of women of reproductive age and primary school–aged children ages 5 to 9. The goal was to improve the handwashing with soap practices of over 500,000 mothers and children.

Studies in 2008 identified which behavioral determinants were correlated with handwashing with soap in an attempt to incorporate a wider spectrum of behavioral determinants into the second phase of the behavior change program. At this point, the majority of the 2,040 mothers who participated in the study understood the campaign message of the first phase, or the importance of using soap when handwashing. Fifty-two percent disagreed with the statement that "water alone is enough." Mothers also understood the link between handwashing with soap and disease prevention, with close to 80 percent agreeing or strongly agreeing that removing dirt and invisible germs requires handwashing with soap. However, research suggested that access to and availability of soap and water in the household is a key determinant for handwashing with soap and had to be planned for.

Based on the assumption that most mothers now understood the importance of handwashing with soap, the second phase of the program aimed to "awaken, fortify, and support" intentions to wash hands with soap. The campaign encouraged mothers to act upon intentions by planning for handwashing, such as designating a certain place for handwashing with soap. The campaign message was delivered through the same communications channels used in the first phase. With technical assistance and guidance from the WSP, local communications and consulting firms and NGOs designed, planned, and carried out different components of the project.

New billboards and radio and television spots were created with the intention of positively reinforcing mothers' and children's commitment to washing hands with soap. From June to December 2009, 92 television and 1,496 radio spots aired. At local soccer games and other community locations, respected community members gave handwashing demonstrations and testimonials of their pledge to wash hands with soap. The 161 events that were held through December 2009 reached an estimated 140,000 people.

Workers from local NGOs also visited homes to discuss with mothers tangible ways of turning into action the intention of washing hands with soap. The 150 trained workers helped mothers plan the necessary steps for setting up a designated handwashing station, including making sure that water and soap were available and accessible.

Of course, the program faced a number of challenges. Engaging local partners, while still ensuring that campaign messages were communicated effectively and consistently, presented some initial challenges. At first, local advertising agencies created negative messages that emphasized germs and disease, rather than positive messages of healthy outcomes from handwashing with soap, as instructed. As a result, the WSP worked closely with local agencies to coordinate advertisements.

Another challenge was making sure that outreach workers who visit homes go beyond offering information, by discussing mothers' obstacles to handwashing with soap and devising practical solutions through careful planning and building of handwashing stations. Performance monitoring and coaching of workers has helped to ensure they do their job effectively.

A lesson learned for changing behavior is that the use or demonstration of a tangible product that facilitates behavior change, such as a sample handwashing station, can be a powerful tool for turning intention into action. This project also exemplifies the importance of continually revising a campaign strategy to account for a project's past successes or failures. In addition to reevaluating the entire campaign message to launch the second phase, throughout this phase certain program elements were further revised to reflect current evaluations. The 2008 campaign advertisements originally portrayed men merely as social supporters; however, later monitoring of the program suggested that a man's role in the family as provider, protector, and role model gives him tremendous influence in promoting handwashing with soap. In fact, half of women surveyed considered their husbands the decision makers in purchasing soap. Thus, program planners recognized the significant role that men play in overcoming barriers to accessibility and availability of soap, and they adjusted the campaign to engage men more in selling the importance of handwashing with soap. Modified communication materials portray men as committed to handwashing with soap, thus fortifying men's intentions to do so and increasing the visibility of their influential role.[29]

Total Sanitation and Sanitation Marketing: East Java, Indonesia[30]

The Global Water Security & Sanitation Partnership (GWSP), formerly called the Water Sanitation Program (WSP), is an international partnership housed at the World Bank that supports low-income people in acquiring affordable, safe, and sustainable access to water and sanitation services.[31] One part of this program has been Total Sanitation and Sanitation Marketing (TSSM) projects in a number of countries.[32] These are based on a three-pronged approach to rapidly increasing the number of people who use sanitary means of disposing of human waste:

- The development of a strategy for changing behaviors, based on consumer research
- The development of an approach to increasing the market for latrines, based on market research
- A community-led campaign for total sanitation— an approach that seeks to make a community completely free of open defecation

TSSM projects also pay particular attention to the monitoring of progress, continuous evaluation of results, and learning as you go. Special emphasis is also placed on creating an enabling environment for the project to meet its goals, by working to enhance the policy, institutional, and financial frameworks within which a sanitation program has to be carried out.

In 2007, a TSSM project was launched in East Java, Indonesia. At the time the project was launched, sanitation coverage was just below 70 percent in urban areas and only about 55 percent in rural areas. The intended project outcome was to provide access to sustainable sanitation services for 1.4 million people in one of the most densely populated places in the world.[30]

This project paid greater attention than many earlier projects to involving the community in the design and development of the project, having the community participate financially in the project, increasing the community's demand for toilets, and ensuring that there would be a sufficient supply of appropriate toilets to meet that demand.[33]

Demand Creation

Districts had to volunteer to participate in the program. One of the first steps in the implementation of the project in East Java, therefore, was to create community-based and household-level demand for improved sanitation.

In order to garner government support of the behavior change program, discussions were held with local and district officials about the economic impact of poor sanitation at the country and district levels and the social and economic returns from investing in sanitation improvements.[30]

To create demand for improved sanitation, the project used the Community-Led Total Sanitation (CLTS) methodology, which mobilizes communities to completely eliminate open defecation. This approach focuses on community-wide sustainable behavioral change, rather than toilet construction for individual households. CLTS efforts try to help communities understand that, regardless of the number of toilets constructed, there is still a risk of disease if even one person continues to defecate in the open. As part of the CLTS approach, communities develop their own solutions to obtain improved sanitation and become free of open defecation.[30] An initial step in this process is mapping village boundaries and indicating where people defecate in the open.[34]

In addition, the program used marketing techniques to improve the demand for sanitation-related products and services, which included advertisements for desirable hygienic behaviors.[34] The program created and marketed, for example, a communication campaign with a character, "Lik Telek," or "Uncle Shit" in the local language, which personifies the open defecation habit. With flies dancing around his head, and a smug smile, Lik Telek goes behind a tree to defecate in the open, while onlookers advise him to use improved sanitation facilities.[35] The districts funded the campaign, which included a series of posters, radio commercials, and an 8-minute video drama.

Improvements in the Supply of Sanitation

The project conducted market research for 18 months to better understand the sanitation market, as well as the demand for sanitation services. Market research revealed that there was no common definition of the ideal sanitation facility among consumers, sanitation suppliers, and engineers. Standards varied greatly and generated an impression that a good sanitation facility was unaffordable. In addition, open defecation into water was considered socially acceptable, convenient, safe, and clean because the feces are considered invisible, carried away by water or eaten by fish.

In light of these findings, the project worked with designers and suppliers to ensure that there would be a common definition of improved sanitation and that various sanitation options would be available, at a range of prices. To popularize a common definition of an ideal sanitation facility, the program created a *WC-ku Sehat*, or "my latrine is healthy/hygienic," thumbs-up sign to identify facilities that meet the improved sanitation criteria. The program also prepared an Informed Choice Catalogue of improved *WC-ku Sehat* sanitation options at varying prices, which displays all possible combinations of belowground, on the ground, and aboveground sections of latrines.[30]

To further strengthen the quantity, quality, and appropriateness of the supply of sanitation, a technological training institute in East Java held mason training and accreditation programs. These aimed to ensure that a qualified mason would be available in every district to work on improved sanitation facilities. As of June 2009, a total of 600 artisans in 10 districts were trained in this way, and an additional 1,110 artisans were to receive training after that.[33]

Achievement of Project Goals

Overall, the program appeared in its first phase to have produced larger benefits than more conventional approaches to sanitation, because of the high level of community involvement and use of research-based strategies for increasing both demand and supply. The community-led approach in East Java yielded a 49 percent increase in access to improved sanitation within an 18-month period. More conventional approaches generally yielded increases of only about 10 to 15 percent over such a period. Moreover, between November 2007 and May 2009, more than 325,000 persons gained access to improved sanitation facilities in 21 districts of East Java. Equally important, again in contrast to the conventional approach, the poorest households in East Java established 715 open defecation–free villages and gained access to improved sanitation at higher rates than higher-income households.

An evaluation was conducted later of the progress of the program up to 2011. By then 1.4 million people had gained access to improved sanitation facilities.[36] In addition, the group that participated in this program was 23 percent more likely to build a toilet and 9 percent less likely to engage in open defecation than the control group. These improvements were associated with a 30 percent drop in diarrhea prevalence in the affected communities.[37] Later estimates suggested that the program averted 220 deaths between 2008 and 2011.[38]

Nonetheless, this later program evaluation showed that the program did not improve equity in the long term. Rather, the majority of families that built toilets were relatively better off. Although the poor gained some benefits from the community-wide impact of better sanitation among some community members, poorer households had no statistically significant increase in toilet use.[37]

The cost per installed toilet was about $65, financed by the following sources[39]:

- $45 was from households
- $14 was financed by the global Water and Sanitation Program
- $5 was from local governments

The United Nations Development Programme (UNDP) estimates that each dollar invested in water and sanitation programs yields $8 in return.[39] Estimates for this program suggest that the program cost $749 per DALY averted. This was only about 25 percent of Indonesia's GDP per capita at the time, which suggests that investment was highly cost-effective.[38]

Lessons Learned

The Indonesia program raises a number of interesting points about efforts to achieve "total sanitation." First is the value of community-led efforts. Second are critical questions about how to ensure that the poor can afford to participate in the program and install and use toilets. The third is the appropriateness of communications that are included in some total sanitation campaigns and whether or not "shaming" should ever be seen as an ethical approach to stopping open defecation.[38]

Concrete Floors for Child Health[40]
The Problem

Diarrhea is one of the top five leading causes of death for children under 5 worldwide, accounting for 750,000 preventable deaths annually. Parasites and worms can lead to micronutrient malnutrition and anemia, in addition to diarrhea. These conditions affect the cognitive development of children, leaving the most disadvantaged even more vulnerable in the long term. Although unsafe water is a common source of such parasites, dirt floors are also known to serve as modes of transmission for infections. Dirt floors are difficult to keep clean and can absorb fecal matter that trails into homes. This is particularly a concern in densely populated slums where sewage systems are deficient.

Although Mexico has seen a reduction in under-5 mortality in the last decade, this improvement has not been experienced equitably. Children who are from rural areas, live in southern states, are part of indigenous communities, or have mothers with low educational attainment are at higher risk for diarrhea and parasitic infections. The built environment and housing are important social determinants of health. Informal housing in urban areas and suboptimal housing in rural areas both pose risks to child health.

Taking Action

After winning the gubernatorial election in Mexico's Coahuila state in 2000, Enrique Martínez y Martínez got to work on his campaign promise of replacing dirt floors with concrete floors across the state. In order to achieve this goal, he started a program called *Piso Firme*, which means "solid floor" in Spanish. Within 5 years, this state-funded initiative provided 34,000 residences with enough cement to replace 540 square feet of dirt floor each with concrete. Once the cement was delivered, people in the community prepared and installed it themselves. To be eligible for the program, households needed to have dirt floors and be low income.

The success of Piso Firme inspired a national scale-up of the program. Mexico already had federal programs with the goal of reducing poverty through cash transfers, public health insurance, deworming campaigns, and improvement of living conditions. The simple, tangible intervention for replacing dirt floors fit nicely into the constellation of these other federal programs. Starting in 2003, Piso Firme began to be replicated by other states. By 2012, 2.2 million homes across the country benefited from the installation of cement floors.

Impact

A key strength of Piso Firme was the accompanying independent impact evaluation of the program funded by Governor Martínez y Martínez's state of Coahuila and the federal government. Researchers from academic settings and the World Bank conducted an evaluation early on in the program that was intended to be shared with the public to ensure transparency and accountability. In order to make sure that the health outcomes being measured were actually linked to the installation of concrete floors and not to other changes in the built environment or programs such as the cash transfers, the researchers used a quasi-experimental design. They compared homes in a city in Coahuila, where the program was first implemented, to comparable homes in a nearby city located in a bordering state, where the program had not yet been implemented.

The findings of the evaluation showed that among families whose dirt floors had been replaced, children under 6 had 13 percent less diarrhea, 20 percent less anemia, and 20 percent fewer parasites. Moreover, these children saw an improvement in cognitive development, as measured by a vocabulary test. A surprising finding that the implementers of the program had not expected was improvement in maternal health. Among families receiving the intervention, mothers saw a 12.5 percent reduction in depression and 10.5 percent reduction in perceived stress. They were pleased that concrete floors were easier to clean and that their children got sick less.

Costs of the Program

When Piso Firme was limited to the state of Coahuila, the cost to implement cement floors was $162 per household. For the 5-year duration of the program, the total cost to the state government was $5.5 million. When the program was scaled-up, the cost of the intervention rose to $460 per household due to transport costs, which were higher for more remote areas. From 2007 to 2013, the federal government spent a total of $1.2 billion on the program. Overall, the program was deemed cost-effective, especially for the cognitive development of children when compared to the conditional cash transfer program called *Oportunidades*, which cost up to $750 per household. While that program led to a 12 percent increase in scores on the Picture Peabody Language Development Test, the Piso Firme intervention led to a 9 percent increase in scores for a lower per-household cost.

Keys to Success

There are multiple factors related to both the design of Piso Firme and the setting in which it was carried out that led to its success. Among the most important were the following:

- The simple, innovative, and tangible nature of the intervention
- Robust independent evaluations guiding program design
- Collaboration between state and federal governments
- Strong political commitment and support
- Sustained funding of the program by the government
- Evidence of effectiveness provided by the impact evaluation
- Compatibility with existing government-funded social impact programs

Future Challenges

The impact of replacing dirt floors with cement on child and maternal health was made clear through Piso Firme. However, the findings may not be generalizable to all populations and settings. For example, the children who benefited most from the intervention were living in urban environments and already had access to clean water and adequate nutrition. In settings where there is lack of access to safe water, sanitation, and hygiene, cement floors may not be as effective in reducing prevalence of diarrhea. Additionally, in thinking about expanding this program to other countries, the cost may be prohibitive for governments in low-income contexts. Nonetheless, this case study shows that simple interventions can be worthwhile for improving child health.

Climate Change and Health

Background

Climate change refers to the increase in the earth's average temperature that has been observed and the consequences that might be associated with this rise in temperature.[41] It is estimated that the earth has warmed by 1.4°F (0.8°C) in the past 100 years.[41] Accompanying the rising temperature has been a change in rainfall levels; an increase in the frequency of extreme weather such as floods, droughts, or heat waves; and the melting of glaciers, warming of the oceans, and the rising of sea levels.[41] The United Nations Secretary-General has said that climate change is the major, overriding environmental issue of our time.[41] Climate change is also considered a significant threat to efforts to improve the health of poor people in the poorest countries.[42]

The Problem: A Range of Future Risks to Health

The United Nations Intergovernmental Panel on Climate Change (IPCC), the leading international body for the assessment of climate change, suggested that climate change thus far has had only a limited impact on human health. The panel further noted that the impacts on health to date have come largely through increased heat-related mortality and decreased cold-related mortality, plus temperature-related changes in the distribution of some waterborne and vector-borne diseases.[43]

The panel also noted, however, a range of future risks to health:

- Declines in the production of some food crops in some locations leading to increases in undernutrition in some settings
- Increases in ill health in low-income countries due to more intense heat waves and fire, as well as increases in food-borne, waterborne, and vector-borne diseases

At the same time, there may be places that can increase food production and see a decline in these diseases. Nonetheless, the panel suggested that the negative impacts of climate change on health in this century will greatly outweigh the positive benefits.[43(p20)]

Taking into account these findings, WHO has estimated that climate change will cause an additional 250,000 deaths per year between 2030 and 2050. Specifically, WHO has estimated that climate change will lead to approximately 38,000 additional deaths annually due to heat exposure in elderly people, 48,000 deaths due to diarrhea, 60,000 deaths due to malaria, and 95,000 deaths due to childhood undernutrition.[44]

The IPCC concluded earlier that it is 95 percent certain that human activities have caused most of the warming of the planet's surface that has occurred since the 1950s.[45] These findings place increased pressure on the global society to act to reverse the observed trends, especially because those predicted to be affected the most by the effects of climate change have contributed least to its causes.[45]

How Does Climate Change Affect Health?

There are many mechanisms through which climate change can affect health. For example, extreme weather patterns such as droughts, flooding, and heat waves can lead to direct increases in mortality as a result of their effect on infrastructure, disruption of daily activities, and severe conditions placed on the human body. Droughts are thought to have the greatest global disaster effects because they often affect large regions.[46] In addition, variable rainfall patterns can result in a lack of a safe water supply, which can compromise hygiene and can lead to increased risk of diarrheal disease.[44] Changes in rainfall can also indirectly affect the nutritional status of populations by altering agricultural production. Higher temperatures contribute to deaths associated with respiratory and cardiovascular disease as the body is subjected to harsher conditions. High temperatures can also exacerbate air pollution levels, which can lead to a greater incidence of asthma cases. Changing weather patterns can influence the balance of ecosystems and biodiversity of a region. Even small changes in rainfall and temperature can alter the distribution of disease carriers, such as mosquitoes, which can then affect the prevalence of vector-borne diseases, such as dengue or malaria.[47] It is anticipated that climate change will also be associated with substantial displacement of populations and a range of impacts on mental health.[48]

Who Is Affected?

All people are at risk of being negatively affected by climate change, and the well-being of billions will be put at risk. Nonetheless, some groups of people are more vulnerable than others.[49] In particular, low-income countries, and in some cases middle-income countries as well, could be affected to a greater extent because areas with weak health infrastructure will be least prepared to respond and adapt to the changes in weather and corresponding changing health and disease patterns. The losses related to climate change are also much less likely to be insured in low-income than in other countries. One estimate, for example, suggested that 99 percent of climate-related losses in low-income countries since 1990 have not been covered by insurance.[50] In addition, it is anticipated that urban areas will be affected to a greater extent by any negative impacts of air pollution or rises in temperature, whereas rural areas will be more affected by changes in weather patterns that affect agricultural production.[44]

Within all countries, children and the elderly will be among the most vulnerable to the diseases climate change is likely to influence. Children will be affected by increased risk of diarrheal disease, malaria, and undernutrition, whereas the elderly will be most affected by increased risk of heat-related conditions and also extreme weather patterns, given their more fragile physical state.[44,51]

What Must Be Done?

Climate change is likely to have high human and economic costs. In fact, WHO estimates that by 2030, the damage to health will be between $2 billion and $4 billion per year.[44] The potential health and economic consequences can be mitigated with cost-effective interventions. The climate change response proposed by the United Nations Environment Programme involves both adaptation strategies that build resilience to climate change in the short run and mitigation strategies that aim to reduce long-term carbon emissions.[52] All mitigation and adaptation strategies offer direct health benefits as a result of either preventing the effects of climate change on health or preparing the health community to better respond to these effects.

In the short term, the public health community can prepare for any negative climate change effects by enhancing public health education surrounding emergency preparedness, warnings of high pollution, and general public health education, including boil water notices during floods, public awareness on vector-borne diseases, and promotion of good hygiene.[53]

In the long term, mitigation efforts revolve around reducing emissions of greenhouse gases, particularly carbon and methane emissions.[54] Assuming a world population of 9 billion by 2050, reductions of more than two-thirds in emissions would be needed to avoid doubling preindustrial revolution levels.[47] Effective control efforts would avoid 0.6 million to 4.4 million deaths related to particulate matter and 0.04 million to 0.52 million ozone-related deaths and can also increase annual crop yields by 30 million to 135 million metric tons due to ozone reductions in 2030 and beyond.[55,56] Benefits of methane emissions reductions have been estimated at $700 to $5,000 per metric ton.[56]

The United Nations Environmental Programme suggests many strategies to control carbon and methane emissions, but given that the largest contributor to greenhouse emissions is the burning of fossil fuels, reducing this activity should be a priority.[54] Fossil fuels can be controlled both directly and indirectly. For example, on a policy level, regulations can be put in place that directly limit the magnitude of emissions or that require manufacturing processes that are more environmentally friendly and less wasteful.[54]

In addition, research and support of energy sources other than fossil fuels must be sustained as a mitigation strategy in order to offer an alternative to the burning of fossil fuels. These commitments need to be made in low- and middle-income countries, as well as in high-income countries, and there have already been successful and cost-effective interventions in resource-poor settings. In Jaipur, India, for example, a 350-bed health facility cut its total energy bill in half between 2005 and 2008 through solar-powered water heaters and lighting. In Brazil, one efficiency initiative reduced the demand for electricity of a group of 101 hospitals by 1,035 kilowatts at a cost savings of 25 percent.[51]

Another mitigation strategy is the halting of deforestation and forest degradation. Agricultural expansion, forest clearing, infrastructure development, destructive logging, fires, and other similar activities contribute almost 20 percent of the global greenhouse gas emissions, the second-leading contributor.[54] These activities can be discouraged through offering alternative economic means for organizations and individuals engaged with them, such as creating carbon markets in which governments or businesses are rewarded for their efforts made to reduce carbon emissions.[54]

Other mitigation strategies can include reducing agricultural waste and inefficiency through investing in new farming and storing technologies, reducing waste associated with the construction industry, investing in improved recycling infrastructure, or promoting sustainable tourism that engages local communities and protects natural ecosystems.[54] A range of actors have stated that interventions must be implemented on the individual, local, national, and international levels in order to best mitigate the looming potential effects of climate change on health.[49]

The 2015 *Lancet* commission on health and climate change[48] also recommended actions along similar lines, as summarized in **TABLE 8-13**.

▶ Future Challenges

Many challenges will be associated with reducing the burden of disease that is related to water supply, sanitation, and hygiene; household air pollution; and ambient

TABLE 8-13 Recommendations of the 2015 *Lancet* Commission on Climate Change

Invest in climate change and public health research

Scale up financing for climate-resilient health systems

Rapidly phase out coal-fired power

Encourage a city-level transition to low-carbon emissions to reduce urban pollution

Establish the framework for a strong, predictable, and international carbon pricing mechanism

Rapidly expand access to renewable energy in low- and middle-income countries

Support accurate quantification of the avoided burden of disease, reduced healthcare costs, and enhanced economic productivity associated with climate change mitigation

Take intersectoral approaches to addressing climate change and its impact on health

Agree and implement an international agreement that supports countries in transitioning to a low-carbon economy

Develop a new, independent group to provide expertise in implementing policies that mitigate climate change and promote public health, and to monitor progress in these over the next 15 years

Data from Watts, N., Adger, W. N., Agnolucci, P., Blackstock, J., Byass, P., Cai, W., . . . Costello, A. (2015). Health and climate change: Policy responses to protect public health. *The Lancet, 386*(10006), 1861–1914.

particulate matter pollution. One important challenge has to do with population growth. The population is continuing to grow in many low- and middle-income countries and will do so for some time. As the population grows, and as increasing numbers of people move to cities, for example, will low- and middle-income countries be able to provide the necessary infrastructure for improved water supply and sanitation?

At the same time, if the economies of low- and middle-income countries grow at a relatively rapid and sustained pace, how will they manage the pollution that is related, for example, to increased use of energy and greater use of automobiles by better-off people? In addition, will relatively poorly governed societies be able to manage and regulate industrial forms of pollution that could further harm air and water quality?

Many of the health impacts related to household air pollution and unsafe water and sanitation exact a larger toll on rural people than on urban people, on the poor rather than the better off, and on women and children. In this light, many countries will need to explore ways to reduce household air pollution and improve the safety of the water supply through community-based approaches. Such approaches will often have to link the public, private, and NGO sectors with communities and will have to explicitly focus on women and children.

Reducing the burden of environmentally related health problems will also require that people be better informed about that burden. At the societal level, people and communities will need to understand more about the links between their health and the environment. At national, regional, local, and family levels, people will also need to be more aware of the solutions to these problems that might be available to them. The need for better and more information about issues and options for addressing them will be especially important among the poor, the poorly educated, the rural, and women.

Another challenge of addressing environmental health issues is that efforts to address them generally require action outside the health sector. Urban water supply systems are usually under the control of public or private companies. Urban sanitation is usually managed by individual cities. In rural areas, water supply and sanitation are most likely to be controlled by communities and individuals. Household air pollution is an issue that can best be addressed by working with families and communities to change the way they cook and the fuel they use for cooking. Ambient air particulate matter pollution comes, among other things, from industrial plants and vehicles, the control of which depends on an array of economic and policy matters beyond the scope of the health ministry.

▶ Main Messages

Environmental health issues have a large impact on the global burden of disease. These impacts occur at the individual, household, community, and global levels. Broadly speaking, about one-quarter of the total global burden of disease is related to environmental factors. This chapter has examined some of the most important environmental health issues: the lack of safe water and sanitation, poor access to handwashing facilities, household air pollution, and ambient particulate matter pollution.

The risks of these environmental factors are greatest for poor women and their children due to their exposure to household air pollution from the burning of solid fuel and to poor-quality water. The risks of environmental impacts on health are greatest in the low-income countries of Africa and Asia. Environmental risk factors are especially important causes of illness and death from diarrhea and acute respiratory infections among young children. They also have a large impact on the burden of disease from certain parasitic infections, such as worms. Given the prominence of these risk factors, it is essential that improvements be made in water, sanitation, and hygiene.

The burden of household air pollution stems largely from cooking on unventilated stoves with solid biomass fuels or coal, as done by a large share of poor people in the world. The sources of ambient air pollution are many, and vehicle emission is among the most important in most cities. Poor sanitation allows pathogens in human waste to spread, but only about 60 percent of the people in the world have access to improved sanitation. Unsafe water carries pathogens. The lack of water prevents people from engaging in appropriate hygiene practices. Poor hygiene practices, including open defecation and the failure to engage in handwashing with soap, are common in low- and middle-income countries, especially among people who lack education.

Data are weak on cost-effective approaches to reducing ambient particulate matter pollution in low- and middle-income countries. However, it appears that a number of measures could be taken to reduce pollution and enhance health, including eliminating leaded gasoline, eliminating two-stroke engines, strengthening emissions standards, and shifting vehicle fuel to natural gas. In Africa and South Asia, the most cost-effective approach to reducing household air pollution will be to promote the use of improved stoves. In East Asia, the most cost-effective approach would be to encourage a shift from biomass fuels and coal to kerosene or gas.

The most cost-effective approach to reducing the burden of water-related diseases, especially diarrhea, is to invest in low-cost sanitation and standposts for water and to promote handwashing with soap. Home water treatment with chlorine also holds potential. Investments in water can have numerous benefits, including saving the time of women who are usually charged with obtaining water and often have to expend large amounts of energy to do so. The provision of water can also contribute to reduction in certain parasitic diseases. However, in the absence of improved hygiene, the provision of improved access to water alone still fails to address an important share of the burden of diarrheal disease.

Study Questions

1. Why are environmental health issues important in global health? Which of them are the most important and why?
2. Why would the burden of disease from household air pollution in low- and middle-income countries be larger than that from ambient particulate matter pollution?
3. In what regions of the world would the burden from household air pollution be the greatest? Why?
4. What are the different ways in which unsafe water is related to the spread of disease? Give some examples of specific diseases that are spread in various water-related ways.
5. What are some of the health problems associated with ambient particulate matter pollution?
6. Why is it important to promote handwashing?
7. What approach would you take in a low-income African country to enhance the access of the poor to better water supplies? Why?
8. How would you try to expand access to low-cost sanitation in Nepal? Why?
9. What would constrain poor people in Nepal from investing their own resources in improved low-cost sanitation? How could those constraints be overcome?

References

1. Cohen, A. J., Brauer, M., Burnett, R., Anderson, H. R., Frostad, J., Estep, K., . . . Forouzanfar, M. H. (2017). Estimates and 25-year trends of the global burden of disease attributable to ambient air pollution: An analysis of data from the Global Burden of Diseases Study 2015. *The Lancet*, *389*(10082), 1907–1918.

2. Institute of Health Metrics and Evaluation (IHME). (n.d.). GBD Compare: Viz Hub. Retrieved from https://vizhub .healthdata.org/gbd-compare/

3. Lopez, A. D., Mathers, C. D., Ezzati, M., Jamison, D. T., & Murray, C. J. L. (2006). Measuring the global burden of disease and risk factors 1990–2001. In A. D. Lopez, C. D. Mathers, M. Ezzati, D. T. Jamison, & C. J. L. Murray (Eds.), *Global burden of disease and risk factors*. New York, NY: Oxford University Press.

4. Friis, R. H. (2007). *Essentials of environmental health*. Sudbury, MA: Jones and Bartlett.

5. Yassi, A., Kjellstrom, T., de Kok, T., & Guidotti, T. L. (2001). *Basic environmental health*. New York, NY: Oxford University Press.

6. McMichael, A. J., Kjellstrom, T., & Smith, K. R. (2001). Environmental health. In M. H. Merson, R. E. Black, & A. Mills (Eds.), *International public health: Diseases, programs, systems, and policies*. Gaithersburg, MD: Aspen.

7. The World Bank. (n.d.). *Environmental health*. Retrieved from http://siteresources.worldbank.org/INTPHAAG/Resources /AAGEHEng.pdf

8. World Health Organization. (n.d.). *Public health, environmental and social determinants of health*. Retrieved from http://www.who.int/phe/en

9. World Health Organization. (2018). *Household air pollution and health: Key facts*. Retrieved from http:// www.who.int/en/news-room/fact-sheets/detail/household -air-pollution-and-health

10. Yassi, A., Kjellstrom, T., de Kok, T., & Guidotti, T. L. (2001). Health and energy use. In *Basic environmental health* (pp. 311–331). New York, NY: Oxford University Press.

11. Yassi, A., Kjellstrom, T., de Kok, T., & Guidotti, T. L. (2001). Air. In *Basic environmental health* (pp. 180–208). New York, NY: Oxford University Press.

12. World Health Organization. (2018). *Drinking water: Key facts*. Retrieved from http://www.who.int/en/news-room /fact-sheets/detail/drinking-water

13. World Health Organization. (2018). *Sanitation: Key facts*. Retrieved from http://www.who.int/en/news-room/fact -sheets/detail/sanitation

14. Cairncross, S., & Valdmanis, V. (2006). Water supply, sanitation, and hygiene promotion. In D. T. Jamison, J. G. Breman, A. R. Measham, et al. (Eds.), *Disease control priorities in developing countries* (2nd ed., pp. 771–792). New York, NY: Oxford University Press.

15. UNICEF. (2017). *Hygiene*. Retrieved from https://data .unicef.org/topic/water-and-sanitation/hygiene/

16. Landrigan, P., Fuller, R., Acosta, N. J. R., Adeyi, O., Arnold, R., Basu, N. N., . . . Zhong, M. (2018). The Lancet Commission on pollution and health. *The Lancet*, *391*(10119), 462–512.

17. World Health Organization. (n.d.). *Air pollution: Ambient air pollution: Health impacts*. Retrieved from http://www.who .int/airpollution/ambient/health-impacts/en/

18. Prüss-Ustün, A., Wolf, J., Corvalán, C., Bos, R., & Neira, M. (2016). *Preventing disease through healthy environments: A global assessment of the burden of disease from environmental risks*. Geneva, Switzerland: World Health Organization.

19. Kjellstrom, T., Lodh, M., McMichael, A. J., Ranmuthugala, G., Shrestha, R., & Kingsland, S. (2006). Air and water pollution: Burden and strategies for control. In D. T. Jamison, J. G. Breman, A. R. Measham, et al. (Eds.), *Disease control priorities in developing countries* (2nd ed., pp. 817–832). New York, NY: Oxford University Press.

20. Bruce, N., Rehfuess, E., Mehta, S., Hutton, G., & Smith, K. (2006). Household air pollution. In D. T. Jamison, J. G. Breman, A. R. Measham, et al. (Eds.), *Disease control priorities in developing countries* (2nd ed., pp. 793–816). New York, NY: Oxford University Press.

21. Feachem, R., Bradley, D., Garelick, H., & Mara, D. (1983). *Sanitation and disease: Health aspects of excreta and wastewater management*. Chichester, UK: John Wiley & Sons.

22. Waterkeyn, J. (2003). *Cost-effective health promotion: Community health clubs*. Paper presented at the 29th WEDC Conference, Abuja, Nigeria.

23. Allan, S. (2003). *The WaterAid Bangladesh/VERC 100% sanitation approach: Cost, motivation and subsidy*. Unpublished Master's thesis, London School of Hygiene.

24. Pruss-Ustun, A., Bartram, J., Clasen, T., Colford, J. M. Jr., Cumming, O., Curtis, V., . . . Cairncross, S. (2014). Burden of disease from inadequate water, sanitation and hygiene in low- and middle-income settings: A retrospective analysis of data from 145 countries. *Tropical Medicine and International Health*, *19*(8), 894–905.

25. Emerson, P. M., Lindsay, S. W., Alexander, N., Bah, M., Dibba, S. M., Faal, H. B., . . . Bailey, R. L. (2004). Role of flies and provision of latrines in trachoma control: Cluster-randomised controlled trial. *The Lancet*, *363*(9415), 1093–1098.

26. United Nations. (n.d). Water. Retrieved from https://www .un.org/en/sections/issues-depth/water/.

27. Ghialane, R., & Thomas, C. (2010). Estimating the scope of household water treatment in low- and medium-income countries. *American Journal of Tropical Medicine and Hygiene*, *82*(2), 289–300.

28. This brief is based on Water and Sanitation Program. (2010). *Senegal: A handwashing behavior change journey*. Retrieved from http://www.wsp.org/wsp/sites/wsp.org/files /publications/WSP_SenegalBCJourney_HWWS.pdf

29. Water and Sanitation Program. (2010). *Involving men in handwashing behavior change in Senegal*. Retrieved from http://www.wsp.org/wsp/sites/wsp.org/files/publications /WSP_InvolvingMen_HWWS.pdf

30. This brief is based largely on Water and Sanitation Program. (2009). *Total sanitation and sanitation marketing project: Indonesia country update. Learning at scale*. Retrieved from http://www.wsp.org/wsp/sites/wsp.org/files/publications /learning_at_scale.pdf

31. Water and Sanitation Program. (n.d.). Home. Retrieved from http://www.wsp.org/

32. The World Bank. (n.d.). *The Global Water Security & Sanitation Partnership*. Retrieved from http://www.worldbank.org/en /programs/global-water-security-sanitation-partnership

33. Water and Sanitation Program. (2009). *Annual report 2009*. Retrieved from http://www.wsp.org/wsp/global-initiatives/Global-Scaling-Up-Handwashing-Project/Annual-Progress-Report-2009

34. Water and Sanitation Program. (n.d.). *Scaling up rural sanitation: Core components*. Retrieved from http://www.wsp.org/global-initiatives/global-scaling-sanitation-project/Sanitation-core-components#applying_total_sanitation

35. Water and Sanitation Project. (n.d.). *Global Scaling Up Sanitation Project second annual progress report. Indonesia, Tanzania and the States of Himachal Pradesh and Madhya Pradesh, India. July 1, 2008 to June 30, 2009*. Retrieved from http://www.wsp.org/sites/wsp.org/files/publications/gsp_annual_progress_report.pdf

36. Pinto, R. (2013). *Results, impacts, and learning from improving sanitation at scale in East Java, Indonesia*. Washington, DC: The World Bank. Retrieved from http://documents.worldbank.org/curated/en/837261468038946470/Results-impacts-and-learning-from-improving-sanitation-at-scale-in-East-Java-Indonesia

37. Cameron, L., Shah, M., & Olivia, S. (2013). *Impact evaluation of a large-scale rural sanitation project in Indonesia*. Policy Research Working Paper No. 6360. Washington, DC: The World Bank. Retrieved from https://openknowledge.worldbank.org/handle/10986/13166

38. Glassman, A., & Temin, M. (2016). A persuasive plea to become "Open Defecation Free": Indonesia's total sanitation and sanitation marketing program. In *Millions saved: New cases of proven success in global health*. Washington, DC: Center for Global Development.

39. Amin, S., Rangarajan, A., & Borkum, E. (2011). *Improving sanitation at scale: Lessons from TSSM implementation in East Java, Indonesia*. Princeton, NJ: Mathematica Policy Research. Retrieved from https://www.mathematica-mpr.com/our-publications-and-findings/publications/improving-sanitation-at-scale-lessons-from-tssm-implementation-in-east-java-indonesia

40. This case is based on Glassman, A., Temin, M., & the Millions Saved Team and Advisory Group. (2016). A solid foundation for child health: Mexico's Piso Firme program. In *Millions saved* (pp. 49–57). Washington, DC: Center for Global Development. Those interested in a more complete account of the case and additional references will want to read the case in *Millions Saved*.

41. Environmental Protection Agency. (2014). *Climate change: Basic information*. Retrieved from http://www.epa.gov/climatechange/basics/

42. The World Bank. (2014). *Climate change overview*. Retrieved from http://www.worldbank.org/en/topic/climatechange/overview#1

43. Intergovernmental Panel on Climate Change. (2014). *Climate change 2014: Impacts, adaptation, and vulnerability. Summary for policymakers* (p.6). UK: Cambridge University Press.

44. World Health Organization. (2018). *Climate change and health: Key facts*. Retrieved from http://www.who.int/news-room/fact-sheets/detail/climate-change-and-health

45. Intergovernmental Panel on Climate Change. (2013). *Climate change 2013: The physical science basis*. Contribution of Working Group I to the fifth assessment report of the Intergovernmental Panel on Climate Change. Cambridge, UK: Cambridge University Press.

46. McMichael, A. J., Woodruff, R. E., & Hales, S. (2006). Climate change and human health: Present and future risks. *The Lancet, 367*, 859–869.

47. Haines, A., Kovats, R. S., Campbell-Lendrum, D., & Corvalan, C. (2006). Climate change and human health: Impacts, vulnerability and public health. *Public Health, 120*, 585–596.

48. Watts, N., Adger, W. N., Agnolucci, P., Blackstock, J., Byass, P., Cai, W., . . . Costello, A. (2015). Health and climate change: Policy responses to protect public health. *The Lancet, 386*(10006), 1861–1914.

49. Costello, A., Abbas, M., Allen, A., Ball, S., Vell, S., Bellamy, R., . . . Patterson, C. (2009). Managing the health effects of climate change. *The Lancet, 37*, 1693–1733. doi: 10.1016/S0140-6736(09)60935-1

50. Watts, N., Amann, M., Ayeb-Karlsson, S., Belesova, K., Bouley, T., Boykoff, M., . . . Costello, A. (2018). The Lancet countdown on health and climate change: From 25 years of inaction to a global transformation for public health. *The Lancet, 391*(10120), 581–630.

51. Neira, M. (2012). *Environmental health and sustainable development*. Geneva, Switzerland: World Health Organization. Retrieved from http://ec.europa.eu/environment/archives/soil/pdf/may2012/02%20-%20Maria%20Neira%20-%20final.pdf

52. United Nations Environment Programme. (n.d.). *Climate change*. Retrieved from https://www.unenvironment.org/explore-topics/climate-change

53. United Nations Environment Programme. (n.d.). *Climate change adaptation*. Retrieved from https://www.unenvironment.org/explore-topics/climate-change/what-we-do/climate-adaptation

54. United Nations Environment Programme. (n.d.). *Climate change mitigation*. Retrieved from https://www.unenvironment.org/explore-topics/climate-change/what-we-do/mitigation

55. Anenberg, S. C. (2012). Global air quality and health co-benefits of mitigating near-term climate change through methane and black carbon emission controls. *Environmental Health Perspectives, 120*, 831–839.

56. Shindell, D., Kuylenstierna, J. C., Vignati, A., van Dingenen, R., Amann, M., Klimont, Z., . . . Fowler, D. (2012). Simultaneously mitigating near-term climate change and improving human health and food security. *Science, 335*(6065), 183–189.

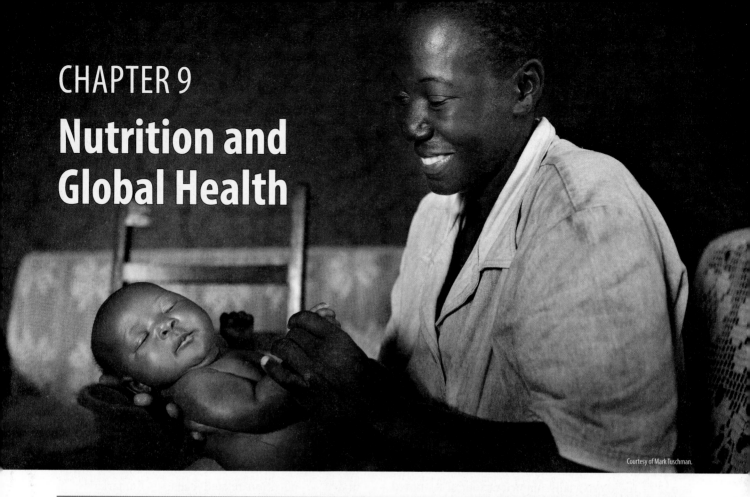

CHAPTER 9
Nutrition and Global Health

Courtesy of Mark Tuschman.

LEARNING OBJECTIVES

By the end of this chapter, the reader will be able to do the following:

- Define key terms related to nutrition
- Describe the determinants of nutritional status
- Discuss nutrition needs at different stages of the life course
- Discuss the burden of nutrition problems globally
- Review the costs and consequences of those burdens
- Discuss measures that can be taken to address key nutrition concerns

▶ Vignettes

Shireen was a 1-year-old who lived in Dhaka, the capital of Bangladesh. Shireen was born with low birthweight. In addition, her family lacked the income needed to provide her with adequate food after she was no longer breastfeeding. Shireen had also repeatedly been ill with respiratory infections and diarrhea, and she was hospitalized again with pneumonia. Despite the best efforts of the hospital, Shireen died after 2 days there.

Ruth lived in Liberia and was pregnant with her first child. Ruth had been anemic for all of her adult life from not having enough iron-rich foods in her diet. She also had no access during pregnancy to iron and folic acid tablets or to foods that were fortified

with vitamins and minerals. Ruth went into labor one evening and delivered the baby with the help of a traditional birth attendant. After the baby was born, however, Ruth began to bleed severely. Her family was not able to get her to a hospital, and Ruth died.

Dorji was 15 years old and lived in the mountains of northern India. Dorji was very short and faced important delays in his cognitive development. Dorji was not the only one in his village with these problems. Dorji lived in an area in which the soils had little iodine. Although the government of India was encouraging the fortification of salt with iodine, such salt was not sold in Dorji's region of the country.

Rachel and her mother lived in Mombassa, a port city in Kenya. Rachel had already received her first polio vaccine, and she would soon get another.

When the children participated in "polio days" they got not only a polio vaccine but also a dose of vitamin A. Until recently, there were many young children in Kenya and elsewhere who were blind due to the lack of vitamin A. Since the polio campaign started and children got extra vitamin A as part of that campaign, however, almost no children had become blind.

Fai Ho was a 7-year-old boy who lived in South China. He was an only child. As his family had done increasingly well economically, they began to eat fewer and fewer traditional foods and more Western and processed foods, such as soft drinks and potato chips. The family also began to watch more television and get less exercise. In addition, whenever the family wanted to do something special with their son, they took him to a fast-food restaurant for a cheeseburger and French fries. Despite the low rates of obesity among children and adults in China traditionally, Fai Ho already had obesity.

▶ The Importance of Nutrition

Some topics in global health have overarching impacts on many different dimensions of well-being. Nutrition is one of these especially important topics. As noted in **TABLE 9-1**, and elaborated on throughout this chapter, nutritional status has a profound relationship with health status.

Nutritional status is fundamental to the growth of young children, their proper mental and physical development, and their health as adults. In addition, because of the impact of nutrition on health, nutritional status is intimately linked with whether or not children enroll in school, perform effectively while there, and complete their schooling. Nutritional status, therefore, has a profound effect on labor productivity and people's prospects for earning income.

Despite the importance of nutrition to health, an exceptional number of people in the world are undernourished. This is especially the case for poor women and children in low-income countries, particularly in South Asia and sub-Saharan Africa. About 14 percent of children under 5 globally were underweight in 2016, with the overwhelming majority of such children living in low- and middle-income countries.[1] Moreover, about 22 percent of children globally are stunted, with especially high rates of stunting in South Asia and sub-Saharan Africa.[2]

Nutritional status is also central to whether young children thrive. A review of maternal and child nutrition in low- and middle-income countries suggested that about 45 percent of all child deaths are attributable to nutrition-related causes.[3] Remarkably, in 2017, that would have been the equivalent of almost 2.4 million deaths that year, or 7,000 nutrition-related child deaths in the world every day.[4] In fact,

TABLE 9-1 Selected Links Between Nutrition and the Health of Mothers and Children

Good maternal nutrition and avoiding obesity is essential for good outcomes of pregnancy for the mother and the child.

Exclusive breastfeeding for 6 months promotes better health and cognitive development for infants than mixing breastfeeding with other foods during that period.

Nutritional deficits in fetuses and in children under 2 years of age may produce growth and developmental deficits in infants and young children that can never be overcome.

About 45 percent of all deaths in children under 5 years worldwide are associated with nutritional deficits.

Underweight and micronutrient deficiencies in children make those children more susceptible to illness, cause illnesses to last longer, and can lead to deaths from diarrhea, measles, pneumonia, and malaria that might have been preventable.

Rapid weight gain in children who were underweight is associated later in life with obesity and noncommunicable diseases.

Obesity in women—and men—is associated with a range of noncommunicable diseases, such as heart disease, stroke, and diabetes.

Data from Black, R. E., Victora, C. G., Walker, S. P., Bhutta, Z. A., Christian, P., de Onis, M., . . . Uauy, R. (2013). Maternal and child undernutrition and overweight in low-income and middle-income countries. *The Lancet, 382*(9890), 427–451.

low birthweight is the 2nd leading risk factor for death of under-5 children globally, child wasting is 3rd, child underweight is 5th, vitamin A deficiency is 9th, and child stunting is 10th.[5]

These issues related to maternal and childhood undernutrition are even more difficult to accept because there are a number of low-cost, but highly effective, nutrition interventions that can dramatically improve nutrition but are not being implemented sufficiently. Many improvements in nutrition can be enabled largely by communication efforts, such as the promotion of breastfeeding, the introduction of appropriate complementary foods, and the eating of foods that are rich in certain micronutrients. Such communication efforts, however, are not put in place frequently enough or effectively enough. The fortification of salt with iodine has been carried out in high-income countries for more than 50 years, but uniodized salt is still sold in many low-income countries. The importance of iron and folic acid to successful outcomes of pregnancy has also been well known for decades,[6] yet many women in low-income countries, like Ruth in the vignette, do not get supplements of iron and folic acid or eat food that is fortified with iron and folate.

At the same time, however, some nutritional issues relate to food insecurity, political instability, and climate variability and are not so amenable to relatively "simple" solutions. Rather, they will require, for example, that actors work together in a coordinated way across a range of sectors to enhance the availability and affordability of more and healthier food.

It is also critical to note that the nutritional picture of the world has changed dramatically in the last few decades. At the same time as so many people are undernourished, about 2.3 billion people—nearly 31 percent of the world's population—are overweight or have obesity.[7] This includes close to 6 percent of the world's under-5 children who are overweight.[8] Obesity was once considered a problem unique to high-income countries. However, the vast majority of people who are overweight and have obesity in the world today live in low- and middle-income countries. In fact, many countries will have to deal simultaneously for some time to come with several different types of malnutrition, including underweight, micronutrient deficiencies, and overweight and obesity.[9]

Overweight and obesity are especially important for several reasons. First, the prevalence of these problems has been increasing in almost all countries. Second, they are closely linked with a number of noncommunicable diseases, such as heart disease, stroke, and diabetes, that exact an enormous toll on people's health and productivity and on the costs of health care. Third, treating these problems can be extremely costly. Finally, prevention of the problems associated with overweight and obesity is complex and involves strategies in a variety of sectors and across individual, local, national, and global spheres.

Nutrition is also central to the achievement of the Sustainable Development Goals. In fact, as you can see in **FIGURE 9-1**, nutrition is related to almost all of these goals. Moreover, this figure makes clear that there are *no* prospects for meeting the SDGs without substantial improvements in nutrition. The hunger goal is completely linked with nutrition, and nutrition deficits are intimately connected to whether or not people are poor. The large number of children who are poorly nourished will challenge the realization of the education goal. In addition, if about 45 percent of all child deaths are related to nutrition, then how can the child mortality goal be met unless nutrition problems are tackled more effectively? The nutritional concerns that are particular to women will constrain their productivity, limit improvements in their economic and social status, preclude gains in the reduction of maternal mortality, and have a deleterious impact on the children to whom they give birth.

In light of the exceptional importance of nutrition to human health, this chapter provides an overview of the most critical matters concerning nutrition globally. First, it introduces you to the most important terms used in discussing nutrition. It then examines the determinants of nutritional status. After that, the chapter explores the most important nutritional needs of people at different stages in their life course. It will then review key issues concerning the nutritional state of the world and the costs and consequences of selected nutrition problems. This is followed by a number of case studies that illustrate key themes covered in this chapter. The chapter concludes by examining some of the challenges of trying to further improve nutritional status worldwide.

This chapter deals with undernutrition *and* overweight and obesity. The sections on undernutrition focus largely on children under 5 and pregnant women. The World Food Programme (WFP) says that "people are considered food secure when they have availability and adequate access at all times to sufficient, safe, nutritious food to maintain a healthy and active life."[10] The chapter comments on, but does not go into detail on, issues related to food security.

▶ Definitions and Key Terms

A number of terms related to nutrition are used throughout this chapter. These terms are defined in **TABLE 9-2**.

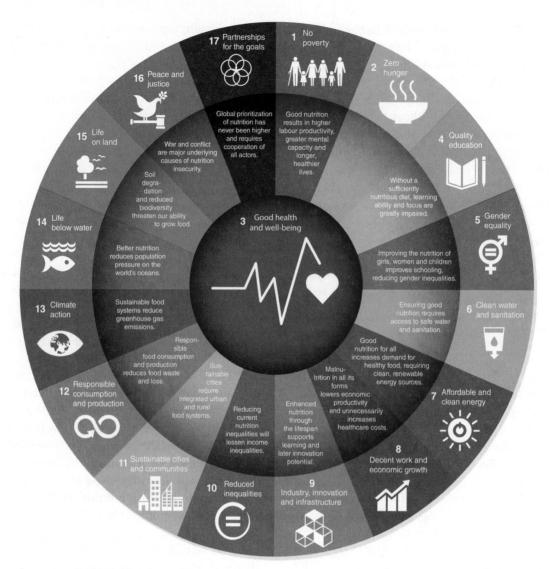

FIGURE 9-1 Nutrition and the SDGs

Reproduced from Food and Agriculture Organization of the United Nations (FAO), International Fund for Agricultural Development (IFAD), UNICEF, World Food Program (WFP), & World Health Organization (WHO). (2018). *The state of food security and nutrition in the world 2018: Building climate resilience for food security and nutrition.* Rome, Italy: FAO.

The term *malnutrition* should be used to refer to those who do not get proper nutrition, whether too little, too much, or of the wrong kind. This is the way that this text uses that term. In addition, people who lack sufficient energy and nutrients are referred to as "undernourished," "stunted," or "wasted," as appropriate. People who have low weight for their age are called "underweight." People who are nourished to the point of being too heavy for their height are said to be "overweight" or to have "obesity," depending on their body mass index.

▶ Data on Nutrition

There are many gaps in the data on nutrition. It is difficult, for example, to find a single consistent data set that addresses issues ranging from low birthweight to micronutrient deficiencies to overweight and obesity, organized by World Bank region or World Bank country income group. In addition, some critical data on nutrition are not broken down into consistent age groups. Moreover, existing data on nutrition are often shown using different regions. Some data is presented by World Health Organization (WHO) regions, but other data may be available by UNICEF regions or World Bank regions. This chapter seeks to be as consistent as possible in its use of data, which is largely taken from the Food and Agriculture Organization of the UN (FAO), UNICEF, WHO, and the World Bank. UNICEF, WHO, and the World Bank have increasingly collaborated in producing such data, which has improved its quality and usefulness.

TABLE 9-2 Key Terms

Anemia—Low level of hemoglobin in the blood, as evidenced by a reduced quality or quantity of red blood cells.

Body mass index (BMI)—Body weight in kilograms divided by height in meters squared (kg/m^2).

Iodine deficiency disorders (IDDs)—The spectrum of IDDs includes goiter, hypothyroidism, impaired mental function, stillbirths, abortions, congenital anomalies, and neurological cretinism.

Low birthweight—Birthweight less than 2,500 grams.

Malnutrition—Various forms of poor nutrition. Underweight or stunting and overweight, as well as micronutrient deficiencies, are forms of malnutrition.

Obesity—Excessive body fat content, commonly measured by BMI. The international reference for classifying an individual as having obesity is a BMI greater than or equal to 30.

Overweight—Excess weight relative to height, commonly measured by BMI among adults. The international reference for adults is as follows:

- 25–29.99 for grade I (overweight)
- 30–39.99 for grade II (obese)
- > 40 for grade III

    For children, overweight is measured as weight-for-height two z-scores above the international reference.

Stunting—Failure to reach linear growth potential because of inadequate nutrition or poor health. Stunting is measured as height-for-age two z-scores below the international reference.

Undernutrition—The three most commonly used indexes for child undernutrition are height-for-age, weight-for-age, and weight-for-height. For adults, underweight is measured by a BMI less than 18.5.

Underweight—Low weight-for-age; that is, two z-scores below the international reference for weight-for-age. It implies stunting or wasting and is an indicator of undernutrition.

Vitamin A deficiency—Tissue concentrations of vitamin A low enough to have adverse health consequences such as increased morbidity and mortality, poor reproductive health, and slowed growth and development, even if there is no clinical deficiency.

Wasting—Weight, measured in kilograms, divided by height in meters squared, that is two z-scores below the international reference.

Z-score—A statistical term, meaning the deviation of an individual's value from the median value of a reference population, divided by the standard deviation of the reference population.

Data from The World Bank. (2006). *Repositioning nutrition as central to development.* Washington, DC: Author. Retrieved from https://siteresources.worldbank.org/NUTRITION/Resources/281846 -1131636806329/NutritionStrategyOverview.pdf

▶ The Determinants of Nutritional Status

Undernutrition

Nutritional status depends on a broad range of factors, which different organizations may seek to portray in a range of ways. **FIGURE 9-2** follows a framework developed by UNICEF for considering the determinants of nutrition.[11] This framework was originally designed to highlight the determinants of undernutrition. However, as we will see later, it is also sheds light on the determinants of overweight and obesity.

In line with this framework, we can consider first the immediate causes of undernutrition. The two most important are inadequate dietary intake and illness.

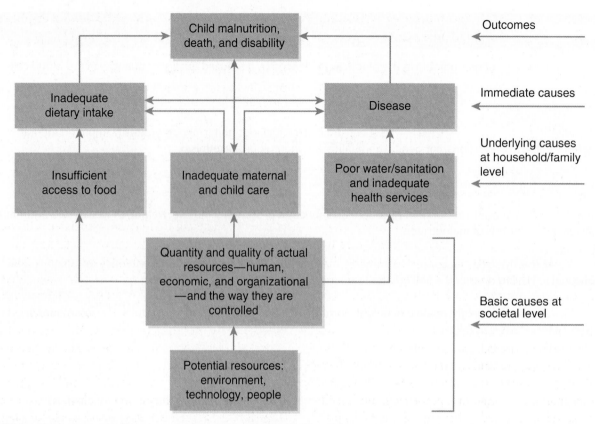

FIGURE 9-2 Determinants of Nutritional Status: The UNICEF Framework

Data from UNICEF. (1998). State of the world's children, 1998. Retrieved from http://www.unicef.org/sowc98/silent4.htm

People may get an insufficient amount of food or not enough of some of the nutrients they need. These factors weaken the body, open the person to illness and infection, and lead to longer and more frequent illness than would otherwise be the case. Inadequate dietary intake becomes part of a vicious cycle of illness and infection, which makes it harder for people to eat, more difficult for them to absorb what they do take in, and actually raises the need for some nutrients. The relationship between infection and nutritional status is very important to keep in mind, especially when considering how to improve the nutritional status of poor children in low- and middle-income countries.

The UNICEF framework also includes a set of underlying causes for inadequate dietary intake and infectious disease that include "inadequate access to food in a household; insufficient health services and an unhealthful environment; and inadequate care for children and women."[11] Whether people get enough food within a household depends on a number of factors, including access to land, the ability to produce food for those living in rural areas, and having access to food and the money to purchase it. In addition, the amount and type of food one gets depend in many families on social position, with women and girls sometimes getting less food or less nutritious food than men and boys get. It is also important to note that

in rural areas in low-income countries, there may be a hungry season, in which families have exhausted the food from their last harvest, have not yet produced the food for the current year, and do not have the income to buy food, even if a market is accessible to them.

The lack of safe water and sanitation is an extremely important cause of diarrheal disease and, therefore, greatly contributes to the cycle of infection and undernutrition. This is made worse when people live in generally unhygienic circumstances, in which food is often handled in unhygienic ways. These are also the circumstances under which people, especially children, are likely to get parasitic infections, such as worms, which sap the energy of children and make it harder for them to absorb what they do eat.

Child caring practices affect the nutritional status of children in similar ways to the manner in which they affect children's health status. If a child is exclusively breastfed for 6 months, if complementary foods that are of sufficient quality and quantity are introduced, and if food and water are handled in hygienic ways, then the nutritional status of young children will be enhanced. In addition, as discussed earlier, the nutrition and health status of the mother is an exceptionally important determinant of whether the child will be born with low birthweight and will thrive thereafter.

Access to appropriate health services is also very important to nutritional status, in a manner similar to its importance for health status. Receiving basic childhood immunizations is an important way to avoid illness and infection. The same is true for vitamin A supplements that are provided by many health services, zinc as an adjunct to oral rehydration therapy for diarrhea, and multiple micronutrient supplementation for pregnant women.[12] Medicines to rid children of worms can also be very important to their nutritional status. Unfortunately, there are still too many health systems that are not capable of effectively providing these services at the scale necessary to cover all who are at risk.

Of course, at the root of nutritional status are the factors that UNICEF calls "basic causes." These relate to the social determinants of health. In a manner similar to the factors that determine health, the root causes of nutritional status also have to do with socioeconomic status, family income, the level of knowledge people have of appropriate health and nutritional practices, and the amount of control that people have over their lives. Governmental and global policies that affect agricultural production, marketing, and distribution as well as education, health, and nutrition programs can have a profound effect on the nutritional status of individuals, communities, and societies.

Overweight and Obesity

Obesity and overweight are caused by genetic, behavioral, and environmental factors that result in weight gain. Weight gain is caused by an increase in total energy intake coupled with a decrease in energy expenditure, and may be partially related to genetic composition. However, the weight gain underlying the rising global rate of obesity is largely due to changes in the food environment, which are broadly driven by global financial and trade liberalization, increased income and socioeconomic status, and urbanization, as discussed further later.

Genes play a role in the development of obesity, as they govern the body's response to changes in its environment. Genetic variations can influence behaviors, such as a drive to overeat or tendency to be sedentary. They also govern metabolism, causing some people to store body fat at higher rates than others.[13] These differences have been documented across racial and ethnic backgrounds and even within families.[13] There is also emerging evidence of gut microbes affecting metabolism and obesity, although this research is still in early stages.[14] Despite this biological role, it is crucial to understand that obesity is a result of the interaction between genetic susceptibility and the unhealthy environmental factors that are discussed further next;

genetic variations just make people more or less susceptible to these environmental factors.[15]

In addition to genetics, there are a number of cultural and region-specific factors that contribute to the prevalence of overweight and obesity. In many cultures, girls are discouraged from participating in physical activity due to cultural and religious notions of gender and modesty.[16,17] Physical activity is also more challenging in regions with hot climates, such as the Arabian peninsula.[18] Furthermore, in some countries, being overweight is considered a sign of health and prosperity; this is especially true in areas with high HIV prevalence.[19]

Genetic and cultural factors associated with overweight are not new. Yet, both overweight and obesity have been increasing in almost all countries. The evidence suggests that these increases have been driven by three macro-level factors related to globalization: global financial and trade liberalization, increased per capita income and socioeconomic status, and increased urbanization.[20] These factors have led to increased availability and consumption of sugar-sweetened beverages and energy-dense, nutrient-poor foods, along with changes in lifestyle and living environment. Together, these are helping to fuel the global obesity epidemic.[21] Market-oriented and liberal agricultural trade policies were increasingly implemented from the 1970s through the 1990s, which altered the price and availability of foods in many countries.[20] In addition, foreign direct investment in a range of countries continues to change the types of foods available, their prices, and the way they are sold and marketed.[22]

Per capita income is rising globally and is expected to continue doing so for some time.[23] Rapid economic growth in low- and middle-income countries is associated with nutritional and lifestyle changes, including increased television viewing and consumption of highly processed foods. In these countries, body weight tends to increase with increased socioeconomic status.[20] On the other hand, in high-income countries, body weight generally decreases with income, as wealthier people tend to have better health education, can afford healthier food choices, and have adequate time for exercise.[24]

There has also been an increase in urbanization in low- and middle-income countries, which in turn leads to overweight and obesity through a multitude of factors. Although in theory urbanization provides greater access to health services and education, which are both preventative measures for obesity, many low- and middle-income countries undergo urbanization at such a rapid pace that essential infrastructure lags behind.[21] Urbanization facilitates obesity through changes in diet, occupation, environment, and behavior, which all contribute directly to increased energy intake and decreased energy expenditure.

Ultimately, these three macro factors—global trade liberalization, increased income, and urbanization—have caused a global increase in energy intake, much of which has stemmed from changes in diet. Across all national income levels, it has been shown that countries that maintain their traditional food culture have less obesity.[25] However, globalization and urbanization have caused a nutrition transition away from traditional diets, opening access to cheap, energy-dense, and nutritionally poor food through fast-food outlets and supermarkets, and a highly caloric, sugar-laden diet prominently featuring animal products. This shift has been accompanied by reduced access to fresh local produce, as urbanization has displaced farmers and farmland.[26]

Fast food has been linked to obesity and its related comorbidities, due to its high calorie content, large portion sizes, highly processed meat, highly refined carbohydrates, sugar-sweetened beverages, and high levels of salt, sugar, and saturated fat.[27] Over the past 40 years, Western fast-food chains have expanded across the globe.[28] McDonald's, for example, one of the world's largest restaurant companies, increased its international presence from 951 outlets in 1987 to over 36,000 outlets in over 100 countries today.[29,30] The spread of multinational and regional supermarkets has also contributed to the obesity epidemic. Although these markets increase access to fresh produce, they also increase access to sugar-sweetened beverages and high-energy, highly processed foods packed with sugar, salt, and saturated fat; in fact, despite supermarket access, many consumers in low- and middle-income countries continue to rely on street fairs and small shops for their produce and use supermarkets as outlets for sugar- and salt-laden packaged foods.[31] Numerous studies have found that the addition of a supermarket to a community does not improve shoppers' diet or weight status,[32,33] and that supermarkets encourage consumers to eat more, regardless of the food.[34] Supermarkets are spreading quickly globally, especially in Latin America but also in Asia, Eastern Europe, and Africa.[31,35]

Accompanying the influx of fast food and supermarkets has been an exponential growth in food marketing and advertising, which creates major shifts in food demand, as marketing leads people to increase their consumption of advertised products.[36] The content of food ads aimed at children especially favors foods of poor nutritional quality,[37] and children are increasingly being exposed to marketing of these unhealthy foods through new media channels, including social media, text messages, phone applications (apps), and branded games.[38]

All of these factors have led to notable trends in diets worldwide. Intake of added sugars has dramatically increased across the globe over the past 4 decades,

largely in the form of sugar-sweetened beverages (SSBs). As national income per capita and the proportion of the population residing in urban areas has increased in low- and middle-income countries, sugar intake has also increased.[39] SSBs are now responsible for 7 percent of total calories and 40 percent of added sugars in the American diet—they are the largest source of added sugars consumed in the United States.[40,41]

Consumption of animal products is also increasing globally. Intake of red and processed meat is associated with weight gain, type 2 diabetes, heart disease, some cancers, and mortality.[42-46] In low- and middle-income countries, daily per capita consumption of protein from animal sources more than doubled from 9 grams in 1961 to 20 grams in 2011, and is expected to reach 25 grams by 2050.[47] There has been a subsequent decrease in global consumption of whole grains, fruits, and vegetables.[15,48]

This global trend toward increasing energy intake has simultaneously been accompanied by a shift toward increased sedentary work, increased sedentary leisure time involving television or other electronic media, and increased use of motorized transport.[49] Current WHO guidelines recommend 150 minutes of moderate-intensity physical activity per week for adults to prevent chronic disease.[50] Yet, the lack of space for outdoor recreation in dense urban areas and fear of urban crime often limit opportunities for physical activity.[51] Additionally, in many low- and middle-income countries, there has been a movement away from jobs with high-energy expenditure such as farming, mining, and forestry, toward employment in less active jobs, including manufacturing and office-based work.[48]

Moreover, urban living is associated with a decrease in sleep duration, which is associated with weight gain in children and adults.[52] Stress, another risk factor for obesity, could be more common in rapidly urbanizing low- and middle-income countries, due to increased work hours and reduced societal support in comparison with traditional village settings.[49]

Technological advances have also encouraged indoor entertainment via television or computer, instead of outdoor recreation.[30] Time spent watching television has been linked to weight gain in children and adults,[53] and a reduction in sedentary behavior has been shown to have beneficial effects on weight, independent of exercise.[54]

▶ Gauging Nutritional Status

The nutritional status of infants and children is largely gauged by measuring and weighing these children and then plotting their weight and height on growth

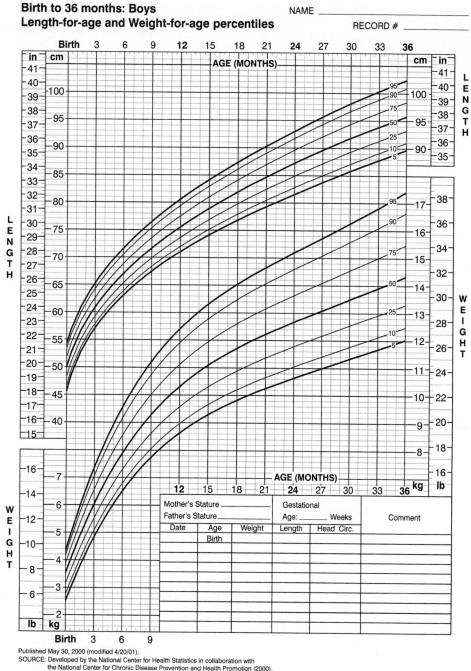

Birth to 36 months: Boys
Length-for-age and Weight-for-age percentiles

NAME _____

RECORD # _____

Published May 30, 2000 (modified 4/20/01).
SOURCE: Developed by the National Center for Health Statistics in collaboration with
the National Center for Chronic Disease Prevention and Health Promotion (2000).
http://www.cdc.gov/growthcharts

FIGURE 9-3 Model Growth Chart

Reproduced from Centers for Disease Control and Prevention (CDC). (2000). *Birth to 36 months: Boys: Length-for-age and weight-for-age percentiles.* Retrieved from http://www.cdc.gov/growthcharts/data/set1clinical/cj41l017.pdf

charts, like the one shown in **FIGURE 9-3**. These growth charts have been standardized internationally. The place of the child on the growth curves indicates how the child is growing compared to the international reference standard.

Table 9-2 showed key terms that relate to measures of nutritional status. Among the most important such measures for infants and children are the following:

- Birthweight—a child has a low birthweight if the child's weight at birth is below 2,500 grams.

- Height-for-age—a child is stunted if his or her height-for-age is two z-scores below the international reference height-for-age.

- Weight-for-age—a child is underweight if his or her weight is two z-scores below the international reference weight-for-age.

- Weight-for-height—a child is wasted if his or her weight, measured in kilograms, divided by height, in meters squared, is more than two z-scores below the international reference.

TABLE 9-3 Key Nutritional Needs, Sources, and Selected Functions

Key Nutritional Needs	Example Sources	Selected Functions
Protein	Milk, eggs, chicken, and beans	Proper growth of children and immune functions
Vitamin A	Liver, eggs, green leafy vegetables, orange and red fruits and vegetables	Proper immune function and prevention of xerophthalmia
Calcium	Milk and dairy products; some green leafy vegetables such as broccoli, kale, mustard greens, and bok choy or Chinese cabbage; almonds, Brazil nuts, and beans	Building strong bones and teeth; clotting blood; sending and receiving nerve signals; reduces problems of hypertension in pregnant women
Folic acid	Leafy green vegetables; fruits; dried beans, peas, and nuts; enriched breads, cereals, and other grain products	Helps body make new cells and is essential for preventing children from being born with neural tube defects
Iodine	Selected seafood, plants grown in iodine-containing soil	Growth and neurological development
Iron	Fish, meat, poultry, grains, vegetables, and legumes	Prevents iron deficiency anemia, prevents low birthweight and premature babies
Zinc	Red and white meat and shellfish	Promotes growth, immune function, and cognitive development

Data from Bhutta, Z. A., Das, J. K., Rizvi, A., Gaffey, M. F., Walker, N., Horton, S., . . . Black, R. E. (2013). Evidence-based intervention for improvement of maternal and child nutrition: What can be done and at what cost? *The Lancet, 382*(9890), 452–477.; Kaiser Permenante. (2016). Essential Nutrients for Everyday. Retrieved from https://m.kp.org/health/care/!ut/p/a0/FchBDslgEADAt _QBmwVayOoNa9-gcNsQUknKtiGo39ceZzDiE6Pwp6zcyy68_R1Slp7bVd69IXPxgRHj0XitjEF2SJxe-TxuvaQtYyBLzniawN3NCFovCi56UjBbM4_uphayHo9a6euH4QdhwOwq/. /; MedlinePlus. (n.d.). Calcium in diet. Retrieved from http://www.nlm.nih.gov/medlineplus/ency/article/002412.htm; MedlinePlus. (n.d.).Folic acid. Retrieved from http://www.nlm.nih.gov/medlineplus/folicacid.html

We usually think of deficits in nutrition as being large and evident; however, it is extremely important to note that this is not necessarily the case. Rather, a large number of the nutritional deficits that exist globally are mild or moderate and may not be very obvious. Nonetheless, even mild and moderate malnutrition can have very negative consequences on the biological development of people, on their health, and on their productivity, and some of these negative effects may be irreversible.

The nutritional status of adults is generally determined on the basis of body mass index (BMI). BMI is the body weight in kilograms, divided by height in meters squared. Although some countries have their own standards, generally, an adult is considered[55]

underweight if their BMI is less than 18.5,

of normal weight if their BMI is 18.5 to 24.99,

overweight if their BMI is 25 to 29.99, or

to have obesity if their BMI is 30 or greater.

▶ Key Nutritional Needs

The Needs of Young Children and Pregnant Women

Many nutrients are important. However, when thinking about the needs of pregnant women and young children, particularly in low- and middle-income countries, several are of paramount importance. These include protein, energy, and the five micronutrients vitamin A, iron, iodine, zinc, and calcium. This section briefly examines each of these topics, and **TABLE 9-3** summarizes the sources of these nutrients and their key impacts.

In order to thrive, people have to take in enough energy and micronutrients to fulfill their physiological needs. When this does not happen, undernutrition results. According to UNICEF, undernutrition is defined as "the outcome of insufficient food intake (hunger) and repeated infectious diseases.

Undernutrition includes being underweight for one's age, too short for one's age (stunted), dangerously thin for one's height (wasted), and deficient in vitamins and minerals (micronutrient malnutrition)."[56(p1)]

Stunting or chronic undernutrition is the result of cumulative deficiencies in dietary intake (inadequate amounts of energy and micronutrients) and recurrent bouts of infectious diseases.[56] This causes linear growth failure, resulting in low height-for-age.[57]

Underweight or low weight-for-age is a composite measure of being too thin (wasted) and too short (stunted). Reducing stunting and wasting are targets for Sustainable Development Goal 2 (Zero Hunger: end hunger, achieve food security and improved nutrition, and promote sustainable agriculture).

Wasting is the outcome of weight loss that is often associated with acute shortages of food and infection. Sometimes wasting is related to shocks such as drought or famine. However, wasting can also be a result of substantial acute energy deficits related to other factors that help to determine nutritional status.

Severe acute malnutrition (SAM) is generally defined by a very low weight-for-height measurement of below minus 3 standard deviations of the median WHO growth standards. Severe acute malnutrition is an extreme form of undernutrition. Wasting, including that associated with severe acute malnutrition, needs to be treated as an emergency.[58]

Undernourishment greatly raises the risk of illness, especially for children. In addition, being malnourished in childhood is associated with decreased intellectual capacity. Somewhat ironically, young children who are malnourished but who rapidly gain weight later in childhood and adolescence are at high risk as adults of nutrition-related chronic diseases such as diabetes, high blood pressure, and high cholesterol.[59]

In addition, undernourished women of short stature have greatly increased risks of dying of pregnancy-related causes. Furthermore, undernourished women have a greatly increased risk of delivering premature or low-birthweight babies. Such babies are, in turn, at much greater risk than full-term babies or babies with a birthweight of over 2,500 grams (5.5 pounds) of growing poorly, not developing properly, or dying.[57] More will be said later about the consequences of undernutrition in children and in pregnant women.

Vitamin A

Vitamin A is found in a variety of plants but mostly in green leafy vegetables, yellow and orange fruits that are not citrus, and carrots. It is also found in some animal products, including liver, milk, and eggs.[57] The lack of vitamin A is associated with the development of a condition known as xerophthalmia. The person with this condition first gets "night blindness." Later, the eye dries out, which can lead to permanent blindness.[60]

What is less well known, however, is that vitamin A is extremely important to the proper functioning of the immune system and to a child's growth. Trials of vitamin A supplements on newborns reduced the risk of deaths from infections by 25 percent and from prematurity by about 66 percent.[61] Deficiency in vitamin A has a profound impact on the severity of certain illnesses and whether a child will survive a bout of pneumonia, malaria, measles, or diarrhea.[57]

Iodine

Iodine is generally found in some types of seafood and in plants that are grown in soil that naturally contains iodine.[62] People who live in mountainous areas often do not get enough iodine in their diets, because they do not consume much seafood and mountainous soils often lack iodine. This was the case, for example, for Dorji in the vignette at the start of this chapter. The lack of iodine is most often associated with a growth on the thyroid, called a goiter, and the failure to develop full intellectual potential.[62] However, iodine deficiency disorders "can also include fetal loss, stillbirth, congenital anomalies, and hearing impairment."[57(p554)] In fact, iodine deficiency most often manifests itself in mild intellectual disabilities,[57] and people with cretinism have an IQ that is on average 10 to 15 points below that of people who do not suffer this deficit.[63] In extreme forms, iodine deficiency may also lead to severe problems of mental development and being both deaf and mute. In fact, iodine deficiency has been a preventable but, nonetheless, major cause of impaired cognitive development in children.[64]

Iron

The most easily absorbable form of iron is found in fish, meat, and poultry. Less absorbable forms can be found in fruits, grains, vegetables, nuts, and dried beans. The lack of iron is most often associated with iron deficiency anemia, which we usually associate with weakness and fatigue. This is especially a problem for adolescent women and pregnant women, because women who are iron deficient have an increased risk of giving birth to a premature or low birthweight baby or of hemorrhaging and dying in childbirth.[65] Iron deficiency is also associated with poor mental development and reduced immune function.[57] In addition, iron is a critical requirement for children in the 6- to 24-month age group to ensure optimal development of their cognitive and motor skills.

Zinc

The best sources of zinc are red and white meat and shellfish.[66] Severe deficiency in zinc is associated with "growth [deficits], impaired immune function, skin disorders, hypogonadism, and cognitive dysfuncion."[57(p554)] Mild to moderate deficiency increases susceptibility to infecion.[58] Indeed, children who receive zinc supplementation when they have diarrhea recover more rapidly than those who do not,[66,67] and zinc deficiency is a major risk factor for morbidity and mortality from diarrhea, pneumonia, and malaria, as discussed later.[57,62]

Folic Acid and Calcium

Folic acid and calcium are especially important for pregnant women and for successful birth outcomes. Folic acid is a B vitamin that helps the body to make new cells. Folic acid is found in leafy green vegetables, some fruits, beans, peas, and nuts, and in enriched products, such as flour. Deficiencies of folic acid in pregnant women are associated with neural tube defects in their children, such as spina bifida.[68] Calcium is generally found in dairy products but can also be acquired from some green leafy vegetables, some fish with small bones, and from some nuts and seeds. Diseases in pregnancy that relate to high blood pressure are among the leading causes of maternal death. Supplementation with calcium has been shown to reduce the risk of hypertensive disorders of pregnancy.[12]

▶ Overweight and Obesity

A balanced, healthy diet is crucial for the prevention of obesity and noncommunicable diseases. A systematic review of dietary recommendations defined by expert panels has identified a number of basic components to a healthy dietary pattern, namely vegetables, fruits, whole grains, legumes, and nuts, with limited amounts of red and processed meat.[69] Such a diet provides a high intake of dietary fiber and micronutrients and a low intake of saturated and trans fats, added sugars, and salt.[69] Various dietary components are playing a large role in the growth of global obesity and overweight. These components are elaborated upon next.

Fats

Monounsaturated and polyunsaturated fats, found in nuts, plant-based oils, and fish, are associated with a number of health benefits. They can help reduce levels of "bad" low-density lipoprotein (LDL) cholesterol in the blood, lowering risk of heart disease, while also providing essential fats that the body cannot manufacture itself: omega-6 and omega-3 fatty acids.[70] On the other hand, saturated and trans fats have been shown to be harmful to cardiovascular health by raising "bad" LDL cholesterol levels; trans fat additionally lowers "good" high-density lipoprotein (HDL) cholesterol levels, making it even more harmful than saturated fat.[71,72] Saturated fats are largely found in red meat and dairy products, but some plant-based foods, such as coconut oil, contain even higher amounts of saturated fat. Although natural trans fats occur in small amounts in certain animal products, artificial trans fats are prominent in processed foods made with partially hydrogenated oils, and are used to extend shelf life.

Sodium

High sodium intake can lead to hypertension, which is a major risk factor for stroke and fatal coronary heart disease.[73] Sodium is found in high quantities in restaurant and processed foods.[73] Evidence suggests that limiting sodium intake to no more than 1.7 grams per day is beneficial in reducing blood pressure; this translates to an overall salt intake of less than 5 grams per day.[74]

Added Sugars

Overconsumption of added sugars (this excludes sugars naturally occurring in milk, fruits, and vegetables) threatens the nutritional quality of diets by providing large amounts of energy without supplying specific nutrients, and has been shown to lead to obesity and type 2 diabetes.[75] The consumption of SSBs in particular has been scientifically shown to promote weight gain, type 2 diabetes, and coronary heart disease.[76-79] Researchers found that adults who drink one SSB or more per day have a 37 percent higher risk of obesity compared to infrequent drinkers, regardless of income or ethnicity.[80] The World Health Organization has called for reducing daily intake of added sugars to less than 10 percent of total energy intake, amounting to 12 teaspoons of added sugars for a diet of 2,000 calories a day.[81]

Dietary Fiber and Refined Carbohydrates

Dietary fiber, sources of which include whole grains, legumes, fruits, and vegetables, has many potential health benefits, including the prevention of obesity, diabetes, cardiovascular diseases, and various cancers.[75] However, whole grains are often processed to produce refined carbohydrates, which effectively removes the majority of fiber and other nutrients from the grain. Most of what remains is starch, which has a high glycemic index and load, and rapidly increases blood glucose. Overconsumption of refined carbohydrates increases the risk of obesity, type 2 diabetes, and heart disease.[82,83]

Examples of refined carbohydrates include white bread, white pasta, and white rice. Studies have shown that for each incremental serving of white rice per day, the type 2 diabetes risk increases by 11 percent.[84,85]

▶ Nutritional Needs Throughout the Life Course

Nutritional needs vary with one's place in the life course. Having outlined some of the most important nutritional needs that concern global health issues, therefore, it will now be valuable to examine how those needs change from pregnancy, through infancy, childhood, adolescence, adulthood, and old age. This will assist us in getting a better understanding of the nature of the nutrition problems globally, the burden of disease related to nutrition, and how this burden might be addressed.

Pregnancy and Birthweight

The nutritional status of a pregnant woman is especially important to the outcome that she will have in pregnancy, both for herself and for her newborn. It is critical that a pregnant woman stay well nourished and healthy. During pregnancy, the woman will need to get a sufficient amount of protein and energy from the food she eats, and it is generally recommended that she consume 300 calories more per day than when she is not pregnant. In addition, iron, iodine, folate, zinc, and calcium will be very important to the health of the woman and her newborn.[86]

The birthweight of a baby is an extremely important determinant of the extent to which a child will thrive and become a healthy adult. Fetuses that do not get sufficient and appropriate nutrition from the mother may suffer a number of problems, including stillbirth, mental impairment, or a variety of severe birth defects. They could also undergo a general failure to grow properly, referred to as **intrauterine growth restriction**. Babies who are born at term but who are low birthweight have a much greater risk of getting diarrhea and pneumonia than babies born above 2,500 grams. Those born with a birthweight from 1,500 to 1,999 grams are 8 times more likely to die from birth asphyxia and infections than those born with a birthweight of 2,000 to 2,499 grams.[61]

Infancy and Young Childhood

An important share of a child's biological development takes place between conception and 2 years of age. This period is often called the "window of opportunity." It is essential to understand that nutritional gaps that arise during this period may produce problems in stature or mental development that may never be overcome. They may also lead to more frequent infection and infections that last longer than would be the case in a better-nourished child. Thus, it is extraordinarily important that infants and young children get a sufficient amount of protein, energy, and fat from their foods. They also need sufficient amounts of iodine, iron, vitamin A, and zinc.

There is very strong evidence worldwide that infants will grow best and stay healthiest if they are exclusively breastfed for the first 6 months of their lives. In fact, it has been estimated that as much as 15 percent of all child deaths have been associated with suboptimal breastfeeding.[3] Indeed, non-exclusive breastfeeding was the 11th most important risk factor for young child death in 2016, and discontinued breastfeeding was the 15th leading risk factor.[5] Children will also thrive best if foods other than breastmilk or infant formula begin to be introduced in hygienic ways around 6 months of age, while breastfeeding continues.[87] Especially in low-income countries in which nutritional deficits are likely to be considerable, such foods will be especially valuable if they are fortified with key vitamins and minerals.

The nutrition needs of the infant continue into young childhood, but the nutritional status of many children faces risks as the child stops breastfeeding, as noted earlier. At this stage, the child's nutritional status depends on the ability of the family to provide an adequate diet and to help the child avoid illnesses and infections. Among the most critical issues concerning childhood nutrition is that stunted children have very little chance to catch up in their growth and that most of the damage done to their development, both physical and mental, cannot be changed.[88]

This fact has enormous implications for public policy aimed at enhancing nutritional status. It means that an important focus of attention in addressing undernutrition and its consequences must be on children from conception to 2 years of age, and it must start by trying to ensure that pregnant women are well nourished and healthy enough to give birth to healthy babies of acceptable birthweight. As previously noted, there is a window of opportunity for ensuring that children grow properly and reach their biological and cognitive potential. This window opens at conception and closes, at least most of the way, around the time the child is 2 years of age.[63]

Adolescence

Adolescent girls who are well nourished grow faster than adolescent girls who are not well nourished. Adolescent girls who are poorly nourished, but still growing, are much more likely than well-nourished girls to give birth to an underweight baby. This may stem from the fact that the fetus and the girl are competing for nutrients in the adolescent who is still growing.[89] Poorly nourished and very small adolescent girls also have more complications of pregnancy than do older girls who are taller. This relates partly to the difficulties of very small women giving birth, because of their size. In addition, all adolescents go through a growth spurt, although children who are stunted are unable to make up in adolescence for their diminished growth. For adolescents to grow properly and become healthy adults they need appropriate protein and energy. They also have particular needs for iodine, iron, and folic acid. Because of their growth during this period, calcium is also especially important for adolescents.[89]

Adulthood and Old Age

Adults need appropriate, well-balanced nutrition to stay healthy and productive. All people, including adults, also need to pay particular attention in their diets to foods that can be harmful to their health, such as foods that contain too much saturated fat, added sugar, or salt. Older adults have special nutritional needs that are very important but often forgotten. The ability of older people to live on their own and to function effectively depends in many ways on their nutritional status; however, many older people lack the income or the support needed to eat properly. Like other adults, they need to get enough protein, energy, and iron and avoid obesity. They also have to pay particular attention to getting enough calcium to reduce the risk of osteoporosis, which is a condition in which bones become fragile and can break.[90]

▶ The Nutritional State of the World

Undernutrition

There has been important progress in reducing the burden of undernutrition over the last 2 decades. The most recent estimates suggest, for example, that the share of children younger than 5 years of age in low- and middle-income countries who are underweight fell from about 25 percent in 1990 to less than 14 percent in 2016.[1] In addition, a number of countries, including Bangladesh, China, Indonesia, Mexico, and Vietnam, made especially rapid progress in reducing levels of undernutrition in their under-5 children over that period.[91] Important progress has been made in addressing micronutrient deficiencies

as well. The number of households using iodized salt, for example, has increased from about 20 percent in 1990 to about 86 percent today.[92] There has also been a dramatic increase in the share of the world's children who receive vitamin A supplements, which now stands above 60 percent in almost all low- and middle-income countries.[93]

Despite this progress, a large number of pregnant women and children in the world are undernourished. In 2016, about 155 million children were stunted and more than 50 million were wasted.[94] Many poor women in the world are also underweight. A large share of the poor women and children in the world also suffer from deficiencies in important micronutrients. Nutritional problems remain a fundamental cause of ill health and of premature death for infants, children, and pregnant women. The economic costs of undernutrition are great. The sections that follow examine the burden of nutrition disorders that relate to undernutrition and review undernutrition as a risk factor for ill health and death.

Low Birthweight

FIGURE 9-4 presents data on low birthweight, which refers to babies born under 2,500 grams. The data are shown for selected UNICEF regions. The data are somewhat dated but still indicative of what we are likely to see today. The most striking points of the figure are the following:

- Even in Latin America and the Caribbean, almost 10 percent of the babies are born with low birthweight.
- The share of low birthweight babies varies between 11 and 14 percent in the UNICEF Africa regions.
- Almost 30 percent of the babies in South Asia are born with low birthweight.

FIGURE 9-5 shows by World Bank region the share of under-5 children who are underweight.

The "good news" is that a relatively small share of children in most regions is underweight. The "bad news," however, is that an exceptionally large share of young children are underweight in sub-Saharan Africa and in South Asia. It is also striking that almost one in three under-5 children are underweight in South Asia, and that this rate is almost 50 percent higher than in sub-Saharan Africa, a region that is poorer than South Asia.

Wasting

In addition to the large number of children who are underweight, it is estimated that about 51 million children globally are moderately or severely wasted.[95]

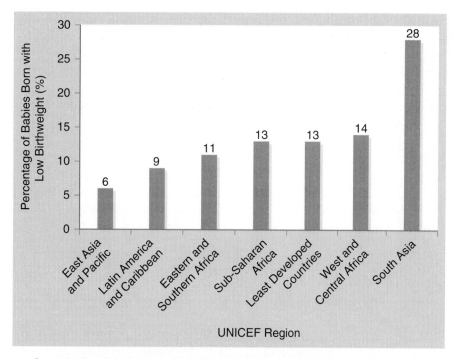

FIGURE 9-4 Prevalence of Low Birthweight, by UNICEF Region, 2008–2012

Data from World Health Organization (WHO). (2014). *Global nutrition targets 2025: Low birth weight policy brief.* Geneva, Switzerland: Author. Retrieved from http://apps.who.int/iris/bitstream/handle/10665/149020/WHO_NMH_NHD_14.5_eng.pdf?ua=1

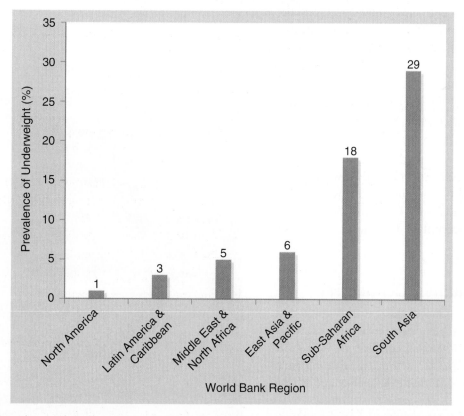

FIGURE 9-5 Prevalence of Underweight in Children Under 5 Years of Age, by World Bank Region, 2017

Data from The World Bank. (n.d.). Data: Prevalence of underweight, weight for age (% of children under 5). Retrieved from https://data.worldbank.org/indicator/SH.STA.MALN.ZS

FIGURE 9-6 shows the rates of wasting by World Bank region.

It is clear from the figure that about 1 in 12 under-5 children are wasted in sub-Saharan Africa and in the Middle East and North Africa region. However, even more exceptional is the fact that the rate of wasting is twice as high in South Asia than in either of these two regions. One in 6 children in South Asia are wasted.

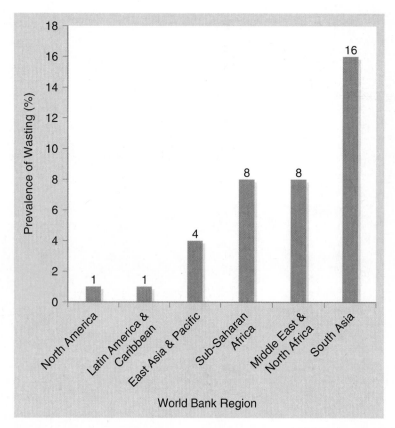

FIGURE 9-6 Prevalence of Wasting in Children Under 5 Years of Age, by World Bank Region, 2017

Data from The World Bank. (n.d.). Data: Prevalence of wasting, weight for height (% of children under 5). Retrieved from https://data.worldbank.org/indicator/SH.STA.WAST.ZS?view=chart

Stunting

Almost 151 million children were also estimated in 2017 to be stunted globally.[95] This was about 22 percent of all under-5 children.[95] As shown in **FIGURE 9-7**, about one-third of all children in sub-Saharan and South Asia are stunted. However, even in the low- and middle-income regions with higher income than sub-Saharan Africa and South Asia, 10 percent to 15 percent of the under-5 children are stunted.

Selected Micronutrient Deficiencies

Unfortunately, there is no consistent and up-to-date data on most micronutrient deficiencies across a wide range of countries, organized consistently by region. **TABLE 9-4** provides some of the best available information on the prevalence of iodine deficiency and of iron deficiency anemia.

TABLE 9-5 provides information on the prevalence of vitamin A deficiency in children under 5 years of age.

It is striking to note the higher prevalence of micronutrient deficiencies in South Asia and sub-Saharan Africa than in other regions. Although the data on vitamin A are not as up to date as we would

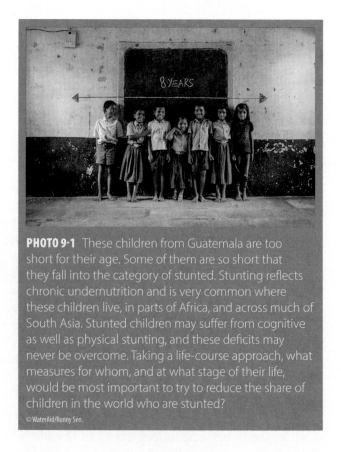

PHOTO 9-1 These children from Guatemala are too short for their age. Some of them are so short that they fall into the category of stunted. Stunting reflects chronic undernutrition and is very common where these children live, in parts of Africa, and across much of South Asia. Stunted children may suffer from cognitive as well as physical stunting, and these deficits may never be overcome. Taking a life-course approach, what measures for whom, and at what stage of their life, would be most important to try to reduce the share of children in the world who are stunted?

© WaterAid/Ronny Sen.

want, they suggest that, despite enormous progress in reducing vitamin A deficiency in low- and middle-income countries, vitamin A deficiency is still a major problem. The high prevalence of iodine deficiency is disappointing because there is such a well-known and low-cost solution to this matter—the iodization of salt. It is also a great concern that iron deficiency anemia remains so prevalent, both among young children and among pregnant women.

Deaths Associated with Undernutrition

Only a small share of the deaths of under-5 children globally is a direct result of undernutrition.[5] However, undernutrition, as discussed earlier, is an exceptionally important risk factor for illness, disability, and death from other causes, including diarrhea, pneumonia, measles, and other communicable diseases.[3] In addition, anemia is a risk factor for more than 25 percent of maternal deaths, and calcium deficiencies contribute to maternal death from preeclampsia.[3]

As noted earlier, about 45 percent of the under-5 child deaths a year can be attributed to nutrition-related causes. This is estimated to be the total number of deaths related to the joint effects of fetal growth restriction, suboptimal breastfeeding, stunting, underweight, wasting, and vitamin A and zinc deficiencies. It was estimated that the nutrition-related deaths could be broken down into approximate percentages as follows[3]:

- 23 percent would be attributable to the joint effects of just fetal growth restriction and suboptimal breastfeeding.
- 34 percent would be attributable to stunting and underweight.
- 12 percent of these deaths would be attributable to wasting.

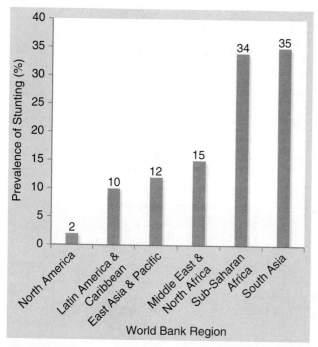

FIGURE 9-7 Prevalence of Stunting in Children Under 5 Years of Age, by World Bank Region, 2017

Data from The World Bank. (n.d.). Data: Prevalence of stunting, height for age (% of children under 5). Retrieved from https://data.worldbank.org/indicator/SH.STA.STNT.ZS?view=chart

	Prevalence of Iodine Deficiency (%)	**Prevalence of Iron Deficiency Anemia (%)**	
Region	**Overall**	**Children < 5**	**Pregnant Women**
Africa	40.0	20.2	20.3
Americas & Caribbean	13.7	12.7	15.2
Asia	31.6	19.0	19.8
Europe	44.2	12.1	16.2
Oceania	17.3	15.4	17.2

TABLE 9-4 Prevalence of Iodine Deficiency and Iron Deficiency Anemia, by UN Region

Note: Iodine deficiency is defined as urine iodine concentration < 100 µg/L (2013); Iron deficiency anemia defined as hemoglobin < 110 g/L (2011)

Data from Black, R. E., Victora, C. G., Walker, S. P., Bhutta, Z. A., Christian, P., de Onis, M., . . . Uauy, R. (2013). Maternal and child undernutrition and overweight in low-income and middle-income countries. *The Lancet, 382*(9890), 427–451.

TABLE 9-5 Prevalence of Vitamin A Deficiency, Children Under 5, Selected Regions, 2013

Region	Prevalence of Vitamin A Deficiency, Children < 5 (%)
Central Asia, Middle East, and North Africa	11%
East and Southeast Asia and Oceania	6%
Latin America and the Caribbean	11%
South Asia	44%
Sub-Saharan Africa	48%
All low-income and middle-income countries	29%

Data from Stevens, G. A., Bennett, J. E., Hennocq, Q., Lu, Y., De-Regil, L. M., Rogers, L., . . . Ezzati, M. (2015). Trends and mortality effects of vitamin A deficiency in children in 138 low-income and middle-income countries between 1991 and 2013: A pooled analysis of population-based surveys. *Lancet Global Health, 3*(9), e528–e536. doi: https://doi.org/10.1016/S2214-109X(15)00039-X

- More than 2.3 percent would be attributable to vitamin A deficiency.
- 1.7 percent would be attributable to zinc deficiency.

Fetal growth restriction is related to low birthweight, as discussed earlier, for babies carried to term. Clearly, any efforts to reduce child deaths will have to focus on addressing these issues, which are fundamental to whether children survive and thrive.[3]

Overweight and Obesity

Once considered a problem unique to high-income Western countries, obesity is now a major contributor to the global burden of disease, affecting people of all ages and incomes around the world.[30,96] Today, 2.3 billion people, nearly 31 percent of the world's population, have obesity or are overweight.[7] In fact, obesity has nearly tripled worldwide since 1975.[7] According to the World Health Organization, overweight and obesity are also responsible for 44 percent of the burden of diabetes, 23 percent of the burden of ischemic heart disease, and 7 percent to 41 percent of the burden of certain cancers.[97] Low- and middle-income countries, including sub-Saharan Africa, India, parts of southeast Asia, China, and most of South America, now collectively carry the majority of the global obesity and chronic disease burden, and are predicted to continue to do so for some time.[98] **FIGURE 9-8** shows the prevalence of obesity in adults in 1975 and 2016.

Among the world's adult population, 39 percent is overweight or has obesity, representing an 81 percent increase since 1975.[7] Broken down by sex, the worldwide proportion of adults who are overweight or have

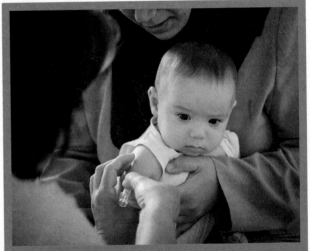

PHOTO 9-2 The young child in this photo is being vaccinated against a number of childhood diseases. There is a "vicious cycle" between infection and undernutrition, and preventing infections is central to ensuring well-nourished children. What measures need to be taken by agencies outside the health sector to try to ensure that young children remain healthy and well-nourished?
© Jasmin Merdan/Moment/Getty Images.

obesity has increased from 20.7 percent to 38.5 percent in men and from 22.7 percent to 39.2 percent in women.[99] As seen in **FIGURE 9-9**, women have higher rates of obesity than men in all of the WHO regions. Of note, an obesity prevalence of over 50 percent (age-standardized) is seen for both men and women in Palau, Nauru, and the Cook Islands, and for women in Kiribati, the Federated States of Micronesia, the Marshall Islands, Niue, Samoa, Tonga, and Tuvalu.[100] All of these countries are in the WHO Western Pacific region. Of all countries in the WHO African region,

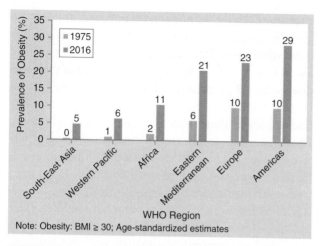

FIGURE 9-8 Prevalence of Obesity in Adults, 1975 and 2016, by WHO Region

Data from World Health Organization (WHO). (2017). Prevalence of obesity among adults, BMI ≥ 30, age-standardized. Retrieved from http://apps.who.int/gho/data/view.main.REGION2480A?lang=en

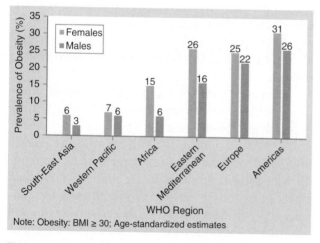

FIGURE 9-9 Prevalence of Obesity in Adults, by Sex and WHO Region, 2016

Data from World Health Organization (WHO). (2017). Prevalence of obesity among adults, BMI ≥ 30, age-standardized. Retrieved from http://apps.who.int/gho/data/view.main.REGION2480A?lang=en

women in South Africa have the highest obesity rate, at 40 percent.[101]

Childhood obesity has emerged as one of the most serious public health challenges of the 21st century, in part because it tends to continue into adulthood, increasing the risk of chronic diseases later in life.[101,50] Globally, 340 million children and adolescents ages 5 to 19 and 41 million children under the age of 5 are overweight or have obesity.[7] Nearly half of these overweight children and children who have obesity under 5 live in Asia.[7] From 1975 to 2016, the prevalence of childhood and adolescent overweight and obesity increased across countries of all income levels: Prevalence in high-income countries increased from 14.4 percent to 35.1 percent for boys and from 14.3 percent to 30.5 percent for girls. For low-income countries, prevalence increased from 0.7

percent to 7.2 percent for boys and from 1.5 percent to 14.1 percent for girls.[102] The increase in childhood obesity has occurred more rapidly than adult rates in several countries, including the United States, Brazil, and China.[15] Particularly high rates of child and adolescent obesity are seen in American, European, and Western Pacific countries, especially among girls.[102] **FIGURE 9-10** provides data on child and adolescent overweight, including obesity.

In terms of individual countries, the United States has the highest proportion of the world's people who have obesity (13 percent), whereas China and India together represent 15 percent of the world's population with obesity. Countries in the Middle East and North Africa, Central America, and island nations in the Pacific and Caribbean have extremely high rates of overweight and obesity, at 44 percent or higher. In terms of world regions, the highest rates of overweight and obesity overall in 2013 were seen in the Middle East and North Africa, where more than 58 percent of men and 65 percent of women were overweight or had obesity. In Central America, more than 57 percent of adult men and more than 65 percent of adult women were overweight or had obesity, with the highest prevalence (greater than 50 percent among both men and women) found in Colombia, Costa Rica, and Mexico. In the Pacific Islands, nearly 44 percent of men and more than 51 percent of women were overweight or had obesity, and in the Caribbean, 38 percent of men and more than 50 percent of women were overweight or had obesity.[103]

Although the overall prevalence of overweight and obesity has increased worldwide over the last 30 to 40 years, there have been large variations in rates. In high-income countries, increases in obesity began in the 1980s, accelerated from 1992 to 2002, and have

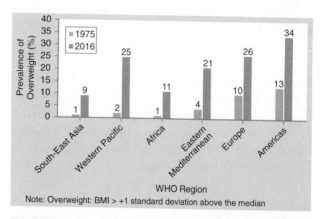

FIGURE 9-10 Prevalence of Overweight, Including Obesity, in Children and Adolescents 5 to 19 Years of Age, by WHO Region, 1975 and 2016

Data from World Health Organization (WHO). (2016). Prevalence of overweight among children and adolescents, BMI > +1 standard deviation above the median, crude. Retrieved from http://apps.who.int/gho/data/view.main.BMIPLUS1CREGv?lang=en

slowed since 2006. Middle Eastern countries such as Saudi Arabia, Bahrain, Egypt, Kuwait, and Palestine are experiencing some of the largest increases in obesity.[103] Over the next 2 decades, the largest proportional increase in overweight and obesity will likely occur in low- and middle-income countries, with predicted increases of 62 percent to 205 percent for overweight and 71 to 263 percent for obesity.[98]

Obesity and overweight are among the leading risks for global deaths. In 2015, high BMI contributed to 4.0 million deaths and 4.9 percent of disability-adjusted life years (DALYs) among adults worldwide.[104] Obesity and overweight are now responsible for more deaths globally than underweight. They are also responsible for more deaths than underweight in all high-income and most middle-income countries.[97]

▶ Nutrition, Health, and Economic Development

Nutrition has an important bearing on the economic development prospects of people, communities, and countries. In some of the early thinking about economic development, many economists saw nutrition as something that people consumed, but they did not see it as a productive investment. However, as you saw earlier and will see again, nutrition is an extremely important contributor to human health and the development of human intellectual and biological potential. It, therefore, has an extremely important link with what people learn, their strength and ability to use their own labor, and other factors relating to their potential productivity. The following comments follow the life course.

First, nutritional deficits can take an enormous toll on maternal health, with important economic consequences. Women are responsible for child care in most low- and middle-income countries. In addition, they often contribute to household income. The death of a woman in the prime of her life, in childbirth, due to undernutrition or deficiencies in iron or vitamin A, can leave poor families with reduced income and needs for child care they cannot meet. In poor families in low-income countries it is common, in fact, for very young children to die not long after their mothers die.

The nutritional status of a woman can also have a major impact on the birthweight of a child and the child's future nutritional status and can lead to neural tube defects.[105] A number of forms of malnutrition contribute to the failure of infants and children to grow or to achieve their full mental potential. Children who are undernourished and small in stature enroll in schools at lower rates or later in age than students who are perceived by their parents to be normal in size. Children who are undernourished have IQs that are lower than students who are properly nourished. These undernourished students are less attentive in class and less able to learn than other students. Children who are undernourished fall ill more than well-nourished children. Thus, they miss more school, learn less from school, and are much more likely than well-nourished children to drop out of school, with the attendant economic consequences.

Nutritional status also plays an important part in the productivity of adults. Numerous studies have shown that improvements in nutritional status, such as eliminating iron deficiency anemia, can improve worker productivity by 5 percent to 15 percent.[106] The contribution of nutrition to maintaining good health also has important economic returns. It helps people avoid disease and the costs associated with treating disease.

Moreover, through its impact on health, nutritional status also has an important bearing on life expectancy. Infants and children who are better nourished live longer than those who are poorly nourished, and they also can contribute to the economy for longer. Adults who are properly nourished get sick less and for shorter periods of time, live longer, and work more years than adults who are not well nourished. Thus, they too can make more contributions to the economy than people who are not well nourished.

A look at social and economic history also speaks to the importance of nutrition to economic development. Studies on the economic development of England showed that improvements in the nutritional status of adults in England in the late 19th century were important to improving the stature and strength of workers, their health, and their economic outputs.[107] Other studies have shown that there is a correlation between height and wages. Rubber tappers in Indonesia significantly improved the amount of rubber they could tap when their anemia was treated with iron supplements, and road construction workers in Kenya were 4 percent to 12.5 percent more productive after getting calorie supplements.[108] Female mill workers in China increased their production efficiency by 17 percent after being given iron supplements for 12 weeks.[109] A major review of nutrition by the World Bank noted that reducing micronutrient deficiencies in China and India could increase their gross domestic product (GDP) by $2.5 billion per year.[63] Other studies have shown that losses from deficiencies in individual micronutrients can cost 1 percent to 2 percent of GDP, and that losses from stunting can be as high as 8 percent to 10 percent of GDP.[105]

Obesity and overweight also take an immense toll on society. First, obesity and overweight are extremely detrimental to health, with economic consequences for individuals and society at large. Obesity and overweight are major risk factors for morbidity and mortality from many noncommunicable diseases, including cardiovascular disease, type 2 diabetes, hypertension, musculoskeletal disorders, and some forms of cancer, including endometrial, breast, and colorectal cancer.[110-112] Obesity and its associated comorbidities have high medical costs that can trap poor households in cycles of debt and illness, exacerbating poverty and perpetuating health and economic inequalities, especially in low- and middle-income countries.[113]

These costs can also be crippling on a national scale. In the United States, 5 percent to 10 percent of all medical spending is used for obesity-related health care, costing an estimated $147 billion to $210 billion annually, and over 25 percent of these costs are paid through public expenditures.[115-117] Expenditures in India and China are rapidly increasing.[118] From 2012 to 2030, diabetes and cardiovascular disease are projected to cost India $2.4 trillion and China $8.74 trillion.[119] It is possible that these costs will overwhelm the health system of China and slow China's economic growth.[120]

Overweight and obesity also affect worker productivity, further burdening society with a loss in economic production. Employees who have obesity are more likely to have higher levels of absenteeism than their lean counterparts due to weight-related health problems.[121] Higher staff turnover and lost earnings due to premature death from obesity-related diseases also result in a loss of worker productivity.[122] The cumulative cost of decreased productivity and increased health care due to noncommunicable diseases (NCDs), for which overweight and obesity are leading risk factors, was estimated to be about $1.4 trillion globally in 2010.[123] It is estimated that between 2011 and 2025, $7.3 trillion in economic production will have been lost in low- and middle-income countries alone due to NCDs.[124] Over the next 2 decades, cardiovascular disease, chronic respiratory disease, cancer, diabetes, and mental health will be responsible for a cumulative output loss of $47 trillion. This loss represents 75 percent of global GDP in 2010.[125]

Finally, obesity can have significant effects on mental health, which can be especially harmful to children and their academic achievement.[126] In many societies around the world, people who are overweight and have obesity experience discrimination in employment, education, and health care due to weight bias.[127] Due to this stigma, obesity and overweight have been shown to cause low self-esteem, anxiety, depression, poor body image, and suicidal thoughts and actions. Bias and bullying in schools, along with their emotional consequences, can seriously hinder academic achievement for children and adolescents who are overweight and have obesity. Adolescents who have obesity are less likely to attend college or attain a degree, thus preventing them from earning as much money later in life and setting them up for a cycle of illness and debt as they age.[128]

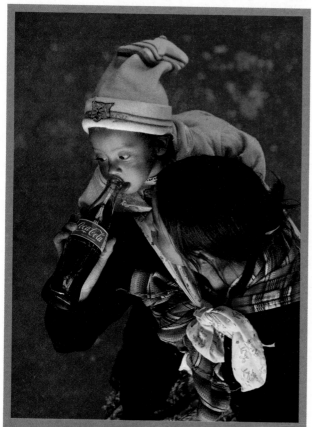

PHOTO 9-3 This Guatemalan mother is helping her child drink Coca-Cola. Global trade liberalization and urbanization have led to a nutrition transition away from traditional diets, increasing access to sugary, nutritionally poor foods and beverages, which in turn promote obesity. The prevalence of childhood overweight and obesity in Guatemala has more than doubled over a 20-year period, from 15 percent in 1996 to 31 percent in 2016.[114] What measures can be taken at the national, local, and individual levels to reduce sugar-sweetened beverage consumption in childhood?
© Marka/Universal Images Group/Getty Images.

▶ Case Studies

Nutrition is a complex issue of immense importance, and addressing nutrition concerns requires action by a range of actors. Thus, five case studies follow that are meant to illustrate many of the themes that have been covered in this chapter. The first discusses South Korea's efforts to encourage the maintenance of traditional diets. The second reviews a program in Brazil for encouraging physical activity. The third examines efforts by Finland to reduce salt consumption. The last two cases examine efforts at addressing critical nutrition issues in the two most populous countries of the world, India and China.

South Korea's Promotion of and Adherence to a Traditional Diet

South Korea's economy grew rapidly after its recovery from the Korean War (1950–1953).[129] This growth was accompanied by changes in lifestyle, including the rapid introduction of a more Western diet; fast-food restaurants in particular were popular among the younger generation, especially after the country hosted the Olympics in 1988.[130] A transition in the primary cause of death from communicable to non-communicable diseases is estimated to have occurred in South Korea around 1970, compared with 1940 for the United States and 1950 for Japan.[131]

Unlike other Asian countries, however, South Korea maintained many of the aspects of its low-fat, high-vegetable traditional diet through its economic and nutrition transition. Based on its level of economic development, a 1998 dietary evaluation found that South Korea had lower than expected levels of fat intake (by 16.7 percentage points) and obesity prevalence, found to be largely due to programs led by the government and private organizations to encourage the retention of the traditional South Korean diet.[129]

Local governments held public educational events and promoted the traditional diet through diverse channels, while the Korea Dietetic Association (KDA), a private organization, provided nutrition education through seminars and obesity camps, aided nutrition services at local health centers, and offered nutrition information for citizens on its website.[129] The KDA also monitored food and nutrition advertising disseminated through mass media and organized national nutrition campaigns.[129] Furthermore, the association held lectures for parents and provided a variety of traditional menus to elementary schools, along with sending letters to students' homes about preserving traditional dietary culture.[132]

A 1998 evaluation of the combination of these efforts revealed that they led to a retention of the traditional Korean diet and subsequent positive health outcomes. Vegetable consumption in South Korea was among the highest in Asia in 1998, composing around 20 percent of total food consumption (280 grams daily per capita).[129] Kimchi remained the most consumed food after rice, accounting for approximately 40 percent of the total vegetable intake.[133] In addition, the daily per capita intake of fruits in South Korea increased significantly during the economic transition period; the increase was especially rapid in the 1990s. In 1998, 197.5 grams of fruits were consumed daily per capita, more than a tenfold increase from the 18.9 grams consumed in 1970.[129]

Daily per capita fat intake in South Korea more than doubled from 16.9 grams in 1969 to 41.5 grams in 1998, and animal fat increased from 30.6 percent of total fat consumed in 1970 to 48.2 percent in 1998.[129] However, the proportion of fat-derived energy was still significantly lower than in other Asian countries, in part due to a traditional cooking style involving small amounts of oil.[130] Furthermore, the majority of meat consumed was cooked in a Korean style, as opposed to a Western style, and was typically accompanied by vegetables.[129]

Obesity rates in South Korea in 1998 remained quite low, at 1.7 percent for men and 3.0 percent for women. These rates were much lower than Western and other Asian countries.[129] Obesity rates in Korea today remain among the lowest in the Organization for Economic Cooperation and Development (OECD), at 5.3 percent of the adult population. However, one in three adults in Korea are overweight,[134] and OECD projections indicate that the obesity rate will increase to 9 percent by 2030.[135]

Through this initiative, South Korea has demonstrated the potential for effective public–private collaboration in the pursuit of a healthy diet. Using a combination of information dissemination and provision of skills, the country was able to adapt its message to contemporary society and successfully retain its traditional diet, slowing the spread of obesity.

Brazil: The Agita São Paulo Program Uses Physical Activity to Promote Health

Starting in the 1970s, Brazil began experiencing rapid economic growth and major socioeconomic shifts, resulting in lifestyle changes promoting obesity and overweight. By 1990, 69.3 percent of the adult Brazilian population led a sedentary lifestyle.[136]

After 2 years of preparatory consultation with the Pan-American Health Organization and other international agencies, the Agita São Paulo Program was launched in 1996 to address São Paulo's growing problem of obesity and overweight. The objective was to increase the level of knowledge among the São Paulo population about the importance of physical activity by 50 percent and the level of actual physical activity by 20 percent over a period of 10 years.[137] School children, the workforce, and the elderly were the main targets. The program concentrated on feasible, low- or no-cost ways to achieve at least 30 minutes of moderate-intensity physical activity per day, most days of the week. The goal was to convince the population that this physical activity could come from routine, daily activities such as walking to and from work or household chores, as opposed to less convenient exercises more likely to cause injury, such as structured fitness programs in gyms or organized sports.[137]

The program was structured as a partnership among government, industry, nongovernment organizations, and academic communities. Coordinated by the Studies Center of the Physical Fitness Research Laboratory of São Caetano do Sul (CELAFISCS), it was largely funded by the São Paulo State Secretariat of Health.[137] It was an extremely cost-effective program: its annual budget ranged from $150,000 to $400,000, representing an investment of less than $0.01 per state inhabitant per year. In contrast, the estimated costs of illness related to a sedentary lifestyle in the state were about $1.00 per person per year.[138]

Agita São Paulo was overseen by a scientific and executive board. The scientific board consisted of Brazilian and international academics and doctors and provided the program's scientific foundation, assessed its implementation, and allowed it to better integrate with the medical community.[137] The executive board included more than 300 governmental, nongovernmental, and private organizations representing a wide range of sectors. These organizations were directly responsible for planning, organizing, and carrying out the program's activities.[139]

The program used three main types of activities to reach its target groups of students, workers, and the elderly: mega-events, actions carried out with partner institutions, and partnerships.[137] Mega-events were intended to reach the majority of cities in São Paolo state and involved at least a million people. Often coinciding with major cultural or seasonal holidays, they raised awareness of the importance of an active lifestyle through their activities and broad media coverage. Different mega-events were tailored to promoting specific activities for students, workers, and the elderly, but the most popular was "Agita Galera" ("Move, Crowd" or "Active Community Day"). It was celebrated across the 6,800 public schools in the state, reaching 6 million students and 250,000 teachers. Schools received a handbook and poster, as well as flyers for students and their families communicating the program's message. Students were also encouraged to prepare their own materials on the subject of physical activity and spread the message of the program in their communities. Partner institutions were also crucial to the program's success. The diversity in focus and type of partners encouraged innovation and a greater exchange of ideas for new activities. Each partner used a variety of pamphlets, manuals, advertising tools, and scientific information to promote physical activity among their employees and the communities they served. Finally, the program partnered with more than 50 municipalities to establish 50 municipal communities throughout the state that each planned, implemented, and monitored physical activities in their area.[137]

Various evaluations of the program were conducted and found positive effects for both increasing physical activity awareness and physical activity itself. Over a 3-year period, recall of the main program objective rose from 9.5 percent to 24 percent across the states. Recall increased with socioeconomic status level, reaching 67 percent of the most educated.[137] Furthermore, people who were aware of the program were more likely to be physically active; 54.2 percent of those familiar with the program were physically active in 2002, versus a rate of 31.9 percent for those who were not familiar with the program.[140] An analysis supported by the World Bank, the Centers for Disease Control and Prevention, and CELAFISCS concluded that the program was a good public health investment, achieving a cost-effectiveness ratio of less than R$50,000 ($12,850)/QALY (quality-adjusted life year).[138]

Agita São Paulo has been a role model for similar local and national programs across Brazil and in other Latin American countries.[138] The World Health Organization has praised it as a model for other low- and middle-income countries, and it has since spurred an international mega-event celebrated annually to promote worldwide physical activity.[137]

Finland Uses Labels to Reduce Salt Consumption

Finland has traditionally had a diet high in salt, as it was used for preservation of food before other methods were available.[141] In the 1970s, Finnish salt intake was estimated to be approximately 12 grams per day (4,800 mg/day sodium), more than twice the amount recommended by the World Health Organization, putting the population at risk for hypertension, stroke, and coronary heart disease.[142] In 1978, this high intake spurred Finland's National Nutrition Council to recommend steps to reduce salt consumption nationally.[143,144] From 1979 to 1982, a community-based intervention to reduce population-wide sodium intake called the North Karelia project was conducted to reduce mortality associated with cardiovascular disease. The project was expanded to cover the entire country after 3 years.

Multiple stakeholders were involved with the project, including health service organizations, schools, nongovernmental organizations, media outlets, and the food industry.[141] Finnish media aided the effort by releasing numerous reports on the harmful health effects of salt, which raised both public and government awareness of salt and lower-sodium alternatives.[145] Health education of consumers and training programs for healthcare professionals, teachers, and caterers on how to reduce salt were also important components of the project.[141]

Building on the momentum from this movement, a number of labeling systems were implemented to inform consumers and discourage them from consuming high amounts of sodium. In 1993, the Ministry of Trade and Industry and the Ministry of Social Affairs and Health implemented salt-labeling legislation for food categories that contribute high amounts of sodium to the diet, such as breads, sausages and other meat products, fish products, butter, soups and sauces, ready-made meals, and spice mixtures containing salt, requiring that such foods be labeled with percentage of salt by weight.[146] The legislation required a "high salt content" label on foods with high levels of sodium, while allowing low-sodium foods to carry a "low salt" label.[143,145] In 2000, the Finnish Heart Association began putting a "Better Choice" label on low-sodium products, and the Pansalt logo was used on products with sodium-reduced, potassium- and magnesium-enriched mineral salts.[143,145] It is estimated that these labeling initiatives caused the industry to reduce the salt content of targeted foods by about 20 percent to 25 percent.[147]

Salt intake was monitored using urinary sodium excretion every 5 years. By 2002, mean sodium intake was 3,900 mg/day for men and 2,700 mg/day for women. Diastolic blood pressure also decreased substantially, by more than 10 mm Hg.[141] This was caused by a combination of consumers choosing lower-sodium products and food companies discontinuing or reformulating their products to avoid high-salt labels through the use of alternatives such as mineral salts.[143,147] There was an 80 percent reduction in death rates from stroke and heart disease among the middle-aged population, contributing to a reduction in overall mortality in Finland and an increase in life expectancy by several years for both men and women.[147]

Tamil Nadu State, India Nutrition Project[148]

Background

The Tamil Nadu Integrated Nutrition Project in India is one of the most important efforts ever undertaken to improve nutritional status on a large scale. This project began in 1980 in the South Indian state of Tamil Nadu. It aimed at improving the nutritional status of poor women and children in the rural areas of the state through a set of well-focused interventions.

These specific goals were set for several reasons. First, the levels of malnutrition among poor women and children in Tamil Nadu were very high at the time the project was conceived. Second, malnutrition persisted despite considerable investments that had already been undertaken to improve nutrition status. Third, studies that had been done on those investments showed that they were not working as planned and were not cost-effective. Rather, the children who needed assistance most were not getting it. In addition, food that was given to children at feeding centers that was meant to be supplementary to their regular diet often replaced their regular food or was taken home and consumed by family members other than the intended children. The form of the food supplement was also difficult for children to eat. Moreover, little attention had been paid to nutrition education for families or to health investments that could complement the investments made in nutrition.

The project design was based on the idea that much of the malnutrition present in Tamil Nadu was because of inappropriate childcare practices, rather than just a lack of money to buy food. Thus, the project focused considerable attention on nutrition education and efforts to improve care and feeding practices for young children. In addition, because deficits at an early age often produce irreversible damage to children's physical and mental development, project interventions focused on pregnant and lactating women and on children younger than 3 years of age.

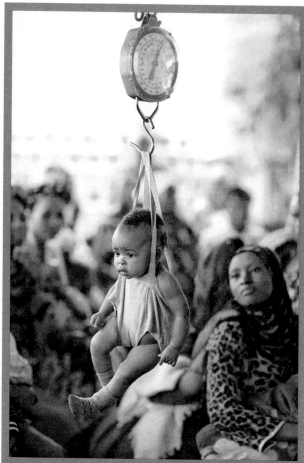

PHOTO 9-4 This is a photo of a young Nigerian being weighed at a community weighing clinic. Monitoring the height and weight of a child is crucial to determine if the child is developing properly. However, growth and weight monitoring must be coupled with early actions to address any deficits that arise in the child's development. What have been the keys to successful efforts to reduce the share of young children who are underweight for their age?
Courtesy of Mark Tuschman.

The Intervention

In line with this approach, the project included a package of services that were delivered by health and nutrition workers that consisted of nutrition education, primary health care, supplementary on-site feeding for children who were not growing properly, vitamin A supplementation, periodic deworming, education of mothers for managing childhood diarrhea, and the supplementary feeding of a small number of women.

An important innovation of the project was that it used growth monitoring of the children as a device for mobilizing community action. Groups of mothers met regularly to weigh their young children. They then plotted their weight-for-age on a growth chart. Together with the community nutrition worker, they

identified which children were not growing properly. A related innovation of great importance was that supplementary feeding was targeted only to the children identified as faltering. In addition, children received food supplements only while they were not growing well. This was done in conjunction with nutrition education for mothers. The intent of this approach was to show that short-term feeding, combined with better childcare practices, could return the child to normal growth. This was a major change compared with previous practice in which supplementary feeding was more universal and longer term.

Impact

The nutrition interventions of the project were largely implemented as planned, but the health efforts were not fully implemented. Nonetheless, through careful evaluation the project was shown to have significantly reduced the levels of malnutrition of the targeted children. These improvements also continued over a substantial time, suggesting that the gains of the project were sustainable. The project was also more cost-effective than other investments that had tried to achieve similar aims in India.

Lessons Learned

This project was pioneering and revealed some very important lessons:

- Growth monitoring, coupled with short-term supplementary feeding of children who are faltering, can be a cost-effective way of improving nutritional status.
- More universal and longer-term feeding of children is not necessary to achieve improvements in nutrition.
- Women can be organized to participate actively in growth monitoring efforts.
- Nutrition education can have a permanent and sustainable impact on child care and child feeding practices, even in the absence of other interventions.

The Challenge of Iodine Deficiency Disease in China[149]
Background

For many years China had the heaviest burden of iodine deficiency in the world. In 1995, 20 percent of children ages 8 to 10 showed signs of goiter. Overall, some 400 million people in China were estimated to be at risk of iodine deficiency disorders, constituting 40 percent of the global total. Fortunately, iodine deficiency can be simply remedied by adding iodine to salt, a cheap and universally consumed food. Implementing this in a relatively poor and vast country like China at that time, however, was far from simple.

The Intervention

Scientific evidence linking iodine deficiency to mental impairment was seen by the Chinese government as a threat to its one-child-per-family policy, since families were concerned about the potential health of the only child they were allowed to have. Thus, the government strengthened its resolve to tackle this widespread health risk. In 1993, China launched the National Iodine Deficiency Disorders Elimination Program, with technical and financial assistance from the donor-funded Iodine Deficiency Disorders Control Project. The public needed to be made aware of the risk of iodine deficiency, especially in regions where goiter was so common that it was regarded as normal. A nationwide public education campaign was launched, using posters on buses, newspaper editorials, and television documentaries to inform consumers and persuade them to switch to iodized salt. Provincial governors ensured that government education efforts reached even the most remote villages. The supply of iodized salt was increased by building 112 new salt iodination factories and enhancing capacity at 55 existing ones. Bulk packaging systems were installed to complement 147 new retail packaging centers, with packaging designed to help consumers easily recognize iodized salt. The sale of noniodized salt was banned, and technological assistance was provided to salt producers to adopt iodination. Salt quality was monitored, both at production, where the amount of iodine added needs to be just right, and in distribution and sales, because iodine in salt dissipates easily, reducing the shelf life of iodized salt. China's nationally controlled network of production and distribution made licensing and enforcement of legislation easier.

The Impact

By 1999, iodized salt was reaching 94 percent of the country, compared to 80 percent in 1995. The quality of iodized salt also improved markedly. As a result, iodine deficiency was reduced dramatically, and goiter rates for children ages 8 to 10 fell from 20.4 percent in 1995 to 8.8 percent in 1999.

Costs and Benefits

At the time of these efforts, fortifying salt with iodine cost about 2 to 7 cents per kilogram, or less than 5 percent of the retail price of salt in most countries. The Chinese government invested approximately $152 million in the program, recovering some of this cost by raising the price of iodized salt. The World Bank, one of several donors, deemed the project extremely cost-effective.

Lessons Learned

China's success in reducing iodine deficiency offers valuable lessons for future efforts to reduce other micronutrient deficiencies such as iron and vitamin A through fortification. The government made a firm and long-standing commitment to tackle the problem and brought about administrative, legal, technical, and sociocultural changes that were needed to do so. Donor coordination was strong and effective and was managed by the Chinese government and the donors themselves, and the major players offered mutual support across all activities. The financing strategy was clearly defined from the start. The salt industry seized the opportunity of the investment in eliminating iodine deficiency to restructure and modernize the industry, gaining a firmer commercial footing and positioning itself to compete in the international market, given its cost advantages.

China's iodination program continues, with special targeting of resources on areas where the consumption of iodized salt is particularly low, usually in poor and remote mountainous regions where residents see iodized salt as too costly, especially when salt can be obtained cheaply from local salt hills, dried lakes, or the sea. Research will be needed to determine the best way to ensure iodine intake in these areas—through price subsidies, iodination of well or irrigation water, or even iodine capsules or injections, in the case of nomadic peoples. A more detailed review of this case is available in *Case Studies in Global Health: Millions Saved*.

▶ Addressing Future Nutrition Challenges

As noted earlier, the world has made progress in the last several decades in addressing key nutrition problems. Nonetheless, the world's nutritional status still faces critical issues in undernutrition, overweight and obesity, and the dietary risks to good health. Problems of undernutrition are especially severe in South Asia and sub-Saharan Africa, and progress against them in many countries has been slow. Problems of overweight and obesity are growing in many low- and middle-income countries, as well as in high-income countries. What steps will have to be taken to speed the world's progress on nutrition?

If the world is to do better in nutrition, it will have to take a number of steps in a variety of domains. First, policymakers who work both globally and in individual countries need to understand the exceptional importance of nutrition to good health and human productivity and act accordingly. About 45 percent of under-5 child deaths globally are associated with nutritional causes. In addition, low-cost, highly effective solutions are available to deal with a number of critical nutrition issues, but they are not being implemented sufficiently. Thus, much greater attention needs to be paid by all concerned parties to nutrition as an underlying issue of human health, well-being, and productivity.

Nutrition does not fit neatly into governmental bureaucracies because it touches many government units, such as agriculture, health, and education. As you know, nutrition status of a population is affected by income, people's knowledge of good nutritional practices, and people's ability to carry out those practices. However, it is also affected, among other things, by agricultural markets, climate, and civil conflict. Thus, governments will also need to ensure that there are government units accountable and responsible for promoting enhanced approaches to nutrition and that a coordinated and intersectoral approach is taken to meet nutrition goals.

Improving government policy and action on nutrition will also require a good understanding of the nature of the nutrition problem in different settings. Nutritional concerns vary considerably by income group, gender, and ethnicity, and solutions to these problems will need to be carefully tailored to local circumstances. Moreover, almost all low- and middle-income countries will have to deal simultaneously with undernutrition and overweight and obesity.

In addition, governments need to work more effectively with the food industry to improve the way in which foods are fortified and to be sure that processed foods are healthy. Legal and financial arrangements need to be made in many countries so that more fortification can take place and the demand for fortified foods will be increased. Similar arrangements will need to be made to limit added sugar, salt, and saturated and trans fats in processed foods. We have also seen the power in Tamil Nadu, for example, of focusing efforts on community-based action, in which affected people are involved in the design, implementation, and oversight of nutrition activities.

Although there is much knowledge of what works in nutrition, there are also other areas in which additional knowledge could fill important gaps. The world needs to continue gathering scientific knowledge about how key nutrition issues can be addressed. It would be very valuable to the world's nutrition status and health if more easy-to-make, nutritious, and inexpensive food supplements were available; if better formulas were available for some of the vitamin and mineral supplements that could be given less frequently, very cheaply, and without side effects; and if additional cost-effective ways were developed for fortifying foods. It will also be essential that today's low- and middle-income countries get a better sense of what works and at what cost to reduce the nutritional risks to good health.

Lastly, it is important for all societies to make the health and nutritional well-being of their citizens a national priority. One way to do this would be to create partnerships of civil society, government, and the private sector that can work together to identify nutrition issues, plan on how they can best be addressed, and then collaborate with each other and with communities to implement solutions to these problems.

As we consider the measures that can be taken to address key nutritional issues, as rapidly as possible and in cost-effective ways, it is essential to consider interventions in three domains:

■ Nutrition-specific interventions—those interventions that can have a direct impact on nutrition, such as promotion of exclusive breastfeeding, micronutrient supplementation, and food fortification.

■ Nutrition-sensitive interventions—those interventions that address the underlying determinants of malnutrition, such as vaccination programs or nutrition programs to enable farmers to increase the yield of crops that they produce.

■ The enabling environment for nutrition—this concerns laws, policies, resources, and institutional issues that relate to the approach countries take to nutrition and how effective they are at formulating, implementing, and monitoring nutrition interventions.[150] This could include, for example, taxing sweetened beverages or foods high in saturated fat.

A number of the volumes of *Disease Control Priorities* (DCP) touch on nutrition, especially those dealing with cardiovascular disease and diabetes; reproductive, newborn, and child health; and adolescent health. **TABLE 9-6** summarizes some of the key nutrition interventions that DCP has recommended as parts of "essential packages" in the areas noted previously.

The sections that follow elaborate on Table 9-6 and speak further about measures for addressing undernutrition and overweight and obesity.

TABLE 9-6 Selected Essential Packages of Nutrition Interventions

Improvement of Maternal and Child Nutrition

Population	Delivery Platform		
	Community Worker or Health Post	Primary Health Center	First-Level and Referral Hospitals
Pregnancy	Micronutrient supplementation		
	Nutrition education		
	Food supplementation		
Postpartum (woman)	Promotion of breastfeeding		
Child	Promote breastfeeding and complementary feeding		
	Provide vitamin A, zinc, and food supplementation		
	Detect and refer severe acute malnutrition	Treat severe acute malnutrition	Treat severe acute malnutrition associated with serious infection

Prevention or Management of Shared Risk Factors for Cardiovascular and Respiratory Disease

Condition	Delivery Platform					
	Fiscal Interventions	Intersectoral Interventions	Public Health Interventions	Community based	Primary Health Center	Referral and Specialized Hospitals
All conditions	Product taxes on sugar-sweetened beverages	School-based programs to improve nutrition and encourage physical activity	Nutritional supplementation for women of reproductive age			
		Ban on trans fatty acids	Use of mass media concerning harms of specific unhealthy foods			

Data from Black, R. E., Walker, N., Laxminarayan, R., & Temmerman, M. (2016). Reproductive, maternal, newborn, and child health: Key messages of this volume. In R. E. Black, R. Laxminarayan, M. Temmerman, & N. Walker (Eds.), *Disease control priorities: Reproductive, maternal, newborn, and child health* (3rd ed., Vol. 2). Washington DC: The World Bank.
Prabhakaran, D., Anand, S., Watkins, D. A., Gaziano, T. A., Wu, Y., Mbanya, J. C., & Nugent, R. (2017). Cardiovascular, respiratory, and related disorders: Key messages and essential interventions to address their burden in low- and middle-income countries. In D. Prabhakaran, S. Anand, T. A. Gaziano, J. C. Mbanya, Y. Wu, & R. Nugent (Eds.), *Disease control priorities: Cardiovascular, respiratory, and related disorders* (3rd ed., Vol. 5). Washington, DC: The World Bank.

Undernutrition

It has already been noted that knowledge and behaviors are important determinants of what foods people eat, how they cook them, and how they consume them. Studies have shown that people can improve what they eat, how they cook, and how they eat their food by improvements in knowledge, even in the absence of improvements in income.[151] Nutrition education needs to be spread much more widely and in more appropriate ways to promote appropriate breastfeeding and complementary feeding and to help people eat better and more nutritious foods.

Growth monitoring and promotion programs, like those in Tamil Nadu, as well as others that were carried out in Honduras, Indonesia, and Madagascar, can also be important to improving nutrition outcomes at low cost. It is especially important that these programs be community-based. In addition, parents—usually mothers—who participate in these programs need to understand the importance of child growth and how they can carry out improved feeding and caring practices, such as exclusive breastfeeding, appropriate introduction of complementary foods, and the management of diarrhea. To succeed, growth monitoring and promotion programs must be coupled with programs for behavior change communication.[152]

The two-way relationship between infection/disease and nutrition status has been noted. Many infections and diseases reduce one's ability to eat or ability to absorb food. At the same time, poor nutritional status reduces immunity to disease. To set the foundation for improvements in the nutritional status of poor people in low- and middle-income countries, especially poor infants, children, and women, it is very important to improve the control of parasitic infections such as hookworm and to control diarrheal diseases, malaria, and vaccine-preventable diseases, such as measles. Of course, doing this will also demand renewed efforts at health education; more effective basic health services, such as immunization; and improvements in water supply and sanitation.

Some people will simply not eat enough food or enough of the right foods, largely because of income gaps. These problems are also the result of, or are compounded by, natural disaster and conflict. Under these circumstances, it may be necessary that people receive food supplements like a high-protein, high-calorie ready-to-use therapeutic food. Alternatively, some people may receive vouchers for food, such as food stamps, which are cash transfers that can be used only to buy certain health and nutrition services or the right to buy certain foods at reduced prices. Cash transfer programs are also being used to promote better nutrition, and smart cards are increasingly taking the place of food stamps or transfers of cash.

Vitamin and mineral supplementation is widespread in the world, is not expensive, and is often used as a way of improving the micronutrient status of large numbers of people, especially infants, children, and pregnant and lactating mothers. These can be given in capsules or syrups. Vitamin A should be given twice per year and should be integrated with child survival and other health services to minimize the cost of distribution.[63] In the last decade or so, vitamin A has been given orally to infants and children during national polio immunization days in many countries. These efforts can be expanded. At the same time, additional and carefully monitored efforts can be made to provide iron and folate to pregnant women. Unfortunately, these efforts have not worked as well as planned and need to be carefully reviewed and refined to enhance both coverage of supplementation and the extent to which women take the pills they do get.

Food fortification is practiced in many countries for a number of micronutrients. In fact, fortification in the industrialized countries has contributed greatly to the disappearance of several deficiencies. The fortification of salt with iodine is a very widespread practice and is very inexpensive, as we have seen in the China case study. About two-thirds of the world now consumes iodized salt, and the impact of fortification of salt could be further expanded through its double fortification with iron, as well as iodine. In addition, many different food products can be fortified. The key to effective fortification is to find a food product that is very widely consumed, for which there are no technical impediments to fortification, and for which fortification is inexpensive.[153] Thus, increasingly one could fortify flour, cooking oil, margarine, soy sauce, and other products, as well as salt. Multiple vitamin and mineral supplements are also being manufactured, which can be sprinkled on children's food to fortify it. Fortification can cost as little as 3 to 5 cents per person reached per year.[63] Clearly, fortification is a good way to harness the resources of commercial marketing networks to enhance the health of the population. Given the difficulties of iron supplementation, it may be that the most effective way of reducing iron deficiency in women is to operate an effective program of fortification for iron and folic acid.

Efforts are also under way for biofortification. The aim of this work is to use technologies to improve the nutritional content of foods, such as rice, yams, or other vegetables.

The latest studies show that young child deaths could be reduced by about 15 percent if the appropriate countries could take to scale a package of specific nutritional interventions, including the following[12]:

- Folic acid supplementation or fortification for pregnant women
- Balanced energy protein supplementation for pregnant women
- Calcium supplementation for pregnant women
- Multiple micronutrient fortification for pregnant women
- Promotion of appropriate breastfeeding practices
- Appropriate complementary feeding
- Supplementation with vitamin A and zinc for children aged 6 to 59 months
- Appropriate management of severe acute malnutrition
- Appropriate management of moderate acute malnutrition

Moreover, the evidence suggests that this package would be highly cost-effective at a cost per DALY averted of about $179.[105] In fact, a range of these and related nutrition interventions are cost-effective or have a high ratio of benefits to costs. **TABLE 9-7** indicates the cost per DALY averted for a number of measures to address undernutrition, as well as the benefit–cost ratio of some nutrition interventions.

These interventions compare favorably in their cost-effectiveness with a range of other health interventions that are cost-effective. The cost-effectiveness of several vaccines and bednets for malaria control, for example, is around $10 per DALY averted. Condom promotion to prevent transmission of HIV has

a cost per DALY averted of about $40. Even the most expensive nutrition interventions, such as food supplements for young children, have a cost-effectiveness that is similar to that of antiretroviral therapy for HIV/AIDS.[105]

These comments on specific nutrition interventions highlight the gains they can produce in cost-effective ways. However, it is also essential to repeat that even at scale these gains can only address a share of key concerns for undernutrition. Addressing them more broadly will require that governments take a coordinated and intersectoral approach to the range of key determinants of the problems of undernutrition.

Overweight and Obesity

The obesity epidemic poses a serious global problem, especially in low- and middle-income countries. Given its scope, it is important to use policy measures across multiple levels to prevent obesity and reverse its trend. Strategies should include efforts on the international, national, local, and individual levels. The involvement of the food industry, healthcare providers, schools, urban planners, the agricultural sector, and the media is also essential.

International organizations can have a large impact on obesity by setting global nutrition and physical activity standards. They can also encourage surveillance, monitoring, and evaluation systems to ensure nutrition standards are met and to identify countries where obesity policies are most needed. In September 2011, the United Nations General Assembly convened a summit on global noncommunicable diseases, identifying key targets for strengthening and

TABLE 9-7   Cost-Effectiveness and Benefit:Cost Ratios of Selected Nutrition Interventions

Cost per DALY Averted
$5–$15 for vitamin A and zinc supplements
$40 for community-based management of severe acute malnutrition
$50–$150 for behavior change interventions taken to scale
$66–$115 for iron fortification
$90 for folic acid fortification

Benefit:Cost Ratios
6:1 for deworming
8:1 for iron fortification of staple foods
30:1 for salt iodination
46:1 for folic acid fortification

Data from Horton, S. (2017). Economics of nutritional interventions. In S. de Pee, D. Taren, & M. Bloem (Eds.), *Nutrition and health in a developing world* (3rd ed., pp.33–45). Totowa, NJ: Humana Press shaping primary prevention to reduce risk factors for NCDs, including obesity.[154] WHO has also done a large amount of work on the subject, including developing best-buy cost-effective interventions to address NCDs. WHO's top recommendations for reducing unhealthy diet and physical inactivity include reducing salt intake through industry reformulation, labeling, and education; banning industry use of trans fat; implementing an SSB tax to reduce sugar consumption; and implementing a public awareness campaign to promote physical activity. To address cardiovascular disease and diabetes, WHO recommends counseling and multidrug therapy for people with a high risk of developing heart attacks and strokes, including those with established cardiovascular disease, and preventive screening and glycemic control for people with diabetes.[155]

On a national scale, there are many opportunities to address obesity. Many governments set dietary guidelines, as well as age-specific physical activity guidelines.[156,157] Additional government campaigns addressing health can be implemented, such as the 2010–2017 Let's Move campaign in the United States, spearheaded by former First Lady Michelle Obama. A comprehensive initiative dedicated to reducing national childhood obesity, Let's Move also established a task force to review programs and policies related to childhood nutrition and physical activity and developed a national action plan with fixed benchmarks.[158] Effective national prevention strategies in low- and middle-income countries are especially important, as many of these countries are still in a nutrition transition, presenting the added challenge of developing policies and programs to address overweight and obesity and undernutrition, while not hindering progress on either issue. There must be coordination and resource allocation across multiple sectors of government to create successful large-scale campaigns.

Aligning national nutrition and agricultural policies with dietary goals can also contribute to reducing obesity and overweight. Policies modifying food prices, such as taxation of unhealthy foods and beverages, can decrease consumption and generate revenue to fund programs that promote health.[159] Over the past 5 years, SSB taxes have been enacted around the world, including in the United Kingdom, South Africa, France, the United Arab Emirates, Mexico, and numerous localities in the United States. Although the full effects of these taxes are yet to be determined, preliminary results have shown that Mexico's 2014 SSB excise tax has decreased per capita sales of SSBs by 7.3 percent and increased per capita sales of plain water by 5.2 percent.[160] Food prices can also be modified

through the removal of subsidies on oils, sugar, and foods from animal sources, increasing product costs globally and leading to reduced consumption, especially among low-income populations.[161] Prices for healthier foods such as fruits and vegetables can simultaneously be decreased through agricultural subsidies, likely increasing consumption with the proper infrastructure in place allowing such products to be accessible.[161] This happened in China in the early 2000s, when subsidies on fruits, vegetables, and soybeans increased production and consumption of these products.[162]

As we saw in Finland, another strategy is for governments to require nutrition labeling on packages listing the caloric and nutrient content of foods to help consumers make healthier, more informed choices; this can also incentivize companies to reformulate products and introduce healthier options.[163] As new research develops, governments can mandate labels to list nutrients of specific concern, such as in Canada, the United States, and Brazil, where trans fat content is required to be listed on food packages.[164-167] Front-of-package labeling systems can be used to convey essential nutritional information simply and prominently using a short label or basic symbols. Using color-coding, these labels can help the consumer identify nutritionally beneficial and harmful foods and beverages just by glancing at the package. For example, the U.K. traffic light front-of-package labeling system shows whether the product has high (colored in red), medium (yellow), or low (green) levels of fat, saturated fat, sugar, and salt.[168] Nutrition-labeling initiatives are growing in popularity among low- and middle-income countries, including Sri Lanka, Vietnam, Brazil, Nigeria, and South Africa.[169] Along similar lines, calorie labeling on menus in restaurant chains with more than 20 locations nationwide was mandated by federal law in the United States in 2018, and preliminary research has shown beneficial effects on industry reformulation of menu items, food choices, and health.[170,171] Educational campaigns must be implemented alongside any type of labeling campaign to raise awareness about the initiative and the reasons for it, so that consumers can understand why the labels are important, where to find them, and what they mean.

Another way to promote healthier eating through nutritional policy is for governments to incentivize production and use of healthier substitutes, such as the use of oil with omega-3 fatty acids instead of partially hydrogenated oils. This requires collaboration between the agricultural and food industry sectors. The food industry, including restaurants, supermarkets, food

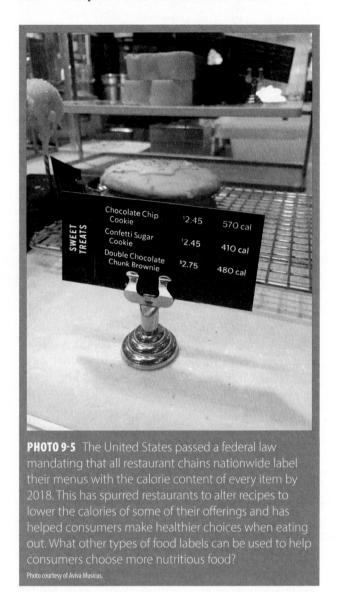

PHOTO 9-5 The United States passed a federal law mandating that all restaurant chains nationwide label their menus with the calorie content of every item by 2018. This has spurred restaurants to alter recipes to lower the calories of some of their offerings and has helped consumers make healthier choices when eating out. What other types of food labels can be used to help consumers choose more nutritious food?

Photo courtesy of Aviva Musicus.

manufacturers, and caterers, can also take voluntary action to reduce sugar, salt, saturated fat, and caloric content from their food over time. Although these initiatives are under way in some high-income countries, similar initiatives should be translated to low- and middle-income countries.[172,173]

Legislation can be used to restrict unhealthy food marketing aimed at children through television, internet, other media, and their environment, thus decreasing their consumption of those products and subsequently decreasing childhood obesity.[174] Zoning laws can also be instituted to limit the number of fast-food restaurants in a given area.[175] Although the World Health Organization has recommended that governments and industry reduce the amount of advertising and marketing of unhealthy foods to children,[176] few countries have taken steps toward this goal.[177]

A healthy food environment in schools can encourage healthier eating for children in general, especially in conjunction with nutritional education for both students and parents.[178] School meal programs can provide healthy, low-cost or free meals to children, simultaneously addressing undernutrition and overweight and obesity. Policies can also be implemented to ban bake sales on school premises and remove vending machines selling sugar-sweetened beverages and less healthy snacks, increasing healthy snacks sold. The amount of physical education required during the school day can also be extended, and food marketing within schools can be eliminated.

The World Health Organization's Global Action Plan for the Prevention and Control of Noncommunicable Diseases 2013–2020 calls for a voluntary global target of a 10 percent relative reduction in the prevalence of insufficient physical activity.[97] To work toward achieving this goal, countries can adopt national physical activity guidelines and education campaigns to encourage over 30 minutes of moderate physical activity on most days of the week, such as we saw in Brazil.[179] Steps can also be taken to reduce television viewing and internet usage via mandatory or voluntary action. For instance, the television network Nickelodeon designates one day a year as a "Worldwide Day of Play," in which they suspend programming across all of their TV channels and websites for 3 hours, encouraging children to "get up, go outside and play."[180] This concept could be extended to other networks for more regular, longer periods of time.

Improving the safety of and access to recreational spaces and facilities through urban planning at the national or regional level is important to encourage an active, pedestrian-friendly community. Governments can promote the use of public transportation and bicycles to increase physical activity levels in cities by providing incentives, such as discounted transportation fares, bike sharing programs, cycling safety classes, and secure bicycle parking.[20] The creation of sidewalks, parks, safe bicycle lanes, and buildings with accessible staircases can also encourage physical activity.

The media have leveraging power to frame obesity as a common challenge and to promote specific policy changes via digital and printed media and social marketing campaigns.[181] Media advocacy in this realm can direct political attention to obesity, generate public debate about policy options, and ultimately persuade the public and lawmakers to support specific policies.[181] The media can also serve to educate the public about the importance of the food environment; this dissemination of nutrition education, in conjunction with environmental, diet, and physical activity changes, has been shown to have positive effects on weight loss and health.[182,183]

Doctors can play a large role in the prevention and treatment of obesity and overweight. Currently, most health professionals are poorly prepared to treat obesity, so medical education efforts need to be directed toward obesity and its associated disease burden, and healthcare providers should be trained to implement behavioral change strategies.[184] As part of standard doctor visits, physicians and other healthcare providers should measure body weight and provide continual nutritional and weight-management advice to encourage a healthy lifestyle.[184] However, it is crucial that health professionals learn to recognize their own weight bias and use appropriate language when working with patients with overweight and obesity.[184] Medical organizations and nongovernmental organizations can also advocate for and influence policy on issues related to health and the environment.[20]

Although food availability and the physical and social environment have a strong influence over choice, it is ultimately the individual who must eat healthily and exercise. It is much easier to prevent weight gain than to lose weight, so prevention is preferable. However, although research has shown that losing weight is very difficult, it is possible for individuals to successfully improve their health by focusing on healthy habits—not weight loss.[185] Individuals should choose a dietary pattern that they can comfortably adhere to that limits energy intake, added sugars, salt, saturated fat, and trans fats.[186] Adults should also get 150 minutes of physical activity a week, and children should exercise for 60 minutes a day.[50]

▶ Main Messages

Undernutrition

Nutritional status is a major determinant of health status. It has an important bearing on the health of pregnant women and on pregnancy outcomes for both mothers and children. It is a major determinant of the birthweight of children, how children grow, and the extent to which their cognitive functions develop properly. Nutrition status is also closely linked with the strength of one's immune system and one's ability to stay healthy.

In addition, nutritional status has an important bearing on people's capacity to learn and on their productivity. Nutritional deficits can seriously hamper the ability of children to attend school, concentrate while they are there, and learn effectively. Numerous studies have shown that workers who are anemic produce less than workers who do not suffer from iron deficiency anemia.

From the global health perspective, the most important concerns related to undernutrition are breastfeeding practices, whether or not people get enough of the right foods to have sufficient energy and protein, and the extent to which people have a sufficient intake of vitamin A, iodine, iron, zinc, and calcium. The importance of these nutrients and micronutrients varies with the place of people in their life course, with needs differing for infants, children, adolescents, pregnant and lactating women, adults, and older adults.

More than 1 billion people in the world today suffer from energy and protein malnutrition and deficiencies in key micronutrients. These problems often stem from people's lack of income to purchase enough food or food of appropriate quality. However, these problems also relate to culture, customs, and eating behaviors. They also are linked to agricultural markets, climate, and civil conflict. Malnutrition of all types disproportionately affects poor people, marginalized people, and females.

Energy and protein malnutrition is associated with low birthweight, being underweight, failing to grow properly, and a weakening of immunity. Vitamin A deficiency is well known for its impact on vision but is also closely associated with general immunity and child growth. The lack of iron is the primary cause of iron deficiency anemia, which leads to weakness and fatigue; however, it is also associated with maternal morbidity and mortality, poor and stunted growth in children, and poor mental development in children. The lack of iodine causes thyroid problems, goiter, and important deficits in mental abilities. Iodine is also essential for proper child growth. The lack of zinc is associated with general immunity, the growth of children, and the development of children's cognitive and motor abilities. About 45 percent of the deaths in the world today of children under 5 years of age are associated with undernutrition.

There are cost-effective solutions to a number of important nutritional concerns. People can wash their hands more frequently with soap to reduce the rate of infections and diarrhea that take such terrible tolls on nutritional status. Efforts can be enhanced to promote exclusive breastfeeding for 6 months, followed by the appropriate introduction of hygienically prepared complementary feeding. Food supplements can be given to those people who are not getting enough protein and energy. Nutritional supplements can be provided for vitamin A and iron. Salt can be fortified with iodine. Pregnant women can receive multivitamins. Zinc can be given along with oral rehydration to reduce the severity of diarrheal disease. Therapeutic feeding can be given to children who suffer from moderate and severe acute malnutrition. Families can also learn, even in the absence of income gains, to improve what they eat. These actions will be most successful if they are tied to approaches that are taken by communities.

It is also critical to remember that the window of opportunity for ensuring that children are well nourished and develop properly is a small one. It begins at conception and lasts until children are about 2 years of age. Damage done to children's development in this period is largely irreversible.

The most critical interventions to deal with undernutrition, therefore, are as follows:

■ Ensure that pregnant women are well nourished and have sufficient amounts of needed micronutrients.
■ Promote exclusive breastfeeding for all children until they are 6 months of age.
■ Encourage the provision of appropriate complementary foods for infants beginning at 6 months of age.
■ Support effective programs in supplementation and fortification, based on nutritional needs at the local level, and embed them in community-based approaches.
■ Fight infection and illness through improved, water, sanitation, and hygiene; immunization; and better health and eating behaviors.
■ Focus on South Asia and sub-Saharan Africa and on poor and marginalized communities elsewhere.

These can be achieved by taking some of the following steps, among others, in the short, medium, and longer run[152]:

Short run
■ Initiate community-based growth monitoring and promotion.
■ Carry out supplementation with vitamin A and iron.
■ Provide zinc for the management of diarrhea.
■ Selectively provide therapeutic food.

Medium run
■ Consolidate community-based growth monitoring and promotion.
■ Implement food supplementation through programs such as vouchers, smart cards, and cash transfers.

■ Fortify locally appropriate foods with needed micronutrients, including completing the agenda on the fortification of salt with iodine.

Long run
■ Improve the education of women and take other appropriate measures to enhance the social standing of women in society.
■ Use technologies to improve the nutritional content of foods.

In addition, countries must take a coordinated intersectoral approach to addressing more broadly the determinants of undernutrition. To enable better nutrition, they must move beyond the important but largely nutrition-specific interventions noted and also address more broadly issues such as these:

■ Water, sanitation, and hygiene
■ Other measures to reduce infection, such as vaccination
■ Enhancing the availability of healthy, nutritious foods
■ Creating mechanisms to reduce vulnerability to food insecurity
■ Enhancing people's ability to pay for healthy, nutritious foods

Overweight and Obesity

The worldwide increase in overweight, obesity, and related chronic diseases has largely been driven by globalization, through a combination of global trade liberalization, economic growth, and rapid urbanization. These factors are causing dramatic changes in diet, lifestyles, and living environments, in turn promoting positive energy balance. Nutritional transitions in low- and middle-income countries involve increases in the consumption of fast food, increased prevalence of supermarkets, and a diet heavy in added sugar and animal products. Coupled with reductions in physical activity, and linked behavioral, cultural, and biological factors, obesity and overweight are increasing at alarming rates, especially in low- and middle-income countries.

A balanced, healthy diet consisting of vegetables, fruits, whole grains, legumes, and nuts is crucial to the prevention of obesity. Such a diet must limit red and processed meats, saturated and trans fats, added sugars, salt, and refined carbohydrates.

Unfortunately, the vast majority of the world is not receiving a healthy diet, as reflected by the 2.3 billion people worldwide who are overweight or have obesity. In high-income countries, poorer people are most at risk for obesity and overweight, whereas in low- and middle-income countries, the wealthier are at a higher risk. Childhood obesity is of particular concern, as 41 million children currently are overweight or have obesity, and will likely continue this trend into adulthood.

Obesity and its related diseases have high costs in terms of health expenditures and quality of life, so prevention strategies are paramount, particularly in low- and middle-income countries that must manage a double burden of malnutrition. Due to the scope and complexity of the obesity epidemic, prevention strategies and policies across multiple levels are needed in order to have a measurable effect. Changes should include high-level global policies from the international community to identify nutritional goals and guidelines. In addition, coordinated efforts by governments, organizations, communities, and individuals will be required to positively influence behavioral and environmental change. Policies and prevention efforts must also involve the industry, media, doctors, farmers, and urban planners.

Some of the most important and cost-effective interventions for addressing overweight, obesity, and the dietary risks to good health include measures that can be taken by governments, by industry, and by individuals:

- Reduce salt intake through industry reformulation of packaged and restaurant foods; government-mandated labeling; expanding lower-sodium offerings in public institutions such as workplaces, schools, and hospitals; and implementing mass-media behavior change campaigns.
- Eliminate trans fats in the food supply through a government-mandated ban, and replace trans fats and saturated fats with unsaturated fats through reformulation, labeling, fiscal policies, or agricultural policies.
- Reduce SSB consumption through taxation.
- Increase public awareness through mass media on diet and physical activity, linked with mass media campaigns organized by government, local health departments, private organizations, and schools.
- Provide counseling and drug therapy for people with a high risk of developing heart attacks and strokes, including those with established cardiovascular disease.
- Provide preventive foot care, retinopathy screening, and effective glycemic control for people with diabetes.

As countries confront undernutrition, overweight, and obesity, it is essential to highlight the fact that addressing nutrition problems of all types will require action in three domains: nutrition-specific, nutrition-sensitive, and areas related to the enabling environment for nutrition.

Study Questions

1. What is the importance of nutrition to the SDGs?
2. What are *stunting* and *wasting*?
3. What are some of the direct and indirect causes of undernutrition?
4. What are some of the direct and indirect causes of overweight and obesity?
5. What are the links between nutrition and health?
6. How are growth charts used to gauge nutrition status?
7. What are the most important micronutrient deficiencies, and what health problems do they cause?
8. Why is anemia a special risk in pregnancy?
9. Why is exclusive breastfeeding for the first 6 months so important?
10. What parts of the world have the worst nutritional problems?
11. What are the links between nutrition and economic development?
12. What are some of the most important cost-effective interventions that could be made to address undernutrition in under-5 children?
13. What are some of the most important cost-effective interventions that could be made to address overweight and obesity?

References

1. The World Bank. (n.d.). *Data: Prevalence of underweight, weight for age (% of children under 5)*. Retrieved from https://data.worldbank.org/indicator/SH.STA.MALN.ZS

2. The World Bank. (n.d.). *Data: Prevalence of stunting, height for age (% of children under 5)*. Retrieved from https://data.worldbank.org/indicator/SH.STA.STNT.ZS

3. Black, R. E., Victora, C. G., Walker, S. P., Bhutta, Z. A., Christian, P., de Onis, M., . . . Uauy, R. (2013). Maternal and child undernutrition and overweight in low-income and middle-income countries. *The Lancet, 382*(9890), 427–451.

4. World Health Organization (WHO). (2018). *Children: Reducing mortality: Key facts.* Retrieved from https://www.who.int/en/news-room/fact-sheets/detail/children-reducing-mortality

5. Institute of Health Metrics and Evaluation (IHME). (n.d.). GBD Compare: Viz Hub. Retrieved from https://vizhub.healthdata.org/gbd-compare/

6. UNICEF & The Micronutrient Initiative. (2004). *Vitamin and mineral deficiency: A global progress report.* Ottawa, Ontario, Canada: The Micronutrient Initiative.

7. World Health Organization (WHO). (2018). *Obesity and overweight.* Retrieved from http://www.who.int/news-room/fact-sheets/detail/obesity-and-overweight

8. United Nations Children's Fund, World Health Organization, & The World Bank. (2017). *UNICEF-WHO-World Bank joint child malnutrition estimates.* New York, NY: UNICEF; Geneva, Switzerland: WHO; Washington, DC: The World Bank.

9. Dietz, W. H. (2017). Double-duty solutions for the double burden of malnutrition. *The Lancet, 390*(10113), 2607–2608.

10. World Food Programme. (n.d.). *What is food security?* Retrieved from https://www.wfp.org/node/359289

11. UNICEF. (1998). *State of the world's children: Focus on nutrition.* New York, NY: Oxford University Press.

12. Bhutta, Z. A., Das, J. K., Rizvi, A., Gaffey, M. F., Walker, N., Horton, S., . . . Black, R. E. (2013). Evidence-based intervention for improvement of maternal and child nutrition: What can be done and at what cost? *The Lancet, 382*(9890), 452–477.

13. Centers for Disease Control and Prevention (CDC). *Public health genomics.* Retrieved from http://www.cdc.gov/genomics/resources/diseases/obesity/index.htm

14. Maruvada, P., Leone, V., Kaplan, L. M., & Chang, E. B. (2017). The human microbiome and obesity: Moving beyond associations. *Cell Host & Microbe, 22*(5), 589–599.

15. Popkin, B. M. (2006). Global nutrition dynamics: The world is shifting rapidly toward a diet linked with noncommunicable diseases. *American Journal of Clinical Nutrition, 84*(2), 289–298.

16. Nakamura, Y. (2002). Beyond the hijab: Female Muslims and physical activity. *Women in Sport & Physical Activity Journal, 11*(2), 21.

17. Langøien, L. J., Terragni, L., Rugseth, G., Nicolaou, M., Holdsworth, M., Stronks, K., . . . Roos, G. (2017). Systematic mapping review of the factors influencing physical activity and sedentary behaviour in ethnic minority groups in Europe: A DEDIPAC study. *International Journal of Behavioral Nutrition and Physical Activity, 14*(1), 99.

18. Sharara, E., Akik, C., Ghattas, H., & Obermeyer, C. M. (2018). Physical inactivity, gender and culture in Arab countries: A systematic assessment of the literature. *BMC Public Health, 18*(1), 639.

19. Matoti-Mvalo, T., & Puoane, T. (2011). Perceptions of body size and its association with HIV/AIDS. *South African Journal of Clinical Nutrition, 24*(1), 40–45.

20. Malik, V. S., Willett, W. C., & Hu, F. B. (2012). Global obesity: Trends, risk factors and policy implications. *Nature Reviews Endocrinology, 9*(1), 13–27.

21. Fuster, V., & Kelly, B. B. (Eds.). (2010). *Promoting cardiovascular health in the developing world: A critical challenge to achieve global health.* Washington, DC: National Academies Press.

22. Hawkes, C., Chopra, M., & Friel, S. (2009). Globalization, trade, and the nutrition transition. In R. Labonté, T. Schrecker, C. Packer, & V. Runnels (Eds.), *Globalization and health: Pathways, evidence and policy* (pp. 235–262). New York, NY: Routledge.

23. Lange, G., Wodon, Q., & Carey, K. (Eds.). (2018). *The changing wealth of nations 2018: Building a sustainable future.* Washington, DC: The World Bank.

24. Caballero, B. A. (2005). A nutrition paradox—Underweight and obesity in developing countries. *New England Journal of Medicine, 352*(15), 1514–1516.

25. Johns, T., & Eyzaguirre, P. B. (2006). Linking biodiversity, diet and health in policy and practice. *Proceedings of the Nutrition Society, 65*(2), 182–189.

26. Wang, Y., Mi, J., Shan, X. Y., Wang, Q. J., & Ge, K. Y. (2007). Is China facing an obesity epidemic and the consequences? The trends in obesity and chronic disease in China. *International Journal of Obesity, 31*(1), 177–188.

27. Pan, A., Malik, V. S., & Hu, F. B. (2012). Exporting diabetes mellitus to Asia: The impact of Western-style fast food. *Circulation, 126*, 163–165.

28. Ritzer, G. (2002). An introduction to McDonaldization. *McDonaldization: The Reader*, 4–25.

29. McDonald's. (2019). *History.* Retrieved from https://corporate.mcdonalds.com/corpmcd/about-us/history.html

30. Misra, A., & Khurana, L. (2008). Obesity and the metabolic syndrome in developing countries. *Journal of Clinical Endocrinology and Metabolism, 93*(11, Suppl. 1), S9–S30.

31. Reardon, T., Timmer, C., Barrett, C., & Berdegue, J. (2003). The rise of supermarkets in Africa, Asia, and Latin America. *American Journal of Agricultural Economics, 85*, 1140–1146.

32. Kimenju, S. C., Rischke, R., Klasen, S., & Qaim, M. (2015). Do supermarkets contribute to the obesity pandemic in developing countries? *Public Health Nutrition, 18*(17), 3224–3233.

33. Abeykoon, A. H., Engler-Stringer, R., & Muhajarine, N. (2017). Health-related outcomes of new grocery store interventions: A systematic review. *Public Health Nutrition, 20*(12), 2236–2248.

34. Hawkes, C. (2008). Dietary implications of supermarket development: A global perspective. *Development Policy Review, 26*(6), 657–692.

35. Wagner, K. H., & Brath, H. (2012). A global view on the development of non communicable diseases. *Preventive Medicine, 54*, S38–S41.

36. Popkin, B. M., Adair, L. S., & Ng, S. W. (2012). Global nutrition transition and the pandemic of obesity in developing countries. *Nutrition Reviews, 70*(1), 3–21.

37. Horgen, K. B., Choate, M., & Brownell, K. D. (2001). Television and children's nutrition. In D. G. Singer & J. L. Singer (Eds.), *Handbook of children and the media* (pp. 447–461). Thousand Oaks, CA: Sage.

38. Tatlow-Golden, M., Verdoodt, V., Oates, J., Jewell, J., Breda, J. J., & Boyland, E. (2017). A safe glimpse within the "black box"? Ethical and legal principles when assessing digital marketing of food and drink to children. *WHO Public Health Panorama, 3*(4), 613–621.

39. Popkin, B. M., & Nielsen, S. J. (2003). The sweetening of the world's diet. *Obesity Research, 11*(11), 1325–1332.

40. U.S. Department of Health and Human Services & U.S. Department of Agriculture. (2015). *Dietary guidelines for Americans: 2015–2020* (8th ed.). Retrieved from http://health.gov/dietaryguidelines/2015/guidelines

41. Centers for Disease Control and Prevention (CDC). (2017). QuickStats: Percentage of total daily kilocalories consumed from sugar-sweetened beverages among children and adults, by sex and income level—National health and nutrition examination survey, United States, 2011–2014. *Morbidity and Mortality Weekly Report, 66*(6), 181. Retrieved from https://www.cdc.gov/mmwr/volumes/66/wr/mm6606a8.htm

42. Mozaffarian, D., Hao, T., Rimm, E. B., Willett, W. C., & Hu, F. B. (2011). Changes in diet and lifestyle and long-term weight gain in women and men. *New England Journal of Medicine, 364*(25), 2392–2404.

43. Pan, A., Sun, Q., Bernstein, A. M., Schulze, M. B., Manson, J. E., Willett, W. C., & Hu, F. B. (2011). Red meat consumption and risk of type 2 diabetes: 3 cohorts of US adults and an updated meta-analysis. *American Journal of Clinical Nutrition, 94*(4), 1088–1096.

44. Bernstein, A. M., Sun, Q., Hu, F. B., Stampfer, M. J., Manson, J. E., & Willett, W. C. (2010). Major dietary protein sources and risk of coronary heart disease in women. *Circulation, 122*(9), 876–883.

45. Bouvard, V., Loomis, D., Guyton, K. Z., Grosse, Y., El Ghissassi, F., Benbrahim-Tallaa, L., . . . Straif, K. (2015). Carcinogenicity of consumption of red and processed meat. *Lancet Oncology, 16*(16), 1599–1600.

46. Pan, A., Sun, Q., Bernstein, A. M., Schulze, M. B., Manson, J. E., Stampfer, M. J., . . . Hu, F. B. (2012). Red meat consumption and mortality: Results from 2 prospective cohort studies. *Archives of Internal Medicine, 172*(7), 555–563.

47. Food and Agriculture Organization of the United Nations. (2017). *The state of food and agriculture, 2013*. Rome, Italy: Author. Retrieved from http://www.fao.org/3/a-I7658E.pdf

48. Popkin, B. M., & Gordon-Larsen, P. (2004). The nutrition transition: Worldwide obesity dynamics and their determinants. *International Journal of Obesity, 28*(Suppl. 3), S2–S9.

49. Hu, F. B. (2008). *Obesity epidemiology*. New York, NY: Oxford University Press.

50. World Health Organization (WHO). (2018). *Global action plan on physical activity 2018–2030: More active people for a healthier world*. Geneva, Switzerland: Author.

51. Sallis, J. F., Slymen, D. J., Conway, T. L., Frank, L. D., Saelens, B. E., Cain, K., & Chapman, J. E. (2011). Income disparities in perceived neighborhood built and social environment attributes. *Health & Place, 17*(6), 1274–1283.

52. Patel, S. R., & Hu, F. B. (2008). Short sleep duration and weight gain: A systematic review. *Obesity, 16*(3), 643–653.

53. Swinburn, B., & Egger, G. (2002). Preventive strategies against weight gain and obesity. *Obesity Reviews, 3*(4), 289–301.

54. Azevedo, L. B., Ling, J., Soos, I., Robalino, S., & Ells, L. (2016). The effectiveness of sedentary behaviour interventions for reducing body mass index in children and adolescents: Systematic review and meta-analysis. *Obesity Reviews, 17*(7), 623–635.

55. World Health Organization (WHO). (2018). *ICD-11 for mortality and morbidity statistics*. Retrieved from https://icd.who.int/browse11/l-m/en

56. UNICEF. (2006). *Progress for children. A report card on nutrition, No. 4*. Retrieved from http://www.unicef.org/progressforchildren/2006n4/index_undernutrition.html

57. Caulfield, L. E., Richard, S. A., Rivera, J. A., Musgrove, P., & Black, R. E. (2006). Stunting, wasting, and micronutrient disorders. In D. T. Jamison, J. G. Breman, A. R. Measham, et al. (Eds.), *Disease control priorities in developing countries* (2nd ed., pp. 551–567). New York, NY: Oxford University Press.

58. World Health Organization (WHO). (2006). *Severe acute malnutrition*. Retrieved from http://www.who.int/nutrition/topics/malnutrition/en/

59. Victora, C. G., Adair, L., Fall, C., Hallal, P. C., Martorell, R., Richter, L., & Sachdev, H. S. (2008). Maternal and child undernutrition: Consequences for adult health and human capital. *The Lancet, 371*(9609), 340–357.

60. GP Notebook. (n.d.). *Xerophthalmia*. Retrieved from http://www.gpnotebook.co.uk/simplepage.cfm?ID=664403984

61. Black, R. E., Allen, L. H., Bhutta, Z. A., Caulfield, L. E., de Onis, M., Ezzati, M., . . . Rivera, J. (2008). Maternal and child undernutrition: Global and regional exposures and health consequences. *The Lancet, 371*(9608), 243–260.

62. Pedersen, T. (2017, April 18). *Facts about iodine*. Retrieved from https://www.livescience.com/37441-iodine.html

63. The World Bank. (2006). *Repositioning nutrition as central to development*. Washington, DC: Author.

64. World Health Organization (WHO). (2015). *Micronutrient deficiencies: Iodine deficiency disorders*. Retrieved from http://www.who.int/nutrition/topics/idd/en/

65. MedlinePlus. (n.d.). *Iron*. Retrieved from http://www.nlm.nih.gov/medlineplus/iron.html

66. World Health Organization (WHO). (2015). *Zinc supplementation in the management of diarrhea*. Retrieved from http://www.who.int/elena/titles/bbc/zinc_diarrhoea/en/

67. Brown, K. H., & Wuehler, S. E. (2000). *The micronutrient initiative*. Ottawa, Ontario, Canada: The Micronutrient Initiative.

68. MedlinePlus. (n.d.). *Folic acid*. Retrieved from http://www.nlm.nih.gov/medlineplus/folicacid.html

69. World Cancer Research Fund. (2018). *Food, nutrition, physical activity and the prevention of cancer: A global perspective*. Washington, DC: Author.

70. American Heart Association. (2018). *Polyunsaturated fat*. Retrieved from http://www.heart.org/en/healthy-living/healthy-eating/eat-smart/fats/polyunsaturated-fats

71. Appel, L. J., Sacks, F. M., Carey, V. J., Obarzanek, E., Swain, J. F., Miller, E. R. III, . . . Bishop, L. M. (2005). Effects of protein, monounsaturated fat, and carbohydrate intake on blood pressure and serum lipids: Results of the OmniHeart randomized trial. *JAMA, 294*(19), 2455–2464.

72. Mozaffarian, D., Micha, R., & Wallace, S. (2010). Effects on coronary heart disease of increasing polyunsaturated fat in place of saturated fat: A systematic review and meta-analysis of randomized controlled trials. *PLoS Medicine, 7*(3), e1000252.

73. World Health Organization (WHO). (2012). *Guideline: Sodium intake for adults and children*. Geneva, Switzerland: Author.

74. World Health Organization (WHO). (2016). *SHAKE the salt habit: The SHAKE technical package for salt reduction*. Geneva, Switzerland: Author.

75. Nishida, C., Uauy, R., Kumanyika, S., & Shetty, P. (2004). The joint WHO/FAO expert consultation on diet, nutrition and the prevention of chronic diseases: Process, product and policy implications. *Public Health Nutrition, 7*(1a), 245–250.

76. Malik, V. S., Popkin, B. M., Bray, G. A., Després, J. P., Willett, W. C., & Hu, F. B. (2010). Sugar-sweetened beverages and risk of metabolic syndrome and type 2 diabetes: A meta-analysis. *Diabetes Care, 33*(11), 2477–2483.

77. Malik, V. S., Willett, W. C., & Hu, F. B. (2009). Sugar-sweetened beverages and BMI in children and adolescents: Reanalyses of a meta-analysis. *American Journal of Clinical Nutrition, 89,* 438–439.

78. Fung, T. T., Malik, V., Rexrode, K. M., Manson, J. E., Willett, W. C., & Hu, F. B. (2009). Sweetened beverage consumption and risk of coronary heart disease in women. *American Journal of Clinical Nutrition, 89*(4), 1037–1042.

79. De Koning, L., Malik, V. S., Kellogg, M. D., Rimm, E. B., Willett, W. C., & Hu, F. B. (2012). Sweetened beverage consumption, incident coronary heart disease and biomarkers of risk in men. *Circulation, 125*(14), 1735–1741.

80. Dhingra, R., Sullivan, L., Jacques, P. F., Wang, T. J., Fox, C. S., Meigs, J. B., . . . Vasan, R. S. (2007). Soft drink consumption and risk of developing cardiometabolic risk factors and the metabolic syndrome in middle-aged adults in the community. *Circulation, 116*(5), 480–488.

81. World Health Organization. (2015). *Guideline: Sugars intake for adults and children.* Geneva, Switzerland: Author. Retrieved from http://apps.who.int/iris/bitstream/10665/149782/1/9789241549028_eng.pdf?ua=1

82. Hu, F. B., & Willett, W. C. (2002). Optimal diets for prevention of coronary heart disease. *JAMA, 288*(20), 2569–2578.

83. Gross, L. S., Li, L., Ford, E. S., & Liu, S. (2004). Increased consumption of refined carbohydrates and the epidemic of type 2 diabetes in the United States: An ecologic assessment. *American Journal of Clinical Nutrition, 79*(5), 774–779.

84. Sun, Q., Spiegelman, D., van Dam, R. M., Holmes, M. D., Malik, V. S., Willett, W. C., & Hu, F. B. (2010). White rice, brown rice, and risk of type 2 diabetes in US men and women. *Archives of Internal Medicine, 170*(11), 961–969.

85. Villegas, R., Liu, S., Gao, Y. T., Yang, G., Li, H., Zheng, W., & Shu, X. O. (2007). Prospective study of dietary carbohydrates, glycemic index, glycemic load, and incidence of type 2 diabetes mellitus in middle-aged Chinese women. *Archives of Internal Medicine, 167*(21), 2310–2316.

86. Ohio State University. (2009). *Nutritional needs of pregnancy and breastfeeding* (Fact Sheet). Retrieved from https://ohioline.osu.edu/factsheet/HYG-5573

87. World Health Organization (WHO). (2017). *10 facts on breastfeeding.* Retrieved from https://www.who.int/features/factfiles/breastfeeding/en/

88. Gillespie, S., & Flores, R. (n.d.). *The life cycle of malnutrition.* Washington, DC: International Food Policy Research Institute. Retrieved from http://ebrary.ifpri.org/cdm/ref/collection/p15738coll2/id/125440

89. Black, R. E., Morris, S. S., & Bryce, J. (2003). Where and why are 10 million children dying every year? *The Lancet, 361*(9376), 2226–2234.

90. National Osteoporosis Foundation. (n.d.). *What is osteoporosis and what causes it?* Retrieved from http://nof.org/articles/7

91. UNICEF. (n.d.). *Nutrition: What are the challenges?* Retrieved from http://www.unicef.org/nutrition/index_challenges.html

92. UNICEF. (2018). *Iodine deficiency.* Retrieved from https://data.unicef.org/topic/nutrition/iodine-deficiency/

93. UNICEF. (2019). *Vitamin A deficiency.* Retrieved from https://data.unicef.org/topic/nutrition/vitamin-a-deficiency/

94. Development Initiatives. (2017). *Global nutrition report 2017: Nourishing the SDGs* (p.10). Bristol, United Kingdom: Author.

95. Development Initiatives. (2018). *2018 global nutrition report: Shining a light to spur action on nutrition.* Bristol, United Kingdom: Author.

96. Finucane, M. M., Stevens, G. A., Cowan, M. J., Danaei, G., Lin, K. K., Paciorek, C. J., . . . Ezzati, M. (2011). National, regional, and global trends in body-mass index since 1980: Systematic analysis of health examination surveys and epidemiological studies with 960 country-years and 9.1 million participants. *The Lancet, 377*(9765), 557–567.

97. World Health Organization (WHO). (2013). *Global action plan for the prevention and control of noncommunicable diseases 2013–2020.* Retrieved from http://apps.who.int/iris/bitstream/10665/94384/1/9789241506236_eng.pdf

98. Kelly, T., Yang, W., Chen, C. S., Reynolds, K., & He, J. (2008). Global burden of obesity in 2005 and projections to 2030. *International Journal of Obesity, 32*(9), 1431–1437.

99. World Health Organization (WHO). (2016). *Prevalence of overweight among adults, BMI ≥ 25, age-standardized.* Retrieved from http://apps.who.int/gho/data/view.main.GLOBAL2461A?lang=en

100. World Health Organization (WHO). (2017). *Prevalence of obesity among adults, BMI ≥ 30, age-standardized.* Retrieved from http://apps.who.int/gho/data/view.main.REGION2480A?lang=en

101. Singh, A. S., Mulder, C., Twisk, J. W., van Mechelen, W., & Chinapaw, M. J. (2008). Tracking of childhood overweight into adulthood: A systematic review of the literature. *Obesity Reviews, 9*(5), 474–488.

102. World Health Organization (WHO). (2016). *Prevalence of overweight among children and adolescents, BMI > +1 standard deviation above the median, crude.* Retrieved from http://apps.who.int/gho/data/view.main.BMIPLUS1CWBv?lang=en

103. Ng, M., Fleming, T., Robinson, M., Thomson, B., Graetz, N., Margono, C., . . . Gakidou, E. (2014). Global, regional, and national prevalence of overweight and obesity in children and adults during 1980–2013: A systematic analysis for the Global Burden of Disease Study 2013. *The Lancet, 384*(9945), 766–781.

104. GBD 2015 Obesity Collaborators. (2017). Health effects of overweight and obesity in 195 countries over 25 years. *New England Journal of Medicine, 377*(1), 13–27.

105. Horton, S. (2017). Economics of *Nutritional Interventions.* In S. de Pee, D. Taren, & M. W. Bloem (Eds.), *Nutrition and Health in a Developing World* (pp. 33-45). New York, NY: Springer Berlin Heidelberg.

106. Hunt, J. M. (2002). Reversing productivity losses from iron deficiency: The economic case. *Journal of Nutrition, 132*(Suppl. 4), 794S–801S.

107. Fogel, R. (1991). *New sources and new techniques for the study of secular trends in nutritional status, health, mortality, and the process of aging.* Cambridge, MA: National Bureau of Economic Research.

108. Wolgemuth, J. C., Latham, M. C., Hall, A., Chesher, A., & Crompton, D. W. (1982). Worker productivity and the nutritional status of Kenyan road construction laborers. *American Journal of Clinical Nutrition, 36*(1), 68–78.

109. Li, R., Chen, X., Yan, H., Deurenberg, P., Garby, L., & Hautvast, J. G. (1994). Functional consequences of iron supplementation in iron-deficient female cotton mill workers in Beijing, China. *American Journal of Clinical Nutrition, 59*(4), 908–913.

110. World Health Organization (WHO). (2009). *Global health risks: Mortality and burden of disease attributable to selected major risks, 2009*. Geneva, Switzerland: Author. Retrieved from http://www.who.int/healthinfo/global_burden_disease /GlobalHealthRisks_report_full.pdf

111. Danaei, G., Ding, E. L., Mozaffarian, D., Taylor, B., Rehm, J., Murray, C. J., & Ezzati, M. (2009). The preventable causes of death in the United States: Comparative risk assessment of dietary, lifestyle, and metabolic risk factors. *PLoS Medicine, 6*(4), e1000058.

112. Prospective Studies Collaboration. (2009). Body-mass index and cause-specific mortality in 900,000 adults: Collaborative analyses of 57 prospective studies. *The Lancet, 373*, 1083–1096.

113. Beaglehole, R., Bonita, R., Horton, R., Adams, C., Alleyne, G., Asaria, P., . . . Watt, J. (2011). Priority actions for the non-communicable disease crisis. *The Lancet, 377*(9775), 1438–1447.

114. World Health Organization (WHO). (2016). *Prevalence of overweight among children and adolescents, BMI > +1 standard deviation above the median, crude*. Retrieved from http://apps.who.int/gho/data/view.main.BMIPLUS1C05 -09v?lang=en).

115. Cawley, J., & Meyerhoefer, C. (2012). The medical care costs of obesity: An instrumental variables approach. *Journal of Health Economics, 31*(1), 219–230.

116. Centers for Medicare and Medicaid Services (CMS). (2016). *National health expenditures 2016 highlights*. Retrieved from http://www.cms.gov/Research-Statistics-Data-and-Systems /Statistics-Trends-and-Reports/NationalHealthExpendData /downloads/highlights.pdf

117. Finkelstein, E. A., Trogdon, J. G., Cohen, J. W., & Dietz, W. (2009). Annual medical spending attributable to obesity: payer-and service-specific estimates. *Health Affairs, 28*(5), w822–w831.

118. Popkin, B., Horton, S., & Kim, S. (2001). The nutrition transition and prevention of diet-related chronic diseases in Asia and the Pacific. *Food and Nutrition Bulletin, 22*(4), 1–58.

119. Bloom, D. E., Cafiero, E. T., McGovern, M. E., Prettner, K., Stanciole, A., Weiss, J., . . . Rosenberg, L. (2013). *The economic impact of non-communicable disease in China and India: Estimates, projections, and comparisons* (NBER Working Paper No. 19335). Cambridge, MA: National Bureau of Economic Research.

120. Popkin, B. M. (2008). Will China's nutrition transition overwhelm its health care system and slow economic growth? *Health Affairs, 27*(4), 1064–1076.

121. Fitzgerald, S., Kirby, A., Murphy, A., & Geaney, F. (2016). Obesity, diet quality and absenteeism in a working population. *Public Health Nutrition, 19*(18), 3287–3295.

122. World Health Organization (WHO). (2000). *Obesity: Preventing and managing the global epidemic* (No. 894). Geneva, Switzerland: Author.

123. Food and Agriculture Organization of the United Nations. (2013). *The state of food and agriculture, 2013*. Rome, Italy: Author. Retrieved from http://www.fao.org/docrep/018 /i3300e/i3300e.pdf

124. World Health Organization, World Economic Forum, & Harvard School of Public Health. (2011). *From burden to "best buys": Reducing the economic impact of non-communicable diseases in low-and middle-income countries*. Retrieved from http://www.who.int/nmh/publications/best_buys_summary .pdf

125. Bloom, D. E., Cafiero, E., Jané-Llopis, E., Abrahams-Gessel, S., Bloom, L. R., Fathima, S., . . . Weinstein, C. (2011). *The global economic burden of non-communicable diseases*. Geneva, Switzerland: World Economic Forum.

126. Kolotkin, R. L., Meter, K., & Williams, G. R. (2001). Quality of life and obesity. *Obesity Reviews, 2*(4), 219–229.

127. Puhl, R., & Suh, Y. (2015). Health consequences of weight stigma: Implications for obesity prevention and treatment. *Current Obesity Reports, 4*(2), 182–190.

128. Friedman, R. R., & Puhl, R. M. (2012). *Weight bias: A social justice issue*. New Haven, CT: Yale University, Rudd Center for Food Policy and Obesity.

129. Lee, M. J., Popkin, B. M., & Kim, S. (2002). The unique aspects of the nutrition transition in South Korea: The retention of healthful elements in their traditional diet. *Public Health Nutrition, 5*(1a), 197–203.

130. Kim, S., Moon, S., & Popkin, B. M. (2000). The nutrition transition in South Korea. *American Journal of Clinical Nutrition, 71*(1), 44–53.

131. Drewnowski, A., & Popkin, B. M. (1997). The nutrition transition: New trends in the global diet. *Nutrition Reviews, 55*(2), 31–43.

132. Korean Dietetic Association. (n.d.). Homepage. Retrieved from http://www.dietitian.or.kr.

133. South Korean Ministry of Health and Welfare. (1999). *Reports on 1969–95, 1998 National Nutrition Survey*. Seoul, South Korea: Ministry of Health and Welfare.

134. Organization for Economic Cooperation and Development. (2017). *Health at a glance 2017: OECD indicators. Paris, France: Author*. Retrieved from http://dx.doi.org/10.1787 /health_glance-2017-en

135. Organization for Economic Cooperation and Development (OECD). (2017). *Obesity update 2017*. Retrieved from https://www.oecd.org/els/health-systems/Obesity -Update-2017.pdf

136. Rego, A., Berardo, F., & Rodrigues, S. (1990). Fatores de risco para doenças crônico não-transmissíveis: Inquérito domiciliar no município de São Paulo, SP (Brasil). Metodologia e resultados preliminares. *Revista de Saúde Pública, 24*, 277–285.

137. Matsudo, S. M., Matsudo, V. R., Araujo, T. L., Andrade, D. R., Andrade, E. L., de Oliveira, L. C., & Braggion, G. F. (2003). The Agita São Paulo Program as a model for using physical activity to promote health. *Revista Panamericana de Salud Pública, 14*(4), 265–272.

138. National Social Marketing Centre. (2012). *ShowCase: Agita São Paulo*. Retrieved from https://www.thensmc.com /resources/showcase/agita-s%C3%A3o-paulo

139. Organización Panamericana de la Salud. (2002). *A multisectoral coalition in health: Agita São Paulo, una coalición multisectorial en salud*. São Paulo, Brazil: Midiograf.

140. Matsudo, S. M., Matsudo, V. R., Araújo, T., Andrade, D., Andrade, E., Oliveira, L., & Braggion, G. (2002). Nível de atividade física da população do estado de São Paulo: Análise de acordo com o gênero, idade, nível sócio-econômico, distribuição geográfica e de conhecimento. *Revista Brasileira de Ciência e Movimento, 10*(4), 41–50.

141. European Commission. (2008). *Collated information on salt reduction in the EU, 2008.* Retrieved from http://ec.europa .eu/health/ph_determinants/life_style/nutrition /documents/compilation_salt_en.pdf

142. World Health Organization & Food and Agriculture Organization. (2003). *Diet, nutrition and the prevention of chronic diseases* (Technical Report Series 916). Geneva, Switzerland: World Health Organization; Rome, Italy: Food and Agriculture Organization.

143. He, F. J., & MacGregor, G. A. (2009). A comprehensive review on salt and health and current experience of worldwide salt reduction programmes. *Journal of Human Hypertension, 23*(6), 363–384.

144. Laatikainen, T., Pietinen, P., Valsta, L., Sundvall, J., Reinivuo, H., & Tuomilehto, J. (2006). Sodium in the Finnish diet: 20-year trends in urinary sodium excretion among the adult population. *European Journal of Clinical Nutrition, 60*(8), 965–970.

145. Karppanen, H., & Mervaala, E. (2006). Sodium intake and hypertension. *Progress in Cardiovascular Diseases, 49*(2), 59–75.

146. Pietinen, P., Valsta, L. M., Hirvonen, T., & Sinkko, H. (2007). Labelling the salt content in foods: A useful tool in reducing sodium intake in Finland. *Public Health Nutrition, 11*(4), 335–340.

147. World Action on Salt & Health. (2009). *Finland: Salt action summary.* Retrieved from http://www.worldactiononsalt .com/worldaction/europe/finland/

148. The World Bank. (1994). *Impact evaluation report: Tamil Nadu Integrated Nutrition Project.* Washington, DC: Author.

149. This case is based on: Levine, R., & What Works Working Group. (2007). *Case studies in global health: Millions saved.* Sudbury, MA: Jones and Bartlett.

150. International Food Policy Research Institute. (2014). *Global nutrition report 2014: Actions and accountability to accelerate the world's progress on nutrition.* Washington, DC: Author.

151. Griffiths, M., Dicken, K., & Favin, M. (1996). *Promoting the growth of children: What works: Rationale and guidance for programs.* Washington, DC: World Bank.

152. Levinson, F. J., & Bassett, L. (2008). *Malnutrition is still a major contributor to child deaths.* Washington, DC: Population Reference Bureau.

153. Lofti, M., Merx, R., Naber, P., & Van der Heuvel, P. (1996). *Micronutrient fortification of foods: Current prospectus, research and opportunities.* Ottawa, Ontario, Canada: International Agriculture Centre.

154. United Nations General Assembly. (2011). *Draft political declaration of the high-level meeting on the prevention and control of non-communicable diseases.* Retrieved from http://www.un.org/en/ga/ncdmeeting2011/pdf/NCD_draft _political_declaration.pdf

155. World Health Organization (WHO). (2017). *Tackling NCDs: Best buys and other recommended interventions for the prevention and control of noncommunicable diseases.* Geneva, Switzerland: Author.

156. U.S. Department of Health and Human Services. (2008). *Physical activity guidelines for Americans.* Retrieved from http://www.health.gov/paguidelines/

157. U.S. Department of Agriculture. (n.d.). *Dietary guidelines from around the world.* Retrieved from https://www.nal.usda .gov/fnic/dietary-guidelines-around-world

158. Let's Move Campaign. (n.d.). *Let's move: America's move to raise a healthier generation of kids.* Retrieved from https:// letsmove.obamawhitehouse.archives.gov/

159. World Health Organization (WHO). (2015). *Fiscal policies for diet and prevention of noncommunicable diseases: Technical meeting report.* Geneva, Switzerland: Author. Retrieved from http://apps.who.int/iris/bitstream/handle /10665/250131/9789241511247-eng.pdf?sequence=1

160. Colchero, M. A., Guerrero-López, C. M., Molina, M., & Rivera, J. A. (2016). Beverages sales in Mexico before and after implementation of a sugar sweetened beverage tax. *PloS One, 11*(9), e0163463.

161. Afshin, A., Micha, R., Webb, M., Capewell, S., Whitsel, L., Prabhakaran, D., . . . Nugent, R. (2017). Effectiveness of dietary policies to reduce noncommunicable diseases. In D. Prabhakaran, S. Anand, & T. Gaziano (Eds.), *Disease control priorities: Cardiovascular, respiratory, and related disorders* (3rd ed., Vol. 5, pp. 101–115). Washington, DC: The World Bank.

162. Zhai, F., Fu, D., Du, S., Ge, K., Chen, C., & Popkin, B. M. (2002). What is China doing in policy-making to push back the negative aspects of the nutrition transition? *Public Health Nutrition, 5*(1a), 269–273.

163. Roberto, C. A., & Khandpur, N. (2014). Improving the design of nutrition labels to promote healthier food choices and reasonable portion sizes. *International Journal of Obesity (2005), 38*(Suppl. 1), S25–S33.

164. Benincá, C., Zanoelo, E. F., de Lima Luz, L. F. Jr., & Spricigo, C. B. (2009). Trans fatty acids in margarines marketed in Brazil: Content, labeling regulations and consumer information. *European Journal of Lipid Science and Technology, 111*(5), 451–458.

165. Skeaf, C. M. (2009). Feasibility of recommending certain replacement or alternative fats. *European Journal of Clinical Nutrition, 63*, S34–S49.

166. Coombes, R. (2011). Trans fats: Chasing a global ban. *BMJ, 343*, d5567.

167. Ratnayake, W. M., L'Abbe, M. R., Farnworth, S., Dumais, L., Gagnon, C., Lampi, B., . . . Lombaert, G. A. (2009). Trans fatty acids: Current contents in Canadian foods and estimated intake levels for the Canadian population. *Journal of AOAC International, 92*(5), 1258–1276.

168. Kmietowicz, Z. (2012). EU law forces UK ministers to rethink food labelling. *BMJ, 344*, e3422.

169. European Food Information Council. (2017). *Global update on nutritional labelling.* Brussels, Belgium: Author. Retrieved from http://www.eufic.org/images/uploads/files/GUNL-2017 -exsummary.pdf

170. Roberto, C. A., Larsen, P. D., Agnew, H., Baik, J., & Brownell, K. D. (2010). Evaluating the impact of menu labeling on food choices and intake. *American Journal of Public Health, 100*(2), 312–318.

171. Bleich, S. N., Wolfson, J. A., Jarlenski, M. P., & Block, J. P. (2015). Restaurants with calories displayed on menus had lower calorie counts compared to restaurants without such labels. *Health Affairs, 34*(11), 1877–1884.

172. UK Department of Health and Social Care. (2012). *Calories to be capped and cut*. Retrieved from http://mediacentre.dh.gov.uk/2012/03/24/calories-to-be-capped-and-cut/

173. Scott, C., Hawkins, B., & Knai, C. (2017). Food and beverage product reformulation as a corporate political strategy. *Social Science & Medicine, 172*, 37–45.

174. Hawkes, C. (2007). Regulating and litigating in the public interest. Regulating food marketing to young people worldwide: Trends and policy drivers. *American Journal of Public Health, 97*(11), 1962–1973.

175. Cooksey-Stowers, K., Schwartz, M. B., & Brownell, K. D. (2017). Food swamps predict obesity rates better than food deserts in the United States. *International Journal of Environmental Research and Public Health, 14*(11), 1366.

176. World Health Organization (WHO). (2010). *Resolution WHA63.14: Marketing of food and non-alcoholic beverages to children*. Sixty-third World Health Assembly, May 21, 2010, Geneva, Switzerland. Geneva, Switzerland: Author. Retrieved from http://apps.who.int/gb/ebwha/pdf_files/WHA63/A63_R14-en.pdf

177. Kraak, V. I., Vandevijvere, S., Sacks, G., Brinsden, H., Hawkes, C., Barquera, S., . . . Swinburn, B. A. (2016). Progress achieved in restricting the marketing of high-fat, sugary and salty food and beverage products to children. *Bulletin of the World Health Organization, 94*(7), 540.

Hawkes, C., Smith, T. G., Jewell, J., Wardle, J., Hammond, R. A., Friel, S., . . . Kain, J. (2015). Smart food policies for obesity prevention. *The Lancet, 385*(9985), 2410–2421.

178. World Health Organization (WHO). (2010). *Global recommendations on physical activity for health*. Geneva, Switzerland: Author.

179. Nickelodeon. (n.d.). *Worldwide day of play*. Retrieved from http://www.worldwidedayofplay.com/

180. Huang, T. T. K., Cawley, J. H., Ashe, M., Costa, S. A., Frerichs, L. M., Zwicker, L., . . . Kumanyika, S. K. (2015, February 18). Mobilisation of public support for policy actions to prevent obesity. *The Lancet, 385*(9985), 2422–2431.

181. Pekka, P., Pirjo, P., & Ulla, U. (2002). Influencing public nutrition for non-communicable disease prevention: From community intervention to national programme—Experiences from Finland. *Public Health Nutrition, 5*(1a), 245–251.

182. Gortmaker, S. L., Peterson, K., Wiecha, J., Sobol, A., Dixit, S., Fox, M. K., & Laird, N. (1999). Reducing obesity via a school-based interdisciplinary intervention among youth: Planet Health. *Archives of Pediatrics and Adolescent Medicine, 153*(4), 409–418.

183. Dietz, W. H., Baur, L. A., Hall, K., Puhl, R. M., Taveras, E. M., Uauy, R., & Kopelman, P. (2015). Management of obesity: Improvement of health-care training and systems for prevention and care. *The Lancet, 385*(9986), 2521–2533.

184. Aamodt, S. (2016). *Why diets make us fat: The unintended consequences of our obsession with weight loss*. New York, NY: Current.

185. Gardner, C. D., Trepanowski, J. F., Del Gobbo, L. C., Hauser, M. E., Rigdon, J., Ioannidis, J. P., . . . King, A. C. (2018). Effect of low-fat vs low-carbohydrate diet on 12-month weight loss in overweight adults and the association with genotype pattern or insulin secretion: The DIETFITS randomized clinical trial. *JAMA, 319*(7), 667–679.

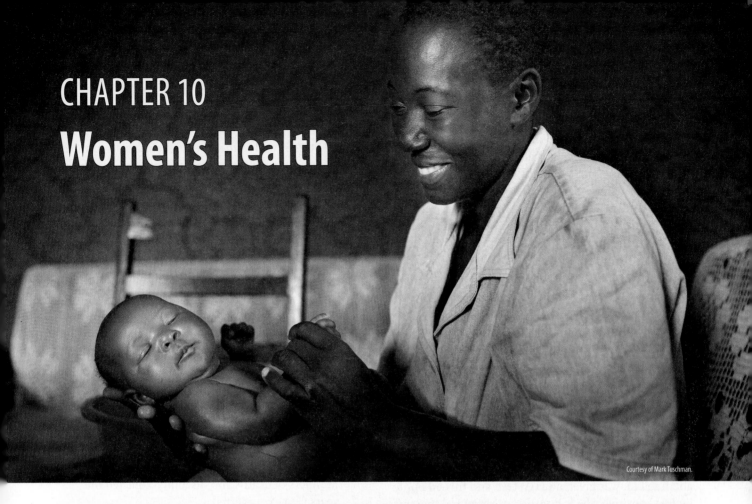

CHAPTER 10
Women's Health

Courtesy of Mark Tuschman.

LEARNING OBJECTIVES

By the end of this chapter, the reader will be able to do the following:

- Describe the importance of women's health to individuals, families, and communities
- Describe the determinants of women's health and how they vary in different settings
- Discuss the burden of disease for women worldwide, with a focus on women in low- and middle-income countries
- Describe critical challenges in improving women's health in low- and middle-income countries
- Describe some success stories in improving women's health and the lessons that can be applied to other women's health efforts

▶ Vignettes

Suneeta was pregnant with her first child. She lived in northern India, where many families prefer to have sons rather than daughters, especially for their firstborn child. Eager to have a son, Suneeta's husband took her to get a sonogram to determine the sex of the baby. When they learned the baby would be a girl, they decided that Suneeta should abort the fetus and try to get pregnant again in hopes of having a boy.

Sarah lived in rural Pakistan and was pregnant with her second child. When she went into labor, Sarah called for the traditional birth attendant, as most women did in her town. As Sarah's labor continued,

she and the birth attendant realized that the labor was complicated. Sarah needed to go to a hospital to deliver the baby. In this part of Pakistan, however, women could not be taken to hospitals without their husband's permission. Sarah's husband was working in another city and was not available to give such permission. Several hours later, Sarah and the baby died at Sarah's home.

Carmen lived in a slum in Guatemala City, Guatemala. She was not married but became pregnant after relations with a man she had met several months before. In her culture, pregnancy without being married was a source of great shame for a woman's family. Fearing the reaction of her family to her pregnancy,

261

Carmen decided to get an abortion. Although abortions are illegal in Guatemala, except to save the life of the mother,[1] they are performed there by both licensed physicians and unlicensed medical practitioners. Carmen could not afford the fee charged by a physician and went instead to an unlicensed abortionist. Carmen's abortion was not performed in a safe and hygienic manner. She bled profusely as a result of the procedure and she died before she could be taken to a hospital.

Elizabeth was a 15-year-old girl in Cape Town, South Africa. She was a good student but came from a poor family and was always short of the money she needed to pay for school supplies, uniforms, and books. John had been eyeing Elizabeth for some time. He was 25 years old, had a good job, and was always interested in spending time with the young ladies at Elizabeth's school. At the start of the second semester, when Elizabeth was trying to get the money for school, John convinced her to sleep with him in exchange for a small amount of money. Elizabeth knew about HIV, but John convinced her that he was healthy and there was no need to use a condom. About a year later, Elizabeth fell ill, was given an HIV test, and turned out to be HIV-positive. She is now on antiretroviral therapy.

Preeti is a 40-year-old woman who lives in Bengaluru, in southern India. She is well educated and comes from a middle-class family. Preeti has tried to "eat healthy" and ensure that her family does the same. Nonetheless, over the years more and more sugary beverages and processed foods have made their way into her family's diet. In fact, Preeti herself weighs substantially more than she would like to, now has obesity, and was recently diagnosed as having type 2 diabetes. With this, she has joined the increasing number of men and women in the world who have diabetes, including in low- and middle-income countries, and including many in middle age.

Rachel is a 60-year-old woman in Monrovia, the capital of Liberia. Rachel completed two years of secondary school and comes from a lower middle-class family. Rachel does not smoke tobacco or consume alcohol. However, over the years Rachel has become more and more sedentary and has had trouble managing her diet in light of the shortages of diverse foods and post-conflict economic difficulties. She also has mild obesity. Rachel was recently diagnosed with hypertension and a form of heart disease. Women in poor countries continue to face a substantial burden of maternal and communicable health conditions. At the same time, however, even in these countries, more and more women, like Rachel, are suffering from and dying from a range of noncommunicable causes, such as cardiovascular disease.

▶ The Importance of Women's Health

FIGURE 10-1, as well as the vignettes, suggests a number of important reasons why women's health issues must be given a prominent place in the global health agenda:

- Being born female can be dangerous to your health, especially in low- and middle-income countries.
- In many societies women are subjected to discrimination and very proscribed roles, both of which can be harmful to their health.
- Women face a number of unique health problems by virtue of their sex and their place in society.
- There are often important and unjustifiable differentials in the health of men and women.
- Morbidity, disability, and premature death of women can have enormous social and economic consequences on the affected women, on their families, and on society more broadly.
- Many relatively low-cost investments in the health of women would result in substantial numbers of deaths and disability-adjusted life years (DALYs) averted.
- Improving the education and health of women and their place in society is one of the most powerful and cost-effective approaches that can be taken to promote social and economic development.

In addition, the health of women is intimately linked with the Sustainable Development Goals (SDGs). **TABLE 10-1** indicates some of the most important such links.

This chapter aims to give the reader a sense of the following:

- The key health challenges facing women in low- and middle-income countries
- Which women are most affected by these challenges
- The most important risk factors for these challenges
- The social and economic consequences of selected health problems for women
- What can be done to address these problems in as cost-effective and fair a manner as possible

The chapter also includes comments on some of the key differences in the health of men and women worldwide. In addition, it contains a number of case studies that illustrate some of its main points. Other aspects of health that relate in particular ways to women are covered elsewhere in the text, specifically in the chapters on nutrition, communicable diseases, and noncommunicable diseases.

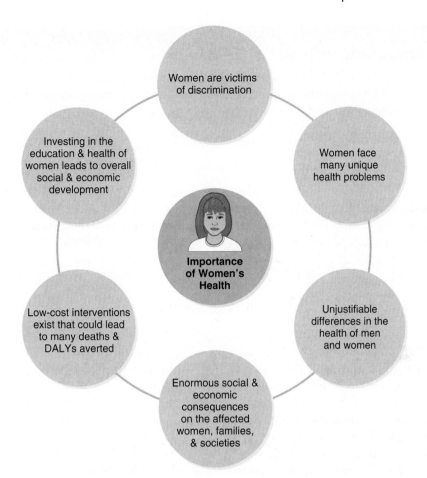

FIGURE 10-1 The Importance of Women's Health

Reproduced with permission from Session 14, Module 4 of Essentials of Global Health, Yale University/Coursera, 2016.

TABLE 10-1 Selected Links Between Women's Health and the SDG Health Targets
Target 3.1 By 2030, reduce the global maternal mortality ratio to less than 70 per 100,000 live births
This is directly linked to the health and well-being of women.
Target 3.2 By 2030, end preventable deaths of newborns and children under 5 years of age, with all countries aiming to reduce neonatal mortality to at least as low as 12 per 1,000 live births and under-5 mortality to at least as low as 25 per 1,000 live births.
Birth outcomes are directly linked to the health and well-being of women, their nutritional status, and their access to reproductive health services and emergency obstetric care of good quality. In addition, if a woman dies in childbirth in a low-income country, her child has only about a 50 percent chance of survival.
Target 3.3 By 2030, end the epidemics of AIDS, tuberculosis, malaria, and neglected tropical diseases and combat hepatitis, waterborne diseases, and other communicable diseases.
Especially in the lower-income countries, these communicable diseases remain important causes of morbidity, disability, and death for women.
Target 3.4 By 2030, reduce by one-third premature mortality from noncommunicable diseases through prevention and treatment and promote mental health and well-being.

(continues)

TABLE 10-1 Selected Links Between Women's Health and the SDG Health Targets	*(continued)*

The noncommunicable diseases and mental health disorders are important causes of morbidity, disability, and death for women everywhere. Women have higher risks and rates of some of these diseases and some mental health disorders and suicide than men do.

Target 3.5: Strengthen the prevention and treatment of substance abuse, including narcotic drug abuse and harmful use of alcohol.

Substance abuse, including the harmful use of alcohol, is an increasingly important cause of morbidity and mortality for women globally. Alcohol is also an important risk factor for a range of health conditions. Substance abuse can also have a deleterious impact on maternal health outcomes. For all of these reasons, and others, addressing substance abuse is fundamental to enhacing the health of women globally.

Target 3.6 By 2020, halve the number of global deaths and injuries from road traffic accidents.

Although men have higher rates of road traffic deaths than women, road traffic accidents are an important cause of disability and death for women as well.

Target 3.7 By 2030, ensure universal access to sexual and reproductive healthcare services, including for family planning, information and education, and the integration of reproductive health into national strategies and programs.

Family planning saves lives. Good quality reproductive health services that can assist families in making choices about family planning and provide maternal health care also save lives.

Target 3.8 Achieve universal health coverage, including financial risk protection, access to quality essential healthcare services, and access to safe, effective, quality, and affordable essential medicines and vaccines for all.

Universal health coverage that is of good quality, reduces out-of-pocket costs for the poor to a minimum, and is fairly prioritized and delivered can have a major impact on the health services most needed to enhance the health and well-being of women in low- and middle-income countries.

Target 3.9 By 2030, substantially reduce the number of deaths and illnesses from hazardous chemicals and air, water, and soil pollution and contamination.

Poor women in low-income countries are especially vulnerable to the detrimental health effects of ambient air pollution, unsafe water, and environmental contaminants.

▶ Key Definitions

As one reviews the most important health issues that affect women worldwide, a number of terms will be used repeatedly. The most important of these are shown in **TABLE 10-2**.

▶ The Determinants of Women's Health

The determinants of a woman's health relate to both **sex** and **gender**. "Sex is biological."[2(p205)] It has to do with being born a female. "Gender is cultural."[2(p205)]

Gender has to do with societal norms about the roles of women and their social position relative to men.[3] Some health issues are primarily determined by biology, such as the fact that women alone get ovarian cancer. Other women's health issues are determined mostly by social factors, such as sex-selective abortion of female fetuses. Most women's health issues, however, are determined by a combination of biological and social determinants, such as the case of Sarah in the opening vignettes, who died in childbirth for a number of biological and social reasons that interacted. Further comments are given now on the biological and social determinants of women's health.

TABLE 10-2 Selected Definitions in Women's Health

Abortion—The premature expulsion or loss of embryo, which may be induced or spontaneous.

Caesarean delivery (section)—The surgical delivery of a fetus through abdominal incision.

Eclampsia—A serious, life-threatening condition in late pregnancy in which very high blood pressure can cause a woman to have seizures.

Family planning—The conscious effort of couples to regulate the number and spacing of births through artificial and natural methods of contraception.

Female genital mutilation—Traditional practices that are all related to the cutting of the female genital organs.

Gestational diabetes—Diabetes that develops during pregnancy because of improper regulation of blood sugar.

Hemorrhage (related to pregnancy)—Significant and uncontrolled loss of blood, either internally or externally, from the body. Antepartum (prenatal) hemorrhage occurs after the 20th week of gestation but before delivery of the baby. Postpartum hemorrhage is the loss of 500 mL or more of blood from the genital tract after delivery of the baby. Primary postpartum hemorrhage occurs in the first 24 hours after delivery.

Maternal death—The death of a woman while pregnant, during delivery, or within 42 days of delivery.

Obstetric fistula—An injury in the birth canal that allows leakage from the bladder or rectum into the vagina, leaving a woman permanently incontinent.

Preeclampsia (previously called toxemia)—A condition characterized by pregnancy-induced high blood pressure, protein in the urine, and swelling (edema) due to fluid retention.

Sepsis—A serious medical condition caused by a severe infection, leading to a systemic inflammatory response.

Sex-selective abortion—The practice of aborting a fetus after a determination that the fetus is an undesired sex, typically female.

Modified from American Diabetes Association. (n.d.). *Gestational diabetes*. Retrieved from http://www.diabetes.org/diabetes-basics/gestational/
MedlinePlus. (n.d.). *Sepsis*. Retrieved from http://www.nlm.nih.gov/medlineplus/ency/article/000666.htm
Planned Parenthood. (n.d.). *Glossary*. Retrieved from http://www.plannedparenthood.org/learn/glossary
Smith, J. R. (2018). Postpartum hemorrhage. *Medscape*. Retrieved from http://emedicine.medscape.com/article/275038-overview
The World Bank. (n.d.). Data: Maternal mortality ratio (modeled estimate, per 100,000 live births). Retrieved from http://data.worldbank.org/indicator/SH.STA.MMRT

Biological Determinants

Women face a number of unique biological risks. One is iron deficiency anemia related to menstruation. Other risks are associated with pregnancy, including complications of pregnancy itself, diseases that may be aggravated by pregnancy, and the effects of some unhealthy lifestyle choices, such as smoking, on pregnancy.[4] During pregnancy, there are a number of conditions, for example, that can cause women to become ill or to die, including hypertensive disorders of pregnancy. In addition, a woman can be left with a number of permanent disabilities related to pregnancy, including uterine prolapse and obstetric fistula. Women can also die of preeclampsia or eclampsia. It is hemorrhage, however, that is the leading cause of maternal mortality. The conditions that can exacerbate pregnancy-related health risks include malaria, hepatitis, tuberculosis, malnutrition, and obesity, as well as certain mental health issues, such as depression. Unsafe abortions lead to significant morbidity and mortality for women. In terms of the effects of lifestyles on pregnancy, it is clear that certain occupations and the use of alcohol, tobacco, and certain drugs are especially important to avoid during pregnancy.[4]

Women are also biologically more susceptible to some sexually transmitted infections than men are, including to the HIV virus.[5] This relates to the fact that women have a greater mucosal area that is exposed during sexual relations than men have. There are also certain health conditions specific to women for biological reasons, such as uterine cancer or ovarian cancer, as mentioned previously. There are other health conditions that affect men, but for which women have a disproportionate share of the burden of disease, such as breast cancer. As women age, they also have a higher rate of heart disease than men have, although it is diagnosed far less frequently.[3]

Social Determinants

The social determinants of women's health are also very important, especially in societies that favor males. These social determinants relate predominantly to gender norms, which assign different roles and values to males and females, usually to the disadvantage of females. In many societies, women's inferior status leads to social, health, and economic problems that men do not face.

The social determinants of health begin even before women are born. In some societies where male preference is very strong, such as in India and in China, some families determine the sex of their unborn children with the use of sonograms and may then abort females, especially for the birth of their first child.[6,7] This was the case for Suneeta in one of the opening vignettes.[8]

Female infants are often breastfed less than boys of the same age and then fed less complementary food when they become toddlers.[9] In addition, young girls in many societies are also fed less than their male siblings. Older women in some cultures feed men first and then eat only the portions that are remaining. Others eat less nutritious food than the men in their family eat. Poor nutrition, often stemming partly from social causes, makes women more susceptible to illness. It also contributes to stunting and small pelvic size, which are hazards to the health of pregnant women and their offspring.

There are a number of critical social issues that relate to women's sexual experiences. The low social status of women in many societies is linked to the physical and sexual abuse of women. Furthermore, male dominance means that women often have a limited choice about when and how to have sexual relations, with whom, and whether or not to use protection. As a result, women are frequently forced to have sex, often at young ages, and many times without a condom or other contraceptives. For these social reasons, women face heightened risks of becoming pregnant, having repeated pregnancies at close intervals, and getting sexually transmitted infections, including HIV/AIDS. In addition, rape is common in many settings, especially in areas of conflict.

A **dowry** is the gift that a bride's family gives to the family of a groom, and another form of violence against women is **dowry death**. The data on mortality for young women in India suggest that there is

a disproportionate number of young married women who accidentally die of burns, which are often alleged to occur when women are cooking. It appears, however, that some of these deaths are not accidental. Rather, the husband's family sometimes perpetrates the burning of the young woman when they are not satisfied with the dowry that she has brought to her marriage.[10]

High levels of depression also appear to be related to the low status of women in different societies and the expectations that those societies have of them. There is also widespread reporting in many societies of general gynecologic discomfort without physical explanation, which may be related to the life stressors many women face.[2]

Especially in low-income populations, there are numerous households that are headed by females who are divorced, separated, or widowed, or by women whose husbands are working elsewhere. The poorest people in a community tend to live in these households. These women also tend to be among the least well-educated people in a community. Low income and limited education negatively impact the health of such women. In addition, divorced or widowed women face severe discrimination in a number of cultures.

The roles that women play in different cultures can also pose important hazards to their health. In many societies, for example, women cook indoors on open fires without adequate ventilation. This is strongly associated with respiratory problems for these women and for their children.

Poverty, lack of or low levels of education, and low social status of women in many societies seriously constrain the access of women to health services. In addition, girls and women who need health services often do not take advantage of such services in a timely way. There are numerous instances, for example, in which women cannot use health services without the permission of a husband or male relative or without having a male relative take them to health services. In some settings, even when women need emergency care, such as during complications of pregnancy, social constraints prevent them from seeking such care when their husbands are unable to take them for treatment, as reflected in the vignette about Sarah.

▶ The Burden of Health Conditions for Females

Having looked at some of the most important biological and social determinants of health for women, we can now look at some of the key health issues that females face, their prevalence, and the critical risk factors for those health conditions. We can also examine how the burden of disease affecting women is different from that which affects men. Much of the literature on the health of women in low- and middle-income countries has focused on reproductive health issues. If one wishes to see improvement in women's health, however, it is extremely important that one take a more holistic view of the burden of disease among women and what can be done to address that burden.

The Leading Causes of Death for Females

TABLE 10-3 shows the 10 leading causes of death for females of all ages by country income group for 2016.

This table suggests that ischemic heart disease, stroke, and COPD are important causes of death for females in low-income countries. However, it also illustrates the exceptional importance for females of all ages in these countries of communicable, maternal, perinatal and nutritional causes, also known as Group I causes. In the upper middle-income countries, noncommunicable diseases are more important causes of death for females than in the lower middle-income countries. Yet, Group I causes remain important causes of death, even in lower middle-income countries. The leading causes of death among females in upper middle-income and high-income countries are overwhelmingly noncommunicable. However, cancers are more important causes of death among females in the high-income countries than in the upper middle-income countries.

TABLE 10-4 shows the 10 leading causes of DALYs for females of all ages by World Bank country income group.

Table 10-4 mirrors Table 10-3 in many respects. The leading causes of DALYs for females in low-income countries are all Group I causes and include protein-energy malnutrition. Noncommunicable causes, including ischemic heart disease, stroke, low back and neck pain, sense organ disorders, and COPD are already among the leading causes of DALYs in lower middle-income countries, although a number of Group I causes remain important for these countries. All of the leading causes of DALYs in upper middle- and high-income countries are noncommunicable, except for injuries in the upper middle-income countries. For both sets of countries it is important to note that depressive disorders are among the leading causes of DALYs. In the high-income countries we also note that Alzheimer's disease is among the leading causes of DALYs.

TABLE 10-5 shows the leading risk factors for deaths for females of all age groups by World Bank country income group.

TABLE 10-3 Leading Causes of Death for Females, All Ages, by World Bank Country Income Group, 2016			
Low-Income		**Lower Middle-Income**	
Rank	**Cause**	**Rank**	**Cause**
1	Lower respiratory infection	1	Ischemic heart disease
2	Ischemic heart disease	2	Stroke
3	Diarrheal diseases	3	Diarrheal diseases
4	Stroke	4	Lower respiratory infection
5	Malaria	5	COPD
6	HIV/AIDS	6	Diabetes
7	Tuberculosis	7	Tuberculosis
8	COPD	8	Alzheimer's disease
9	Neonatal encephalopathy	9	Malaria
10	Neonatal preterm birth	10	Chronic kidney disease

(continues)

TABLE 10-3 Leading Causes of Death for Females, All Ages, by World Bank Country Income Group, 2016   (continued)

Upper Middle-Income		High-Income	
Rank	Cause	Rank	Cause
1	Ischemic heart disease	1	Ischemic heart disease
2	Stroke	2	Alzheimer's disease
3	Alzheimer's disease	3	Stroke
4	COPD	4	Lung cancer
5	Diabetes	5	COPD
6	Lung cancer	6	Lower respiratory infections
7	Lower respiratory infections	7	Breast cancer
8	Hypertensive heart disease	8	Colorectal cancer
9	Chronic kidney disease	9	Chronic kidney disease
10	Breast cancer	10	Diabetes

Data from Institute of Health Metrics and Evaluation (IHME). (n.d.). GBD Compare: Viz Hub. Retrieved from https://vizhub.healthdata.org/gbd-compare/

TABLE 10-4 Leading Causes of DALYs for Females, All Ages, by World Bank Country Income Group, 2016

Low-Income		Lower Middle-Income	
Rank	Cause	Rank	Cause
1	Malaria	1	Ischemic heart disease
2	Lower respiratory infections	2	Diarrheal diseases
3	Diarrheal diseases	3	Lower respiratory infections
4	HIV/AIDS	4	Stroke
5	Neonatal encephalopathy	5	Dietary iron deficiency
6	Neonatal preterm birth	6	Neonatal preterm birth
7	Tuberculosis	7	Malaria
8	Protein-energy malnutrition	8	Low back and neck pain
9	Congenital defects	9	Sense organ diseases
10	Meningitis	10	COPD

Upper Middle-Income		High-Income	
Rank	**Cause**	**Rank**	**Cause**
1	Ischemic heart disease	1	Low back and neck pain
2	Stroke	2	Ischemic heart disease
3	Low back and neck pain	3	Alzheimer's disease
4	Sense organ diseases	4	Stroke
5	Depressive disorders	5	Skin diseases
6	Diabetes	6	Sense organ diseases
7	Skin diseases	7	Migraine
8	Migraine	8	Depressive disorders
9	COPD	9	Diabetes
10	Road injuries	10	Lung cancer

Data from Institute of Health Metrics and Evaluation (IHME). (n.d.). GBD Compare: Viz Hub. Retrieved from https://vizhub.healthdata.org/gbd-compare/

Table 10-5 suggests the importance for all country income groups of high blood pressure and high fasting plasma glucose. However, in the lower-income countries, as we would expect, unsafe water, unsafe sanitation, and handwashing are also key risk factors. Household air pollution is also important in the lower-income countries, as are factors related to child growth failure and low birthweight. Unsafe water, household air pollution, and low birthweight are also important risk factors in lower middle-income countries. However, the other leading risk factors concern high blood pressure, diet, ambient particulate matter pollution, and impaired kidney function. As we move to countries with higher incomes, the risk factors overwhelmingly relate to diet, ambient particulate matter, and smoking.

As noted earlier, it is essential if one is to enable better health that one understand the following:

- The burden of disease for particular groups
- The risk factors for that burden
- Who is most affected by that burden

Only then can one determine in a data-driven manner what measures should be taken on a priority basis to reduce the burden of disease in fair and cost-effective ways.

It is true that maternal deaths are overwhelmingly preventable, occur largely in the poorest populations in the poorest countries, and are an important reflection of the extent to which different societies are inclusive and concerned about the well-being of their people, including their females. Thus, one must be especially concerned about reproductive and maternal health issues.

Yet, as noted earlier, to enhance the health of females globally, one must focus on women's health in a manner that goes beyond reproductive health. There remains an important number of women globally for whom the greatest risks are to Group I causes. However, there is a growing burden of disease from noncommunicable diseases that will also have to be addressed if the health of females, especially poorer females in low- and lower middle-income countries, is to be improved.

▶ Leading Causes of Death and DALYs, Males and Females Compared

TABLE 10-6 shows the leading causes of death by sex for all ages by World Bank country income group. **TABLE 10-7** shows the leading causes of DALYs by sex for all ages by World Bank country income group.

TABLE 10-5 Leading Risk Factors for Deaths for Females, All Ages, by World Bank Country Income Group, 2016

Rank	Low-Income	Lower Middle-Income	Upper Middle-Income	High-Income
1	High blood pressure	High blood pressure	High blood pressure	High blood pressure
2	Household air pollution	High fasting plasma glucose	High body mass index	High body mass index
3	Low birthweight and short gestation	Ambient particulate matter	High fasting plasma glucose	High fasting plasma glucose
4	Child growth failure	High total cholesterol	High total cholesterol	Smoking
5	Unsafe sex	High body mass index	Ambient particulate matter	High total cholesterol
6	Ambient particulate matter	Household air pollution	Smoking	Impaired kidney function
7	High fasting plasma glucose	Unsafe water	High sodium	Low whole grains
8	Unsafe water	Low birthweight and short gestation	Low whole grains	Ambient particulate matter
9	Unsafe sanitation	Impaired kidney function	Impaired kidney function	High sodium
10	Handwashing	Low fruit	Low nuts and seeds	Low physical activity

Data from Institute of Health Metrics and Evaluation (IHME). (n.d.). GBD Compare: Viz Hub. Retrieved from https://vizhub.healthdata.org/gbd-compare/

TABLE 10-6 Leading Causes of Death, All Ages, by Sex and World Bank Country Income Group, 2016

Rank	Low-Income		Lower Middle-Income	
	Female	Male	Female	Male
1	Lower respiratory infection	Lower respiratory infections	Ischemic heart disease	Ischemic heart disease
2	Ischemic heart disease	Diarrheal diseases	Stroke	Stroke
3	Diarrheal diseases	Ischemic heart disease	Diarrheal diseases	COPD
4	Stroke	Tuberculosis	Lower respiratory infection	Lower respiratory infections
5	Malaria	HIV/AIDS	COPD	Diarrheal diseases
6	HIV/AIDS	Malaria	Diabetes	Tuberculosis

7	Tuberculosis	Stroke	Tuberculosis	Road injuries
8	COPD	Neonatal encephalopathy	Alzheimer's disease	Diabetes
9	Neonatal encephalopathy	Road injuries	Malaria	Chronic kidney disease
10	Neonatal preterm birth	Protein-energy malnutrition	Chronic kidney disease	HIV/AIDS

	Upper Middle-Income		**High-Income**	
Rank	**Female**	**Male**	**Female**	**Male**
1	Ischemic heart disease	Ischemic heart disease	Ischemic heart disease	Ischemic heart disease
2	Stroke	Stroke	Alzheimer's disease	Lung cancer
3	Alzheimer's disease	COPD	Stroke	Stroke
4	COPD	Lung cancer	Lung cancer	Alzheimer's disease
5	Diabetes	Road injuries	COPD	COPD
6	Lung cancer	Liver cancer	Lower respiratory infections	Lower respiratory infections
7	Lower respiratory infections	Alzheimer's disease	Breast cancer	Colorectal cancer
8	Hypertensive heart disease	Stomach cancer	Colorectal cancer	Prostate cancer
9	Chronic kidney disease	Lower respiratory infections	Chronic kidney disease	Self-harm
10	Breast cancer	Chronic kidney disease	Diabetes	Chronic kidney disease

Data from Institute of Health Metrics and Evaluation (IHME). (n.d.). GBD Compare: Viz Hub. Retrieved from https://vizhub.healthdata.org/gbd-compare/

TABLE 10-7 Leading Causes of DALYs, All Ages, by Sex and World Bank Country Income Group, 2016

	Low-Income		**Lower Middle-Income**	
Rank	**Female**	**Male**	**Female**	**Male**
1	Malaria	Lower respiratory infections	Ischemic heart disease	Ischemic heart disease
2	Lower respiratory infections	Malaria	Diarrheal diseases	Lower respiratory infections

(continues)

TABLE 10-7 Leading Causes of DALYs, All Ages, by Sex and World Bank Country Income Group, 2016   (*continued*)

	Low-Income		Lower Middle-Income	
Rank	**Female**	**Male**	**Female**	**Male**
3	Diarrheal diseases	Diarrheal diseases	Lower respiratory infections	Diarrheal diseases
4	HIV/AIDS	HIV/AIDS	Stroke	Road injuries
5	Neonatal encephalopathy	Neonatal encephalopathy	Dietary iron deficiency	Stroke
6	Neonatal preterm birth	Tuberculosis	Neonatal preterm birth	Neonatal preterm birth
7	Tuberculosis	Neonatal preterm birth	Malaria	COPD
8	Protein-energy malnutrition	Protein-energy malnutrition	Low back and neck pain	Tuberculosis
9	Congenital defects	Meningitis	Sense organ diseases	Neonatal encephalopathy
10	Meningitis	Neonatal sepsis	COPD	Malaria
	Upper Middle-Income		**High-Income**	
Rank	**Female**	**Male**	**Female**	**Male**
1	Ischemic heart disease	Ischemic heart disease	Low back and neck pain	Ischemic heart disease
2	Stroke	Stroke	Ischemic heart disease	Low back and neck pain
3	Low back and neck pain	Road injuries	Alzheimer's disease	Lung cancer
4	Sense organ diseases	Low back and neck pain	Stroke	Stroke
5	Depressive disorders	Lung cancer	Skin diseases	Sense organ diseases
6	Diabetes	COPD	Sense organ diseases	Diabetes
7	Skin diseases	Sense organ diseases	Migraine	Road injuries
8	Migraine	Liver cancer	Depressive disorders	Self-harm
9	COPD	Diabetes	Diabetes	COPD
10	Road injuries	Interpersonal violence	Lung cancer	Skin diseases

Data from Institute of Health Metrics and Evaluation (IHME). (n.d.). GBD Compare: Viz Hub. Retrieved from https://vizhub.healthdata.org/gbd-compare/

When we examine deaths, we see the importance of ischemic heart disease and stroke for males and females in all country income groups. We also see the importance of cancers in upper middle- and high-income countries and how the importance of different cancers varies by sex and country income group. In addition, road injuries are consistently a higher ranked cause of death for males than for females. This relates largely to the fact that males drive more than females do in most low- and middle-income countries. In the low- and lower middle-income countries in which tuberculosis (TB) is still prevalent, it is a higher ranked cause of death for males than for females. This relates to the fact that males have a higher incidence rate of TB, for reasons that have not been fully explained. From the lower middle-income countries up, diabetes and Alzheimer's disease are higher ranked causes of death for females than for males.

When we look at the leading causes of DALYs for females and males, we again see the importance for both sexes of ischemic heart disease and stroke. However, we also see the higher ranking for females than for males of dietary iron deficiency, skin diseases, depressive disorders, back and neck pain, and Alzheimer's disease. As we would expect, considering the patterns of death, the DALYs attributable to road injuries and TB are higher ranked for males than for females.

▶ Selected Health Burdens for Females

The next section explores a number of health issues that are of particular concern for females, especially low-income females in low- and lower middle-income countries.

Sex-Selective Abortion

How common is sex-selective abortion worldwide? How many unborn children are affected? Sex-selective abortion appears to be more prevalent in India and China than in any other country.[11] A number of studies have been done of this phenomenon, and one study estimated that close to 10 million female fetuses were aborted in India over a recent 20-year period due to a preference for male offspring.[12] A more recent study concluded that India now has between 300,000 and 600,000 abortions of female fetuses each year, about 2 percent to 4 percent of all pregnancies with a female fetus. The study further concluded that from 2001 to 2010, 3 million to 6 million female fetuses were aborted due to sex-selection.[8]

An important consequence of sex-selective abortion is the skewed ratios of males to females in a number of countries. Naturally, one would expect that there would be about 105 males born for every 100 females. However, in India on average between 2013 and 2015, there were only 900 females born for every 1,000 males who were born. This varied from 967 in Kerala state, which is well-known for the relatively equal place of females in that society, to 831 in Haryana state, where the standing of females and the education level of the population is much lower than in Kerala. In addition, the ratio of females to males has been falling. There were, for example, 909 females born for every 1,000 males born in India in 2011.[13] It was estimated that in China in 2016, only 870 females were born for every 1,000 males. This is the lowest ratio of female-to-male births in the world.[14] This phenomenon used to be the case in a number of other countries, including Singapore and South Korea, but the sex ratios at birth in those countries are now closer to what one would naturally expect.[15]

There is considerable evidence worldwide that both family size and preferences for males generally decrease as income and education rise. Nonetheless, for much of India and China, as incomes and education have risen and as technology has become more available, some families have used their income, knowledge, and access to technology—ultrasound in this case—to express their preference for males by engaging in sex-selective abortion. In India, this takes place especially after the first-born child is a female.[8] The one-child policy in China, which was in effect for many years until recently, has almost certainly exacerbated the expression of male preference.

Female Genital Mutilation

Female genital mutilation (FGM) is sometimes called female genital cutting (FGC) or is referred to as female genital mutilation/cutting. The World Health Organization (WHO) has grouped female genital mutilation into four types, generally varying from excision of the prepuce, the fold of skin surrounding the clitoris, to excision of part or all of the external genitalia and the stitching and narrowing of the vaginal opening. There are also a variety of related practices, including pricking of the genitalia or using chemicals to narrow the vaginal opening.[16]

WHO has recently estimated that almost 200 million females worldwide have been cut, predominantly in 30 countries in which FGM is concentrated.[17] These countries are generally in west, east, or northeastern

Africa and selected countries in the Middle East and Asia. It was estimated until recently that half of the girls who undergo FGM will be cut before they are 5 years of age and the remainder will be cut before they are 15 years of age. The cutting is generally done with razor blades, knives, or glass.

WHO has also suggested that as many as 3 million girls annually may be at risk of FGM.[17] In some countries, such as Egypt, Guinea, and Somalia, female genital mutilation has been practically universal among women who are 15 to 49 years old. However, there are other countries in Africa, such as Cameroon, Niger, and Uganda, in which only a small share of the women have had FGM. Female genital mutilation is very closely related to ethnicity. In addition, the higher the level of education of the mother, the less likely the daughter is to be cut.[18]

The practice of FGM appears to be diminishing in Africa, but staying around the same level in Asia. In fact, the most recent study of FGM prevalence suggested that the prevalence of FGM has fallen substantially in Africa over the last 2 to 3 decades[19]:

- From 71 percent in 1995 to 8 percent in 2016 in East Africa
- From 74 percent in 1996 to 25 percent in 2017 in West Africa
- From 58 percent in 1990 to 4 percent in 2015 in North Africa

When FGM is performed initially, it can result in terrible pain or shock. It is also associated with infection because the instruments used for cutting are not always clean, as well as with acute hemorrhage. Over the longer term, it can lead to the retention of urine, infertility, and obstructed labor. Studies have shown that those more severely cut are more likely than others to have postpartum hemorrhage, caesarean section, and long stays in hospital. In addition, the babies of such women are more likely than babies born to mothers who have not undergone FGM to need resuscitation immediately after birth, to be stillborn or to die a neonatal death.[20] If infection and hemorrhage linked to the act of FGM are not addressed in a timely and appropriate manner, FGM can also lead to death.[16]

Sexually Transmitted Infections

This section briefly addresses sexually transmitted infections (STIs) other than HIV. It is important as one reviews this section to note that women are more biologically susceptible to sexually transmitted infections and their impact because they have more exposed mucosal surfaces, because they often show no symptoms of those diseases, and because their roles in society make them less likely to get treated for sexually transmitted infections than men.

WHO estimates that each year there are over 350 million new infections with one of four STIs: chlamydia, gonorrhea, syphilis, and trichomoniasis. WHO further estimates that more than 500 million people worldwide have an infection with herpes simplex virus (HSV) and that more than 250 million women are infected with human papilloma virus (HPV). It has also been estimated that almost 900,000 pregnant women are infected with syphilis.[21]

The Global Burden of Disease Study includes estimates of the burden of disease from STIs other than HIV. That study suggests that in 2016 these infections were responsible for the following percentages of DALYs in females[22]:

- 1 percent of DALYs in low-income countries
- 0.5 percent of DALYs in lower middle-income countries
- 0.2 percent of DALYs in upper middle-income countries
- Less than 0.1 percent of DALYs in high-income countries

Females in sub-Saharan Africa have a burden of disease from STIs, other than HIV, that is 3 to 5 times higher than the burden females face in the other World Bank regions.[22]

From the limited studies available, the prevalence of chlamydia, gonorrhea, and syphilis appears to vary widely. Earlier studies done in China showed that rates of chlamydia in different parts of China ranged from 1 percent to 24 percent.[23] Studies done in other parts of Asia indicated that the prevalence of syphilis ranged from almost negligible to about 15 percent.[23] Studies done in sub-Saharan Africa have shown ranges for chlamydia from 2 percent to 30 percent, for gonorrhea from 2 percent to 32 percent, and for syphilis from almost negligible to 23 percent.[23]

Young people are at special risk of STIs because they are often forced to have sex, their sexual relations are often unplanned, and they may not have the power or skills to use a condom.[20]

The risk factors for a woman getting an STI are well known and include young age when engaging in sexual relations, often because of child marriage, especially in Asia and sub-Saharan Africa; multiple sexual partners; sex with high-risk partners, including partners considerably older than the woman; and inability to use a condom. The use of alcohol and drugs is also associated with unprotected sex, as is unequal power between the woman and the man who are engaging in sexual relations.

Sexually transmitted infections other than HIV that are not treated in a timely and appropriate manner can have a number of long-lasting effects on the health of women. These include pelvic inflammatory disease, chronic pain, ovarian abscesses, ectopic pregnancies, and infertility.[23] When pregnant women cannot get STIs treated in appropriate and timely ways, it can lead to fetal wastage, stillbirths, low birthweight babies, eye and lung damage in babies, and congenital abnormalities.[23] In fact, recent estimates suggest that syphilis in pregnancy results in 305,000 fetal and neonatal deaths annually.[24] In addition, the complications of syphilis can lead to the death of the infected person.[23] HPV is associated with cervical cancer[23]; there are an estimated 530,000 cases of HPV a year and HPV causes about 270,000 cervical cancer deaths a year.[21] Chlamydia bears special mention because it is nine times more prevalent in women than in men.[3] Chlamydia is very prevalent in low-income countries and is associated with chronic conjunctivitis, reproductive tract infections, genital ulcer disease, and infertility.[3]

Violence and Sexual Abuse Against Women

Violence and sexual abuse against women occur with remarkable frequency throughout the world. Violence is usually episodic, it is often not reported, and it is often associated with sexual abuse.[9] Sexual abuse can include rape, sexual assault, sexual molestation, sexual harassment, and incest.[25] It is very hard to get reliable data on violence and sexual abuse against women. However, a 2006 UNAIDS study suggested that 10 percent to 50 percent of women worldwide have been abused physically by an intimate partner

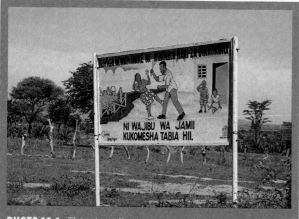

PHOTO 10-1 This sign discourages violence against women. Changing norms about intimate partner violence is very difficult to do. Are there examples from any country of widespread change in such norms? If so, what factors contributed to such change? If not, why not?
Courtesy of Mark Tuschman.

at least once in their lives. The UNAIDS study also noted that "between 20–48% of adolescent girls aged 10–25 report their first sexual encounter was forced."[26] Another study on intimate partner violence indicated that "one-third of women have been beaten, coerced into sex, or subjected to extreme emotional abuse."[27(p159)] The most recent WHO estimates of intimate partner violence suggest the following[28]:

- About 35 percent of all women have been subject to sexual violence and or physical violence from an intimate partner or nonpartner.
- About 30 percent of all women worldwide have been subject to intimate partner violence, although in some regions this is close to 40 percent.
- Thirty-eight percent of all women who are murdered are murdered by intimate partners.
- Seven percent of all women have been subjected to sexual violence by someone who was not an intimate partner.

In addition, there have been a number of conflicts in which rape has been used systematically, as a "weapon of war."[29]

Violence and abuse against women have a number of negative consequences for the health of women. These include injuries, unwanted pregnancies, STIs, depression, and sometimes permanent disability or death.[4] The risk factors for whether or not a woman will suffer intimate partner violence can be complicated, are often a result of many factors, and are not well-documented. However, it appears that such violence is associated with factors such as young age of the male partner, a history of violence of the male partner, low socioeconomic status of the male and female involved, proximity to drugs or alcohol, social isolation, and gender inequality. The likelihood of violence is heightened in conflict and post conflict situations.[30]

Maternal Morbidity and Mortality

WHO estimates that about 300,000 maternal deaths occurred in 2015, meaning deaths that occur during pregnancy, during childbirth, or until 42 days after the baby is born.[31,32] From 1990 to 2015, it is estimated that the number of maternal deaths that occur annually declined by about 44 percent, which represented a decline of about 2.3 percent annually over that period. Although this was important progress, it was less than the rate of annual decline that was needed to achieve the Millennium Development Goal (MDG) concerning maternal mortality.[31]

About 99 percent of these maternal deaths occur in low- and middle-income countries. Sub-Saharan

Africa accounts for more than half of these deaths and South Asia for about one-third of them.[31] One-third of the maternal deaths occur in India and Nigeria. Ten countries account for almost 60 percent of all maternal deaths: India, Nigeria, Democratic Republic of the Congo, Ethiopia, Pakistan, Tanzania, Kenya, Indonesia, Uganda, and Bangladesh.[33]

TABLE 10-8 shows the maternal mortality ratio by World Bank region and country income group and the lifetime chance of maternal death in those regions and income groups.

The risk of maternal death is a stark reflection of the disparities in the health status between different countries and within those countries. The maternal mortality ratio in sub-Saharan Africa is more than 40 times that in North America. A woman in South Asia faces a lifetime risk of a maternal death that is more than 20 times that in North America. For a woman in sub-Saharan Africa that risk is more than 100 times greater. The maternal mortality ratio in low-income countries is around 30 times the ratio in high-income countries. Women in low-income countries face a lifetime risk of maternal death that is about 80 times greater than the risk faced by women in high-income countries.

FIGURE 10-2 illustrates the maternal mortality ratio by country in 2015.

One can see in Figure 10-2 the substantial number of countries in sub-Saharan Africa that have a maternal mortality ratio above 300 per 100,000 live births, including a large number with ratios above 500. Afghanistan and Yemen, both very poor countries, are the only countries outside sub-Saharan Africa with maternal mortality ratios above 300.

Birth is the time of greatest risk for the mother and the baby. Studies suggest that 42 percent of maternal deaths happen during birth or the first day after birth[34] and that between 50 percent and 71 percent of maternal deaths occur in the postpartum period, with most of those occurring in the first week after birth.[4]

There are both indirect and direct causes of maternal death. About 28 percent of maternal deaths are from obstructed labor and indirect causes, meaning diseases that complicate pregnancy or that are

TABLE 10-8 Maternal Mortality Ratio and Lifetime Risk of Dying a Maternal Death, by Region and World Bank Income Group, 2015

Region	Maternal Mortality Ratio	Lifetime Risk of Dying a Maternal Death (1 in X)
Sub-Saharan Africa	547	36
South Asia	182	200
Middle East and North Africa	91	350
Latin America and the Caribbean	69	670
East Asia and Pacific	63	860
Europe and Central Asia	25	1,900
North America	13	4,100
Income Group		
Low-Income	495	41
Lower Middle-Income	253	130
Upper Middle-Income	55	970
High-Income	17	3,300

Reproduced from WHO, UNICEF, UNFPA, The World Bank, and the United Nations Population Division. (2015). *Trends in maternal mortality: 1990 to 2015*. Geneva, Switzerland: World Health Organization.

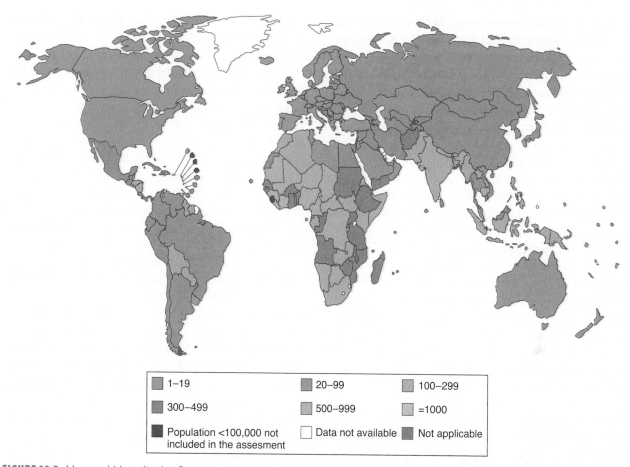

FIGURE 10-2 | 1–19 | | 20–99 | | 100–299 |

Legend:
- 1–19
- 20–99
- 100–299
- 300–499
- 500–999
- =1000
- Population <100,000 not included in the assesment
- Data not available
- Not applicable

FIGURE 10-2 Maternal Mortality by Country, 2015

Reproduced from WHO, UNICEF, UNFPA, The World Bank, and the United Nations Population Division. (2015). *Trends in maternal mortality: 1990 to 2015*. Geneva, Switzerland: World Health Organization.

complicated by pregnancy. These include malaria, anemia, HIV/AIDS, and cardiovascular disease.[4] The importance of these problems depends on the presence of these diseases in different communities and how effective the health system is in responding to them. About 70 percent of maternal deaths stem from direct causes, including hemorrhage, infection, and hypertensive disorders. Unsafe abortion is also an important contributor to maternal death.[31,35] **FIGURE 10-3** indicates the major causes of maternal death and the share of maternal deaths in low- and middle-income countries that are associated with them.

There are a number of risk factors for maternal death. Among the first are the nutritional status and general health status of the mother. Similarly, being of short stature is an important risk factor for maternal death. There is also a very strong correlation between maternal death and the level of education and income of the mother. Clearly, well-educated women with comfortable incomes do not suffer many maternal deaths, while uneducated and poor women do suffer such deaths. Maternal death also varies with ethnicity and location, with rural women being at greater risk than urban dwellers. The risk of maternal death is also

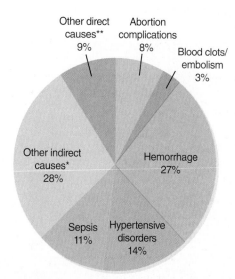

Other direct causes** 9%
Abortion complications 8%
Blood clots/ embolism 3%
Other indirect causes* 28%
Hemorrhage 27%
Other indirect causes* 28%
Sepsis 11%
Hypertensive disorders 14%

** Other direct causes include complications of delivery, obstructed labor, and "other direct causes"
* Other indirect causes include HIV-related causes, preexisting medical condition that are exacerbated during pregnancy, and "other indirect causes"

FIGURE 10-3 Maternal Death by Cause, Low- and Middle-Income Countries, Percentage Distribution

Data from Say, L., Chou, D., Gemmil, A., Tunçalp, Ö., Moller, A. B., Daniels, J., . . . Alkema, L. (2014). Global causes of maternal death: A WHO systematic analysis. *Lancet Global Health, 2*(6), e323–e333.

associated, among other things, with childbirth by adolescents,[9] women having their first child,[36] women having more than five children,[36] and childbirth at ages older than 35 years.[36] Short intervals between the births of subsequent children are also a risk factor for maternal death. Having a birth attended by a skilled healthcare provider and having access to emergency obstetric care are important to successful outcomes of pregnancy. In addition, consumption of alcohol, tobacco, and drugs during pregnancy can be harmful to both mother and child. Malaria and HIV/AIDS also pose substantial risks to pregnancy outcomes.

Maternal deaths are also more likely when women face what has been called "the three delays," which can occur at various levels: "the delay in deciding to seek care; the delay in identifying and reaching a medical facility; the delay in receiving appropriate care at health facilities."[37] This framework is discussed again later in the chapter.

Unsafe Abortion

A critical issue concerning abortions is whether they are safe or unsafe. WHO defines safe abortion as those abortions that are performed "by trained healthcare providers, with proper equipment, correct technique, and sanitary standards."[4] Unsafe abortions are essentially the opposite of that definition—performed by an untrained provider, with inappropriate equipment, poor technique, and unhygienic conditions.[4]

The latest estimates suggest that about 25 percent of all pregnancies end with an induced abortion and that about 56 million induced abortions took place each year between 2010 and 2014. The rate of induced abortion is higher in low- and middle-income countries than in high-income countries. Each year there are about 35 induced abortions for every 1,000 women of reproductive age, 15 to 44 years of age.[38]

It is thought that about 55 percent of all abortions are safe but that around 45 percent are unsafe. Almost all of the unsafe abortions take place in low- and middle-income countries. Moreover, it is estimated that 75 percent of the abortions in Africa and Latin America are unsafe, and that about one-third of all unsafe abortions are carried out in what WHO calls "dangerous" conditions.[38]

Fewer than 1 woman per 100,000 who has a safe abortion will die as a result of the abortion. The mortality rate for unsafe abortions, however, is at least 100 times greater, although it varies widely by country, from about 30 per 100,000 such abortions to about 520 per 100,000.[4,38] About 7 million women a year are admitted to hospitals as a result of unsafe abortion, and it has been estimated that between 5 and 13 percent of all maternal deaths can be attributed to unsafe abortions.[38] **FIGURE 10-4** indicates the share of all abortions by region that are unsafe.

Obstetric Fistula

An obstetric fistula is a condition in which a hole opens up in a woman between the bladder and the vagina or between the rectum and the vagina. It is usually the result of prolonged or failed childbirth.

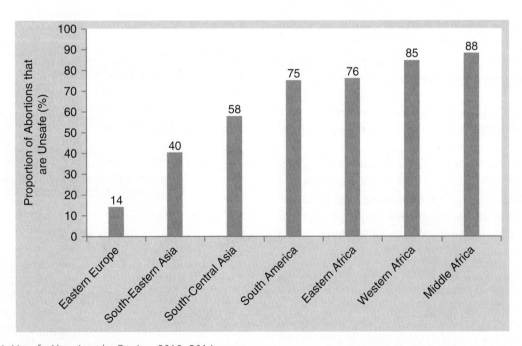

FIGURE 10-4 Unsafe Abortions by Region, 2010–2014

Data from Ganatra, B., Gerdts, C., Rossier, C., Johnson Jr, B. R., Tunçalp, Ö., Assifi, A., . . . Bearak, J. (2017). Global, regional, and subregional classification of abortions by safety, 2010–14: Estimates from a Bayesian hierarchical model. *The Lancet, 390*(10110), 2372–2381.

As a consequence, urine or feces leak through the vagina. Obstetric fistula can have severe social and economic consequences, because women with fistula are often terribly stigmatized or abandoned.[39]

It is difficult to get good estimates of the number of women who suffer from obstetric fistula every year. Studies suggest that for every 100,000 births, between 50 and 80 women in sub-Saharan Africa, North Africa, and west and South Asia, and about 30 women in Latin America and China, suffer a fistula.[40] At these rates, about 50,000 to 100,000 women each year will suffer a fistula.[41] It is thought that about 2 million women worldwide are living with fistula.[41]

The risk factors for fistula are those that are linked with an obstructed delivery, which is the precipitating factor for a fistula. These include undernutrition, young age at first birth, and having had multiple births. In addition, female genital mutilation and some traditional practices that damage the birth canal can also cause prolonged labor and lead to fistula. Fistula can also result from trauma, such as rape or sexual violence. The lack of access to emergency obstetric care and the failure to make use of such care, if available, also contribute to the prevalence of fistula.[41]

▶ The Costs and Consequences of Women's Health Problems

Women's health issues have enormous social costs. Violence against girls and women tends to isolate them socially. When a woman dies in childbirth, the social impacts are enormous. In most societies, women are the primary caregivers for children; therefore, when a mother dies, the death usually has a profound impact on the health of her children, with young children often dying soon thereafter. The social costs of some problems are particularly high. For example, women who have obstetric fistula are often socially isolated from their community.

Women are stigmatized for a variety of communicable diseases as well, such as TB, HIV/AIDS, and some of the neglected tropical diseases. There are also exceptional economic costs related to women's nutritional and health conditions, but these are not often given the attention they deserve. The costs of violence against women, especially in low-income countries, have not been studied carefully, but they are substantial. A study in Chile, for example, suggested that the costs of domestic violence were equal to 2 percent of Chile's gross domestic product (GDP). A similar study in Nicaragua indicated that such violence cost 1.6 percent of GDP. A review of intimate partner violence in the United States indicated that it led, in a single year, to 2 million injuries and about $6 billion in costs.[30]

The economic costs of maternal health conditions are also high but not well-documented. They also often fail to take account of morbidity associated with maternal health and not just mortality. These morbidities can seriously constrain women's productivity both in and outside the home. They can also significantly reduce the income that women can earn. When a woman dies a premature maternal death, the economic losses are substantial, given the many years that the woman could have engaged in care of her family and worked inside and outside the home. In addition, the death of a mother will likely damage the future prospects for economic well-being and economic contributions of any children who survive her. Illness associated with maternal conditions seriously constrains women's productivity and reduces the income they can contribute to their family. Similarly, depression in women also has high economic costs.

▶ Case Studies

Two case studies follow. The first case study examines maternal mortality in Sri Lanka. This case is significant because many other countries have made only modest progress over the last 20 years in reducing maternal mortality and have not been able to put into place what has been learned elsewhere. The second case examines the well-known story of efforts in Bangladesh to encourage family planning.

Maternal Mortality in Sri Lanka[42]
Background

Sri Lanka has had an impressive history of public-sector commitment to education and health, even when its income per capita was low. The female literacy rate in Sri Lanka for many years was more than double the South Asian average, and free health services have been available in rural areas since the 1930s.[42] Another unusual strength of Sri Lanka is that it has a good civil registration system that has recorded maternal deaths since about 1900.[43]

Interventions

Sri Lanka has taken a number of steps to reduce maternal deaths. First, Sri Lanka improved access to health services. Starting in the 1930s, Sri Lanka established health facilities throughout the country that were staffed by medical officers. In addition, Sri Lanka expanded secondary and tertiary facilities in the 1950s and around the same time established a working ambulance service.

Second, as early as the 1940s, Sri Lanka introduced policies to expand the number of midwives, who were the frontline workers dealing with pregnant women and childbirth. The focus on midwifery and on promoting easy access to higher-level health services in Sri Lanka has contributed to a wide acceptance by women and their families of giving birth with the assistance of a trained midwife at home or in the hospital. Midwives in Sri Lanka today serve a population of 3,000 to 5,000 people, and they provide an invaluable link between the local community and the health system.

Another step that Sri Lanka took to reduce maternal deaths was to make use of its civil registration data to identify what areas of the country had the most significant problems with maternal mortality. On this basis, the government was able to target its efforts to especially vulnerable groups, including women who were isolated both physically and socially, such as on retlatively isolated tea estates. The government coupled these efforts with continuous activities, starting in the 1960s, to ensure that the quality of maternal health services was always appropriate. The lessons learned from individual maternal deaths, for example, were disseminated throughout the health system so that the quality of services could be improved and errors in dealing with obstetric problems could be reduced.

At the same time, the government made considerable progress in other health areas. This included efforts to improve health by improving sanitation and by measures to combat malaria and hookworm. These actions also contributed to improved health and lowered maternal mortality rates.

Impact

As a result of these efforts, Sri Lanka halved maternal deaths every 6 to 12 years between 1935 and 2008. This meant a decline in the maternal mortality ratio from between 500 and 600 maternal deaths per 100,000 live births in 1950 to 29 per 100,000 more recently.[44,45] Skilled medical practitioners now attend 97 percent of the births in Sri Lanka, compared with 30 percent in 1940.

One very important point to note about Sri Lanka is that it has achieved better maternal health outcomes than many countries that have higher per capita incomes or spend more on health than Sri Lanka. Low-cost, but dedicated and well-trained health personnel, including midwives, helped make the expansion of access to health care in Sri Lanka affordable.

Lessons

Sri Lanka's success in reducing maternal deaths can be attributed to widespread access to maternal health care, including emergency obstetric care, built upon a strong health system that provides free services to the entire population. The professionalism and broad use of midwives, the systematic use of health information to identify problems and guide decision making, and targeted quality improvements for vulnerable groups were also ingredients for success. Sri Lanka's tradition of public-sector commitment to human development created conditions where gains were reinforced by good education, an emphasis on gender equity, the promotion of family planning, and a coordinated network of health services. Although factors such as the introduction of antibiotics and national efforts against malaria helped lower maternal mortality ratios, it was the step-by-step actions of the government rather than better living conditions alone that led to most of the improvements in maternal health. Sri Lanka's success offers important lessons for other low- and middle-income countries that have unacceptably high levels of maternal deaths. Detailed information on this case is available in *Case Studies in Global Health: Millions Saved.*[46]

Reducing Fertility in Bangladesh
Background

Despite the existence of several family planning methods, more than 150 million women in low- and middle-income countries who wish to limit or space childbearing do not use contraception. In Bangladesh, where more than half the women have been illiterate until recently and where cultural traditions favor large families, each woman had, on average, almost seven children in the mid-1970s, thereby jeopardizing her health and that of her children. For a country with the world's highest population density and where almost 80 percent of the people lived in poverty, it became clear that lowering population growth would be very important.

The Intervention

In 1975, the government of Bangladesh launched a program to reduce the national birth rate. The program had four components. First, young, married women were trained as outreach workers to visit women at home and offer information and contraceptive services. The number of these family welfare assistants (FWAs) eventually exceeded 40,000. Their outreach surpassed all expectations, with virtually all Bangladeshi women having been contacted at least once by an FWA, including many women isolated by cultural practices, geographical location, or poor transportation. The second element of the program was the provision of a wide range of family planning methods through a well-managed distribution system. The third component was the establishment of thousands of family planning clinics in rural areas to which outreach workers could refer clients for long-term family planning methods such as sterilization. The fourth element was the information, education, and communication (IEC) campaign. The IEC program successfully tailored its message to achieve different aims, such as persuading men to talk to their wives about contraception and winning social acceptance for FWAs by creating a story about a compelling soap opera heroine who eventually becomes an FWA. In fact, the IEC campaign's remarkable success has inspired similar mass media initiatives in other countries such as Kenya, Tanzania, and Brazil.[47]

The government's program evolved substantially over time, benefiting greatly from the existence of the Matlab Health Research Center that has operated for more than 40 years as a site for large-scale research on the operation of health, nutrition, and family planning programs. Within villages in the Matlab area, researchers have tested various approaches to the delivery of health services. Matlab evaluations have shaped maternal and child health programs in Bangladesh and in many other countries.

The Impact

The program resulted in virtually all women in Bangladesh becoming aware of family planning options. Contraceptive use increased from 8 percent in the mid-1970s to about 50 percent by 2007, and fertility declined from 6.3 births per woman in the early 1970s to about 3.3 in the mid-1990s.[48] Although other factors such as increased education and employment opportunities for women also increased demand for contraception, the family planning program has been shown to have had an independent effect on attitudes and behaviors.[49]

Costs and Benefits

The program is estimated to have cost about $100 million to $150 million per year, with more than half the funding coming from the United States Agency for International Development (USAID), the United Nations Development Programme (UNDP), the World Bank, and other agencies. Efforts are underway to increase program efficiency. The most expensive program component is that of FWAs, who were once critical to program success but are now valued by clients more as a convenience than as an essential source of information.[50] Research suggests that the most cost-effective strategy for the continued promotion of family planning is a fixed site approach that provides health and family planning services from clinics, complemented with targeted outreach to hard-to-reach clients.[51] However, some of those involved in women's health believe that "doorstep delivery" by FWAs would continue to be cost-effective if the FWAs delivered not only family planning but also other messages on sexual and reproductive health, such as safe motherhood, STIs, and HIV/AIDS. They also note the benefits of the FWAs as role models for women's status in rural areas.[25]

Lessons Learned

The success of the program can be attributed to four main factors. The first was political commitment on the part of Bangladesh and the international agencies involved. The second was the broad use of FWAs, who carried the program's message into almost every home, however isolated. The third was the excellent use of mass media strategies to target audiences and change behavior. The fourth was the research and data provided by the Matlab Center that helped to constantly identify problems and improve the program. Although the program still faces a number of challenges, Bangladesh is one of the few low-income countries to have reduced fertility rapidly without resorting to coercive measures. More detailed information on this case is available in *Case Studies in Global Health: Millions Saved.*[46]

▶ Addressing Future Challenges

The Place of Women in Society

The health of females is a powerful reflection of biological susceptibility and gender norms that assign certain roles, restrictions, and values to females, compared to males. It also reflects the fact that the health systems in many countries have profound gender gaps and cannot or do not serve effectively the health needs of females. In this light, improving the health of females, especially in low- and middle-income countries, will require attention to an array of social and public health measures.

One future challenge will be to improve the nutritional status of females, because it is poor nutrition *in utero* and from infancy that can later lead to women becoming stunted, not reaching their full biological potential, and experiencing a variety of health conditions.

Another challenge that is central to the long-term improvement in the health of females is access to education. The empowerment of females socially is strongly associated with their level of education. Empowerment will improve the status of females and reduce the extent to which discrimination against them hurts their health. In addition, education improves access to important health information that can make a difference in women's and children's health. The education of females is among the most powerful contributors to overall development, as well.

Major changes must also be made in the perception that communities have of female roles and the health of females. This will require significant efforts at the level of communities and populations as a whole to put greater value on women's health. This will help to reduce the abortion of female fetuses and ensure that women in obstructed labor do not die because they lack appropriate and timely medical attention.

A continuing challenge will also be to put greater emphasis on the health of females as people, rather than as just women who give birth. This would encourage policymakers to take a number of steps that are essential to improving the health of females globally, including gaining a better understanding of the health conditions affecting females and what can be done about them and making the health of females central to all health efforts. In addition, in many cultures, females are constrained in dealing with male medical workers, so it is also very important to train more female health workers and to deploy them appropriately to the places where they are most needed.

Addressing the Burden of Disease

More broadly speaking, it is clear that women, especially in the low- and middle-income countries, continue to suffer from an unacceptable burden of Group I causes: communicable diseases, nutritional deficiencies, and maternal causes. At the same time, however, women in those same countries face a growing burden of noncommunicable diseases, which have already been the leading causes of deaths and DALYS in high-income countries for a substantial period of time.

Enhancing the health of women, especially poorer women in low- and middle-income countries, will require a multifaceted approach. First must be the enhancement of nutritional status. Second must be the effective implementation of cost-effective approaches to reduce the burden of communicable diseases. Third, there must be much greater access to family planning, to prenatal care of appropriate quality, and to emergency obstetric care of good quality. Efforts will also have to be made to stem the growth of and the existing burden of noncommunicable diseases. This must include a package of efforts related to improving diet, reducing hypertension, treating diabetes, and preventing heart disease and stroke through cost-effective interventions.

FIGURE 10-5 summarizes selected measures for addressing some of the most important general health burdens that women face in low- and middle-income countries.

Cardiovascular and Cerebrovascular Disease
• Control hypertension
• Reduce obesity
• Address diabetes
• Increase physical activity

Mental Health
• Improve women's status in society and reduce gender disparities
• Offer community-based psychosocial support
• Implement an effective system for referrals
• Increase availability of modern generic drugs

Malaria
• Promote use of bednets
• Promote indoor residual spraying
• Provide intermittent preventative treatment to pregnant women
• Confirm diagnosis and treat with ACT

HIV/AIDS
• Delay sexual debut & reduce the number of partners
• Promote condom use
• Male medical circumcision
• Test & treat

Tuberculosis
• Encourage case-finding in women
• Raise cure rates
• Implement patient-centered TB care
• Treat drug-resistant TB

Sexually Transmitted Infections
• Delay age of sexual debut
• Empower women to negotiate safe sex
• Promote girls' education
• Promptly diagnose and treat STIs

Female Genital Mutilation
• Mobilize and educate communities to change social norms
• Take account of local cultural, geographical, ethnic, and socioeconomic factors influencing practices

FIGURE 10-5 Selected Interventions to Improve Women's Health

▶ Further Measures to Enhance the Health of Women

The next section comments further on measures that can be taken to deal with some of the particular health problems discussed previously, such as female genital mutilation, sexually transmitted infections, violence against women, and other reproductive health issues, including maternal mortality, unsafe abortion, and fistula.

Female Genital Mutilation

It is important to ensure that efforts to promote change are specifically tailored to local practices and to local beliefs. Linking these efforts with other measures that promote female empowerment, female education, and female control over economic resources will also be needed. FGM is intimately linked with deep-seated local beliefs and traditions that vary with ethnicity, education, income, and location. Only by taking account of these underlying issues will one be able to address FGM.[16]

Violence Against Women

We have already discussed the extent to which violence against women is usually a result of a complex set of factors and the interactions among them. Although there is increasing evidence on the factors linked to violence against women, there is little evidence about what works to reduce such violence and what the most cost-effective approaches are to doing so, especially in low- and middle-income countries.

Some studies have shown that protecting women against violence through legislation, as has been done in the United States and some other high-income countries, can have important positive effects in some settings. Shelters for abused women can also be used to reduce violence against them. Ensuring that the police, judges, and healthcare personnel are trained to deal with violence against women in more sensitive and more effective ways has also been useful. It also appears that many nongovernmental organizations can deal with violence against women as effectively and at a lower cost than some government services can.[30]

Other studies have shown that a combination of measures adapted to local circumstances best addresses the constellation of factors that put women at risk of violence. Some of the most important of these measures are noted in **TABLE 10-9**.

A study based on a review of literature about violence against women in low- and middle-income countries suggests that the most successful programs of the small number that have been evaluated appear to be "participatory, engage multiple stakeholders, support critical discussion about gender relationships and the acceptability of violence, and support greater communication and shared decision making among family members, as well as non-violent behaviour."[52(p1555)]

Sexually Transmitted Infections

Sexually transmitted infections are important to women's health not only because of the morbidity and mortality associated with them, particularly among women in sub-Saharan Africa, but also because they increase the chance of getting or transmitting HIV/AIDS. It is critical, therefore, that the burden of these diseases

---

TABLE 10-9 Selected Measures to Reduce Intimate Partner Violence
Prevention and education campaigns to increase awareness of intimate partner violence and change cultural norms about violence against women
Treatment for those who engage in intimate partner violence
Programs to strengthen ties to family and jobs
Couples counseling
Shelters and crisis centers for battered women
Mandatory arrest for offenders

Modified with permission from Rosenberg, M. L., Butchart, A., Mercy, J., Narasimhan, V., Waters, H., & Marshall, M. S. (2006). Interpersonal violence. In D. T. Jamison, J. G. Breman, A. R. Measham, et al. (Eds.), *Disease control priorities in developing countries* (2nd ed., pp. 755–770). New York, NY: Oxford University Press.

be addressed. Some comments follow about addressing three of the most common STIs other than HIV among women: syphilis, gonorrhea, and chlamydia.

The goals of any program for reducing these sexually transmitted infections must be to reduce infection, reduce the complications of infections, and reduce the spread of STIs to infants when they are born.[23] It is much more cost-effective to prevent these diseases and to treat them before they lead to complications than it is to treat them later. Achieving these goals requires that young women initiate their first sexual relations at later ages; be able to refuse unwanted sex, even from their husbands; have relations with fewer partners; use condoms; and have any STIs diagnosed early and treated properly.

Meeting these aims will also require that young people get "the information and skills for making good decisions"; have access to "a range of health services that help them to act on those decisions"; and "live within a social, legal, and regulatory framework that supports health behaviors and protects young people from harm."[53(p153)]

The successes in reducing STIs other than HIV to date have focused on a common set of health system interventions and capacities. First, the health system must have an ability to carry out surveillance of STIs. Second, there needs to be a health education program, targeted to those people most at risk of infection. Third, appropriately trained health workers need to be able to provide proper treatment of infection. Fourth, a system of partner notification must be in place so that the partners of the infected individuals can also be tested and treated, if necessary. Finally, there must be an effective program for access to health services, including condom use, generally referred to as "condom promotion."[23]

For example, Sweden has made important strides in reducing chlamydia. Sweden offered free diagnosis coupled with a major health education campaign in schools, partner notification, and condom promotion. Linked to this, Sweden was able to reduce the prevalence of gonorrhea 15-fold and cut the prevalence of chlamydia by one-half over a 15-year period. Zambia also made good progress in reducing the burden of sexually transmitted infections by expanding the number of STI clinics, improving the training of health educators and clinicians, and expanding health education.[23] South Africa's "Love Life" initiative focuses on improving the sexual health of adolescents ages 12 to 17 years. Some reviews of this program suggest that it is associated with "better understanding of health risks, delayed debut of sexual relations, fewer partners, more assertive behavior regarding condom use, and better communication with parents about sex."[53(p154)]

Maternal Mortality

We have already seen that about 300,000 women die each year of maternal causes, and that as many as around 40,000 of those deaths are related to unsafe abortion. There is also considerable morbidity related to pregnancy. The fact that childbirth itself is such a risk in some settings is usually a result of the three delays: a delay in deciding to seek care, a delay in identifying problems and transporting the woman to a hospital, and a delay in providing appropriate and high-quality emergency obstetric care in the hospital. There is also considerable disability, illness, and death related to unsafe abortion.

Addressing maternal mortality requires a life course approach that takes account of a range of social, nutritional, health, and health systems issues. In very broad terms, it will be important to take the following measures, among others, to reduce maternal mortality:

- Enhance the nutritional status of adolescent girls, who would ideally marry and give birth later, engage in family planning, and have fewer births that are more widely spaced than is now the case
- Reduce the demand for abortion and the number of risky births through more accessible and good-quality family planning services and reduce the risks of unsafe abortion by making abortion legal and safe if a country so desires or ensuring, at least, the provision of safe postabortion care
- Ensure that mothers-to-be are healthy and well nourished, get appropriate and good-quality prenatal care, and that this care takes account of the risks, among other things, of gestational diabetes, pre-eclampsia and eclampsia, TB, HIV, other sexually transmitted diseases, and malaria
- Provide skilled attendance at delivery and good-quality emergency obstetric care

These and other points central to reducing maternal mortality are elaborated upon below.

Unsafe Abortion

Most of the disability, morbidity, and mortality associated with abortion are the result of unsafe abortion, mostly in low- and middle-income countries in which abortion is legally restricted. To address the effects of unsafe abortion, it is essential that the health system in these settings be able to provide hygienic and appropriate postabortion care at the lowest level of the health system possible. This means that they must be able to deal effectively with sepsis, hemorrhage, and shock. This may require a hospital stay, antibiotics, the ability to perform anesthesia, and the ability to transfuse blood.[9] Vacuum aspiration is a more cost-effective way to deal with incomplete abortion than to depend on the more surgical dilation and curettage approach. The drug misoprostol may also be a cost-effective means for dealing with an incomplete abortion in low-resource settings or could be used as a complement to vacuum aspiration. However, the use of the drug, which can be used to induce abortion, raises political issues in a number of settings.[54] Prevention of unsafe abortion is also important, including universal access to family planning and services, including after abortion.[9]

In countries in which abortion laws are more liberal, it is essential that services be widely available so that women do not turn to unsafe abortion providers. Women also need to know that legal abortion is available. In addition, it is critical that legal abortions are safe and hygienic and that services be available to deal with any postabortion complications. In these cases, including countries in Eastern Europe and Japan in which abortion is a common method of family planning, it is important that counseling be available about different types of family planning methods.[9]

Family Planning

"Family Planning Saves Lives" is the name of a long-standing publication and a phrase of considerable importance.[55] Indeed, because pregnancy and abortion are such important risks for disability,

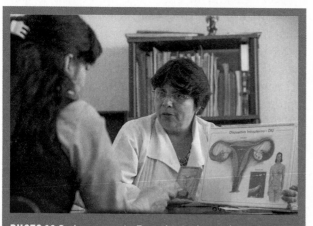

PHOTO 10-2 A woman in Ecuador is shown here counseling another woman about family planning methods. Ecuador is a middle-income country, and the facilities for this counseling session are much nicer than would be the case in many low- and lower middle-income countries. What does the evidence say about the effectiveness and cost-effectiveness of one-on-one counseling for family planning, as in this picture, compared to counseling in groups?

Courtesy of Mark Tuschman.

illness, and death, one way to avoid these problems is to reduce unwanted pregnancy through the promotion and widespread availability of family planning. In fact, it has been suggested that in countries with high maternal mortality ratios, as many as one-third of the maternal deaths could be avoided through an effective family planning program.[9] The importance of family planning is highlighted by the fact that many women in the world today would like to delay or avoid pregnancy or space their births, but they do not have the access to family planning needed to do this. Studies done in sub-Saharan Africa, for example, suggest that 20 percent of the women in the region who would like to avoid pregnancy do not have access to family planning.

There are permanent methods of family planning that include sterilization of either males or females, although only about 8 percent of the total number of sterilizations worldwide are among men.[56] There are also long-term methods of family planning, including intrauterine devices and implants. Short-term methods include contraceptive pills, injectables, and barrier methods, such as condoms or diaphragms. In addition, exclusive breastfeeding for at least 6 months—before the mother's menstrual period returns—acts as a natural contraceptive. There are also methods for natural family planning that focus on periodic abstinence.

A number of countries, including Bangladesh, Brazil, Colombia, South Korea, and Vietnam, have made important progress in promoting the use of family planning. The experience from these countries suggests that an effective family planning program has to include information, education, and communication to promote informed choices by families about family planning; the need for a good selection of family planning technologies; the use of many points of service in both the public and private sectors; services that are free or inexpensive enough for the poor to afford them; and health workers who are trained to work on family planning with knowledge and sensitivity, especially female health workers for women who are reluctant to see male health workers.[57] There is considerable evidence that social marketing is an effective tool for promoting family planning as well. Social marketing refers to the use of commercial marketing techniques to sell health-related measures, such as family planning.

Family planning is a cost-effective investment in reducing maternal death, but it is not clear which approach to family planning programs is most cost-effective compared to other approaches. The high rate of maternal death in sub-Saharan Africa and South Asia suggest that these are the two regions in which family planning would be most cost-effective to reduce maternal morbidity, disability, and mortality.[58] In addition, total fertility remains very high in many parts of sub-Saharan Africa and some parts of South Asia. It continues to be accompanied, as well, by young age of marriage, first birth, and closely spaced births.

Complications of Pregnancy

The risks of complications of pregnancy increase when the general health of the mother is not good. Thus, the nutritional status of the mother is very important. In addition, malaria is very dangerous for pregnant women, especially in sub-Saharan Africa. HIV/AIDS, TB, and diabetes also complicate pregnancy outcomes for both women and their children.

Some of the conditions that affect pregnancy outcomes can be identified during prenatal care. However, although it is important for pregnant women to

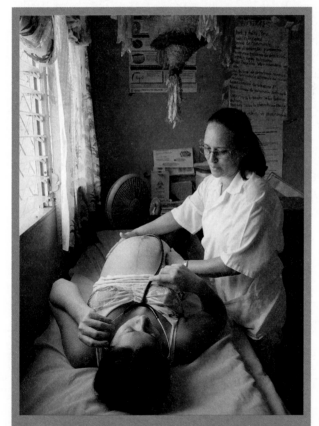

PHOTO 10-3 An Ecuadorian midwife is shown here giving a prenatal exam to a woman whose pregnancy appears to be quite advanced. As you can see in the photo, the pregnant woman is listening to her baby's heartbeat. Prenatal care is important to try to identify some of the most common complications of pregnancy early, such as diabetes and hypertension-related disorders of pregnancy. However, what other measures are needed to try to ensure a safe delivery for the mother and the child? By whom should these measures be taken?
Courtesy of Mark Tuschman.

get regular medical exams during their pregnancy—and WHO recommends four such visits—some complications of pregnancy cannot be foreseen during those checkups. Thus, it is also critical to ensure that a skilled healthcare provider attends births in order to handle the complications of pregnancy and refer the pregnant woman to a facility where the complications can be addressed appropriately. In addition, it is important that communities have transportation to urgently get women to emergency obstetric care when there are complications of pregnancy and that health services be able to address the complications with high-quality care.

Studies show that there are several cost-effective packages of services that can reduce maternal death due to complications of pregnancy. **TABLE 10-10** highlights the findings of an important recent study on the suggested contents of a package of maternal care services.

The same study suggested a package of services for enhancing reproductive health, which is shown in **TABLE 10-11**.

Of course, it is critical that appropriate services of good quality be available. However, it is also essential that there be a demand for such services from the people who need them. This is especially important in places where there are substantial barriers to overcoming the first and second delays of identifying a problem with the delivery and transporting the woman to a place where she can get emergency obstetric care. A number of countries have initiated conditional cash transfer schemes to encourage all women to have births in hospitals. These schemes are meant to overcome the social and economic constraints to hospital deliveries. Parts of India, for example, are implementing conditional cash transfer programs that offer a payment to the person attending the birth for bringing the woman to the hospital for delivery and offer the family a payment for coming for a hospital-based delivery. In many settings, there is a risk that increased demand for hospital-based delivery will not improve maternal outcomes unless there is an improvement in the quality of care. It will be important in such settings to couple incentives to increase the demand for services with other incentive programs to improve the amount and quality of emergency obstetric services.

▶ Main Messages

As discussed by a well-known scholar and practitioner of women's health, "being born female is dangerous for your health."[2(p205)] Some of the health conditions that women face are biologically determined. Others

TABLE 10-10 Essential Interventions for Maternal Health			
	Delivery Platform		
	Community Workers or Health Post	**Primary Health Center**	**First-Level and Referral Hospitals**
Pregnancy	Preparation for safe birth and newborn care; emergency planning		
	Micronutrient supplementation		
	Nutrition education		
	Intermittent preventive treatment of malaria in pregnancy		
	Food supplementation		
	Education on family planning	Management of unwanted pregnancy	
	Promotion of HIV testing	Screening and treatment for HIV and syphilis	
		Management of miscarriage or incomplete abortion and postabortion care	
		Antibiotics for preterm/premature rupture of membranes	
		Management of chronic medical conditions (hypertension, diabetes mellitus, and others)	
		Tetanus toxoid	
		Screening for complications of pregnancy	
		Initiate antenatal steroids (as long as clinical criteria and standards are met)	Antenatal steroids
		Initiate magnesium sulfate (loading dose)	Magnesium sulfate
		Detection of sepsis	Treatment of sepsis
			Induction of labor postterm

(*continues*)

TABLE 10-10 Essential Interventions for Maternal Health (continued)

	Delivery Platform		
	Community Workers or Health Post	**Primary Health Center**	**First-Level and Referral Hospitals**
			Ectopic pregnancy case management
			Detection and management of fetal growth restriction
Delivery	Management of labor and delivery in low-risk women by skilled attendant	Management of labor and delivery in low-risk women, including initial treatment of obstetric and delivery complications prior to transfer	Management of labor and delivery in high-risk women, including operative delivery (comprehensive emergency and newborn obstetric care)
Postpartum	Promotion of breastfeeding		

Black, R. E., Walker, N., Laxminarayan, R., & Temmerman, M. (2016). Reproductive, maternal, newborn, and child health: Key messages of this volume. In R. E. Black, R. Laxminarayan, M. Temmerman, & N. Walker (Eds.), *Disease control priorities: Reproductive, maternal, newborn, and child health* (3rd ed., Vol. 2). Washington, DC: The World Bank.

are socially determined. Some result from the interplay between biological and social determinants of health. The inferior social status of women in many cultures, however, is reflected in certain health conditions that women face and in some of the differentials that favor men between the health of men and the health of women.

As one looks globally at the health of women, it is important to think broadly of their health and go beyond the traditional focus on reproductive health issues. In low-income countries, Group I causes, including HIV/AIDS, TB, malaria, and maternal causes continue to be the leading causes of deaths of females 15 to 49 years of age. The same causes are of special importance for females of that age group in lower middle-income countries, but ischemic heart disease and stroke rise in importance in this group. As one moves to upper middle-income countries, HIV/AIDS continues to be important, but road injuries, ischemic heart disease, stroke, and breast cancer are also in the top five causes of death. In high-income countries, self-harm is the leading cause of death in this age group, and breast cancer, drug use disorders, road injuries, and ischemic heart disease are also in the top five causes of death. Clearly, maternal causes remain an important cause of female death. However,

reducing premature deaths of females, especially in low- and middle-income countries, will require a focus on a number of Group I causes, self-harm, and the growing burden in those countries of noncommunicable diseases.

Improving the health status of females, especially poor women in low- and middle-income countries, will also require attention to some of the specific issues noted earlier in the chapter. One is nutrition. Another is sex-selective abortion. A third is discriminatory healthcare practices toward young girls that cause these girls to suffer higher rates of mortality before age 5 than boys. Sexually transmitted infections are an important cause of DALYs for women in the reproductive age group, especially in sub-Saharan Africa. Female genital mutilation is a practice that is widespread, especially in parts of Africa, and it is associated with important morbidity and disability for women. Violence against women is also a central cause of ill health for women.

About 300,000 women die each year of maternal causes; about 40,000 of these deaths are due to unsafe abortions. Complicated labor that is not properly attended can also lead to problems, such as fistula, from which an estimated 2 million women suffer worldwide. The risk of maternal morbidity, disability,

TABLE 10-11 Essential Interventions for Women's Reproductive Health

	Delivery Platform		
	Community Workers or Health Post	Primary Health Center	First-Level and Referral Hospitals
Information and Education	Sexuality education		
	Nutrition education and food supplementation		
	Promotion of care-seeking for antenatal care and delivery		
	Prevention of sexual and reproductive tract infections	Detection and treatment of sexual and reproductive tract infections	
	Prevention of female genital mutilation (may be for daughters of women of reproductive age)	Management of complications following female genital mutilation	
	Prevention of gender-based violence	Post-gender-based violence care (prevention of sexually transmitted infection and HIV, emergency contraception, support and counseling)	
	Information about cervical cancer and screening	Screening and treatment of precancerous lesions, referral of cancers	Management of cervical cancer
Service Delivery	Folic acid supplementation		
	Immunization (human papillomavirus, hepatitis B)		
	Contraception (provision of condoms and hormonal contraceptives)	Tubal ligation, vasectomy, and insertion and removal of long-lasting contraceptives	Management of complicated contraceptive procedures

Black, R. E., Walker, N., Laxminarayan, R., & Temmerman, M. (2016). Reproductive, maternal, newborn, and child health: Key messages of this volume. In R. E. Black, R. Laxminarayan, M. Temmerman, & N. Walker (Eds.), *Disease control priorities: Reproductive, maternal, newborn, and child health* (3rd ed., Vol. 2). Washington, DC: The World Bank.

and mortality is increased by having a stunted mother, young age at marriage, young age at first birth, having more than five children, and having closely spaced pregnancies. The lack of access to family planning and the demand for it is at the foundation of some of these

problems. This is particularly the case in some places in South Asia and much of sub-Saharan Africa, where total fertility remains high and the coverage of family planning remains low. Increasing the uptake of family planning to delay the age at first birth, increase birth intervals, and reduce the number of births per woman would save lives, especially in low- and middle-income countries with weak emergency obstetric care.

The costs of women's health problems are very substantial. In many societies, women are the primary caregivers to children, and when the health of the mother suffers, there is often a negative effect on the health of the children as well. In addition, women play important economic roles in many families, and the morbidity, disability, and mortality associated with particular problems of women's health have substantial economic implications.

Some countries, such as Sri Lanka, have been able to improve the health of women at relatively low levels of expenditure by making wise choices about investments in health and education. These included increasing female education, providing widespread access to midwives, and ensuring adequate backup for the midwives at hospitals.

The quest for universal health coverage in an increasing number of countries should enhance the health of females. Improving the health of females in the future will also require that health systems provide a cost-effective package of services, including nutrition, family planning, prenatal care, deliveries attended by skilled healthcare providers, emergency transportation of women who are having complicated labors, and emergency obstetric services of appropriate quality at a hospital. A number of countries are now undertaking a variety of efforts, including incentive programs, to try to increase the demand for such services and the supply of these services at an appropriate level of quality. In the long run, it will be important to change the gender roles that favor males, promote the education and empowerment of females, promote their prospects for earning income, and educate communities to better understand the health conditions that females face and the measures that can be taken to address them. These measures could help, among other things, to reduce sex-selective abortion, female infanticide, and violence against women, and avoid the three delays that are associated with maternal morbidity, disability, and mortality. They would also promote more attention to the overall health of females and measures to reduce in cost-effective and fair ways the leading burdens of disease that females face.

Study Questions

1. Why can it be said that "being born female is dangerous to your health"?
2. Why should we pay particular attention to the health of females?
3. In what ways do gender issues affect the health of females?
4. What are some of the key differences in the burden of disease between males and females?
5. What are the sources of those differences?
6. What are the three delays, and why are they important?
7. What steps do countries need to take to deal with the complications of unsafe abortions?
8. What measures might be taken to reduce intimate partner violence?
9. How could one reduce the risk to women of sexually transmitted infections?
10. What are some of the most cost-effective investments that should be made to improve the health of women in low-income countries?

References

1. Prada, E., Restler, E., Sten, C., Dauphinee, L., & Ramirez, L. (2005). *Abortion and postabortion care in Guatemala: A report from health care professionals and health facilities* (Occasional Report No. 18). New York, NY: Guttmacher Institute. Retrieved from http://www.guttmacher.org/pubs/2005/12/30/or18.pdf
2. Murphy, E. M. (2003). Being born female is dangerous for your health. *American Psychologist, 58*(3), 205–210.
3. Buvinic, M., Medici, A., Fernandez, E., & Torres, A. C. (2006). Gender differentials in health. In D. T. Jamison, J. G. Breman, A. R. Measham, et al. (Eds.), *Disease control priorities in developing countries* (2nd ed., pp. 195–210). New York, NY: Oxford University Press.
4. World Health Organization (WHO). (2005). *The world health report 2005: Make every mother and child count.* Geneva, Switzerland: Author.
5. Quinn, T. C., & Overbaugh, J. (2005). HIV/AIDS in women: An expanding epidemic. *Science, 308*(5728), 1582–1583.
6. Abeykoon, A. T. P. L. (1995). Sex preference in South Asia: Sri Lanka an outlier. *Asia-Pacific Population Journal, 10*(3), 5–16.
7. Gu, B., & Roy, K. (1995). Sex ratio at birth in China, with reference to other areas in East Asia: What we know. *Asia-Pacific Population Journal, 10*(3), 17–42.
8. Jha, P., Kesler, M. A., Kumar, R., Ram, F., Ram, U., Aleksandriwicz, L., . . . Banthia, J. K. (2011). Trends in selective abortions of girls in India: Analysis of nationally representative birth histories from 1990 to 2005 and census data from 1991 to 2011. *The Lancet, 377*, 1921–1928.
9. Tinker, A. (1994). *A new agenda for women's health and nutrition.* Washington, DC: The World Bank.
10. Rov, K. (1999). *Encyclopaedia against women & dowry death in India.* New Delhi, India: Anmol Publications.

11. Gendercide Watch. (n.d.). *Case study: Female infanticide.* Retrieved from http://www.gendercide.org/case_infanticide.html

12. Jha, P., Kumar, R., Vasa, P., Dhingra, N., Thiruchelvam, D., & Moineddin, R. (2006). Low female-to-male sex ratio of children born in India: National survey of 1.1 million households. *The Lancet, 367*(9506), 211–218.

13. Office of the Registrar General & Census Commissioner, India. (2015). Estimates of fertility indicators. In *SRS statistical report 2015* (Ch. 3). Retrieved from http://www.censusindia.gov.in/vital_statistics/SRS_Report_2015/7.Chap%203-Fertility%20Indicators-2015.pdf

14. World Economic Forum. (n.d.). *The global gender gap report: China.* Retrieved from http://reports.weforum.org/global-gender-gap-report-2016/economies/#economy=CHN

15. Central Intelligence Agency (CIA). (n.d.). *The world factbook field listing: Sex ratio.* Retrieved from https://www.cia.gov/library/publications/the-world-factbook/fields/351.html

16. UNICEF. (2005). *Female genital mutilation/cutting: A statistical exploration 2005.* New York, NY: UNICEF.

17. World Health Organization (WHO). (2018). *Female genital mutilation.* Retrieved from http://www.who.int/news-room/fact-sheets/detail/female-genital-mutilation

18. UNICEF. (2014). *Female genital mutilation/cutting: A statistical overview and exploration of the dynamics of change.* York, NY: UNICEF.

19. Kandala, N.-B., Ezejimofor, M. C., Uthman, O. A., & Komba, P. (2018). Secular trends in the prevalence of female genital mutilation/cutting among girls: A systematic analysis. *BMJ Global Health, 3*(5), e000549. doi: 10.1136/bmjgh-2017-000549

20. Glasier, A., Gulmezoglu, A. M., Schmid, G. P., Moreno, C. G., & Look, P. F. V. (2006). Sexual and reproductive health: A matter of life and death. *The Lancet, 368*, 1595–1607.

21. World Health Organization (WHO). (2016). *Sexually transmitted infections (STIs).* Retrieved from http://www.who.int/en/news-room/fact-sheets/detail/sexually-transmitted-infections-(stis)

22. Institute of Health Metrics and Evaluation (IHME). (n.d). GBD Compare: Viz Hub. Retrieved from https://vizhub.healthdata.org/gbd-compare/

23. Rowley, J., & Berkley, S. (1998). Sexually transmitted diseases. In C. J. L. Murray & A. D. Lopez (Eds.), *Health dimensions of sex and reproduction* (pp. 19–110). Geneva, Switzerland: World Health Organization.

24. World Health Organization (WHO). (2013). *Sexually transmitted infections (STIs).* Retrieved from http://apps.who.int/iris/bitstream/10665/82207/1/WHO_RHR_13.02_eng.pdf

25. World Health Organization (WHO). (2017). *Violence against women.* Retrieved from http://www.who.int/mediacentre/factsheets/fs239/en/

26. UNAIDS. (n.d.). *Violence against women and AIDS.* Retrieved from http://data.unaids.org/GCWA/GCWA_BG_Violence_en.pdf

27. Williams, J. (2004). Women's mental health: Taking inequality into account. In J. Tew (Ed.), *Social perspectives in mental health: Developing social models to understand and work with mental distress* (pp. 151–167). London, United Kingdom: Jessica Kingsley.

28. World Health Organization, London School of Hygiene and Tropical Medicine, & South African Medical Research Council. (2013). *Global and regional estimates of violence against women.* Geneva, Switzerland: World Health Organization.

29. UNICEF. (n.d.). *Sexual violence as a weapon of war.* Retrieved from http://www.unicef.org/sowc96pk/sexviol.htm

30. Rosenberg, M. L., Butchart, A., Mercy, J., Narasimhan, V., Waters, H., & Marshall, M. S. (2006). Interpersonal violence. In D. T. Jamison, J. G. Breman, A. R. Measham, et al. (Eds.), *Disease control priorities in developing countries* (2nd ed., pp. 755–770). New York, NY: Oxford University Press.

31. World Health Organization (WHO). (2018). *Maternal mortality.* Retrieved from http://www.who.int/mediacentre/factsheets/fs348/en/

32. Last, J. M. (2001). *A dictionary of epidemiology* (4th ed.). New York, NY: Oxford University Press.

33. World Health Organization, UNICEF, World Bank Group, UNFPA, & United Nations. (2015). *Trends in maternal mortality: 1990 to 2015—Estimates by WHO, UNICEF, UNFPA, World Bank Group and the United Nations Population Division.* Geneva, Switzerland: World Health Organization.

34. Lawn, J. E., Lee, A. C., Kinney, M., Sibley, L., Carlo, W. A., Pau, V. K., . . . Darmstadt, G. L. (2009). Two million intrapartum-related stillbirths and neonatal deaths: Where, why, and what can be done? *International Journal of Gynaecology and Obstetrics, 107*, S5–S19.

35. Say, L., Chou, D., Gemmil, A., Tunçalp, Ö., Moller, A. B., Daniels, J., . . . Alkema, L. (2014). Global causes of maternal death: A WHO systematic analysis. *Lancet Global Health, 2*(6), e323–e333.

36. AbouZahr, C. (1998). Antepartum and postpartum hemorrhage. In C. J. L. Murray & A. D. Lopez (Eds.), *Health dimensions of sex and reproduction: The global burden of sexually transmitted diseases, HIV, maternal conditions, perinatal disorders, and congenital anomalies* (pp. 165–190). Cambridge, MA: Harvard School of Public Health.

37. Measure Evaluation. (2014). *Safe motherhood.* Retrieved from http://www.cpc.unc.edu/measure/prh/rh_indicators/specific/sm

38. World Health Organization (WHO). (2018). *Preventing unsafe abortion.* Retrieved from http://www.who.int/en/news-room/fact-sheets/detail/preventing-unsafe-abortion

39. Royal College of Midwives. (2010). *Obstetric fistula: A silent tragedy.* London, United Kingdom: The Royal College of Midwives Trust.

40. AbouZahr, C. (1998). Prolonged and obstructed labor. In C. J. L. Murray & A. D. Lopez (Eds.), *Health dimensions of sex and reproduction: The global burden of sexually transmitted diseases, HIV, maternal conditions, perinatal disorders, and congenital anomalies* (pp. 243–266). Cambridge, MA: Harvard School of Public Health.

41. Health & Development International. (2005). *Obstetric fistula as a catalyst: Exploring approaches for safe motherhood.* Meeting report, Atlanta, GA, October 3–5, 2005.

42. This case study is largely based on Pathmathan, I., Lijestrand, J., Martins, J. M., Rajapaksa, L. C., Lissner, C., de Silva, A., . . . Singh, P. J. (2003). *Investing in maternal health: Learning from Malaysia and Sri Lanka.* Washington, DC: The World Bank.

43. Wickramasuriya, G. A. W. (1939). Maternal mortality and morbidity in Ceylon. *Journal of the Ceylon Branch of the British Medical Association, 36*(2), 79–106.

44. United Nations. (2003). *Human development report.* New York, NY: Author.

45. The World Bank. (2014). *Data: Maternal mortality ratio (modeled estimate per 100,000 live births.* Retrieved http://data.worldbank.org/indicator/SH.STA.MMRT

46. Levine, R., & What Works Working Group. (2007). *Case studies in global health: Millions saved.* Sudbury, MA: Jones and Bartlett.

47. Manoff, R. (1997). Getting your message out with social marketing. *American Journal of Tropical Medicine and Hygiene, 57*(3), 260–265.

48. Mitra, S. N., Al-Sabir, A., Cross, A. R., & Jamil, K. (1997). *Bangladesh demographic and health survey 1996–1997.* Dhaka, Bangladesh: National Institute for Population Research and Training.

49. Barkat-e-Khuda, Roy, N. C., & Rahman, D. M. (2000). Family planning and fertility in Bangladesh. *Asia-Pacific Population Journal, 15*(1), 41–54.

50. Janowitz, B., Holtman, M., Johnson, L., & Trottier, D. (1999). The importance of field workers in Bangladesh's family planning programme. *Asia-Pacific Population Journal, 14*(2), 23–36.

51. Routh, S., & Barkat-e-Khuda. (2000). An economic appraisal of alternative strategies for the delivery of MCH-FP services in urban Dhaka, Bangladesh. *International Journal of Health Planning and Management, 15*(2), 115–132.

52. Ellsberg, M., Arango, D. J., & Morton, M., Gennari, F., Kiplesund, S., Contreras, M., & Watts, C. (2015). Prevention of violence against women and girls: What does the evidence say? *The Lancet, 385*(9977), 1555–1566.

53. (2006). Providing interventions. In D. T. Jamison, J. G. Breman, A. R. Measham, et al. (Eds.), *Priorities in Health* (pp. 129–154). Washington, DC: The International Bank for Reconstruction and Development / The World Bank.

54. Barot, S. (2014). Implementing postabortion care programs in the developing world: Ongoing challenges. *Guttmacher Institute.* Retrieved from https://www.guttmacher.org/pubs/gpr/17/1/gpr170122.html

55. Smith, R., Ashford, L., Gribble, J., & Clifton, D. (2009). *Family planning saves lives* (4th ed.). Washington, DC: PRB.

56. Jamison, D. T. (2006). Maternal and perinatal conditions. In D. T. Jamison, J. G. Breman, A. R. Measham, et al. (Eds.), *Disease control priorities in developing countries* (2nd ed., pp. 499–529). New York, NY: Oxford University Press.

57. Graham, W. J., Cairns, J., Bhattacharya, S., Bullough, C. H. W., Quayyum, Z., & Rogo, K. (2006). Maternal and perinatal conditions. In D. T. Jamison, J. G. Breman, A. R. Measham, et al. (Eds.), *Disease control priorities in developing countries* (2nd ed., pp. 499–530). New York, NY: Oxford University Press.

58. Jamison, D. T., Breman, J. G., Measham, A. R., Alleyne, G., Claeson, M., Evans, D. B., . . . Musgrove, P. (Eds.). (2006). *Priorities in health.* Washington, DC: The World Bank.

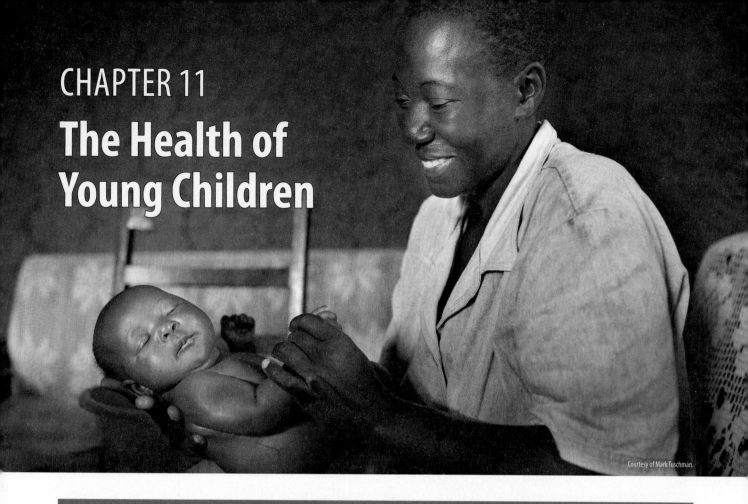

Courtesy of Mark Tuschman.

CHAPTER 11
The Health of Young Children

LEARNING OBJECTIVES

By the end of this chapter, the reader will be able to do the following:

- Describe the most important causes of illness and death among young children globally
- Discuss the key risk factors for child morbidity and mortality
- Describe the most cost-effective interventions for reducing childhood illness and death
- Discuss the importance of immunization, progress made in expanding immunization coverage, and the challenges to global immunization efforts
- Discuss some of the constraints to further enhancing the health of young children in low- and middle-income countries and what might be done to address them

▶ Vignettes

Nassiba was born in a remote part of Tajikistan. At 3 years of age, she became very ill with measles. She died before her parents could get her to a health center. Nassiba's birth was never registered because the registration center was far from her home and her parents could not afford the registration fee. When Nassiba died, her death was not recorded either. According to the national records, she never existed.

Esther was born in Cape Town, South Africa, to an HIV-positive mother. At the time of Esther's birth, the health system did not offer drugs to prevent the transmission of HIV from mother to child. A few months later, Esther showed signs of HIV infection.

Tirtha was born in far western Nepal 7 months ago. She was the fourth child in her family. She was eating some baby foods as well as breastfeeding. One day Tirtha developed persistent diarrhea and became feverish. Her mother wanted to take Tirtha to the health center, but it was 2 hours away, so she decided to see how Tirtha was feeling the next day. The next morning Tirtha was dead from dehydration.

Juan was born in the highlands of Bolivia to an indigenous family. The family did what they could to keep the new baby warm, but it was very cold in the mountains. Several days after birth, Juan began to breathe heavily. The family called the community health worker for assistance. The health worker treated Juan for pneumonia with an antibiotic that she had just learned to use through a community-based program for saving newborn lives. She also gave the family advice about taking care of the baby. The last child born to the family had died of pneumonia, but Juan survived.

▶ The Importance of Child Health

There are a number of reasons why the health of young children deserves its own chapter. First, it has been estimated that about 5.4 million children under 5 years of age died in 2017.[1(p2)] This is equal to almost 15,000 children under 5 who died *each day* that year. The second reason to pay special attention to child health is that an overwhelming share of these deaths are preventable. Young children, for example, almost never die in high-income countries,[2] and it has been estimated that more than half of child deaths each year could be avoided through known, simple, and low-cost interventions.[3] Third, children have a special place in the global health agenda because they are so vulnerable. The measures needed to ensure that they are born healthier, breastfed properly, immunized on schedule, and raised in safe, nurturing, and hygienic conditions, for example, can be taken only by others who care for

them. Their vulnerability also raises important ethical issues about the responsibility of adults to ensure the health and survival of children.

Child health is also closely linked with poverty. If children had access to safer water and better sanitation, then many of them would not succumb to diarrhea. If their families had more education, especially their mothers, then families would be better equipped to ensure that their children are better cared for. If families had more income, then they would have greater access to health, education, and other social services that would also serve children well.

There has been substantial progress in reducing the number of under-5 children who die each year globally, as shown in **FIGURE 11-1**.

However, despite this progress, the health of young children is also of particular concern because some parts of the world have not made sufficient progress in enhancing child health. This has been especially true in parts of sub-Saharan Africa and South Asia, as can also be seen in Figure 11-1.[4]

For all these reasons, children are featured prominently in the Sustainable Development Goals (SDGs), as noted in **TABLE 11-1**.

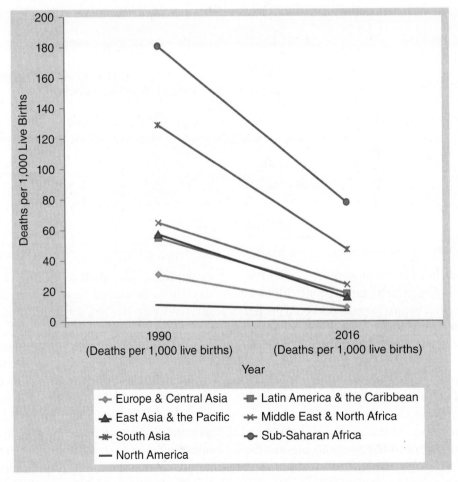

FIGURE 11-1 Declines in Under-5 Child Mortality, by World Bank Region, 1990–2016

Data from The World Bank. (n.d.). *Mortality rate*, under-5 (per 1,000 live births). Retrieved from http://data.worldbank.org/indicator/SH.DYN.MORT/countries/1W-Z4-ZQ-Z7?display=graph

TABLE 11-1 Selected Links Between the Health of Young Children and the SDG Health Targets

Target 3.1 By 2030, reduce the global maternal mortality ratio to less than 70 per 100,000 live births.

Reducing maternal mortality will help to reduce child mortality.

Target 3.2 By 2030, end preventable deaths of newborns and children under 5 years of age, with all countries aiming to reduce neonatal mortality to at least as low as 12 per 1,000 live births and under-5 mortality to at least as low as 25 per 1,000 live births.

This target is directly related to the health and well-being of young children.

Target 3.3 By 2030, end the epidemics of AIDS, tuberculosis, malaria, and neglected tropical diseases and combat hepatitis, waterborne diseases, and other communicable diseases.

Communicable diseases continue to take an enormous toll on young children, especially in the poorest countries, in sub-Saharan Africa and in South Asia. Hepatitis B is also a major issue for young children in parts of the world such as East Asia. Addressing this target effectively could have a major impact on the health and well-being of young children.

Target 3.4 By 2030, reduce by one-third premature mortality from noncommunicable diseases through prevention and treatment and promote mental health and well-being.

The noncommunicable diseases and mental health disorders are important causes of morbidity, disability, and death for women everywhere. Women have higher risks and rates of some of these diseases and some mental health disorders and suicide than men do. Addressing this target would help improve birth outcomes. It would also enhance the ability of mothers and families to nurture their children better, improving young child health and development.

Target 3.6 By 2020, halve the number of global deaths and injuries from road traffic accidents.

As children get older and societies move along the epidemiological transition, road traffic accidents become an increasingly large share of child deaths. Reducing road traffic accidents would have an important impact on child health.

Target 3.7 By 2030, ensure universal access to sexual and reproductive healthcare services, including for family planning, information and education, and the integration of reproductive health into national strategies and programs.

Family planning saves lives. Good quality reproductive health services that can assist families in making choices about family planning will enhance the health of women and of the children born to them. Providing better maternal health services also saves lives of both mothers and children. Healthier mothers are also better able than unhealthy mothers to care for their children and ensure better child development.

Target 3.8 Achieve universal health coverage, including financial risk protection, access to quality essential healthcare services and access to safe, effective, quality, and affordable essential medicines and vaccines for all.

Universal health coverage that is of good quality reduces out-of-pocket costs to the poor to a minimum. In addition, if it is fairly prioritized and delivered, it can have a major impact on the health services most needed to enhance the health and well-being of mothers-to-be in low- and middle-income countries. Moving toward universal coverage would also have an important impact on improving the services that can directly enhance the health of young children.

Target 3.9 By 2030, substantially reduce the number of deaths and illnesses from hazardous chemicals and air, water, and soil pollution and contamination.

Poor children in low-income countries are especially vulnerable to the detrimental health effects of ambient air pollution, unsafe water, and environmental contaminants. Meeting this target would have an important impact on morbidity and mortality among young children.

This chapter highlights the most important issues concerning the health of young children in low- and middle-income countries. It will review the burden of disease for these children, with important comments on their first month of life. It will assess the risk factors for illness and death that occur in children under 5 years of age. It then examines measures that can be taken to reduce the burden of disease in young children. The chapter concludes with a review of some of the key challenges to further improving the health of young children in low- and middle-income countries. A number of case studies illustrate key concepts that are discussed in the chapter.

This chapter focuses on the most important causes of illness and death in children: causes related to the deaths of neonates, plus pneumonia, diarrhea, malaria, the neglected tropical diseases, and vaccine-preventable diseases. This chapter is about children under 5 years of age, largely in low- and middle-income countries. The chapter generally refers to them as "young children" or "children."

It is also important to note that the chapter does not discuss stillbirths. The World Health Organization (WHO) defines a stillbirth as "a baby born with no signs of life at or after 28 weeks' gestation."[5] Stillbirths are a very important issue, one that WHO has called an "invisible public health priority."[5] It was earlier estimated that 2.6 million babies are stillborn each year, almost all of them in low- and middle-income countries.[5] Readers who are interested can review this issue in greater detail, starting with materials from WHO and a *The Lancet* series that extensively covered stillbirths.[6]

As one considers the health of young children, it is critical to remember that a range of interventions is needed to ensure that young children develop to their full biological and intellectual potential. It is also important to remember that without these interventions, a substantial portion of young children, especially in low- and middle-income countries, will never achieve their full potential. Health *is* central to early childhood development. The health sector can also serve as a platform for a range of early child development interventions. However, achieving the highest levels of early child development will also require, among other things, a package of good nutrition, a nurturing environment, safety and security, and early learning that is provided at appropriate times along the life course. Nonetheless, reviewing early childhood development more broadly is beyond the scope of this chapter, and

readers are encouraged to examine, among other literature, the 2016 *Lancet* series on early childhood development.[7]

▶ Key Terms

Some of the key indicators used in measuring and analyzing global health issues, which will be used extensively in this chapter, include the **neonatal mortality rate**, **infant mortality rate**, and **under-5 child mortality rate**.

In this chapter, we also speak of three different phases of the lives of young children:

Neonatal: Referring to the first month of life

Infant: Referring to the first year of life

Under-5: Referring to children 0 to 4 years old

In addition, you will read about some of the most important causes of disease, disability, and death in children under 5 years, as shown in **TABLE 11-2**.

▶ Note on Data

This chapter takes its data from a number of sources. Some of the basic data are taken from publications of the United Nations (U.N.) Interagency Group for Child Mortality Estimation, whose latest report was issued in 2018.[1] Other data come from WHO, UNICEF, the World Bank, and the Global Burden of Disease Study 2016.[8] The chapter also takes data and considerable information from various *The Lancet* publications and from *Disease Control Priorities, Third Edition* (DCP3).[9] To be consistent with data on the burden of disease in the rest of the text, most data have been updated to 2016. However, because the recent estimations of child mortality include data for 2017, some data are also shown for that year.

▶ Mortality and the Burden of Disease

Mortality

As noted earlier, about 5.4 million children under 5 years of age died worldwide in 2017.[1(p2)] About 99 percent of these deaths took place in low- and middle-income countries. The risk of dying decreases with the age of the young child, with the first hours, days, and weeks being the riskiest. Related

TABLE 11-2 Selected Terms Relating to Causes of Child Illness and Death
Asphyxia—A condition of severely deficient oxygen supply.
Diarrhea—A condition characterized by frequent and watery bowel movements.
Hookworm—A parasite that lives in the intestines of its host, which may be a mammal such as a dog, cat, or human. Two species of hookworm commonly infect humans, *Ancylostoma duodenale* and *Necator americanus*.
Malaria—A disease of humans caused by blood parasites of the species *Plasmodium falciparum, vivax, ovale, knowlesi,* or *malariae* and transmitted by *Anopheles* mosquitoes.
Pertussis—A highly contagious bacterial disease that is one of the leading causes of vaccine-preventable death. Pertussis is also known as whooping cough.
Pneumonia—An inflammation, usually caused by infection, involving the alveoli of the lungs. Pneumonia is one of several lower respiratory tract infections.
Polio—An infectious disease caused by poliovirus that can lead to paralysis.
Sepsis—A serious medical condition caused by a severe infection, leading to a systematic inflammatory response.
Tetanus—A bacterial infection usually contracted through a puncture wound with an unclean object. Neonates acquire tetanus when their umbilical cord is contaminated, often when cut with an unsterile object.

Definitions are based on the definitions and discussions found in: The Free Dictionary. Medical Dictionary. Retrieved from https://medical-dictionary.thefreedictionary.com
These definitions also take account of the discussions of WHO fact sheets related to each term.

to this, the breakdown of these deaths by age and by percentage of total deaths of under-5 children is shown here[1(p6)]:

0 to 28 days – 2.5 million – 46 percent

1 month to 11 months – 1.5 million – 28 percent

1 to 4 years – 1.4 million – 26 percent

Moreover, estimates also suggest that more than one-third of the children who died in the first 28 days died in the first day of life.[4]

FIGURE 11-2 depicts the neonatal mortality rate by World Bank region in 2016.

FIGURE 11-3 shows neonatal mortality rate by country income group in 2016.

Figure 11-2 clearly shows the substantial differences in rates by region. As expected, the highest rates are in sub-Saharan Africa and South Asia, with rates seven times the rate in the best-off regions. Figure 11-3 portrays the strong correlation between country income group and the neonatal mortality rate. On average, a child born in a low-income country has a nine times greater chance of dying in its first 28 days than a child born in a high-income country. The low rates of neonatal death in high-income countries highlight the fact that almost all of these deaths are avoidable. The correlation between country income and neonatal mortality also highlights the aim of public policy on this matter—to try to ensure that countries reduce neonatal and young child deaths as fast as possible, at least cost, even while the level of country income remains relatively low.

FIGURE 11-4 shows the infant mortality rate by World Bank region.

FIGURE 11-5 shows the infant mortality rate by country income group.

The pattern for infant mortality is similar to that for neonatal mortality, with sub-Saharan Africa having the highest rate and South Asia having the second-highest rate. In this case, however, sub-Saharan Africa has a rate about 9 times greater than

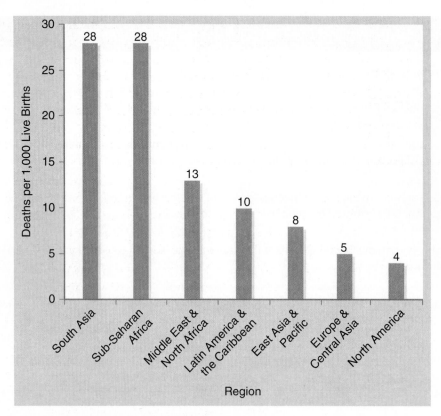

FIGURE 11-2 Neonatal Mortality Rate, by World Bank Region, 2016

Data from The World Bank. (n.d.). Data: *Mortality rate, neonatal* (per 1,000 live births). Retrieved from https://data.worldbank.org/indicator/SH.DYN.NMRT?end=2016&start=1960

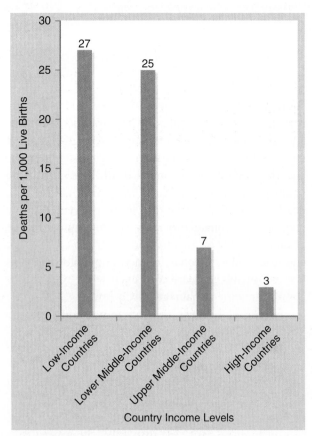

FIGURE 11-3 Neonatal Mortality Rate, by World Bank Country Income Group, 2016

Data from The World Bank. (n.d.). Data: *Mortality rate, neonatal* (per 1,000 live births). Retrieved from https://data.worldbank.org/indicator/SH.DYN.NMRT?end=2016&start=1960

North America, and South Asia has a rate more than 6 times the rate in North America. The data on the infant mortality rate by country income groups also follow the same pattern as those for neonatal mortality. The low-income countries have an average infant mortality rate that is 5 times higher than that of the high-income countries.

FIGURE 11-6 shows the rates of under-5 child mortality by World Bank region.

FIGURE 11-7 shows the rates of under-5 child mortality by country income group.

The under-5 child mortality rate for sub-Saharan Africa is substantially higher than for any other region, including South Asia, and is more than 11 times the rate for North America. South Asia again has the second-highest rate, in this case almost 7 times more than the rate in North America. The low-income countries have an average infant mortality rate that is 12 times that of the high-income countries.

FIGURE 11-8 shows neonatal, infant, and under-5 child mortality side by side for each World Bank region.

This figure makes a number of very important points:

- Sub-Saharan Africa has the highest rates for all indicators.

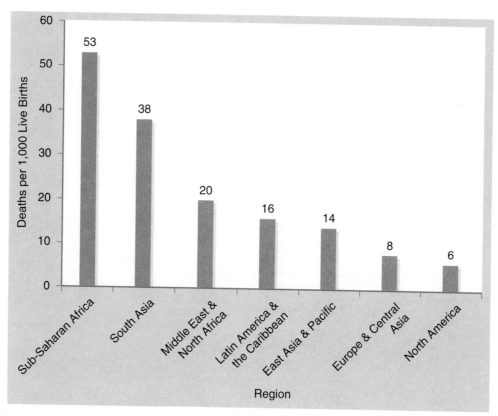

FIGURE 11-4 Infant Mortality Rate, by World Bank Region, 2016

Data from The World Bank. (n.d.). Data: *Mortality rate, infant* (per 1,000 live births). Retrieved from https://data.worldbank.org/indicator/SP.DYN.IMRT.IN

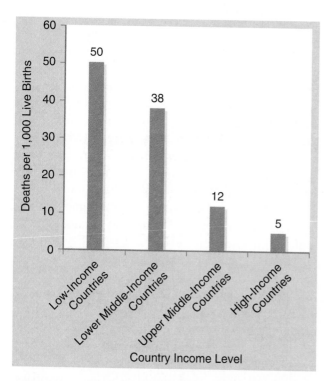

FIGURE 11-5 Infant Mortality Rate, by World Bank Country Income Group, 2016

Data from The World Bank. (n.d.). Data: *Mortality rate, infant* (per 1,000 live births). Retrieved from https://data.worldbank.org/indicator/SP.DYN.IMRT.IN

- South Asia has the second-highest rates for all indicators.
- The rates tend to vary directly with the income group of the region.
- In general, the higher the income group of the region, the more likely it is that children who die before they are 5 years old will die as neonates.
- Nonetheless, in some regions there is still a significant risk of dying from the 1st month of life to the 12th month of life and from 1 to 4 years of age. In South Asia, about 21 percent of under-5 deaths are among children 1 year to 4 years of age. In sub-Saharan Africa, almost 32 percent of all under-5 deaths are among children 1 to 4 years of age.
- South Asia has an anomalous pattern of child deaths. It appears that South Asia has a much higher share of total deaths among neonates than one might predict, suggesting an area in which South Asia needs to make much more progress.
- In sub-Saharan Africa, uniquely, there are almost equal risks of dying in each of the

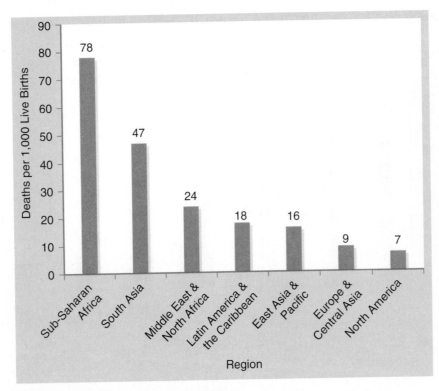

FIGURE 11-6 Under-5 Mortality Rate, by World Bank Region, 2016

Data from The World Bank. (n.d.). *Mortality rate: Under-5* (per 1,000 live births). Retrieved from https://data.worldbank.org/indicator/SH.DYN.MORT?end=2016&start=1960

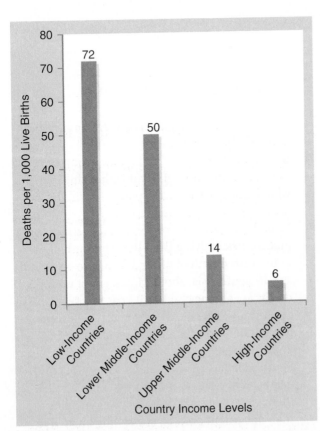

FIGURE 11-7 Under-5 Mortality Rate, by World Bank Country Income Group, 2016

Data from The World Bank. (n.d.). *Mortality rate: Under-5* (per 1,000 live births). Retrieved from https://data.worldbank.org/indicator/SH.DYN.MORT?end=2016&start=1960

periods shown—those living past the first month and those living past the first year still face substantial risks of dying between their first and fifth years.

As one would expect, the rates of infant and child mortality vary *within countries* by a number of factors, including income, education, and location. A study conducted by UNICEF several years ago showed that in sub-Saharan Africa, children from the lowest-income quintile had almost twice the risk of dying before they were 5 years of age as children in the highest-income quintile. In the East Asia and Pacific, South Asia, and the Middle East and North Africa regions, the poorest quintile children were almost three times more likely to die before they were 5 years old as those in the highest-income quintile.[10]

The differences by rural or urban location were less severe but still important. Rural populations in Latin America and the Caribbean were about 1.7 times more likely to die before their fifth birthday than urban populations, whereas those in South Asia were 1.5 times more likely, and those in sub-Saharan Africa were about 1.4 times more likely to die.[10]

For all low- and middle-income countries, under-5 children of mothers with no primary education were about twice as likely to die before they were

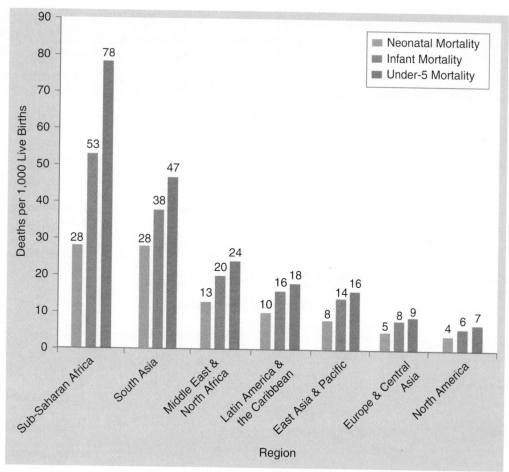

FIGURE 11-8 Neonatal, Infant, and Under-5 Child Mortality Rates, by World Bank Region, 2016

Data from The World Bank. (n.d.). *World development indicators: Mortality.* (per 1,000 live births). Retrieved from http://data.worldbank.org/indicator/SH.DYN.MORT/countries/1W-Z4-ZQ-Z7?display=graph

5 years of age, compared to children of mothers with a secondary education or higher. In most regions, other than South Asia, boys were more likely to die before they were 5 than girls. In the East Asia and Pacific region, however, boys and girls were equally likely to die before they were 5. [10]

The Burden of Disease for Young Children

Globally, the leading causes of death for children under 5 years of age are shown in **TABLE 11-3** by World Bank region.

TABLE 11-4 shows the leading causes of death for children under 5 years of age by country income group.

These tables highlight several points:

- In all regions, preterm birth complications and congenital defects remain among the most important causes of under-5 child death.
- In all regions, other causes of death among newborns, such as neonatal encephalopathy, neonatal

sepsis, and "other neonatal disorders," are also major causes of death.

- Sub-Saharan Africa has a unique pattern of the leading causes of death for under-5 children, with the top cause being malaria and the next two causes also being communicable diseases.
- In the two poorest regions, protein-energy malnutrition is among the leading causes of death.
- The higher the income group of the region, the more likely under-5 children who die will die of conditions related to birth, such as congenital anomalies.

FIGURE 11-9 shows the percentage share of different causes of death of under-5 children globally.

Almost all of the under-5 deaths that occur annually are in low- and middle-income countries. As these countries have made progress in reducing under-5 child deaths, the leading causes of death globally have shifted toward prematurity and other issues around the period of birth, such as "intrapartum complications,"

TABLE 11-3 Ten Leading Causes of Under-5 Deaths, by World Bank Region, 2016

	East Asia & Pacific	Europe & Central Asia	Latin America & the Caribbean	Middle East & North Africa
1.	Preterm birth complications	Congenital defects	Congenital defects	Preterm birth complications
2.	Congenital defects	Preterm birth complications	Preterm birth complications	Congenital defects
3.	Lower respiratory infections	Lower respiratory infections	Lower respiratory infections	Lower respiratory infections
4.	Neonatal encephalopathy	Neonatal encephalopathy	Neonatal encephalopathy	Diarrheal diseases
5.	Neonatal sepsis	Other neonatal disorders	Neonatal sepsis	Neonatal sepsis
6.	Other neonatal disorders	Neonatal sepsis	Other neonatal disorders	Conflict and terrorism
7.	Diarrheal diseases	Diarrheal diseases	Diarrheal diseases	Neonatal encephalopathy
8.	Drowning	Sudden infant death syndrome	Foreign body	Other neonatal disorders
9.	Road injury	Foreign body	Protein-energy malnutrition	Road injury
10.	Meningitis	Drowning	Meningitis	STDs

	North America	South Asia	Sub-Saharan Africa
1.	Preterm birth complications	Lower respiratory infections	Malaria
2.	Congenital defects	Preterm birth complications	Lower respiratory infections
3.	Other neonatal disorders	Neonatal encephalopathy	Diarrheal diseases
4.	Neonatal encephalopathy	Other neonatal disorders	Neonatal encephalopathy
5.	Sudden infant death syndrome	Diarrheal diseases	Preterm birth complications
6.	Mechanical forces	Congenital defects	Neonatal sepsis
7.	Neonatal sepsis	Neonatal sepsis	Congenital defects
8.	Interpersonal violence	Meningitis	Protein-energy malnutrition
9.	Road injuries	Neonatal hemolysis	Meningitis
10.	Lower respiratory infections	Protein-energy malnutrition	Other neonatal disorders

Institute of Health Metrics and Evaluation (IHME). (n.d.). GBD Compare: Viz Hub. Retrieved from https://vizhub.healthdata.org/gbd-compare/

TABLE 11-4 Ten Leading Causes of Under-5 Deaths, by World Bank Country Income Group, 2016

Low-Income Countries	Lower Middle-Income Countries	Upper Middle-Income Countries	High-Income Countries
1. Malaria	Lower respiratory infections	Preterm birth complications	Congenital defects
2. Lower respiratory infections	Preterm birth complications	Congenital defects	Preterm birth complications
3. Diarrheal diseases	Neonatal encephalopathy	Lower respiratory infections	Other neonatal disorders
4. Neonatal encephalopathy	Malaria	Neonatal encephalopathy	Neonatal encephalopathy
5. Preterm birth complications	Diarrheal diseases	Other neonatal disorders	Sudden infant death syndrome
6. Protein-energy malnutrition	Congenital defects	Neonatal sepsis	Neonatal sepsis
7. Neonatal sepsis	Other neonatal disorders	HIV/AIDS	Lower respiratory infections
8. Congenital defects	Neonatal sepsis	Diarrheal diseases	Road injuries
9. Other neonatal disorders	Meningitis	Road injuries	Endocrine, metabolic, blood, immune disorders
10. Meningitis	Protein-energy malnutrition	Drowning	Mechanical forces

Data from Institute of Health Metrics and Evaluation (IHME). (n.d.). GBD Compare: Viz Hub. Retrieved from https://vizhub.healthdata.org/gbd-compare/

for example, birth asphyxia, congenital anomalies, sepsis, and meningitis. Nonetheless, a number of communicable causes that generally affect the child most after the neonatal period are also among the leading causes of death. These include pneumonia, diarrhea, malaria, measles, and HIV/AIDS. It is also important to note that injury is a leading cause of death of under-5 children.

It is especially important for the formulation of policies addressing the deaths of under-5 children to understand the causes of death at different times between birth and the end of the child's fourth year. **FIGURE 11-10** examines the causes of death among neonates globally.

Beyond the importance of preterm birth complications and congenital anomalies, it is important to note the share of neonatal deaths attributable to intrapartum complications, birth asphyxia, sepsis, and pneumonia. As discussed later, low-cost measures are available that can be carried out at the community level to prevent most such deaths.

FIGURE 11-11 shows the percentage distribution, by cause, of deaths in the post-neonatal period.

With the exception of meningitis, the leading causes of post-neonatal death are similar to those for under-5 children more broadly. It is important to note the significance of communicable causes beyond meningitis: malaria, pneumonia, diarrhea, HIV/AIDS, and measles. The significance of injury deaths must also be noted.

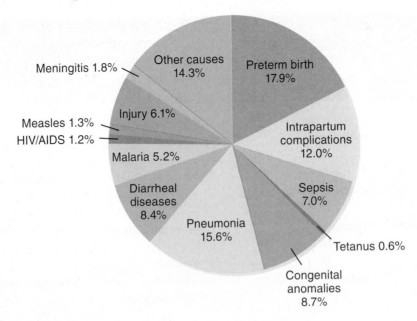

FIGURE 11-9 Percentage Distribution of Under-5 Child Deaths Globally, by Cause, 2016

Data from UNICEF. (2017). *Child mortality estimates*. Retrieved from https://data.unicef.org/topic/child-survival/under-five-mortality/#data

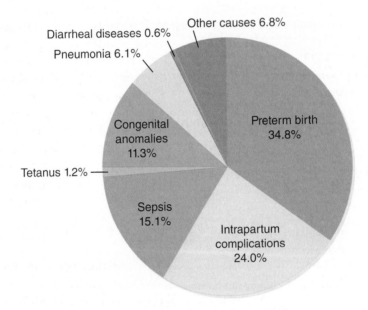

FIGURE 11-10 Percentage Distribution of Neonatal Deaths Globally, by Cause, 2016

Data from UNICEF. (2017). *Child mortality estimates*. Retrieved from https://data.unicef.org/topic/child-survival/under-five-mortality/#data

Additional Comments on Selected Causes of Morbidity and Mortality of Young Children

Pneumonia

Acute respiratory infections are very common causes of sickness and death in children younger than 5 years of age in low- and middle-income countries where children average three to six acute respiratory infections per year. These cases are more severe and cause higher rates of death in low- and middle-income countries than in high-income countries. The most common acute respiratory infections are upper respiratory tract infections, such as the common cold and ear infections.[11]

The common lower respiratory infections are pneumonia and bronchiolitis. Pneumonia is caused by bacteria, viruses, and fungi. The most common forms of bacterial pneumonia are caused by *Streptococcus pneumoniae* (pneumococcus) and *Haemophilus influenzae*, type b (Hib).[11] The most common

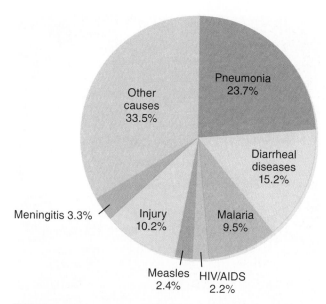

FIGURE 11-11 Percentage Distribution of Post-Neonatal Under-5 Child Deaths (1–59 months) Globally, by Cause, 2016

Data from UNICEF. (2017). *Child mortality estimates*. Retrieved from https://data.unicef.org/topic/child-survival/under-five -mortality/#data

form of viral pneumonia is caused by respiratory syncytial virus. *Pneumocystis jirovecii* is a common form of pneumonia among children who are infected with HIV and the most significant cause of their death from pneumonia.[12] As noted earlier, pneumonia is the leading infectious cause of death globally of children under 5 years of age.

The most common way for pneumonia to be transmitted is via airborne droplets. However, it can also be transmitted through blood, especially around the time of birth.[12] Children who are sick with pneumonia may have fever, cough, wheezing, and difficulty breathing. Pneumonia can be diagnosed at the community level in resource-poor settings by the detection of rapid breathing of the sick child or the drawing in of the chest wall of the child during breathing, rather than its expansion, as is the case in a healthy person. Children who have bacterial pneumonia need to be treated with antibiotics, but only about one-third of the children who should receive such antibiotics actually get them. Most children with pneumonia can be treated in the community, but very sick and very young children need to be treated in the hospital.[12]

Most healthy children can fight off infection. However, children whose immune systems are compromised by undernutrition or by not being exclusively breastfed for 6 months are at greater risk of pneumonia. Illnesses such as HIV/AIDS and measles can also predispose a child to pneumonia. Certain environmental conditions, such as crowded living conditions,

household air pollution from cooking with biomass fuels, and exposure to secondhand smoke, are also risk factors for a child developing pneumonia.[13]

Diarrhea

Diarrhea is the second leading infectious cause of young child deaths, as noted earlier, and is caused by a number of different infectious agents, including bacteria, viruses, protozoa, and helminths.[14] Diarrhea is transmitted by what is known as the "fecal–oral" route of transmission, from the stool of one individual, eventually to the mouth of another. This is generally the result of unsafe water, poor sanitation, and poor hygiene.[14]

Dehydration, loss of nutrition and wasting, and damage to the intestines are all consequences of severe diarrhea.[14] Rapid dehydration due to diarrhea can be quickly fatal. In one study, infants with persistent diarrhea and severe malnutrition were at 17 times greater risk of dying than infants with mild malnutrition.[14] Children under 3 years of age in low-income countries suffer three episodes of diarrhea a year, on average.[15] Children younger than 5 years of age in low- and middle-income countries have around three to four cases of diarrhea per year, with infants 6 to 11 months of age having almost twice as many cases. As noted earlier, this is the age during which children usually stop exclusive breastfeeding and are at most risk of being exposed to unsafe water and foods.[14]

Malaria

Malaria is transmitted by the bite of one of several varieties of mosquito. It is an acute illness that arises in susceptible individuals 10 to 15 days after being bitten. Malaria should be diagnosed with either a blood smear or a rapid diagnostic test. It should be treated with artemisinin-based combination therapy (ACT) only upon a confirmed diagnosis, but there are still significant gaps in following this approach.[16]

Malaria has an enormous impact on the morbidity and mortality of young children. The overwhelming majority of the 435,000 deaths a year that are caused by malaria occur among young children in sub-Saharan Africa.[17] In addition, the morbidity associated with malaria in these children is staggering. One estimate suggested that people in endemic areas of sub-Saharan Africa have almost five episodes of malaria a year.[18] Moreover, the most severe form of malaria, cerebral malaria, has a case fatality rate of close to 20 percent, meaning that 20 percent of the children who get the disease die from it. Beyond the direct consequences of malaria on children are the indirect consequences. Malaria is associated with premature birth and intrauterine growth restriction, which are linked with low birthweight and reduced chances of survival.[18]

HIV/AIDS

One route of HIV transmission is from mother to child. This can take place either during birth or through breastfeeding. A newborn has a 15 percent to 45 percent chance of being infected with HIV from an HIV-positive mother who is not receiving antiretroviral therapy. This rate, however, can be reduced to 5 percent or lower by following established protocols for the reduction of mother-to-child transmission.[19] Children who are HIV-positive and who are not treated with antiretroviral therapy have about a one-third risk of dying during their first year of life and a one-half risk of dying by their second birthday. However, starting treatment by their 12th week of life can reduce their chances of death by 75 percent.[20]

As the rates of new HIV infections among women have generally declined globally, and the use of antiretroviral drugs and other methods to prevent mother-to-child transmission has increased, fewer newborns have been infected with HIV. Nonetheless, in 2017, it was estimated that there were still 180,000 newborns infected with HIV,[21] and more than 90 percent of them were in sub-Saharan Africa.[20] As noted earlier, about 1.2 percent of the deaths of children under 5 globally are a result of HIV infection.

Measles

Measles is discussed further both in the section on immunization and in a case study on global efforts to reduce the burden of measles. For now, it is important to understand that measles is an acute respiratory infection that is spread through droplets in the air or contact with the nasal or throat secretions of an infected person. The initial symptoms are a runny nose, watery eyes, and white spots inside the cheeks. Later, a rash will break out, eventually spreading to the hands and feet.[22] Measles is highly contagious. The U.S. Centers for Disease Control and Prevention (CDC) says that, in the absence of vaccination, 90 percent of the people who come in contact with an infected person will contract measles.[23]

Measles can lead to complications including pneumonia, diarrhea, encephalitis, and blindness. Children who are younger than 5 years of age and either vitamin

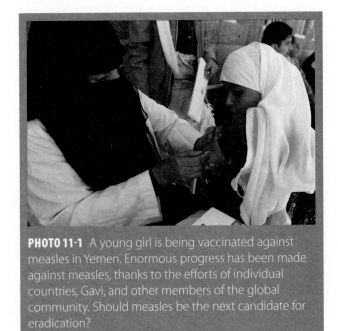

PHOTO 11-1 A young girl is being vaccinated against measles in Yemen. Enormous progress has been made against measles, thanks to the efforts of individual countries, Gavi, and other members of the global community. Should measles be the next candidate for eradication?
© Mohammed Huwais/AFP/Getty Images.

A deficient or HIV-infected are more vulnerable to measles complications and are at higher risk of death than other children their age. Studies in sub-Saharan Africa suggest that between 0.5 percent and 10 percent of children who get measles will die from it.[23]

There has been an enormous amount of progress in increasing vaccination against measles in low- and middle-income countries and in reducing measles infections and deaths. In fact, such deaths decreased by 80 percent globally between 2000 and 2016, with over 550,000 measles deaths in 2000 and close to 90,000 in 2016.[24] Nonetheless, as noted earlier, measles is still among the leading killers of under-5 children globally, accounting for about 1.3 percent of their deaths. The role of vaccination in preventing measles and other diseases is discussed later in the chapter.

Soil-Transmitted Helminths

Soil-transmitted helminths are generally thought of as "worms" that infect humans. The most common such infections come from roundworm, hookworm, and whipworm. About 270 million children of preschool age and another almost 560 million children of school age live in areas of intense transmission of these parasites.[25] These infections can lead to severe morbidity, such as iron deficiency anemia, and are also associated with impaired physical and mental development in childhood.[26] Moreover, the burden of several species of worms is highest in children around 6 or 7 years of age.[27] About 70 percent of the children at risk are receiving antihelminthic medicines.[25]

Additional Comments on Neonatal Mortality

There has been important progress in reducing the deaths of children younger than 5 years, as discussed earlier. However, there has been less progress in reducing the neonatal death rate. Of the 5.4 million children under 5 years of age who died in 2017, about 2.5 million, or 46 percent of them, died in the first month of life, and almost all of them lived in low- and middle-income countries.[1(p2)]

If the world is to further reduce child death rates, then it will have to reduce neonatal death rates. If the world is to do that, it will have to focus more precisely on when child deaths take place, where they take place, and why they occur. More than one-third of the children who die in their first month of life will actually die on their first day of life.[28] About 73 percent of the deaths that take place in the first month of life actually take place in the first week of life. Clearly, every day that a child lives increases the likelihood that he or she will stay alive. This may help to explain why children in a number of cultures are not named until after their first month of life. It may also help to explain why so many births are not registered with civil authorities, as was the case for Nassiba in the vignette that opened this chapter.

In thinking about neonatal deaths, just as in thinking about the deaths of all infants and children under 5 years, we must remember the relationship between the health of the mother and the health of the baby. Between 60 percent and 80 percent of neonatal deaths occur in low-birthweight babies. This generally reflects the poor health and nutritional status of the mother, including her being undernourished or having malaria, for example.[29] We also need to remember that an enormous number of child lives could be saved if the gap in child deaths between the richest and poorest segments of society were narrowed, even *within* most low- and middle-income countries.

▶ Risk Factors for Neonatal, Infant, and Young Child Deaths

Why do so many children get sick and die of preventable causes? As mentioned earlier, an important part of the risks has to do with the social determinants of health. Poverty, for example, contributes to poor health and is a major underlying cause of morbidity and mortality among children. Where there is poverty, there is often inadequate nutrition. Where there is poverty, there is less access to safe water and sanitation, health services, and education. All of these are important determinants of child health. As noted earlier, there is a very strong correlation between family income and the likelihood that a neonate, an infant, or a child will survive. There is a similar correlation between the health and the educational status of the mother and the prospects that a child will survive birth and the first 5 years of life.

In fact, *The Millennium Development Goals Report 2006*, in commenting on progress toward the Millennium Development Goal of reducing child morbidity and mortality, revealed that higher household income and education for mothers doubled child survival rates. In families where the mother had no education or only primary education, child mortality averaged 157 deaths per 1,000 live births, whereas in families where the mother had secondary education or higher, mortality rates were close to 50 percent lower, at 82 per 1,000 live births.[30]

The health of the mother is also a critical determinant of the health of the newborn. The risks to the mother and child increase if the mother is a teenager or an older woman, if the woman has had only a short birth interval between her last child and the next one, if the woman is of short stature, or if the woman is herself poorly nourished or suffering from malaria. These factors contribute to prematurity and low birthweight, both of which are important predictors of the well-being and survival of the child.[31]

The survival of a newborn is also closely linked with whether the birth took place in an appropriate healthcare setting and is attended by a trained healthcare provider.[32] A baby's chances of survival increase

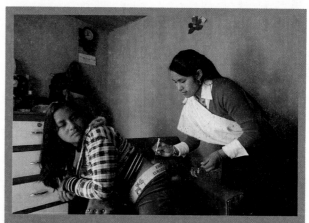

PHOTO 11-2 This is a picture of a woman making a prenatal visit in Ecuador. What measures must be taken to promote the births of healthier babies in settings where women may be undernourished, have their first birth when they are very young, and give birth at home without a skilled attendant?
Courtesy of Mark Tuschman.

greatly when the baby is born in a setting that can deal with obstetric emergencies. The chances of survival also increase if the delivery is attended by a skilled birth attendant who can resuscitate babies who need it and can help counsel families about keeping babies warm and initiating breastfeeding early.

The environmental circumstances under which the child lives are also fundamental to well-being. Household air pollution is an important risk factor for respiratory diseases. Living in zones that are endemic for malaria and other diseases also poses a risk to young children. The lack of access to clean water and sanitation is linked with diarrheal disease and soil-transmitted helminths, among other problems. Moreover, the risk of unsafe hygiene increases greatly as the child begins to eat complementary foods and is no longer exclusively breastfed. We have also seen that better-educated families have more awareness about health risks, as well as safe behaviors that can improve their children's health and chances of survival.

Nutritional status has a profound impact, indirectly through the mother, and directly on the health and survival prospects of neonates, infants, and children younger than 5 years of age. As a critical study noted[33(p2227)]:

- "Infants aged 0–5 months who are not breastfed have five-fold and seven-fold increased risks of death from pneumonia and diarrhea, respectively, compared to infants who are exclusively breastfed."
- "35% of all child deaths are due to the effect of underweight status on diarrhea, pneumonia, measles, and malaria and relative risks of maternal body mass index for fetal growth restriction and its risks for selected neonatal causes of death."
- "In children with vitamin A deficiency, the risk of dying from diarrhea, measles, and malaria is increased by 20 to 24%. Likewise, zinc deficiency increases the risk of mortality from diarrhea, pneumonia, and malaria by 13 to 21%."

Wars and conflicts take a significant toll on children and are regrettable risk factors for child morbidity and mortality, particularly in sub-Saharan Africa and the Middle East. UNICEF estimated that in a typical 5-year war, under-5 mortality increases 13 percent.[34] In addition, the highest rates of neonatal death occur in conflict-ridden countries or countries just emerging from conflict, such as Liberia and Sierra Leone.[29]

Of course, family knowledge about health-seeking behaviors, the ability of families to actually seek appropriate health services, and their ability to get services of appropriate quality in a timely manner are

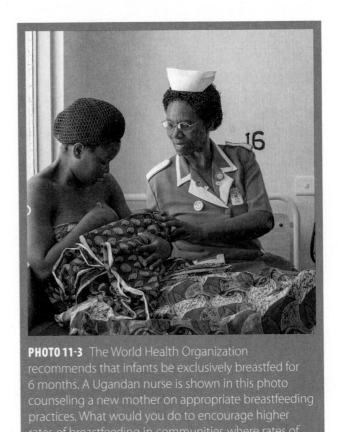

PHOTO 11-3 The World Health Organization recommends that infants be exclusively breastfed for 6 months. A Ugandan nurse is shown in this photo counseling a new mother on appropriate breastfeeding practices. What would you do to encourage higher rates of breastfeeding in communities where rates of exclusive breastfeeding are low?
Courtesy of Mark Tuschman.

also critical to whether children survive and thrive. As discussed further later, there are a number of low-cost and highly effective interventions that can reduce the burden of childhood deaths. There are, for example, vaccines that can prevent some pneumonia and diarrhea and that can greatly reduce the burden of other vaccine-preventable diseases, such as measles. Families can be taught to diagnose pneumonia, and community health workers can be taught to treat it with antibiotics. Oral rehydration can prevent deaths from diarrhea. Sleeping under a bed net can reduce the burden of malaria. Antiretroviral therapy can reduce mother-to-child transmission of HIV. Additionally, there are a range of nutrition interventions that are also low-cost and highly effective and that can enhance maternal and child health.

▶ The Costs and Consequences of Child Morbidity and Mortality

One cannot measure direct losses in productivity that relate immediately to the morbidity and mortality of young children. There are, however, enormous costs and consequences to these illnesses. Some of them are short-term and relate to the family. Others are medium- or longer-term and relate to the child directly.

First, the direct and indirect costs of caring for a sick child can be very high. As noted earlier in this chapter, the average child in Africa is infected with malaria every 40 days. In addition, the average child in low- and middle-income countries will get three to six cases per year of acute respiratory infection and two to three cases of diarrhea. In this light, it is not surprising that families spend considerable parts of their limited financial resources on buying medical care for a sick child.[14] Moreover, caregivers devote special attention to the child who is ill, which prevents them from engaging in their normal income-earning activities.

Second, the medium- and long-term consequences of some childhood illnesses can be very high. Problems associated with prematurity, low birthweight, intrauterine growth restriction, and congenital abnormalities can lead to permanent disability and the associated costs to families and to society. A study on diarrheal disease in Brazil concluded that intelligence test scores were "25 to 65 percent lower in children with an earlier history of persistent diarrhea."[14(p375)] The complications of measles can lead to encephalitis and blindness, as indicated earlier. By causing anemia, growth restriction, and the slowing of mental development, helminthic infections reduce children's enrollment, attendance, and performance in school and have consequences for later productivity.[27]

Finally, there is a range of social costs and consequences associated with childhood illness and death. Many poor families in low-income countries, knowing the odds are high that their newborn will die, have very high fertility to compensate for these deaths. In other words, in the hope of ensuring that the number of children they want will survive, they have more children than they would have otherwise.

▶ Immunization: A Best Buy in Global Health

The Unique Importance of Immunization in Child Health

In a discussion of child health, immunization merits special attention because it is one of the most successful and cost-effective child health interventions that is available. Effective national immunization programs are essential to reduce under-5 morbidity and mortality globally. In fact, each year, routine immunization prevents between 2 million and 3 million deaths and protects up to 100 million people against illness and disability.[35,36]

Immunization provides a range of direct and indirect benefits. The direct benefits include the prevention of illness in the immunized individual, reducing the health costs the immunized person would face if they fell ill from the disease for which they are immunized, and preventing the loss of productivity of the ill person and people who have to care for them. The indirect or "broader" benefits of immunization are also extensive. By preventing illness, vaccines contribute to healthy child development and higher cognitive skills in the child, and reduce losses in productivity later in life. By reducing healthcare costs, immunization allows families to save and invest money that encourages broader economic and social development. Through **herd immunity**, vaccines protect the health of unvaccinated people, conferring important health, economic, and social benefits on them as well.[37] In addition, because immunization prevents illnesses that are typically treated with antibiotics, immunization decreases the use of antibiotics and the risk of the development of antibiotic-resistant pathogens, which are more difficult and expensive to treat than drug-susceptible pathogens.

Recognized as a "best buy in global health," national immunization programs are investments in the individuals, families, communities, and countries in which they operate. Immunization makes economic sense. Studies have suggested, for example, that scaling up existing vaccines in 72 of the poorest countries could save 6.4 million lives and avert $6.2 billion in treatment costs and $145 billion in productivity losses between 2011 and 2020.[38] Routine immunization generates economic benefits that derive from both productive human capital and from medical costs averted by preventing disease.[39]

Immunization also improves life expectancy, and research suggests that a 5-year improvement in life expectancy results in 0.3 to 0.5 percent more annual growth in income per capita.[40,41] In addition, immunization prevents families of sick children from incurring the direct costs of treatment and hospitalization and the indirect costs associated with caregiving, such as inability to participate in the labor market while caring for a sick child. Moreover, in areas where the under-5 mortality rate is high, fertility rates also tend to be high as parents seek to ensure that some of their children will survive to adulthood. When population health improves and fertility rates drop, the age distribution becomes more favorable to economic growth, through the **demographic dividend**.

Global Immunization Efforts

The international community has developed a variety of programs and initiatives to promote child health through immunization. The most significant of these programs has been the Expanded Programme on Immunization (EPI). In 1974, the World Health Assembly launched EPI with the objective of vaccinating children throughout the world.[42] In its first phase, EPI focused on six diseases: tuberculosis (TB), poliomyelitis (polio), diphtheria, tetanus, pertussis (whooping cough), and measles. At the time EPI was created, only about 5 percent of the world's children were vaccinated against these six diseases, which were targeted by four vaccines.[43] EPI recommended vaccinating all eligible children from birth to 12 months against these diseases and giving pregnant women tetanus toxoid vaccinations.

Countries throughout the world progressively adopted EPI until the 1980s when the program became universal. When EPI was created in 1974, WHO established a standardized vaccine schedule that included four vaccines against six diseases: Bacillus Calmette-Guérin (BCG) for TB; diphtheria-tetanus-pertussis (DTP); oral polio (OPV); and measles vaccine. For the first 20 to 30 years after EPI was created, global immunization efforts consistently included these four vaccines and six antigens. Starting around the year 2000, however, scientific advances in the vaccines themselves and in logistics and storage, combined with a renewed global commitment to immunization, began to increase the number of introductions of new and underused vaccines (NUVIs), even in low- and middle-income countries.[44] Over time, EPI recommended that all children also be immunized against rubella, hepatitis B (HepB), *Haemophilus influenzae* b (Hib), rotavirus, pneumococcal pneumonia, and human papillomavirus (HPV). Antigens to protect against these diseases are now included in a range of different vaccine combinations. This includes the pentavalent vaccine, which has antigens against five childhood diseases: diphtheria, tetanus, pertussis (whooping cough), hepatitis B, and *Haemophilus influenzae* type b (Hib).[45]

TABLE 11-5 shows the antigens that WHO recommends for children in all countries and those that are recommended for children residing in certain regions at risk for particular vaccine-preventable diseases.

The main strategic document for global vaccine efforts is the Global Vaccine Action Plan (GVAP), which was launched in 2011 and covers the period to 2020. The member states of the World Health Assembly endorsed GVAP. This plan builds upon the success of earlier efforts and seeks to achieve key milestones in discovery, development, and delivery of life-saving vaccines to the world's most vulnerable populations. GVAP lays out specific targets against which progress in immunization can be measured.[46]

Financing Immunization

From the beginning of EPI, it was clear that many countries would require financial assistance with the costs of their national immunization programs.[42,47] In 1977, therefore, the Pan American Health Organization (PAHO) created the PAHO Revolving Fund for Vaccine Procurement. This fund, which pooled the resources of 41 countries, allowed those countries to bargain as a group to buy large quantities of high-quality vaccines, syringes, and related supplies at the lowest possible price and then distribute them among the individual countries. This purchasing system helped enable the vaccination of tens of millions of children in the Americas and avert millions of deaths from vaccine-preventable disease.[48] The fund promotes self-sufficiency by using economies of scale to bring prices down to affordable levels. As of several years ago, PAHO member states covered 95 percent of vaccination costs from their own national budgets.[48]

The Global Alliance for Vaccines and Immunization (GAVI), now officially titled Gavi, The Vaccine Alliance, was established in 2000. Gavi was created to help address the large number of children globally who were not being vaccinated at the time with the six basic antigens. It also was established to deal with the exceptionally slow pace with which many low- and middle-income countries adopted the "newer" vaccines, such as the HepB, Hib, and pneumococcal vaccines. Gavi was "seeded" with a $750 million grant from the Bill & Melinda Gates Foundation.[49]

Gavi is a public–private partnership that works to promote and strengthen immunization programs in low- and middle-income countries. It aims to assist countries in being able to manage and finance national vaccination programs over time, without external financial support. Toward these aims, Gavi assists countries in financing procurement of vaccines and related supplies and strengthening their capacity to deliver vaccines to those who need them in a timely, high-quality, and sustainable way.[49]

Gavi has also sought to influence markets for vaccines and related products by encouraging lower prices on existing vaccines and the development of new vaccines. Gavi has also supported the development and implementation of more efficient procurement

TABLE 11-5 WHO Recommended Vaccines

Antigen	Related Disease
Recommended for All Children	
BCG	Tuberculosis
Hepatitis B	Hepatitis B
Polio	Polio
Haemophilus influenzae type b (Hib)	Pneumonia
Pneumococcal	Pneumococcal disease
Rotavirus	Diarrhea
Measles	Measles
Rubella	Rubella
Human papillomavirus (HPV)	HPV
Recommended for Children Residing in Certain Regions	
Japanese encephalitis	Japanese encephalitis
Yellow fever	Yellow fever
Tick-borne encephalitis	Encephalitis

World Health Organization (WHO). (2018). *WHO recommendations for routine immunization*: Summary tables. Retrieved from https://www.who.int/immunization/policy/immunization_tables/en/

mechanisms.[50] Gavi has done this partly through novel financing mechanisms, such as the International Finance Facility for Immunisation, which is discussed in Chapter 18. Gavi estimates that it has assisted countries since 2000 in immunizing more than 700 million children, associated with saving about 10 million lives.[49]

Countries are eligible to seek Gavi support based on their average Gross National Income (GNI) per capita over the last 3 years. The threshold for 2018 was $1,580 per capita. On that basis, 47 countries were eligible for Gavi financing in 2018. As countries approach the income threshold for support, Gavi works with them to transition out of Gavi assistance.[51]

A study covering 73 Gavi-supported countries over the 2011 to 2020 period estimated that, for every $1 spent on immunization, $18 would be saved in healthcare costs, lost wages, and lost productivity due to illness. The estimated return on investment rose to

$48 per $1 spent when taking into account the benefits of people living longer and healthier lives.[52]

Progress in Immunization Coverage

TABLE 11-6 highlights some of the key areas in which progress has been made in achieving universal coverage of the vaccines that are recommended for all children.

In many respects, progress has been exceptional over the last 2 decades. The number of children who are not vaccinated in low- and middle-income countries has decreased by almost 2 million. The number of children receiving three doses of DTP was the highest ever, as was the share of children receiving the second dose of the measles vaccine. The number of low- and middle-income countries introducing at least one underutilized vaccine has continued to grow. Three more countries eliminated neonatal tetanus. In addition, there were only 15 cases of wild poliovirus in the world in 2018.[53]

TABLE 11-6 Selected Progress in Immunization Coverage, 2017/2018

The number of undervaccinated children fell by 1.8 million between 2000 and 2017.

More children received DTP3 than ever.

Despite humanitarian emergencies in 8 of 22 countries, the WHO Eastern Mediterranean region achieved a DTP3 coverage rate of 81%.

Globally, 88% of the world's children are immunized with BCG against TB.

Haiti achieved elimination of neonatal tetanus, making the Americas free of neonatal tetanus.

The WHO Western Pacific region achieved its lowest level of measles incidence, and two countries have eliminated rubella.

The Africa region has expanded funding for immunization by 130% since 2010.

The number of new wild polio infections declined from 22 in 2017 to 15 in 2018, and the number of new cases of circulating vaccine-derived polio fell from 96 to 32.

Five more countries introduced a new or underutilized vaccine.

Fewer countries experienced vaccine stock-outs.

Data from World Health Organization (WHO). (2018). *2018 assessment report of the global vaccine action plan*. Geneva, Switzerland: Author. Retrieved from https://www.who.int/immunization /sage/meetings/2018/october/2_Draft2018GVAP_Ass_Rep.pdf?ua=1; World Health Organization (WHO). (2018, September 21). *Global and regional immunization profile*. Retrieved from https:// www.who.int/immunization/monitoring_surveillance/data/gs_gloprofile.pdf?ua=1

Continuing Gaps in Coverage

Despite enormous progress in expanding coverage of the recommended vaccines, there remain a number of critical gaps in achieving universal coverage. **TABLE 11-7** highlights some of the key gaps.

First, there are almost 20 million children in low- and middle-income countries who are undervaccinated. About 60 percent of these children live in nine, mostly very populous, countries, including Angola, Democratic Republic of Congo, Ethiopia, India, Indonesia, Iraq, Nigeria, Pakistan, and South Africa. Second, the rates of coverage with the third DTP vaccine is disturbingly low in some countries, such as 25 percent in Equatorial Guinea, 26 percent in South Sudan, 41 percent in Chad, and 43 percent in Nigeria. In addition, four regions suffered measles outbreaks, and two regions suffered outbreaks of diphtheria. While five regions are targeted for rubella elimination by 2020, only one region has achieved it so far. Moreover, although the number of polio cases has declined, eradication of polio remains immensely challenging.[53]

Gaps in vaccination coverage are explained by a number of variables. Low-income countries may lack the health infrastructure, human resources, and financing to maintain a predictable and sustainable national immunization program. The success of national immunization programs may also be inhibited by armed conflict, natural disasters, gaps in vaccine-preventable disease surveillance, and inadequate safety measures.[42] Critical challenges to universal coverage are discussed in the next section.

Critical Challenges to Universal Vaccine Coverage

Today, there remain a number of critical challenges to universal childhood immunization. **TABLE 11-8** cites some of the key challenges, a few of which are elaborated in this section.

Some of these challenges have to do with the "basics" of immunization. These center on healthcare infrastructure, human resources, and financing. Despite substantial progress in most countries, some low- and middle-income countries still lack the healthcare infrastructure or human resources necessary to run a successful national immunization program on their own. Some countries may also have difficulty forecasting the number of vaccines they need or procuring and distributing them in a timely way.[53]

TABLE 11-7 Selected Gaps in Vaccine Coverage, 2017/2018

19.9 million children were undervaccinated in 2017.

11 countries that previously achieved 90% DTP3 coverage in the past failed to reach this target in 2017.

A substantial number of countries, including some in sub-Saharan Africa and some conflict-ridden countries in the Middle East and North Africa, have rates of DTP3 coverage below 50%.

Measles outbreaks occurred in 2017 in four WHO regions, and measles is again endemic in all WHO regions.

Measles incidence increased from 19 cases per million to 25 cases per million.

Coverage of the first measles dose plateaued below the desired level, and despite progress, coverage of the second dose was still only 65%.

Only one WHO region is free of rubella.

Vaccine hesitancy exists in almost all countries.

The world is not on track to meet a number of key targets from the Global Vaccine Action Plan.

New vaccine introductions are at risk of stalling.

Data from World Health Organization (WHO). (2018). *2018 assessment report of the global vaccine action plan*. Geneva, Switzerland: Author. Retrieved from https://www.who.int/immunization /sage/meetings/2018/october/2_Draft2018GVAP_Ass_Rep.pdf?ua=1

TABLE 11-8 Selected Challenges to Achieving Universal Immunization Coverage

Capacity gaps in national vaccine programs, including in technical, financial, and human resource domains

Vaccine hesitancy

The fragility of gains achieved to date

The need for high and consistent levels of coverage, especially in "the last mile" of efforts to eradicate polio and given the infectiousness of measles

National ownership and commitment

Complacency in the face of progress and the lack of visibility of some diseases in some settings

Gaps in equity and the coverage of the most "difficult to reach"

The financing of immunization in middle-income countries, including after a transition from Gavi financing

Political conflict and the fragility of some states

The need for research and development on new and more effective vaccines and on innovative delivery technologies

Threats to global cooperation

Data from World Health Organization (WHO). (2018). *2018 assessment report of the global vaccine action plan*. Geneva, Switzerland: Author. Retrieved from https://www.who.int/immunization /sage/meetings/2018/october/2_Draft2018GVAP_Ass_Rep.pdf?ua=1

Complacency is another risk to universal coverage of recommended vaccines. Children continue to be born. Thus, vaccine programs have to be sustained indefinitely. A failure to do so can lead to a rise in cases of vaccine-preventable diseases or serious outbreaks of such diseases.[53]

There have also been growing problems in many countries with vaccine hesitancy, a delay in accepting or an unwillingness to accept available vaccines. Since the development of the first vaccines, there have been issues with people who did not wish to be vaccinated, often because of a lack of understanding of the safety and efficacy of the vaccine or due to mistaken notions of such safety and efficacy.[54] However, substantial hesitancy has now arisen in a number of countries, often in high-income countries and often among well-educated people, fueled by a lack of understanding of scientific facts concerning vaccines or an unwillingness to accept those facts. This has also been exacerbated by social media networks of "anti-vaxxers." These networks started after an article in 1998 suggested a link between the measles vaccine and autism in children. Despite the fact that this article was withdrawn, the author of the article lost his medical license, and repeated studies have shown there is *no* link between vaccines and autism, the anti-vaxx movement is quite loud in its opposition to recommended approaches to childhood vaccination. WHO suggests that vaccine hesitancy can best be addressed by a multi-pronged approach that examines the specific hesitancy issues in different settings, creating evidence-based solutions to dealing with hesitancy, and carefully evaluating the impact of those interventions. WHO also reminds us that analysis of hesitancy has to carefully distinguish between barriers to access and barriers to acceptance.[55]

We are also living in a world that is volatile in a number of ways, some of which threaten vaccine programs. Political and civil conflict such as in Afghanistan, Iraq, and Syria poses immense barriers for immunization. Economic disarray and the decline of fragile states, such as in Venezuela, South Sudan, or the Central African Republic, can do the same. In addition, the migration that accompanies conflict can also pose enormous barriers to universal vaccine coverage.[53]

▶ Case Studies

Given the importance of immunization, three case studies follow on that topic. The first looks at efforts to eliminate polio from the Americas. The second examines progress against measles. The last case examines a program for vitamin A supplementation in Nepal. This supplementation is often given in conjunction with mass polio immunization. You can read more about polio in the Americas and Nepal's vitamin A program in *Case Studies in Global Health: Millions Saved.*[56]

Eliminating Polio in Latin America and the Caribbean

Background

In 1952, Jonas Salk discovered the inactivated polio vaccine. Mass immunizations between 1955 and 1961 led to a 90 percent drop in infections in the Western Hemisphere.[57] Ten years later, in 1962, Albert Sabin developed an oral polio vaccine that cost less, was easier to administer, and reduced the multiplication of the virus in the intestine.

The new oral polio vaccine became part of a package of six childhood vaccines included in EPI, launched by WHO in 1974. Latin America adopted EPI in 1977, and the coverage of oral polio vaccine reached 80 percent within just 7 years. Between 1975 and 1981, the incidence of polio was nearly halved, and the number of countries reporting polio cases dropped from 19 to 11.[58]

Intervention

Encouraged by the remarkable progress against polio, PAHO launched a program to eradicate polio from Latin America and the Caribbean. Many international organizations joined together in the program, and regional and country-level Interagency Coordinating Committees were established to oversee the program. Thousands of health workers, managers, and technicians were trained to implement the strategy for the eradication of polio, which included reaching every child with oral polio vaccination, identification of new polio cases, and aggressive control of any outbreaks. If polio was to be eradicated, then the campaign against it would build on the lessons learned from the smallpox eradication campaign.[59]

Impact

The last case of polio in the Latin America and the Caribbean region was reported in Peru in 1991. Polio re-emerged briefly in the year 2000 when 20 vaccine-associated cases were reported in Haiti and the Dominican Republic, but no cases have been reported since 2000.

Costs and Benefits

The polio campaign in the Latin American and Caribbean region cost $120 million in its first 5 years—$74 million from national sources and $46 million from international donors—and $10 million annually from donor sources thereafter. Taking into account the costs of treating polio and its disabling consequences, the investment paid for itself in only 15 years.[60] The program also generated vast improvements in the region's health infrastructure, and it advanced overall goals for immunization.

Lessons Learned

The success of eliminating polio from Latin America and the Caribbean in only 6 years was a result of exemplary political commitment, interagency and regional coordination, and tremendous social and community mobilization. The re-emergence of polio in 2000 alerted the region to the need for continued vaccination and surveillance. The success in Latin America and the Caribbean prompted the global effort to eradicate polio that was launched in 1988.[61] The importance of building trust with local leaders and working closely with communities is one of many lessons from the polio campaign in the Americas that is being adopted in the Global Polio Eradication Initiative.

Measles: Progress and Challenges

Background

There has been substantial progress against measles in the last decade, with measles deaths falling globally from 548,000 in 2000, to 158,000 in 2011,[62] to about 90,000 in 2016.[24] Nonetheless, measles was the 9th largest killer of children under 5 years of age globally in 2016. In addition, measles was the 10th leading cause of death of children under 5 years of age in sub-Saharan Africa and in East Asia and the Pacific and the 11th leading cause in South Asia.[8] There have also been an increasing number of outbreaks in high-income countries, reflecting declines in coverage of the measles vaccine associated with the anti-vaxx movement.[53] This case study discusses what measles is, the vaccine against it, trends in the burden of disease, global goals, and the barriers the world faces in trying to address measles.

The Measles Virus

Measles is a highly contagious viral disease. In the absence of being vaccinated, about 90 percent of those exposed to the virus will contract measles, as noted earlier. The measles virus typically grows in the cells that line the back of the throat and lungs.[22] The virus that causes measles is transmitted by coughing and sneezing, as well as by close contact with infected nasal or throat secretions.[22] The virus continues to be active and contagious in the air or on infected surfaces for up to 2 hours.[22] It can be transmitted by an infected person from 4 days before symptoms start to occur to 4 days after the onset of symptoms.

The first sign of measles is usually high fever, which begins about 10 to 12 days after exposure to the virus.[22] In the initial stage of the virus, the symptoms include a runny nose, a cough, red and watery eyes, and small white spots inside the cheeks.[22] A rash will appear about 14 days after exposure to the virus and will last about 5 to 6 days.[22] The greatest risk of a severe reaction to measles is among poorly nourished young children, children with insufficient vitamin A, or those whose immune systems have been weakened by HIV/AIDS or other diseases.[22]

The Measles Vaccine

The measles vaccine is safe, effective, and inexpensive—it costs less than $1.00 to purchase and deliver[62] in low-income countries. The measles vaccine is often combined with a rubella vaccine, with the result known as "MR" vaccine. WHO recommends that each child receive two doses of the vaccine to ensure immunity and to prevent further outbreaks.[22] In countries where there is ongoing transmission of measles, WHO recommends the first dose be given to children when they are 9 months of age.[63] The second dose can be given through routine immunization programs or supplementary immunization.[64] Even with only one dose of the vaccine, however, there is an 85 percent chance that the child will develop immunity to the measles virus.[22]

Trends in the Burden of Disease

Despite the availability of a safe and cost-effective vaccine, about 15 percent of the children who should receive the first dose each year do not.[53] In addition, in 2017 there were measles outbreaks in four of the six WHO regions.[53]

Any person who is not immune to measles can become infected. The most notable complications from measles include blindness, encephalitis, severe diarrhea and related dehydration, ear infections, and severe respiratory infections such as pneumonia.[22] Unvaccinated pregnant women are also at high risk of measles complications.[22] People who survive the measles virus remain immune for the rest of their lives.[22]

More than 95 percent of measles-related deaths occur in low-income countries, and death rates from measles can reach 10 percent in settings with high rates of undernutrition and poor health systems.[22] People who live in areas experiencing or recovering from a natural disaster or conflict are also at greater risk of contracting measles. This is largely because damage to health infrastructure and health services constrains routine immunizations and results in overcrowding in residential camps—both of which greatly increase the risk of infection.[22]

Global Goals

A Measles & Rubella Initiative that began in 2000 represents a collaborative effort of WHO, UNICEF, the American Red Cross, the Centers for Disease Control and Prevention, and the United Nations Foundation to achieve measles and rubella control goals.[22] Since 2000, the Measles & Rubella Initiative has reached over 1 billion children through mass vaccination campaigns.[22]

In 2012, the Measles & Rubella Initiative launched a new Global Measles and Rubella Strategic Plan, which covers the period 2012 to 2020.[62] The plan aims to eliminate measles and rubella in at least five WHO regions by 2020.[22] The plan focuses on five concepts: to achieve 95 percent coverage with two doses of vaccines, monitor the disease using effective surveillance, develop and maintain outbreak preparedness, build public confidence and demand for immunization, and perform the necessary research and development to improve vaccination.[62]

Outstanding Challenges

There are a number of critical challenges to eliminating measles globally. First is the highly infectious nature of measles. This means that elimination requires a very high level of vaccine coverage and that this coverage must be sustained. This becomes more critical in the face of urbanizing populations that are globally becoming more dense. Second, all countries need to act in harmony on vaccinating their populations against measles, but not all countries see the threat that measles poses. This has become more complicated, as noted earlier, by the anti-vaxx movement in North America and Europe. This has also become more complicated by the fragile nature of some states. Third, as also noted earlier, many countries have not yet developed the capacity to implement measles vaccination effectively, and there are large pockets, especially in several large countries, of unimmunized children. Nor have they developed the ability to contain periodic outbreaks of measles. Further progress against measles could also be constrained by competing priorities for both funding and technical capacity, such as the need to complete the eradication of polio.[65-67]

Some of these challenges can be seen in the developments pertaining to measles in the Americas. Successful measles elimination strategies were implemented in member countries of PAHO in 2000, and endemic measles transmission was successfully halted in the Americas in 2002.[68] Unfortunately, however, there was an outbreak of measles in the Americas in 2017, related to the economic chaos and decline of the health system in Venezuela. It then spread to Brazil, Ecuador, Columbia, and Peru.[69]

Gavi has been an active partner in work against measles and has supported the financing of measles vaccine, syringes, and operational costs.[64] By the end of 2017, Gavi had supported the immunization of more than 52 million children with a second dose of measles and rubella-containing vaccine. Even as Gavi has supported catch-up campaigns against measles and rubella, it has also worked with countries to make immunization against measles and rubella a regular part of their routine immunization programs.[70]

Reducing Child Mortality in Nepal Through Vitamin A

Background

Vitamin A deficiency is a leading determinant of child mortality in low- and middle-income countries. Until the last decade or so, vitamin A deficiency compromised the immune systems of nearly 40 percent of the children in low- and middle-income countries and led to almost 1 million deaths each year. Additionally,

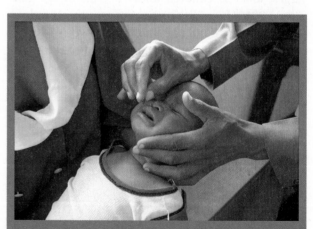

PHOTO 11-4 There has been enormous progress in many countries in distributing vitamin A supplements to young children, often in association with campaigns for mass polio vaccination. This has helped to lower rates of illness and death that are related to vitamin A deficiencies. What can be done to increase vitamin A in children's diets in low-income countries, especially among poor families?

© Wendy Stone/Corbis Historical/Getty Images.

it contributed significantly to the burden of disease caused by malaria, diarrheal disease, acute respiratory infections, and measles.[71]

Vitamin A deficiency was especially important in Nepal, with 2 percent to 13 percent of preschool-aged children experiencing xerophthalmia, a form of blindness caused by vitamin A deficiency. Economic and geographic barriers helped to explain this high prevalence rate. First, difficult terrain made it hard to grow or access the types of food that supply vitamin A. Second, 38 percent of the Nepali population lived in absolute poverty, many of whom were socially excluded lower-caste families, who frequently lacked the means to pay for nutritious foods.

Intervention

Prior to the late 1980s, it was widely held that micronutrient deficiencies were a result of diarrhea and other infant illnesses, rather than a cause of them. Yet, as early as the 1970s, Alfred Sommer noticed in conjunction with studies in Indonesia that vitamin A deficiency appeared to be linked with child death. A later randomized controlled trial conducted in Nepal by Keith West and Sommer indicated that periodic vitamin A supplementation could reduce mortality in children ages 6 to 60 months by as much as 30 percent.[72]

In light of these research findings and Nepal's excessive infant mortality rate, the Nepalese Ministry of Health initiated a plan of action on vitamin A in 1992. The ministry worked closely with other government agencies and nongovernmental organizations (NGOs) to develop a pilot program to deliver vitamin A capsules throughout Nepal. A technical assistance group was created to assist the health ministry in running the program. His Majesty, the King of Nepal, also demonstrated long-term commitment to this effort by incorporating Nepal's National Vitamin A Program into the Ten Year National Program of Action.

This program aimed to reduce child morbidity and mortality by prophylactic supplementation of high-dose vitamin A capsules to children 6 to 60 months of age, twice each year; the treatment of xerophthalmia, severe malnutrition, and prolonged diarrhea; and the promotion of behavior change to increase dietary intake of vitamin A and promote exclusive breastfeeding for the first 6 months of a baby's life.

The action plan on vitamin A focused on expanding the intervention in phases as Nepal's administrative capacity for the program was strengthened. The program was expanded to 32 priority districts at a rate of 8 districts per year over 4 years. From 1993 to 2001, the program was brought to Nepal's remaining 43 districts. Children and new mothers in districts where the

National Vitamin A Program was not yet established received one dose of vitamin A as part of national immunization campaigns. Once the National Vitamin A Program was operating in their district, the children received vitamin A supplementation twice a year.

Nepal's public health system faced severe problems at the time the vitamin A program was developed, from low utilization rates by people who had no confidence in the system to absenteeism by health workers. Consequently, the vitamin A intervention was revised to build upon and improve the existing networks of female community health volunteers (FCHVs) who helped deliver primary health care and family planning services to the villages of Nepal. Before the intervention, there were 24,000 FCHVs throughout 58 districts. However, many were not respected in their communities and had little incentive to remain committed to volunteering. The leader of the program's technical assistance group, Ram Shrestha, changed the way FCHVs were viewed by communities and by themselves by focusing on notions of respect, recognition, and opportunity. Shrestha challenged deeply rooted gender biases by giving women responsibilities valued by their families and communities and the opportunity to make a difference.

A few years later, the number of FCHVs had more than doubled to 49,000 strong, and they were able to reach 3.7 million children twice a year with vitamin A capsules. By directly administering the capsules, the FCHVs served as a critical bridge between the public health sector and the community. Families were urged to bring their children to the distribution site, and many government sectors began to integrate messages about the importance of vitamin A into their programs.

Impact

An evaluation of the program indicated that under-5 mortality decreased by almost 48 deaths per 1,000 births, on average. Higher literacy rates among women, improved weight and nutritional status of children, and better vaccination rates were also associated with success. About 134,000 deaths were averted between mid-1995 and mid-2000 as a result of Nepal's vitamin A program.[73] Although it took nearly 8 years to achieve nationwide distribution, program coverage never dropped below 90 percent in districts once they were covered.

Costs and Benefits

Compared to other micronutrient supplement programs, which can cost up to about $5 per child,[74] the vitamin A supplement program in Nepal was a relatively inexpensive approach to ease the burden of a national problem. The cost of the program per child covered was approximately $0.81 to $1.09 for a child receiving one capsule and $0.68 to $1.65 for a child receiving two capsules of vitamin A.[75] Additionally, given the 7,500 lives saved annually, the expanded program in 2000 was estimated to cost $345 per death averted or $11 to $12 per DALY averted.[76]

Lessons Learned

The success of Nepal's vitamin A supplementation program demonstrates how a technical innovation, when paired with an equally innovative operational plan, can result in a major population impact. Rather than trying to restructure the health system to accommodate the vitamin A program, Shrestha adapted the vitamin A program to the preexisting network of FCHVs and then refined it in such a way that it could be successful. This approach also reinforced a multisectoral effort by involving the government, NGOs, and communities. Other key factors associated with this successful effort were partnership building, regular monitoring of quality, straightforward and effective public messages, and clarity of objectives and operational strategy. These lessons are all the more important given that this successful effort took place in a very low-income country with extremely weak governance and poor administrative capacity.

▶ Addressing Key Challenges in Child Health

As noted earlier, there has been important progress in the last 30 years in reducing morbidity and mortality of children younger than 5 years of age. In 1990, 1 of every 11 children born died before their fifth birthday. In 2017, that number had decreased to 1 in 26. Moreover, the pace of such reduction increased from 2000 to 2017, compared to the period of the 1990s.[77]

Despite this progress, the challenges to improving the health of children in low- and middle-income countries remain substantial. First, much less progress has been made in reducing neonatal deaths than in reducing post-neonatal deaths.[1] Second, progress in reducing child deaths has remained insufficient in the two regions with the highest rate of such deaths—sub-Saharan Africa and South Asia. In addition, given demographic patterns, sub-Saharan Africa is the only region with more under-5 children than in 1990, and this is the region where progress in reducing the under-5 mortality rate has been the lowest.[4]

In addition, many interventions that are known to be low-cost and effective at reducing morbidity and mortality in young children are not being implemented where they are needed most. Many mothers-to-be and mothers are not well-nourished and are not receiving appropriate prenatal care. A large number of births in low-income countries take place without the help of a skilled birth attendant who can assist the mother and, for example, resuscitate the baby if needed. Many families still do not use oral rehydration therapy (ORT) when their child gets diarrhea. Too often, the pneumonia that kills young children is not diagnosed or treated appropriately or in a timely way. Insecticide-treated bed nets, which are known to reduce the transmission of malaria, are still not as widely used as they should be. There are also major gaps in the early diagnosis and appropriate treatment of malaria in children.

Additionally, a large proportion of neonatal deaths in low- and middle-income countries could be avoided with simple technologies that can be effectively implemented in low-income settings.[32] In fact, almost two-thirds of the child deaths that occur every year could be prevented by the effective implementation of measures such as these, that are both low-cost and effective.[33]

Moreover, there remain important gaps in addressing the social determinants of poor child health and many of the key risk factors, such as undernutrition, water, sanitation, hygiene, and education. There are also only a small number of low-income countries that have taken a coordinated approach across government agencies to address these risk factors.

What can be done to increase the uptake of these approaches, especially in South Asia and sub-Saharan Africa? What can be done to decrease as quickly as possible the rate of neonatal deaths, again, largely in these two regions? Can measures be taken that will help children from low-income families with little education die as rarely as children from better-off and better-educated families?[78] The following section examines some of what has been learned about cost-effective interventions to prevent child deaths and how these efforts can be scaled up more rapidly. Some of the comments will be organized around the life cycle. Others will be organized by type of intervention. Additional comments on intersectoral approaches to addressing child health are provided in Chapter 19.

Critical Child Health Interventions
An Overview of Key Interventions

There are several ways to think coherently about the interventions needed to reduce preventable illness and deaths among children under 5 years of age. One is to take a life-course approach, as shown in **FIGURE 11-12**.

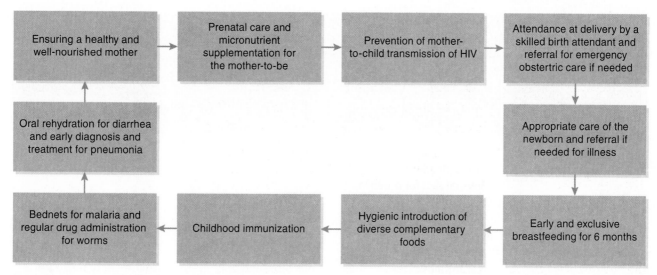

FIGURE 11-12 Key Interventions Along the Life Course

In this case, we can think of the timing for different interventions[79,80]:

- Pre-pregnancy
- During pregnancy
- During labor, birth, and in the first week after birth
- In the postnatal period of infancy
- Between 1 and 5 years of age

In addition, it is critical to think about what interventions are needed during each of these periods.[79,80]

It is also essential to consider what the critical impediments would be to implementing those interventions[81]:

- Which are the most difficult interventions to implement and take to scale?
- What are the key gaps in implementing them—insufficient financing, the lack of human resources, weaknesses in service delivery?
- What can be learned from the experiences of those countries that have done well in reducing newborn and young child deaths?

It is also valuable to understand that the world has adopted the Every Newborn Action Plan, which has five strategic objectives[80]:

- Strengthen and invest in care during the crucial period of labor, childbirth, and the first days of life
- Improve the quality of maternal and newborn care
- Reach every woman and every newborn baby and reduce inequities
- Harness the power of parents, families, and communities for change

- Count every newborn baby—improve measurement and accountability, including birth and death registration

In thinking about newborns and children who survive the neonatal period, it will also be essential to consider what causes children to get sick and die, which children get these conditions, the risk factors for these conditions, and what can be done at the least cost to address these problems in fairly distributed ways. To ensure the survival and well-being of children in the post-neonatal period, it will be imperative to pay particular attention to pneumonia, diarrhea, sepsis and other infections, malaria, HIV/AIDS, and soil-transmitted helminths.

An Essential Package of Interventions for Child Health

DCP3 has recently recommended an "essential package" of interventions for addressing critical issues in the health of newborns and young children in low- and middle-income countries.[9,82] This was part of a study of reproductive, maternal, newborn, and child health. These packages are shown in **TABLE 11-9**. The interventions are noted by the delivery platform from which they should be offered: the community worker or health post, a primary health center, or a first-level or referral hospital.

This DCP3 study suggests that progress in reducing child morbidity and mortality could be accelerated by the adoption of the proposed packages. The proposed interventions are deemed to be highly cost-effective. In addition, when examining the cost–benefit ratios of the interventions to 2035, they yielded a return of 7 to 11 dollars for every dollar spent.[9(p1)]

TABLE 11-9 Essential Package of Interventions for Child Health

	Delivery Platform		
	Community Worker or Health Post	**Primary Health Center**	**First-Level and Referral Hospitals**
Newborn Health	Promotion of exclusive breastfeeding Thermal care for preterm newborns	Kangaroo mother care	Full supportive care for preterm newborns
	Neonatal resuscitation		
	Oral antibiotics for pneumonia	Injectable and oral antibiotics for sepsis, pneumonia, and meningitis	Treatment of newborn complications, meningitis, and other very serious infections
		Jaundice management	
Child Health	Promote breastfeeding and complementary feeding		
	Provide vitamin A, zinc, and food supplementation		
	Immunizations		
	Cotrimoxazole for HIV-positive children		
	Education on safe disposal of children's stools and handwashing		
	Distribute and promote use of insecticide-treated nets (ITNs) or indoor residual spraying (IRS)		
	Detect and refer severe acute malnutrition	Treat severe acute malnutrition	Treat severe acute malnutrition associated with serious infection
	Detect and treat serious infections without danger signs with integrated community case management (iCCM); refer if danger signs	Detect and treat serious infections with danger signs with integrated management of childhood illness (IMCI)	Detect and treat serious infections with danger signs with full supportive care

Reproduced form Black, R. E., Walker, N., Laxminarayan, R., & Temmerman, M. (2016). Reproductive, maternal, newborn, and child health: Key messages of this volume. In R. E. Black, R. Laxminarayan, M. Temmerman, & N. Walker (Eds.), *Disease control priorities: Reproductive, maternal, newborn, and child health* (3rd ed., Vol. 2). Washington, DC: The World Bank.

The study also highlighted the importance of contraception. It suggested that, at current rates of pregnancy, stillbirths, and newborn and young child deaths, meeting 90 percent of the unmet need for family planning could annually avert 67,000 maternal deaths, 440,000 neonatal deaths, 473,000 child deaths, and 564,000 stillbirths from avoided pregnancies.[9(p1)]

The study further suggested that the biggest impact on deaths, including maternal deaths, would come from the following[9(p1)]:

- The provision of contraception
- Management of labor and delivery
- Care of preterm births
- Treatment of severe infectious diseases, including pneumonia, diarrhea, malaria, and neonatal sepsis
- Management of severe acute malnutrition

The study also suggested that the proposed packages, including interventions for maternal health, would be affordable, costing less than $4 per person per year in low-income countries. It further indicated that efforts at the community level and primary health center level could, if taken to scale, avert almost 80 percent of the deaths that could be averted by the entire package, including at the hospital level. Of course, ensuring quality delivery of these packages in countries with the least capacity would require strengthening of the health system and its delivery mechanisms, through task shifting; household visitation, community mobilization, and service delivery; financial incentives to families and providers; and supervision and accreditation.[9(p2)]

The comments that follow elaborate briefly on interventions to enhance child health.

The Mother-to-Be and the Mother[83]

Delaying marriage and first birth is critical in settings where women give birth as teenagers and tend to have many births with short birth intervals. In these settings, birth spacing and reducing total fertility would encourage healthier mothers and babies.

Prenatal care can help ensure that women are properly nourished and are taking prenatal micronutrient supplements. This care can also help detect problems related to hypertension or diabetes that are important to the health of the mother and the child. Mothers can also be treated during pregnancy for malaria, which can have a deleterious impact on the growth of the fetus and on child birthweight. In certain settings, measures can also be taken to help women with difficulties carrying the baby to term, seeking to avoid stillbirths and prematurity.

A substantial number of pregnant women are infected with HIV/AIDS, particularly in parts of central and southern Africa. Prenatal care can assist in diagnosing HIV infection in a pregnant woman and referring her for antiretroviral therapy for her own health and to avoid mother-to-child transmission. Measures to prevent HIV infection among women and mothers-to-be are the most cost-effective ways to ensure that HIV/AIDS is not transmitted from mothers to their children. However, if a mother is HIV-infected, then providing drug therapy to the mother and the newborn to prevent transmission can also be cost-effective.[84]

It is also important to have a skilled birth attendant at delivery. Proper monitoring of labor and the fetus can improve pregnancy and birth outcomes. In addition, if the labor is complicated, then access to emergency obstetric care can reduce risks to both mother and child. Preventing infection is also important to the mother and child. Ensuring that the mother is vaccinated against tetanus is also critical to the prospects for child survival.[29] Early postnatal visits can also reduce neonatal deaths.[85]

The Newborn

As discussed earlier, most child deaths in the first month of life will be from the complications of prematurity, asphyxia, or sepsis. A number of cost-effective measures can be taken to address these problems. They focus on essential newborn care for all newborns, extra care for small babies, and emergency care. These measures are summarized in **TABLE 11-10**.[29] Low-income countries do not need to adopt expensive, high-technology solutions to reduce their neonatal death rates in the near future.

In terms of essential care of newborns, skilled attendance at delivery is crucial to save both newborn lives and the lives of mothers. It is imperative for the health of the baby, for example, that the delivery attendant cut the umbilical cord in a hygienic manner and practice other infection controls. In addition, the baby needs to be kept warm and not bathed for the first 24 hours. The attendant should also be trained and have the equipment needed to resuscitate the baby if necessary, and efforts are under way for that to be done in the simplest possible way in low-income settings. Attendance at delivery is also an appropriate time for a trained practitioner to counsel the family about exclusive breastfeeding and recognizing the danger signs to the baby's health that require immediate attention, such as pneumonia.[29]

Some babies need extra care. If the baby is born prematurely or is of low birthweight, then it is

TABLE 11-10 Interventions for Essential Newborn Care, Extra Care for Small Babies, and Newborn Emergency Care

Essential Newborn Care

- Early and exclusive breastfeeding
- Warmth provision and avoidance of bathing during the first 24 hours
- Infection control, including cord care and hygiene
- Postpartum vitamin A provided to mothers
- Eye antimicrobial to prevent ophthalmia, inflammation of the eye, or conjunctiva
- Information and counseling for home care and emergency preparedness
- Neonatal resuscitation if not breathing at birth

Extra Care for Small Babies

- Extra attention to warmth, feeding support, infection prevention, skin care, and early identification and management of complications
- Kangaroo mother care
- Vitamin K injection
- Monitored safe oxygen use

Emergency Care

- Providing supportive care for severe infections, neonatal encephalopathy (brain disease), severe jaundice or bleeding, seizure management, respiratory distress syndrome (RDS), and neonatal tetanus where appropriate

Modified from Lawn, J. E., Zupan, J., Begkoyian, G., & Knippenberg, R. (2006). Newborn survival. In D. T. Jamison, J. G. Breman, A. R. Measham, et al. (Eds.), *Disease control priorities in developing countries* (2nd ed., pp. 531–549). Washington, DC: Oxford University Press; Additions made from Howson, C. P., Kinney, M. V., McDougall, L., & Lawn, J. E. (2012). *Born too soon: The global action report on preterm birth.* Geneva, Switzerland: World Health Organization.

especially important that the baby be kept warm and fed properly and that any complications be managed quickly and appropriately. In high-income countries, premature babies would be kept in an incubator. This option rarely exists for the children of poor families in low-income countries. However, a study done in India[86] showed that the neonatal mortality rate among babies born between 35 and 37 weeks, or moderately premature babies, was reduced by 87 percent by the provision of special sleeping bags to keep the baby warm, coupled with the promotion of breastfeeding and early treatment of infections.

Another effort at keeping otherwise healthy premature and low-birthweight babies warm is kangaroo mother care (KMC). KMC involves skin-to-skin contact between a mother (and others) and her newborn, frequent and exclusive or nearly exclusive breastfeeding, and early discharge from the hospital.[87] KMC can meet a baby's needs for warmth, breastfeeding, stimulation, safety, and affection.[88] First, the baby, wearing only a diaper, is kept warm through contact with the mother's skin. Second, the skin-to-skin contact between the mother and baby enhances their psychological bond, which improves health and development. Third, the baby can nurse on demand, which helps low-birthweight babies to gain weight, among other benefits, such as protection from infection.[89] KMC can be started at a health facility and continued at home, with proper follow-up and support.[88]

Studies of KMC have shown that it can reduce by 50 percent the mortality of babies born weighing less than 2,000 grams. It has also been associated with reductions in sepsis and infections by 60 percent. It has been shown to reduce hypothermia and lower respiratory diseases, while improving weight gain, head circumference, and exclusive breastfeeding. It also appears to confer long-term benefits on maternal and child bonds and on child development.[90]

Despite these efforts, some babies will become infected and will require emergency care. The question of providing antibiotics to neonates who have infections is a challenging one in many settings. In many places, only physicians are legally allowed to prescribe antibiotics. Yet, physicians may not be accessible, particularly in rural and impoverished settings that will have the highest rates of neonatal mortality. There is evidence that community health workers can be trained to safely give antibiotics to neonates who have infections that are life-threatening.[29,86,91]

Managing Pneumonia and Diarrhea in Infants and Young Children

Pneumonia is the leading infectious killer of under-5 children, and diarrhea is the second-leading infectious cause of their deaths. Such deaths are almost completely avoidable. In this light, WHO and UNICEF have outlined a plan to eliminate preventable deaths

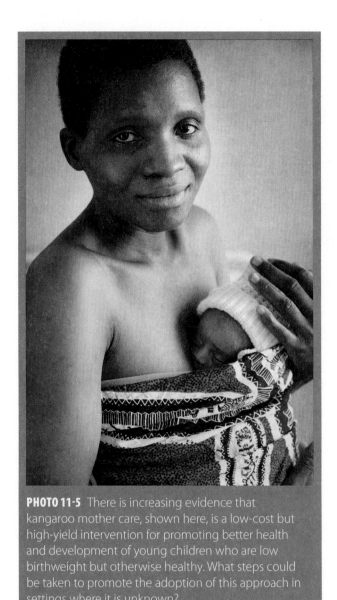

PHOTO 11-5 There is increasing evidence that kangaroo mother care, shown here, is a low-cost but high-yield intervention for promoting better health and development of young children who are low birthweight but otherwise healthy. What steps could be taken to promote the adoption of this approach in settings where it is unknown?
Courtesy of Mark Tuschman.

from pneumonia and diarrhea by 2025. They refer to this as the Integrated Global Action Plan for Pneumonia and Diarrhea.[91]

The plan is based on the notion that children are dying needlessly of pneumonia and diarrhea because of the failure to reach them with well-known, low-cost, and highly effective interventions. A key bottleneck to reaching these children has been that such services have too often been carried out piecemeal rather than in a more integrated manner. As noted earlier, for example, only about 30 percent of children with suspected pneumonia receive appropriate antibiotics, and only about 35 percent of children with diarrhea are given oral rehydration therapy.[91]

To reduce pneumonia and diarrheal deaths, the action plan suggests that national governments take an integrated approach across all government and partner organizations to deliver a series of interventions that follow the Protect, Prevent, and Treat Framework as outlined in **FIGURE 11-13**.

The premises of this approach are to protect children through good health practices; to prevent children from becoming ill using immunization, HIV/AIDS prevention, and the provision of a healthy environment; and to treat them at an appropriate level of quality if they do fall ill.[91]

As discussed repeatedly in the text, there are many reasons why exclusive breastfeeding until children are 6 months of age is so important, and one of them is to avoid diarrhea in settings that are not hygienic. As children move to complementary foods, a number of measures can be taken to reduce their risk of diarrheal disease. The first, of course, is to engage in better personal hygiene and more hygienic food preparation. Second, complementary foods that are fortified can help children meet their requirements for micronutrients.[16]

Some immunizations, as discussed earlier, can directly affect pneumonia and diarrhea, such as the pneumococcal vaccine, the Hib vaccine, and the rotavirus vaccine. However, other vaccines protect children indirectly. Ensuring that children are immunized against measles, for example, can help to reduce deaths from diarrhea. It has been estimated, in fact, that measles immunization could eliminate 6 percent to 26 percent of diarrheal deaths in children younger than 5 years.[16] Improving water supply and sanitation can be very important to reducing diarrhea in children. Unfortunately, the infrastructure to do so can be very expensive, and health benefits are gained mainly when communities adopt safer water and sanitation systems, coupled with improvements in hygiene, rather than just having them adopted by individual families.[29]

When young children do get the types of diarrhea that do not require antibiotics, two very cost-effective measures can be taken to manage the illness. First is the household use of ORT. Second is supplementation with zinc, because such supplements have been shown to reduce the duration and severity of diarrhea.

Community-Based Approaches to Improving Child Health

As you have seen throughout the text, many of the measures that are needed to reduce the burden of illness and death in neonates, infants, and young children have to do with appropriate knowledge and behavior of individuals and families. You have also read that studies that have been done in a number of places show that home- and community-based approaches to improving health behaviors and providing basic health services with the help of trained members

PROTECT

Children by establishing good health practices from birth

- Exclusive breastfeeding for 6 months
- Adequate complementary feeding
- Vitamin A supplementation

PREVENT

Children becoming ill from pneumonia and diarrhea

- Vaccines: pertussis, measles, Hib, PCV and rotavirus
- Handwashing with soap
- Safe drinking-water and sanitation
- Reduce household air pollution
- HIV prevention
- Cotrimoxazole prophylaxis for HIV-infected and exposed children

Reduce pneumonia and diarrhoea morbidity and mortality

TREAT

Children who are ill from pneumonia and diarrhea with appropriate treatment

- Improved care seeking and referral
- Case management at the health facility and community level
- Supplies: Low-osmolarity ORS, zinc, antibiotics and oxygen
- Continued feeding (including breastfeeding)

FIGURE 11-13 The UNICEF/WHO Protect, Prevent, and Treat Framework for Pneumonia and Diarrhea

Adapted from UNICEF & World Health Organization (WHO). (2013). *Ending preventable child deaths from pneumonia and diarrhoea by 2025* (p. 6). Geneva, Switzerland: Author.

of the community can lead to significant gains in health. For example, a very large share of all primary healthcare services are delivered in Bangladesh by a community-based NGO called BRAC.

The role of the family and community is key to newborn health. Community awareness and the engagement of women's groups have been highly effective in improving the health and survival of newborns. In one project in rural Bolivia, the involvement of local women's groups in raising awareness of maternal, fetal, and neonatal issues led to increased use of prenatal and postnatal health services, more traditional birth assistants at childbirth, and an overall 62 percent reduction of perinatal mortality. In another study in rural Nepal, working with local women's groups was key to motivating increased hygiene and health-seeking behavior, which contributed to a 30 percent reduction in neonatal mortality.[29]

In fact, family- and community-based approaches to promoting hygiene, including handwashing and umbilical cord care, keeping the newborn warm, and exclusively breastfeeding, are important home measures that could lead to an estimated 10 percent to 40 percent reduction in neonatal mortality. Home-based supplementary feeding, using a dropper or a cup, is another important measure to ensure the survival of low-birthweight babies, who account for 60 percent to 80 percent of neonatal deaths.[29]

TABLE 11-11 is a summary of measures that families can take, even in low-income communities, to protect the health of their young children. You can see in the table the extent to which families, if they had better knowledge of good health practices and community support to engage in them, could promote important

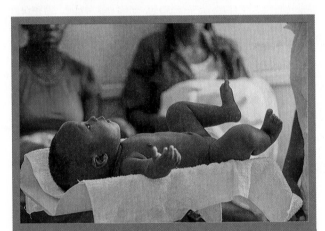

PHOTO 11-6 It is essential to healthy child growth and development that the height and weight of young children be monitored regularly. Are there approaches to growth monitoring and promotion that can be used to mobilize communities around better nutrition and child caring practices?

Courtesy of Mark Tuschman.

reductions in child morbidity and mortality. Low-income people in low- and middle-income countries are not likely to experience rapid increases in formal education, income, or social and political voice. Thus, it will be very important to take community-based approaches to help families improve their knowledge and practice of good health behaviors.

▶ Main Messages

Approximately 5.4 million children around the world died in 2017 before they reached their fifth birthday. This is equal to almost 15,000 young child deaths every

TABLE 11-11 Twelve Key Family Health Practices

1. **Exclusive breastfeeding.** Breastfeed infants exclusively for up to 6 months. (Mothers that are HIV-positive require counseling about possible alternatives to breastfeeding.)
2. **Complementary feeding.** Starting at about 6 months of age, feed children freshly prepared energy- and nutrient-rich complementary foods, while continuing to breastfeed up to 2 years or longer.
3. **Micronutrients.** Ensure that children receive adequate amounts of micronutrients (vitamin A, iron, and zinc, in particular), either in their diet or through supplementation.
4. **Hygiene.** Safely dispose of feces, including children's feces, and wash hands after defecation, before preparing meals, and before feeding children.
5. **Immunization.** Take children as scheduled to complete a full course of immunizations (BCG, DPT, OPV, and measles) before their first birthday.
6. **Malaria and use of bed nets.** Protect children in malaria-endemic areas by ensuring that they sleep under insecticide-treated bed nets.
7. **Psychosocial development.** Promote mental and social development by responding to a child's needs for care and through talking, playing, and providing a stimulating environment.
8. **Home care for illness.** Continue to feed and offer more fluids, including breastmilk, to children when they are sick. Home care for sick children includes several practices that are enumerated individually in this list of 12 key family practices, such as continuing feeding and offering more fluids, oral rehydration therapy, treatment of fever, prompt care-seeking, and compliance with a health provider's advice.
9. **Home treatment for infections.** Give sick children appropriate home treatment for infections.
10. **Care-seeking.** Recognize when sick children need treatment outside the home and seek care from appropriate providers.
11. **Compliance with advice.** Follow the health worker's advice about treatment, follow-up, and referral.
12. **Antenatal care.** Ensure that every pregnant woman has adequate antenatal care. (This includes having at least four antenatal visits with an appropriate healthcare provider and receiving the recommended doses of the tetanus toxoid vaccination. The mother also needs support from her family and community in seeking care at the time of delivery and during the postpartum and lactation period.)

World Health Organization (WHO). (2004). *Family and community practices that promote child survival, growth, and development: A review of the evidence.* Geneva, Switzerland: Author.

day globally. About 47 percent of the deaths take place in the first 28 days; 28 percent in the post-neonatal period; and 24 percent between the first and fourth years.

As we learned in the vignettes that opened the chapter, the chances of survival for a newborn, an infant, and a young child are vastly different across different settings. The discrepancies within an individual country can be as wide as differences between countries. High-income countries have, on average, about 5 deaths per 1,000 live births for children younger than 5 years. However, the rate in low-income countries is 50 deaths per 1,000 live births, or 10 times higher than the rate in high-income countries. However, in some of the most fragile states the rate can go above 80, as it does in the Central African Republic and in Sierra Leone.[92]

The largest cause of death of under-5 children globally is prematurity, which killed almost 18 percent of all of those children who died before reaching age 5 in 2016. Other conditions related to birth, such as birth asphyxia and birth trauma, were responsible for 12 percent of the deaths, and congenital anomalies for almost 9 percent.

Pneumonia is the most important infectious killer of children who are younger than 5 years of age and is responsible for about 16 percent of their deaths. The second most important infectious cause of illness and death among children is diarrheal disease, followed by sepsis, malaria, measles, and HIV/AIDS.

The social determinants of health have a major impact on the health of young children. Poverty is a significant underlying factor of morbidity and mortality among children, as is the lack of education for mothers.

Nutritional status is also a powerful determinant of whether a child lives and thrives. About 45 percent of all deaths of children under 5 years of age are related to children being undernourished. This undernourishment may stem from poor maternal nutrition, suboptimal breastfeeding, infection, or insufficient energy, protein, and the lack of key micronutrients in the child's diet.

Inadequate water and sanitation and poor hygiene practices are major risk factors for childhood illness and death. Household air pollution is also a major risk factor.

There are well-known, proven, and cost-effective interventions for substantially reducing the deaths of neonates, infants, and young children. Their deaths do not stem from a failure of knowing what to do. Rather, they stem mostly from a failure to reach all children with these interventions.

The key interventions can be oriented in a life-course approach—those important before pregnancy; during pregnancy, birth, and shortly after birth; those needed in the post-neonatal period; and those most important for the young child. The following will be among the most important interventions:

- Ensuring the health and proper nourishment of the mother
- Providing access to modern contraceptives
- Prenatal care and micronutrient supplementation for the mother-to-be
- Prevention of mother-to-child transmission of HIV/AIDS
- Attendance at delivery by a skilled birth attendant and referral for emergency obstetric care if needed
- Appropriate care of the newborn, special measures for low birthweight babies, and referral if needed for illness
- Early and exclusive breastfeeding for 6 months
- Hygienic introduction of diverse complementary foods
- Childhood immunization
- Bed nets for malaria and regular drug administration for worms
- Oral rehydration for diarrhea and early diagnosis and treatment for pneumonia

Study Questions

1. What are the most important causes of child death globally?
2. How do causes of death differ for neonates, infants, and young children?
3. Why are there different levels of child illness and death in different parts of the same country?
4. What is the link between nutrition and child health?
5. How does the health of young children in low-income countries vary with the income of the family?
6. How does the health of young children in low-income countries vary with the mother's level of education?
7. What is the importance to neonatal health of having a skilled birth attendant at delivery?
8. What are some of the most cost-effective interventions for saving the lives of newborns?
9. What are some of the most cost-effective interventions for saving the lives of children younger than 5 years?
10. What measures can families take, even in the absence of additional income or health services, to keep their children healthy?

References

1. The United Nations Interagency Group for Child Mortality Estimation. (2018). *Levels and trends in child mortality.* New York, NY: UNICEF.
2. The World Bank. (n.d.). *Data: Mortality rate, under 5 (per 1,000 live births).* Retrieved from http://data.worldbank.org/indicator/SH.DYN.MORT/countries?display=map
3. World Health Organization (WHO). (2018). *Children: Reducing mortality* (Fact sheet no. 178). Retrieved from http://www.who.int/mediacentre/factsheets/fs178/en/
4. UNICEF. (2013). *Committing to child survival: A promise renewed—Progress report 2013.* New York, NY: Author.
5. World Health Organization (WHO). *Stillbirths.* Retrieved from http://www.who.int/maternal_child_adolescent/epidemiology/stillbirth/en/
6. The Lancet. (2011, April 15). *Stillbirths 2011.* Retrieved from http://www.thelancet.com/series/stillbirth
7. The Lancet. (2016, October 4). *Advancing early childhood development: From science to scale.* Retrieved from https://www.thelancet.com/series/ECD2016
8. Institute of Health Metrics and Evaluation (IHME). (n.d.). GBD Compare: Viz Hub. Retrieved from https://vizhub.healthdata.org/gbd-compare/
9. Black, R. E., Laxminarayan, R., Temmerman, M., & Walker, N. (Eds.). (2016). *Disease control priorities: Reproductive, maternal, newborn, and child health* (3rd ed., Vol. 2). Washington, DC: The World Bank.
10. UNICEF. (2010). *Progress for children: Achieving the MDGs with equity.* New York, NY: Author.
11. Simoes, E. A. F., Cherian, T., Chow, J., Shahid-Salles, S., Laxminarayan, R., & John, T. J. (2006). Acute respiratory infections in children. In D. T. Jamison, J. G. Breman, A. R. Measham, et al. (Eds.), *Disease control priorities in developing countries* (2nd ed., pp. 483–497). New York, NY: Oxford University Press.
12. World Health Organization (WHO). (2014). *Pneumonia* (Fact sheet no. 331). Retrieved from http://www.who.int/mediacentre/factsheets/fs331/en/
13. World Health Organization (WHO). (2016). *Pneumonia.* Retrieved from https://www.who.int/en/news-room/fact-sheets/detail/pneumonia
14. Keusch, G. F., Fontaine, O., Bhargava, A., Boschi-Pinto, C., Bhutta, Z. A., Gotuzzo, E., . . . Laxminarayan, R. (2006). Diarrheal diseases. In D. T. Jamison, J. G. Breman, A. R. Measham, et al. (Eds.), *Disease control priorities in developing*

countries (2nd ed., pp. 371–387). New York, NY: Oxford University Press.

15. World Health Organization (WHO). (2017). *Diarrhoeal disease: Key facts.* Retrieved from: https://www.who.int/en/news-room/fact-sheets/detail/diarrhoeal-disease

16. World Health Organization (WHO). (2014). *Malaria* (Fact sheet no. 94). Retrieved from http://www.who.int/mediacentre/factsheets/fs094/en/

17. World Health Organization (WHO). (2018). *Malaria.* Retrieved from https://www.who.int/news-room/fact-sheets/detail/malaria

18. Breman, J. G., Mills, A., Snow, R. W., Mulligan, J. A., Lengeler, C., Mendis, K., . . . Doumbo, O. K. (2006). Conquering malaria. In D. T. Jamison, J. G. Breman, A. R. Measham, et al. (Eds.), *Disease control priorities in developing countries* (2nd ed., pp. 413–431). New York, NY: Oxford University Press.

19. World Health Organization (WHO). (n.d.). *HIV/AIDS mother-to-child transmission of HIV.* Retrieved from http://www.who.int/hiv/topics/mtct/en/

20. UNAIDS. (2014). *The gap report.* Geneva, Switzerland: Author.

21. Avert. (n.d.). *Global HIV and AIDS statistics.* Retrieved from https://www.avert.org/global-hiv-and-aids-statistics

22. World Health Organization (WHO). (2015). *Measles* (Fact sheet no. 286). Retrieved from http://www.who.int/mediacentre/factsheets/fs286/en/

23. Centers for Disease Control and Prevention (CDC). (n.d.). *Measles (Rubeola): Transmission of measles.* Retrieved from https://www.cdc.gov/measles/about/transmission.html

24. World Health Organization (WHO). (2018). *Immunization, vaccines, and biological: Measles.* Retrieved from https://www.who.int/immunization/diseases/measles/en/

25. World Health Organization (WHO). (2018). *Soil-transmitted helminth infections.* Retrieved from https://www.who.int/en/news-room/fact-sheets/detail/soil-transmitted-helminth-infections

26. World Health Organization (WHO). *Intestinal worms.* Retrieved from http://www.who.int/intestinal_worms/more/en/

27. Hotez, P. J., Bundy, D. A. P., Beegle, K., Brooker, S., Drake, L., de Silva, N., . . . Savioli, L. (2006). Helminth infections: Soil-transmitted helminth infections and schistosomiasis. In D. T. Jamison, J. G. Breman, A. R. Measham, et al. (Eds.), *Disease control priorities in developing countries* (2nd ed., pp. 467–482). New York, NY: Oxford University Press.

28. UNICEF. (2015). *Neonatal mortality rates are declining in all regions but more slowly in sub-Saharan Africa.* Retrieved from http://data.unicef.org/child-mortality/neonatal

29. Lawn, J. E., Zupan, J., Begkoyian, G., & Knippenberg, R. (2006). Newborn survival. In D. T. Jamison, J. G. Breman, A. R. Measham, et al. (Eds.), *Disease control priorities in developing countries* (2nd ed., pp. 531–549). New York, NY: Oxford University Press.

30. United Nations. (2006). *The millennium development goals report 2006.* New York, NY: Author.

31. Lawn, J. E., Blencowe, H., Oza, S., You, D., Lee, A. C., Waiswa, P., . . . Cousens, S. N. (2014, May 20). Every newborn: Progress, priorities, and potential beyond survival. *The Lancet, 384,* 189–205.

32. Darmstadt, G. L., Bhutta, Z. A., Cousens, S., Adam, T., Walker, N., & de Bernis, L. (2005). Evidence-based, cost-effective interventions: How many newborn babies can we save? *The Lancet, 365*(9463), 977–988.

33. Black, R. E., Morris, S. S., & Bryce, J. (2003). Where and why are 10 million children dying every year? *The Lancet, 361*(9376), 2226–2234.

34. UNICEF. (2005). *State of the world's children 2005.* New York, NY: Author.

35. United Nations. (n.d.). *We can end poverty: Millennium Development Goals and beyond 2015.* Retrieved from http://www.un.org/millenniumgoals/childhealth.shtml

36. UNICEF. (n.d.). *Immunization.* Retrieved from http://www.unicef.org/immunization/

37. Gavi. (n.d.). *The value of vaccination.* Retrieved from https://www.gavi.org/about/value/

38. World Health Organization (WHO). (2014). *Global immunization data.* Geneva, Switzerland: Author. Retrieved from http://www.who.int/immunization/monitoring_surveillance/global_immunization_data.pdf

39. World Health Organization (WHO). (2013). *Global vaccine action plan 2011–2020.* Geneva, Switzerland: Author. Retrieved from http://www.who.int/immunization/global_vaccine_action_plan/GVAP_doc_2011_2020/en/

40. Bärnighausen, T., Berkley, S., Bhutta, Z. A., Bishai, D. M., Black, M. M., Bloom, D. E., . . . Walker, D. (2014). Reassessing the value of vaccines. *The Lancet Global Health, 2*(5), e251–e252. Retrieved from http://www.thelancet.com/journals/langlo/article/PIIS2214-109X%2813%2970170-0/fulltext?rss=yes

41. Deogaonkar, R. (2012). Systematic review of studies evaluating the broader economic impact of vaccination in low and middle income countries. *BMC Public Health, 12*(1), 878.

42. Nshimirimana, D., Mihigo, R., & Clements, C. J. (2013). Routine immunization services in Africa: Back to basics. *Journal of Vaccines and Immunization, 1*(1), 6–12.

43. Chan, M. (2014). Beyond expectations: 40 years of EPI. *The Lancet, 383*(9930), 1697–1698. Retrieved from http://www.thelancet.com/pdfs/journals/lancet/PIIS0140673614607510.pdf

44. Wang, S., Hyde, T. B., Mounier-Jack, S., Brenzeld, L., Favine, M., Gordon, W. G., . . . Durrheim, D. (2013). New vaccine introductions: Assessing the impact and the opportunities for immunization and health systems strengthening. *Vaccine, 31,* 122–128. Retrieved from http://www.sciencedirect.com/science/article/pii/S0264410X12015927

45. Gavi. (n.d.). *Pentavalent vaccine support.* Retrieved from https://www.gavi.org/support/nvs/pentavalent/

46. Cherian, T., & Okwo-Bele, J.-M. (2014). The decade of vaccines global vaccine action plan: Shaping immunization programmes in the current decade. *Expert Review of Vaccines, 13*(5), 573–575. Retrieved from http://informahealthcare.com/doi/abs/10.1586/14760584.2014.897618

47. World Health Organization (WHO). (2001). *Expanded program on immunization (EPI) in the Africa region: Strategic plan of action 2001–2005.* Harare: Zimbabwe WHO.

48. Pan American Health Organization. (2014). *About PAHO Revolving Fund: Why we need it.* Retrieved from http://www.paho.org/hq/index.php?option=com_content&view=article&id=9562&Itemid=40717&lang=en&limitstart=1

49. Gavi. (n. d.). *Gavi's mission.* Retrieved from https://www.gavi.org/about/mission/

50. Gavi. (n.d.). *Gavi's strategy.* Retrieved from https://www.gavi.org/about/strategy/

51. Gavi. (n.d.). *Countries eligible for support.* Retrieved from https://www.gavi.org/support/sustainability/countries-eligible-for-support/

52. Ozawa, S., Clark, S., Portnoy, A., Grewal, S., Brenzel, L., & Walker, D. G. (2016). Return on Investment in childhood immunizations in low- and middle-income countries, 2011–2020. *Health Affairs, 35*(2). doi: 10.1377/hlthaff.2015.1086

53. World Health Organization (WHO). (2018). *2018 assessment report of the global vaccine action plan.* Geneva, Switzerland: Author. Retrieved from https://www.who.int/immunization/sage/meetings/2018/october/2_Draft2018GVAP_Ass_Rep.pdf?ua=1

54. College of Physicians of Philadelphia. (2018). *History of anti-vaccination movements.* Retrieved from https://www.historyofvaccines.org/content/articles/history-anti-vaccination-movements

55. World Health Organization (WHO). (n.d.). *Immunization, vaccines and biological: Addressing vaccine hesitancy.* Retrieved from https://www.who.int/immunization/programmes_systems/vaccine_hesitancy/en/

56. Levine, R., & What Works Working Group. (2007). *Case studies in global health: Millions saved.* Sudbury, MA: Jones and Bartlett.

57. Henderson D. A., de Quadros, C. A., Andrus, J., Olive, J.-M., & Guerra de Macedo, C. (1992). Polio eradication from the Western Hemisphere. *Annual Review of Public Health, 13,* 239–252.

58. de Quadros, C. A. (2000). Polio. In J. Lederberg (Ed.), *Encyclopedia of microbiology* (2nd ed., Vol. 3, pp. 762–772). San Diego, CA: Academic Press.

59. Gawande, A. (2004, January 12). The mop-up: Eradicating polio from the planet. *The New Yorker,* pp. 34–40.

60. Musgrove, P. (1988). Is the eradication of polio in the western hemisphere economically justified? *Bulletin of the Pan American Sanitary Bureau, 22*(1), 67.

61. Global Polio Eradication Initiative. (2003). *Progress 2003.* Retrieved from http://www.who.int/biologicals/publications/meetings/areas/vaccines/polio/2003_global_polio_%20eradication_initiative-progress.pdf?ua=1

62. Measles and Rubella Initiative. (2013). *Moving faster than measles and rubella.* Retrieved from http://www.measlesrubellainitiative.org/wp-content/uploads/2013/07/MRI-Fact-Sheet-FINAL-JULY9.pdf

63. World Health Organization (WHO). (2018). *Table 1: Summary of WHO Position Papers—Recommendations for routine immunization.* Retrieved from http://www.who.int/immunization/policy/Immunization_routine_table1.pdf?ua=1

64. Gavi Alliance. (n.d.). *Measles vaccine.* Retrieved from http://www.gavialliance.org/support/nvs/measles/

65. Epi Monitor. (n.d.). *Experts identify the six most daunting challenges for the global measles eradication program.* Retrieved from http://epimonitor.net/Six_Challenges_for_Measles_Eradication.htm

66. Holzmann, H., Hengel, H., Tenbusch, M., & Doerr, H. W. (2016). Eradication of measles: remaining challenges. *Medical Microbiology and Immunology, 205*(3), 201–208. doi: 10.1007/s00430-016-0451-4

67. Minetti, A., Kagoli, M., Katsulukuta, A., Huerga, H., Featherstone, A., Chiotcha, H., . . . Luquero, F. J. (2013). Lessons and challenges for measles control from unexpected

68. Pan American Health Organization (PAHO). (n.d.). *Verification of measles and rubella elimination in the Americas.* Retrieved from http://www.paho.org/hq./index.php?option=com_docman&task=doc_view&gid=19677&Itemid=

69. Fraser, B. (2018). Measles outbreak in the Americas. *The Lancet, 392*(10145), 373.

70. Gavi. (n.d.). *Measles and measles-rubella vaccine support.* Retrieved from https://www.gavi.org/support/nvs/measles-rubella/

71. World Health Organization (WHO). (2002). *The world health report 2002: Reducing risks, promoting healthy life.* Geneva, Switzerland: Author.

72. West, K. P. Jr., Pokhrel, R. P., Katz, J., LeClerq, S. C., Khatry, S. K., Shrestha, S. R., . . . Sommer, A. (1991). Efficacy of vitamin A in reducing preschool child mortality in Nepal. *The Lancet, 338*(8759), 67–71.

73. Rutstein, S. O., & Govindasamy, P. (2002). *The mortality effects of Nepal's vitamin A distribution program.* Calverton, MD: ORC Macro.

74. Caulfield, L. E., Richard, S. A., Rivera, J. A., Musgrove, P., & Black, R. E. (2006). Stunting, wasting, and micronutrient disorders. In D. T. Jamison, J. G. Breman, A. R. Measham, et al. (Eds.), *Disease control priorities in developing countries* (2nd ed., pp. 551–568). New York, NY: Oxford University Press.

75. Fiedler, J. L. (1997). *The Nepal national vitamin A program: A program review and cost analysis.* Bethesda, MD: Partnerships for Health Reform Project, Abt Associates.

76. Fiedler, J. L. (2000). The Nepal national vitamin A program: Prototype to emulate or donor enclave? *Health Policy and Planning, 15*(2), 145–156.

77. UNICEF. (2018). *Data: Under-five mortality.* Retrieved from https://data.unicef.org/topic/child-survival/under-five-mortality/

78. Victora, C. G., Wagstaff, A., Schellenberg, J. A., Gwatkin, D., Claeson, M., & Habicht, J. P. (2003). Applying an equity lens to child health and mortality: More of the same is not enough. *The Lancet, 362*(9379), 233–241.

79. Bhutta, Z. A., Das, J. K., Bahl, R., Lawn, J. E., Salam, R. A., Paul, V. K., . . . Walker, N. (2014). Can available interventions end preventable deaths in mother's newborn babies, and stillbirths, and at what cost? *The Lancet, 384,* 347–370.

80. Mason, E., McDougall, L., Lawn, J. E., Gupta, A., Claeson, M., Pillay, Y., . . . Chopra, A. (2014). From evidence to action to deliver a healthy start for the next generation. *The Lancet, 384,* 455–467.

81. Dickson, K. E., Simen-Kapeu, A., Kinney, M. V., Huicho, L., Vesel, L., Lackritz, E., Lawn, J. E. (2014). Every newborn: Health-systems bottlenecks and strategies to accelerate scale-up in countries. *The Lancet, 384,* 438–454.

82. Black, R. E., Levin, C., Walker, N., Chou, D., Liu, L., & Temmerman, M. (2016). Reproductive, maternal, newborn, and child health: Key messages from *Disease Control Priorities 3rd Edition. The Lancet, 388,* 2811–2824.

83. Unless otherwise noted, this section is based primarily on the interventions noted in Bhutta et al., Mason et al., and Dickson et al. (references 79, 80, and 81).

84. Bertozzi, S., Padian, N. S., Wegbreit, J., DeMaria, L. M., Feldman, B., Gayle, H., . . . Isbell, M. T. (2006). HIV/AIDS

large outbreak, Malawi. *Emerging Infectious Diseases, 19*(2), 202–209.

prevention and treatment. In D. T. Jamison, J. G. Breman, A. R. Measham, et al. (Eds.), *Disease control priorities in developing countries* (2nd ed., pp. 331–369). New York, NY: Oxford University Press.

85. Lawn, J. E., Cousens, S., & Zupan, J. (2005). 4 million neonatal deaths: When? Where? Why? *The Lancet, 365*(9462), 891–900.

86. Bang, A. T., Bang, R. A., Baitule, S. B., Reddy, M. H., & Deshmukh, M. D. (1999). Effect of home-based neonatal care and management of sepsis on neonatal mortality: Field trial in rural India. *The Lancet, 354*(9194), 1955–1961.

87. World Health Organization (WHO). (2003). *Kangaroo mother care: A practical guide.* Geneva, Switzerland: Author.

88. Conde-Agudelo, A., Belizán, J. M., & Diaz-Rossello, J. L. (2007). Kangaroo mother care to reduce morbidity and mortality in low birthweight infants (Review). *Cochrane Collaboration.* Retrieved from http://apps.who.int/rhl /reviews/CD002771.pdf

89. Osman, N. (2009, October 13). "Kangaroo" incubation urged for Indonesia's pre-mature babies. *Jakarta Globe.* Retrieved from http://www.thejakartaglobe.com/national/kangaroo -incubation-urged-for-indonesias-premature-babies/335372

90. Vesel, L., Bergh, A.- M., Kerber, K. J. Valsangkar, B., Mazia, G., Moxon, S. G., . . . Lawn, J. E. (2015). Kangaroo mother care: A multi-country analysis of health system bottlenecks and potential solutions. *BMC Pregnancy and Childbirth, 15*(Suppl. 2), S5.

91. UNICEF & World Health Organization. (2013). *Ending preventable child deaths from pneumonia and diarrhoea by 2025.* Geneva, Switzerland: Author.

92. The World Bank. (n.d.). *Data: Mortality rate, infant (per 1,000 live births).* Retrieved from https://data.worldbank .org/indicator/SP.DYN.IMRT.IN

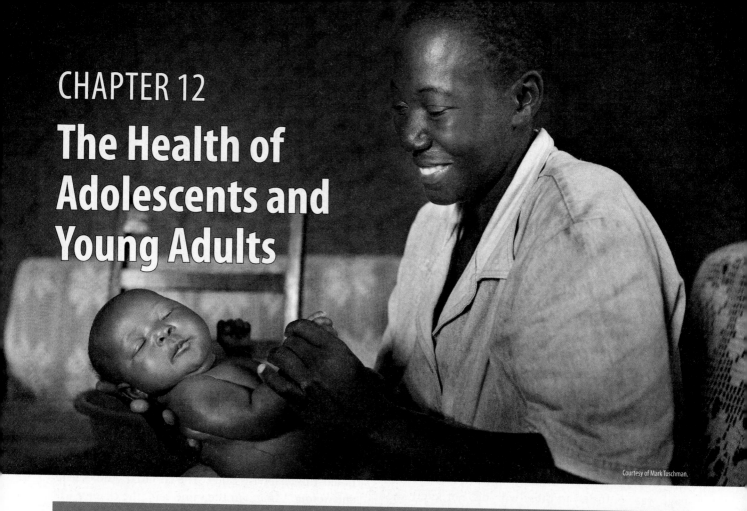

CHAPTER 12
The Health of Adolescents and Young Adults

Courtesy of Mark Tuschman.

LEARNING OBJECTIVES

By the end of this chapter, the reader will be able to do the following:

- Discuss the importance of the health of adolescents and young adults
- Review the leading causes of death, the burden of disease, and key risk factors and social determinants for these groups
- Review the health, social, and economic consequences of key health problems among adolescents and young adults
- Outline some of the main steps that could be taken to reduce the burden of disease and deaths in adolescents and young adults

▶ Vignettes

Carmen is a 16-year-old girl in El Salvador. Although premarital sex is socially unacceptable in her community, Carmen became sexually active at 14. At 16, she became pregnant. As a result, she dropped out of high school and went to live with relatives in the countryside until she had her baby. It will be very difficult for Carmen to return to school, and her economic prospects have been severely damaged by giving birth at such a young age.

Rachel is a 15-year-old girl in South Africa. She is one of many people her age born to an HIV-positive mother before South Africa made much progress in

stopping mother-to-child transmission of HIV. Rachel has been taking drugs against this disease for as long as she can remember. In the last few years, however, she has found it more and more difficult to remember to take her drugs on time. She also worries constantly that her peers will know that she is HIV-positive.

John was an 18-year-old boy in Chicago, Illinois, in the United States. He had gone most of the way through secondary school but did not complete it. There are few jobs in Chicago for young people without a secondary school diploma, and John spent much of his time "hanging around" with friends of a similar background. Over time, John joined a youth gang and made some money by selling small amounts of illegal drugs, some of which he occasionally used himself. At 19, John was murdered while selling drugs on a street corner near his home, becoming one of many adolescent victims of interpersonal violence worldwide.

Rashmi is a 14-year-old girl in Punjab state in India. She is hardworking and very intelligent but always feels great pressure to meet the expectations of her family and community. She worries all the time about how she can do all her chores at home, help earn money for the family, do well in school, and then marry the young man her family will choose for her. Lately, her body has gone through a number of changes that she does not understand, and she has begun to feel more and more overwhelmed about all that she has to do. In the last few months, in fact, she has found herself very happy at some times but very sad at other times. She feels like something is wrong but does not know what it is or what to do about it.

Juan was 21 when he was killed in a car crash outside Lima, Peru. Juan had just gotten his driver's license when the accident occurred at a busy intersection where several roads came together, and the signage was confusing to those who did not know the area. Juan failed to understand that he could turn left only on the green left arrow and turned into the path of an oncoming car. The collision spun his car around, and it was then hit by another car on the driver's side. Juan was severely injured and died in the hospital the next day.

▶ Key Terms and Definitions

There is important debate about what age groups should be considered when one examines the health of "adolescents." Traditionally, "adolescence" was considered the period between puberty and marriage and parenthood.[1] Indeed, as noted in **TABLE 12-1**, the World Health Organization (WHO) considers adolescents to be people between 10 and 19 years of age.[2] Nonetheless, the end points of this period are not as clear as they were earlier. They also vary by different cultural groups. Thus, the most recent study of importance on "adolescents" covered the age range of 10 to 24 years.[1]

There is little debate, however, about the importance of disaggregating this age range into several different groups if one is to get the best possible understanding of the health of "young people" across their life course. With this in mind, the 10- to 24-year period is broken down into three groups:

TABLE 12-1 Key Terms
■ The World Health Organization defines **adolescent** as a person between the ages of 10 and 19 years.
■ The United Nations defines **youth** as a person between the ages of 15 and 24 years.
■ The United Nations *Convention on the Rights of the Child* defines **child** as a person under the age of 18 years.

Data from United Nations. (n.d.). *Definition of youth*. Retrieved from http://www.un.org/esa/socdev/documents/youth/fact-sheets/youth-definition.pdf; Data from United Nations Office of the High Commissioner for Human Rights. (1989). *Convention on the rights of the child*. Retrieved from http://www.ohchr.org/EN/ProfessionalInterest/Pages/CRC.aspx; Modified from World Health Organization (WHO). (2018). *Adolescents: health risks and solutions*. Retrieved from http://www.who.int/mediacentre/factsheets/fs345/en/

10–14: early adolescence

15–19: older adolescence

20–24: young adulthood

To be consistent with this terminology while respecting the important differences in the age groups noted, this chapter is titled "The Health of Adolescents and Young Adults." In the same vein, the chapter will consistently speak of "early adolescence," "older adolescence," and "young adulthood." When the chapter speaks of all three groups together, it will speak of "adolescents and young adults." The chapter will occasionally also refer to only the 10 to 19 age group as "adolescents."

▶ The Importance of the Health of Adolescents and Young Adults

The health of adolescents and young adults deserves special attention for several reasons. First, adolescents and young adults make up 24 percent of the global population.[3] They also make up a larger share of the population in low- and middle-income countries than in high-income countries. These groups constitute almost 32 percent of the population of Nigeria, for example, but only around 17 percent of the population of Germany.[3] Second, the burden of disease for adolescents and young adults is a unique one and needs to be addressed directly, rather than together with that of younger children. This is particularly so, for example, when one considers issues of sexuality and reproductive health, mental health, interpersonal violence, and road safety. Third, the period of adolescence and young adulthood is one during which important health behaviors are established, and it is critical to ensure that adolescents and young adults adopt healthy behaviors. The health of future adult populations, for example, will depend, to a large extent, on whether or not adolescents and young adults drive safely; avoid early marriage, excess alcohol consumption, and tobacco smoking; and consume healthy diets while getting appropriate physical activity. Finally, as shown in **TABLE 12-2**, there are critical links between the Sustainable Development Goals (SDGs) and the health of adolescents and young adults.

This chapter examines the most critical issues in the health of adolescents and young adults with a focus on these populations in low- and middle-income countries. The chapter begins by examining the burden of disease for adolescents and young adults, key risk factors for those burdens, and the costs and consequences of the most important health issues among these groups. A case study illustrates an intervention addressing some critical health issues among adolescent girls in Malawi. The chapter concludes with comments on how the most important health burdens among adolescents and young adults might be addressed in cost-effective and fair ways.

▶ Data on the Health of Adolescents and Young Adults

The data on the burden of disease in this chapter come largely from the Global Burden of Disease Study 2016.[4] Other data are taken from a major 2014 report on the health of adolescents produced by WHO[5] and the report of a recent *The Lancet* commission on adolescent health.[1] The chapter also builds on the volume on child and adolescent health and development in *Disease Control Priorities, Third Edition*.[6]

It is important to note, however, that there have been important gaps in data on the health of adolescents and young adults. Much of the focus in global health has been on children under 5 years of age, and much of the available data on child health have referred to that age group as well. In addition, it has been difficult to find data for ages 10 to 19. However, attention to adolescents and young adults has been increasing, and the availability of data on these age groups has also increased.

▶ Adolescence and Young Adulthood as Transitional and Critical Periods

During the years of adolescence and young adulthood, children undergo rapid biological, psychological, and social changes. These include hormonal changes and the onset of puberty. Psychologically, adolescence is a phase of rapid increase in cognitive and emotional development in various regions of the brain. However, the brain does not fully develop until people are about 25 years of age, and, as adolescents age, they become more able to control their impulses and make more rational decisions. Younger adolescents are heavily influenced by their peers, and as adolescents get older they reduce their dependence on their parents.[5,7] Some of the key changes that children undergo as they move from early adolescence to young adulthood are noted in **TABLE 12-3**.

Another important point to consider about adolescence is that the period of adolescence has been getting longer. Puberty comes earlier for most boys and girls than it did in the past, and they also marry and assume mature social roles later than was historically the case.[7]

▶ Key Health Burdens of Adolescents and Young Adults

The section that follows discusses the key health burdens that adolescents and young adults face.

Deaths and DALYs

As shown in **TABLE 12-4**, the leading causes of death among adolescents and young adults vary by age, sex, and country income group. In lower-income countries, we see the continuing importance of communicable causes, especially in earlier and older adolescence. These include intestinal infectious diseases, diarrheal diseases, tuberculosis (TB), lower respiratory infections, and HIV/AIDS. In low- and lower middle-income countries, we also see the importance for females of maternal causes. As one moves to higher-income countries and older age groups, one notes a shift away from the causes above and toward causes such as road injuries, self-harm, interpersonal violence, and certain cancers.

TABLE 12-5 notes the five leading causes of disability-adjusted life years (DALYs) by age group

TABLE 12-2 Selected Links Between the Health of Adolescents and Young Adults and the SDG Health Targets

Target 3.1 By 2030, reduce the global maternal mortality ratio to less than 70 per 100,000 live births.

Young age at first birth is an important risk factor for maternal mortality. Reducing early marriage is important to achieving this target.

Target 3.2 By 2030, end preventable deaths of newborns and children under 5 years of age, with all countries aiming to reduce neonatal mortality to at least as low as 12 per 1,000 live births and under-5 mortality to at least as low as 25 per 1,000 live births.

Birth outcomes are directly linked to the health and well-being of women, their nutritional status, and their access to reproductive health services and emergency obstetric care of good quality. In addition, if a woman dies in childbirth in low-income countries, her child has only about a 50 percent chance of survival. Achieving this target will require, among other things, better nutrition and enhanced reproductive health services for adolescents and young adults and a reduction in early marriage.

Target 3.3 By 2030, end the epidemics of AIDS, tuberculosis, malaria, and neglected tropical diseases and combat hepatitis, waterborne diseases, and other communicable diseases.

Older adolescents and young adults are an important risk group for HIV. Reducing the burden of HIV/AIDS will require enhanced prevention and treatment among these groups.

Target 3.4 By 2030, reduce by one-third premature mortality from noncommunicable diseases through prevention and treatment and promote mental health and well-being.

The health behaviors of adolescents and young adults are central to the extent to which they will suffer from noncommunicable diseases later. Thus, it is critical that these groups avoid tobacco consumption, not engage in excess consumption of alcohol, have a healthy diet, and get sufficient physical activity. In addition, adolescents and young adults are at special risk of mental health disorders. Measures need to be taken to reduce these risks and to diagnose and address such problems earlier and to reduce the burden of self-harm.

Target 3.5 Strengthen the prevention and treatment of substance abuse, including narcotic drug abuse and harmful use of alcohol.

Adolescents and young adults are an especially vulnerable group for substance abuse and harmful use of alcohol. Achieving this goal will require careful attention to reducing the risk factors for such behaviors and providing evidence-based public health responses to them.

Target 3.6 By 2020, halve the number of global deaths and injuries from road traffic accidents.

Older adolescents and young adults are at high risk for road traffic injuries. Measures need to be taken to reduce these risks.

Target 3.7 By 2030, ensure universal access to sexual and reproductive healthcare services, including for family planning, information and education, and the integration of reproductive health into national strategies and programs.

This target is especially important for older adolescents and young adults who have high risks of HIV/AIDS, other sexually transmitted diseases, and early pregnancy. Services need to be delivered in ways that are sensitive to these groups.

Target 3.8 Achieve universal health coverage, including financial risk protection, access to quality essential healthcare services, and access to safe, effective, quality, and affordable essential medicines and vaccines for all.

Given the number of adolescents and young adults and their health risks, enhancing access to and the quality of universal health coverage is critical to enhancing their health. However, this, too, will need to be done in ways that are inclusive of these groups and sensitive to their particular needs.

TABLE 12-3 Major Biological and Psychological Changes Along the Life Course from Early Adolescence to Young Adulthood

Early Adolescence: 10–14 Years

Biological: Puberty and its effects on body morphology and sexual and brain development.

Psychological: Low resistance to peer influences, low levels of future orientation, and low risk perception, often leading to increases in risk-taking behavior and poor self-regulation. Identity formation and development of new interests, including emerging interest in sexual and romantic relationships.

Late Adolescence: 15–19 Years

Biological: Pubertal maturation, especially in boys. Continued very active brain development, particularly in terms of the development of the prefrontal cortex and the increased connectivity among brain networks.

Psychological: Continued development of executive and self-regulatory skills, leading to greater future orientation and an increased ability to weigh the short-term and long-term implications of decisions. Many adolescents enjoy greater autonomy, even if they still live with their families.

Young Adulthood: 20–24 Years

Biological: Maturation of the prefrontal cortex, end of high brain plasticity, and final organization of the adult brain.

Psychological: Enhanced reasoning and self-regulatory functions. Generally, adoption of adult roles and responsibilities, including entering the workforce or tertiary education, marriage, childbearing, and economic independence.

Modified from Office of Adolescent Health, U.S. Department of Health & Human Services. (n.d.). *Adolescent development e-learning module.* Retrieved from http://www.hhs.gov/ash/oah/resourcesand-publications/learning/ad_dev/index.html; Patton, G. C., Sawyer, S. M, Santelli, J. S., Ross, D. A., Afifi, R., Allen, N. B., . . . Viner, R. M. (2016). Our future: A *Lancet* commission on adolescent health and wellbeing. *The Lancet,* 387(10036), 2427.

and sex, globally, for adolescents and young adults. This table highlights the importance of several causes:

- Skin diseases for all of the groups
- Self-harm for almost all of the age groups
- Road injuries and interpersonal violence for males
- Migraines, anxiety disorders, and depressive disorders and dietary iron deficiency for females
- The continuing importance of HIV/AIDS for 10- to 14-year-old females and 15- to 19-year-old males

As we would expect, mortality rates rise as one goes from early adolescence to young adulthood. As we would also expect, mortality rates vary by region and country income groups. The lower the income level of the country, in general, the higher the mortality rate of any age group.[8]

Some other key facts concerning differences by sex and age group are as follows:

- Almost 11 percent of deaths of 10- to 14-year-old males are from road injuries, another 11 percent from diarrheal and other intestinal infectious diseases, and almost 9 percent from drowning.
- Almost 13 percent of deaths among 10- to 14-year-old females are from diarrheal and other intestinal infectious diseases, almost 7 percent from road injuries, and another almost 7 percent from malaria.
- About 19 percent of the deaths among 15- to 19-year-old males are from road injuries, 10 percent from interpersonal violence, and 7 percent from self-harm.
- About 10 percent of the deaths among 15- to 19-year-old females are from self-harm, 9 percent from maternal disorders, and 8 percent from road injuries.
- For 20- to 24-year-old males, almost 20 percent of deaths are from road injuries, 12 percent from interpersonal violence, and 10 percent from self-harm.
- For 20- to 24-year-old females, about 13 percent of all deaths are due to maternal disorders, 10 percent to self-harm, and 8 percent to road injuries.[4]

TABLE 12-4 Five Leading Causes of Death Among Adolescents and Young Adults, by Sex, Age Group, and World Bank Country Income Group, 2016

Low-Income Countries

	Ages 10–14	Ages 15–19	Ages 20–24
	Males	*Males*	*Males*
1	HIV/AIDS	HIV/AIDS	Road injuries
2	Malaria	Road injuries	Tuberculosis
3	Diarrheal diseases	Tuberculosis	HIV/AIDS
4	Meningitis	Diarrheal diseases	Interpersonal violence
5	Lower respiratory infections	Interpersonal violence	Diarrheal diseases
	Females	*Females*	*Females*
1	HIV/AIDS	HIV/AIDS	HIV/AIDS
2	Malaria	Diarrheal diseases	Tuberculosis
3	Diarrheal diseases	Tuberculosis	Diarrheal diseases
4	Lower respiratory infections	Road injuries	Maternal hemorrhage
5	Meningitis	Malaria	Indirect maternal deaths

Lower Middle-Income Countries

	Ages 10–14	Ages 15–19	Ages 20–24
	Males	*Males*	*Males*
1	Intestinal infectious diseases	Road injuries	Road injuries
2	Road injuries	Self-harm	Self-harm
3	Drowning	HIV/AIDS	Conflict and terror
4	Malaria	Conflict and terror	Interpersonal violence
5	HIV/AIDS	Intestinal infectious diseases	Tuberculosis
	Females	*Females*	*Females*
1	Intestinal infectious diseases	Self-harm	Self-harm
2	HIV/AIDS	HIV/AIDS	HIV/AIDS
3	Malaria	Diarrheal diseases	Maternal hemorrhage
4	Diarrheal diseases	Road injuries	Tuberculosis
5	Lower respiratory infections	Intestinal infectious diseases	Road injuries

Upper Middle-Income Countries

	Ages 10–14	Ages 15–19	Ages 20–24
	Males	*Males*	*Males*
1	Road injuries	Road injuries	Road injuries
2	Drowning	Interpersonal violence	Interpersonal violence
3	Leukemia	Self-harm	Self-harm
4	Interpersonal violence	Drowning	Drowning
5	Congenital defects	HIV/AIDS	Conflict and terror
	Females	*Females*	*Females*
1	Road injuries	Road injuries	Road injuries
2	Drowning	HIV/AIDS	HIV/AIDS
3	Leukemia	Self-harm	Self-harm
4	Congenital defects	Interpersonal violence	Interpersonal violence
5	Lower respiratory infections	Leukemia	Leukemia

High-Income Countries

	Ages 10–14	Ages 15–19	Ages 20–24
	Males	*Males*	*Males*
1	Road injuries	Road injuries	Road injuries
2	Self-harm	Self-harm	Self-harm
3	Congenital defects	Interpersonal violence	Interpersonal violence
4	Leukemia	Drug use disorders	Drug use disorders
5	Drowning	Drowning	Drowning
	Females	*Females*	*Females*
1	Road injuries	Road injuries	Road injuries
2	Congenital defects	Self-harm	Self-harm
3	Leukemia	Interpersonal violence	Drug use disorders
4	Other neoplasms	Other neoplasms	Interpersonal violence
5	Brain cancer	Congenital defects	Other neoplasms

Data from Institute of Health Metrics and Evaluation (IHME). (n.d.). GBD Compare: Viz Hub. Retrieved from https://vizhub.healthdata.org/gbd-compare/

TABLE 12-5 Five Leading Causes of DALYs, by Age Group and Sex, Globally, 2016

	Ages 10–14	Ages 15–19	Ages 20–24
	Males	*Males*	*Males*
1	Skin diseases	Road injuries	Road injuries
2	Conduct disorder	Skin diseases	Interpersonal violence
3	Dietary iron deficiency	Interpersonal violence	Self-harm
4	Road injuries	Self-harm	Skin diseases
5	Drowning	HIV/AIDS	Drug use disorders
	Females	*Females*	*Females*
1	Skin diseases	Skin diseases	Skin diseases
2	Dietary iron deficiency	Migraine	Migraine
3	Migraine	Depressive disorders	Depressive disorders
4	Anxiety disorders	Dietary iron deficiency	Dietary iron deficiency
5	HIV/AIDS	Self-harm	Self-harm

Data from Institute of Health Metrics and Evaluation (IHME). (n.d.). GBD Compare: Viz Hub. Retrieved from https://vizhub.healthdata.org/gbd-compare/

Risk Factors and Social Determinants

TABLE 12-6 shows the leading risk factors globally for deaths for 10- to 14-year-olds, 15- to 19-year-olds, and 20- to 24-year-olds. The overwhelming majority of 10- to 14-year-olds who die are in low- and middle-income countries. They also continue to die, as we saw, of mostly preventable, communicable causes. Thus, we should not be surprised to see that the most important risk factors for their deaths are those related to the poor circumstances in which they live—including unsafe water and sanitation. However, unsafe sex is also an important risk factor and is related to the importance of HIV/AIDS among this group, most of which was acquired from their mothers.

As one moves to the older age groups, the most important risk factors are increasingly related to behaviors, such as unsafe sex and alcohol use. However, occupational injury is also important, especially in low- and lower middle-income countries with poor working conditions. Unsafe water and sanitation also remain important, especially in the 15- to 19-year-old group.

It is important to note that the health of some populations of adolescents and young adults is more vulnerable than others. For instance, those who are marginalized due to their sexuality or ethnicity, those who live in rural areas, those who live in areas of conflict or natural disasters, and those who are incarcerated face greater risks to their health and well-being than other adolescents and young adults do.[5]

In addition, some of the differences in risk factors between males and females can be attributed to gender disparities. For instance, fewer adolescent girls are enrolled in or complete secondary school, and they are consequently less informed on health issues.[9] Young men, however, face much greater risks than women from war, interpersonal violence, and traffic accidents. In all age groups and regions, in fact, the mortality rate for adolescent males is higher than that for adolescent females, with the exception of Africa.[9] Among drivers, the risk of getting killed on the road for young men is three times that of their female counterparts, due to sociocultural reasons and a greater propensity for risk-taking.[10]

TABLE 12-6 Five Leading Risk Factors for Deaths Among Adolescents and Young Adults, by Age Group, Globally, 2016

	Ages 10–14	Ages 15–19	Ages 20–24
1	Unsafe water	Unsafe sex	Alcohol use
2	Unsafe sex	Alcohol use	Unsafe sex
3	Unsafe sanitation	Occupational injury	Occupational injury
4	Handwashing	Unsafe water	Unsafe water
5	Household air pollution	Unsafe sanitation	Drug use

Data from Institute of Health Metrics and Evaluation (IHME). (n.d.). GBD Compare: Viz Hub. Retrieved from https://vizhub.healthdata.org/gbd-compare/

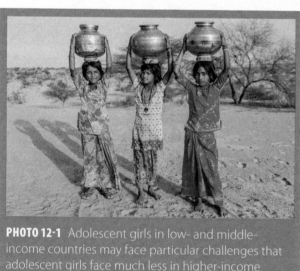

PHOTO 12-1 Adolescent girls in low- and middle-income countries may face particular challenges that adolescent girls face much less in higher-income countries. Some of these can have an important impact on their health and well-being. These can include very time-consuming home-related chores, such as shown in this picture, taken in rural Rajasthan state, India; being married off at a young age; or family barriers to girls continuing their schooling. In traditional societies in low- and lower middle-income countries, what are some of the measures that can be taken to give girls greater opportunities to reach their full potential?
© Hadynyah/E+/Getty Images.

Clearly, the social determinants of health are exceptionally important for adolescents and young adults. Studies have shown that national wealth, income inequality, and access to education are among the most important social determinants of health of adolescents and young adults.[11] In addition, safe and supportive families, peers, and schools are also critical to helping adolescents and young adults develop physically, mentally, and socially. It also appears that exposure to social and other media can have an influence on their behaviors and health.[11]

Additional Comments on Selected Causes of Deaths and DALYs Among Adolescents and Young Adults

Some of the major causes of deaths and DALYs among adolescents and young adults are elaborated upon next.

Early Pregnancy and Childbirth

FIGURE 12-1 shows the older adolescent fertility rate across the World Bank regions. This figure clearly portrays that older adolescent fertility in sub-Saharan Africa and Latin America and the Caribbean is substantially higher than in any other region. In sub-Saharan Africa, in fact, it is six times higher than in the region with the lowest rate and three times higher than in South Asia. High fertility rates among this group pose grave risks to young women because the risks of dying of maternal causes are higher for women in low-resource settings, especially those who are undernourished and of short stature and who give birth at young ages, with short birth intervals, and in places where maternal health services are weak.

As we have seen, complications from pregnancy and childbirth are the leading cause of deaths among females aged 15 to 19 years in many low- and middle-income countries, where 95 percent of births occur.[12] In the WHO Africa region, where birth rates are high, adolescent females aged 15 to 19 years are 1.5 times more likely to die compared to their male counterparts aged 15 to 19 years.[9] In addition, about 3 million girls aged 15 to 19 years undergo unsafe abortions yearly, and some of these lead to maternal death.[12]

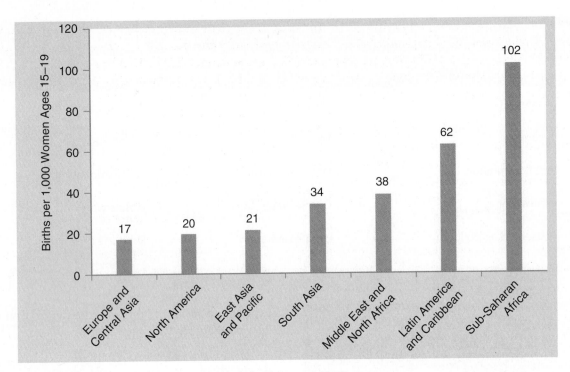

FIGURE 12-1 Adolescent Fertility, Ages 15–19, by World Bank Region, 2016

Data from The World Bank. (2016). Data: Adolescent fertility rate (births per 1,000 women ages 15–19). Retrieved from https://data.worldbank.org/indicator/SP.ADO.TFRT

Anemia

Many young people enter adolescence having suffered from undernutrition and stunting. This is especially so in those parts of the world that are most deficient nutritionally for children, including South Asia, sub-Saharan Africa, the indigenous parts of the Americas, and the poorer and less food-secure parts of other low- and middle-income regions. Iron deficiency anemia, in particular, continues to be an important part of the burden of disease for 10- to 14-year-olds. In fact, it is the leading cause of DALYs among males and females in this age group globally.[4]

HIV/AIDS and Other Sexually Transmitted Infections

It is estimated that more than 2 million adolescents, aged 10 to 19 years, are living with HIV/AIDS. In addition, although the total number of HIV-related deaths has decreased by 30 percent since its peak, estimates suggest that HIV/AIDS-related deaths among adolescents are increasing, mostly in the WHO Africa region. This could be a result of HIV-positive children who survive past childhood but may not be receiving all of the care that they require in adolescence. Among all 15- to 24-year-olds in sub-Saharan Africa, only 10 percent of males and 15 percent of females know their HIV status.[13] In some countries, up to 60 percent of all new HIV infections occur among 15- to 24-year-olds. Adolescence is the period when most people initiate sexual

activity. Adolescent girls are at particular risk both biologically and socially of becoming infected with HIV. In addition, adolescents and young adults face risks of engaging in alcohol and drug use that can also lead to unsafe sexual practices and the transmission of HIV.[12]

Adolescent girls, aged 10 to 19 years, especially in low- and some middle-income countries, face particular risks not only for HIV but also for other sexually transmitted infections. These include their immature reproductive and immune systems, gender norms that discriminate against them, age differences with male sexual partners, and pressure in some settings to engage in transactional sex or prostitution. In addition, in many high-income countries and much of sub-Saharan Africa, more than a third of adolescent girls have had sexual intercourse. Although condom use has increased in high-income countries among adolescents, data show that young women in 19 African countries used a condom in less than a third of their last sexual encounters. Accordingly, most sexually transmitted infections globally occur in people younger than 25 years of age. WHO estimates that 340 million new cases of syphilis, gonorrhea, chlamydia, and trichomoniasis occur each year, and it is thought that the prevalence of sexually transmitted infections is rising in most countries.[14]

Other Communicable Diseases

Deaths and disabilities from communicable diseases like measles have decreased significantly, due largely to the increased coverage of childhood vaccinations.

However, as noted earlier, communicable diseases such as diarrhea, lower respiratory infections, meningitis, and TB remain among the leading causes of mortality of adolescents and young adults. As also shown earlier, malaria is a leading cause of DALYs for early and older adolescents.

TB is a major cause of death for older adolescents and young adults in those parts of sub-Saharan Africa where HIV/AIDS and TB have the highest prevalence rates. TB is also a major cause of adolescent death in South Asia, which also has among the highest prevalence rates of adult TB in the world.[15] The global community is now paying greater attention to the risks of developing active TB disease among young children and adolescents and to their needs for effective TB treatment. This has been a major issue because of the difficulty of diagnosing TB in young children and the lack until recently of pediatric formulations of some TB drugs.

Noncommunicable Diseases

As noted earlier, the behaviors in which adolescents and young adults engage have a significant impact on their health as adults, including what and how much they eat, their levels of physical activity, and whether they drink alcohol or smoke tobacco.

Adolescents and young adults globally are increasingly eating foods high in sugar, salt, and saturated fats, as well as engaging in insufficient physical activity. An increasing share of adolescents now have obesity. In a range of countries for which there are data, fewer than one in four adolescents meet the recommended guidelines for physical activity, and in some countries as many as one in three adolescents now has obesity. It is especially important to note that in many countries this obesity exists side by side with a substantial share of children who suffer from underweight, stunting, and micronutrient deficiencies.[5]

In many high-income countries, the prevalence of cigarette smoking is decreasing among adolescents and young adults. In many low- and middle-income countries, however, the prevalence of cigarette smoking is increasing, as tobacco companies focus an increasing amount of attention on selling their cigarettes in these settings. The gap between male and female prevalence of cigarette smoking is also closing in some settings, as an increasing share of females smoke.

FIGURE 12-2 portrays the prevalence of tobacco smoking among 13- to 15-year-old males and females for a selected group of countries. As shown in the figure, about 50 percent of both males and females smoke in Argentina, which has the highest prevalence for these age groups among the countries surveyed. In Indonesia about 40 percent of the males aged 13 to 15 years smoke tobacco, although the prevalence of female smoking in Indonesia remains low.[5]

As also noted earlier, excessive drinking is a major risk factor, both directly and indirectly, for a range of health issues. Besides being a risk factor for mental health problems and a number of other conditions, alcohol consumption reduces self-control and increases risky behavior, such as unsafe sex, unsafe driving, and violence.[16] Estimates suggest that about 5 percent of all deaths of people aged 15 to 29 years of age are due to alcohol.[17] **FIGURE 12-3** indicates the percentage of adolescents aged 15 to 19 years who are current drinkers, former drinkers, or lifetime abstainers, by WHO region and globally. The figure makes clear the extent to which alcohol consumption is an important risk factor for adolescents, except in the Eastern Mediterranean and South-East Asia WHO regions.

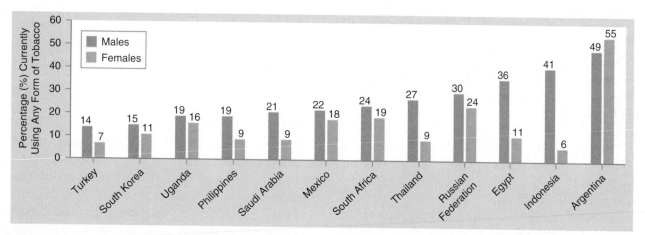

FIGURE 12-2 Prevalence of Tobacco Use Among Males and Females, Ages 13–15, for Selected Countries, 2012

Data from World Health Organization (WHO). (2014). *Health for the world's adolescents: A second chance in the second decade.* Geneva, Switzerland: Author. Retrieved from http://apps.who.int/adolescent/second-decade/

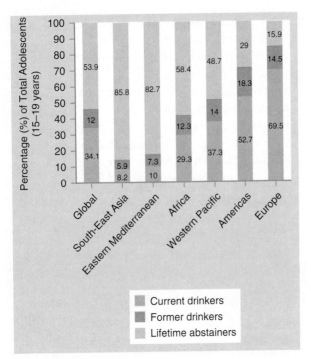

FIGURE 12-3 Percentage of Current Drinkers, Former Drinkers, and Lifetime Abstainers Among Adolescents, Ages 15–19, by WHO Region and Globally

Data from World Health Organization (WHO). (2014). *Global status report on alcohol and health 2014.* Geneva, Switzerland: Author.

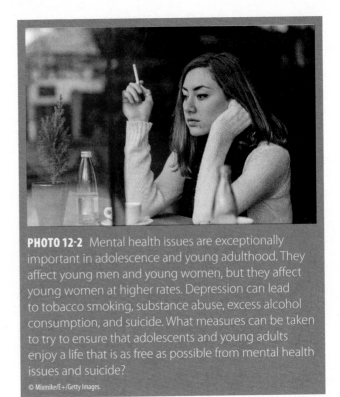

PHOTO 12-2 Mental health issues are exceptionally important in adolescence and young adulthood. They affect young men and young women, but they affect young women at higher rates. Depression can lead to tobacco smoking, substance abuse, excess alcohol consumption, and suicide. What measures can be taken to try to ensure that adolescents and young adults enjoy a life that is as free as possible from mental health issues and suicide?
© Mixmike/E+/Getty Images.

Mental Health

Most mental disorders begin before age 25,[1] and mental health is a fundamental issue for adolescents and young adults. It has been estimated that between 10 percent and 20 percent of all adolescents suffer from mental health problems.[18] As noted earlier, anxiety disorders are among the leading causes of DALYs in females aged 10 to 14 years, and depressive disorders are among the leading causes of DALYs among females ages 15 to 19 and 20 to 24. Self-harm is also a leading cause of DALYs among females and males ages 15 to 19 and 20 to 24.[4] Eating and conduct disorders are also common among adolescents. Although symptoms of around half of all mental health disorders in adulthood have their onset by age 14, most go unnoticed or untreated, but still affect adolescents' potential and development.[12] Those with mental disorders often face stigma, isolation, and discrimination, reducing their access to health care and education. Other risk behaviors that relate to mental health problems include violent behavior, unsafe sexual behavior, and substance abuse.[19]

The risk factors for mental health problems among adolescents are numerous and start with genetics and the health of the mother. At the earliest stages, they include having an adolescent parent, being an unintended birth, being born after a short birth interval, and having a parent who married a blood relative. They also include, for example, poor physical health and nutritional status of the child, growing up without caregivers, being orphaned, or growing up in an institution. In addition, they include exposure to harmful substances, violence, conflict, or abuse. Gender disparity, discrimination, immigrant status, or being displaced can also be risk factors for mental health problems.[18]

Studies have also shown that experiences of school-age children can be important risks for mental health problems in adolescence and later. Beyond those mentioned already, such experiences can include being the victim of bullying, family dysfunction, pathological use of the internet, adolescent pregnancy, and being a child soldier.[18]

Suicide, as noted earlier, deserves special mention when considering the health of adolescents and young adults. It is the leading cause of death among 15- to 19-year-olds and 20- to 24-year-olds globally. It is among the five leading causes of deaths among older adolescents and young adults in all country income groups, except in lower-income countries.[4]

Transport Injuries

Transport injuries are the third leading cause of death among those aged 10 to 14 years, the second leading cause among those aged 15 to 19 years, and the second leading cause among those aged 20 to 24 years.[4] Around 330 adolescents die every day, and close to 400,000 young people under the age of 25 die every year from a road injury.[12] From the ages of 10 to 14 to the ages of 20 to 24, there is a sixfold increase in

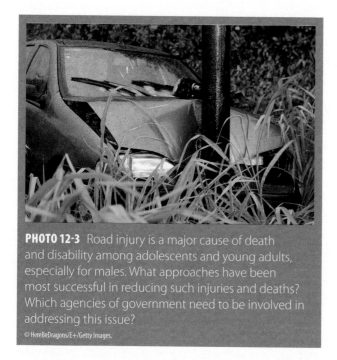

PHOTO 12-3 Road injury is a major cause of death and disability among adolescents and young adults, especially for males. What approaches have been most successful in reducing such injuries and deaths? Which agencies of government need to be involved in addressing this issue?
© HereBeDragons/E+/Getty Images.

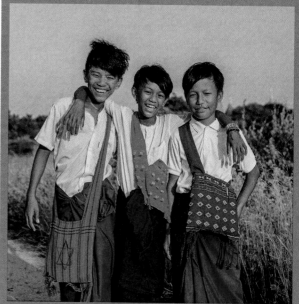

PHOTO 12-4 Despite the happy appearance of these adolescent males from rural Nepal, they, too will face an array of challenges as they move to adulthood. How will they pay for their further schooling? Will there be well-paying and fulfilling jobs for them? Where will they have to go for those jobs? How will they deal with social pressures that might include pressure to smoke, drink alcohol, or engage in relations with women? What are the best approaches to ensuring that they will mature in a way that enhances their physical and mental health?
© Hadynyah/E+/Getty Images.

traffic-related deaths.[9] Many of these deaths happen in low- and middle-income countries not only among passengers in automobiles but also among pedestrians, bicyclists, and motorcyclists.

Violence

Interpersonal violence is a leading cause of adolescent mortality, resulting in an estimated 180 deaths every day.[12] Moreover, interpersonal violence is among the five leading causes of deaths among 15- to 19-year-olds in all World Bank regions, except for sub-Saharan Africa, for which is it is sixth, and South Asia, for which it is eighth. In the Latin America and the Caribbean region of the World Bank, interpersonal violence is the leading cause of death of adolescents 15 to 19 years of age.[4] Among adolescent males, around one in three deaths in the low- and middle-income countries in the WHO Americas region is attributed to violence. Thirty percent of 15- to 19-year-old girls are victims of violence by a partner.[12]

▶ Economic and Social Consequences of Health Issues Among Adolescents and Young Adults

Health issues among adolescents and young adults have profound consequences socially and economically, as well as on health. First, it is clear that maintaining the health of adolescents and young adults is central to maintaining the gains that have occurred in the health of young children. More and more children are living longer and healthier lives as progress has been made, among other things, against vaccine-preventable diseases and malaria. This progress can be undone if adolescents and young adults face important health issues that take their lives away or lead to major illness or disability.

Second, the health of adolescents and young adults and behaviors in which they engage set a foundation for their health as adults. Adolescent pregnancy can diminish the chances that a girl will complete schooling or that her child will become a well-educated, healthy, and productive adult. Obesity during adolescence or young adulthood, for example, can have a permanent effect on the health and productivity of an adult. Most people who take up smoking tobacco, drinking alcohol, and using illegal drugs start such behaviors in adolescence, and these behaviors are difficult to stop as adults.

Other burdens of disease among adolescents and young adults also have substantial costs. The social and economic costs of HIV/AIDS are well known, and adolescent girls are among those at greatest risk of being infected with HIV. Tuberculosis is a major cause of morbidity and death among adolescents in

Africa, and TB leads to months of lost work, even if treated effectively. Road traffic injuries, the leading cause of death among adolescents and young adults globally, can lead to substantial and long-lasting disabilities, as well as many years of life lost. Mental health issues often start in adolescence, go on for much or all of a person's life, and have enormous social and economic costs to individuals, their families, and societies.

▶ Case Study

The case study that follows examines Malawi's attempt to reduce the health risks to young women by using incentives to keep them in school longer.

Cash Transfer Program for Adolescent Girls in Malawi

Malawi, one of the world's poorest countries, faces a high burden of HIV/AIDS. The adult prevalence of HIV is over 10 percent, and females, especially adolescent girls, are particularly vulnerable.[20] Women in Malawi are at highest risk of contracting HIV between ages 15 and 24 years.[21] Interventions that reduce young women's risk of becoming infected with HIV have the potential to significantly reduce HIV prevalence in the general population.

Low educational attainment and economic dependence on men are widely understood to be important risk factors for HIV infection among adolescent girls.[22] In low-resource settings, adolescent girls often engage in transactional sex with older men to pay for school fees and other day-to-day expenses. Cash transfer programs have the potential to reduce the incentive for adolescent girls to engage in such risky transactional sex and ultimately reduce the number of new HIV infections among young women.

In the rural Zomba district of Malawi, a randomized trial was conducted to assess the effect of a cash transfer program on HIV prevalence among young women. Over 1,000 young, unmarried women (ages 13 to 22 years) participated in the program. Half of them were randomly assigned to receive conditional cash transfers, with school attendance required to receive payments. The other half received unconditional cash transfers and did not have to attend school to receive their payments. Those who were going to get payments were randomly assigned by lottery to receive monthly payments ranging from $1 to $5. Participants completed behavioral risk assessments at baseline and 12 months later. Eighteen months after baseline, their HIV status was tested.

After the 18-month program, participants of the cash transfer program had a significantly lower HIV prevalence rate of 1.2 percent, compared to 3.0 percent in the control group who got no cash transfer payment. The study also showed that there was no significant difference in the effect between the conditional and unconditional cash transfer programs. This suggests that, where monitoring school attendance is difficult, even unconditional cash transfers can have the desired effect on health. The program also found that the cash transfers significantly reduced the number of sexual encounters girls had, especially with older men. This evidence supports the notion that cash transfers can reduce HIV prevalence by reducing the need for young women to engage in transactional sex with older men.

In response to this study and other similar studies in the region, conditional cash transfer programs are being scaled up significantly in Malawi. UNAIDS and the World Bank have pledged funds to help the Malawian government expand its existing cash transfer program. Similar efforts are also being expanded in neighboring countries, including South Africa, Botswana, and Kenya.[23]

The conditional cash transfer program in Malawi highlights the importance of helping to address the underlying causes of risk behavior, such as economic need. It also suggests that unconditional cash transfer programs may be as effective as conditional cash transfer programs.

▶ Improving the Health of Adolescents and Young Adults in Low- and Middle-Income Countries

Adolescents and young adults are unique groups, with particular burdens of disease related to a specific set of risk factors and social determinants. It is critical, therefore, that policymakers pay particular attention to the period of adolescence and young adulthood. They also need to take a life-course perspective to the health of adolescents and young adults, seeing it as one stage in a series of age categories that people pass through as they go through life. It will also be important for policymakers to collect data specific to adolescents and young adults, breaking that data down into early adolescence, 10 to 14 years; older adolescence, 15 to 19 years; and young adulthood, 20 to 24 years. This would provide an enhanced basis for analyzing and acting on adolescent and young adult health issues. Evidence also suggests that approaches to improving adolescent and young adult health will be more effective if these groups participate in the identification of program needs.[7]

The importance of social determinants to the well-being of adolescents and young adults also argues for a broad-based approach to addressing their health needs. Thus, it will be important for policymakers to take an approach to adolescent and young adult health that integrates interventions at the community, family, and school levels. Improving the health of adolescents and young adults will also require an integrated approach across sectors. This will have to include, for example, enhancing educational opportunities, especially for girls, and managing the economy in ways that promote employment for the large numbers of adolescents and young adults making their way into the labor force in many countries.[11]

Health authorities lack control over many of the factors that concern road traffic injuries and morbidity and mortality from interpersonal violence. Thus, programs to enhance the health of adolescents and young adults will also have to be intersectoral. Those responsible for road safety will need to take measures that can address the risks for adolescent and young adult drivers, including, for example, improving licensing requirements, taking a stepwise approach to their driving rights, and enforcing drunk driving laws. Governments will also need to take measures to promote home and school environments that reduce the risks of adolescent and young adult violence, such as promoting better child nutrition, better parental caring behaviors, and welcoming school environments. Gun control can also reduce violence among adolescents and young adults.[11]

A recent study in Indian secondary schools, in fact, may suggest an approach to enhancing school environments in a manner that improves the health and well-being of secondary students. A multi-component intervention was delivered to entire schools by lay counselors or teachers in selected schools in the Indian state of Bihar. Each of these approaches was compared with the other and to the life skills program taught in government secondary schools. The intervention using lay counselors was associated with improvements in the school climate and in a number of health outcomes, including depressive disorders, bullying, knowledge of reproductive health, and attitudes toward gender equality.[24]

There are also a number of measures that health systems can take to help address health issues among adolescents and young adults. First, by adopting universal health coverage, health systems can reduce the barriers to care that many adolescents and young adults

face. Second, health systems can take measures to be more friendly to adolescents and young adults. They can train providers in the needs of adolescents and young adults and create settings that encourage adolescents and young adults to seek care. Health authorities can also lead efforts within countries to enact and enforce laws that reduce risk to adolescents and young adults, such as those concerning road safety and the use of tobacco, alcohol, and drugs. Many health systems have focused adolescent and young adult health almost exclusively on sexual and reproductive health. However, such services need to expand their focus and address a broader range of health concerns, as is clear from the burden of disease among adolescents and young adults.[5]

Health interventions in specific areas also need to take into account the particular needs of adolescents and young adults. Efforts to promote family planning and reduce maternal deaths, for example, must pay attention to early marriage, adolescent pregnancy, and short birth intervals among young mothers. Efforts to reduce new HIV infections among adolescents and young adults will have to take into account, among other things, the early sexual debut of many adolescents, multiple sexual partners, transactional sex among young females, access to condoms, and the risks that alcohol and substance abuse pose for unsafe sexual practices. In addition, policies on alcohol and tobacco must always include efforts to limit sales to minors.

WHO has developed guidelines for health services and interventions that can address the health needs and risks that adolescents face. The recommended services are summarized in **FIGURE 12-4**. These services and interventions are meant to complement the broader approach taken to reduce risk, reduce harm, and treat adolescent and young adult health problems in specific areas.[5] WHO guidelines for offering support and treatment for tobacco cessation for adolescents, for example, must be seen in the context of efforts to tax tobacco, prohibit the advertising of tobacco products, reduce the number of places that people can smoke, and prohibit the sale of tobacco to minors. Thus, the figure also includes some comments on the broader policy measures that are needed in specific areas.

The recent *Lancet* commission expanded on the WHO framework in a number of ways. First, it outlined measures to address the health of adolescents and young adults. Second, it categorized proposed measures into a range of types, such as those that are structural, community-based, focused on social marketing, or that take place within families, schools, or health services. **TABLE 12-7** summarizes some of the main points of the package of services proposed by the commission.

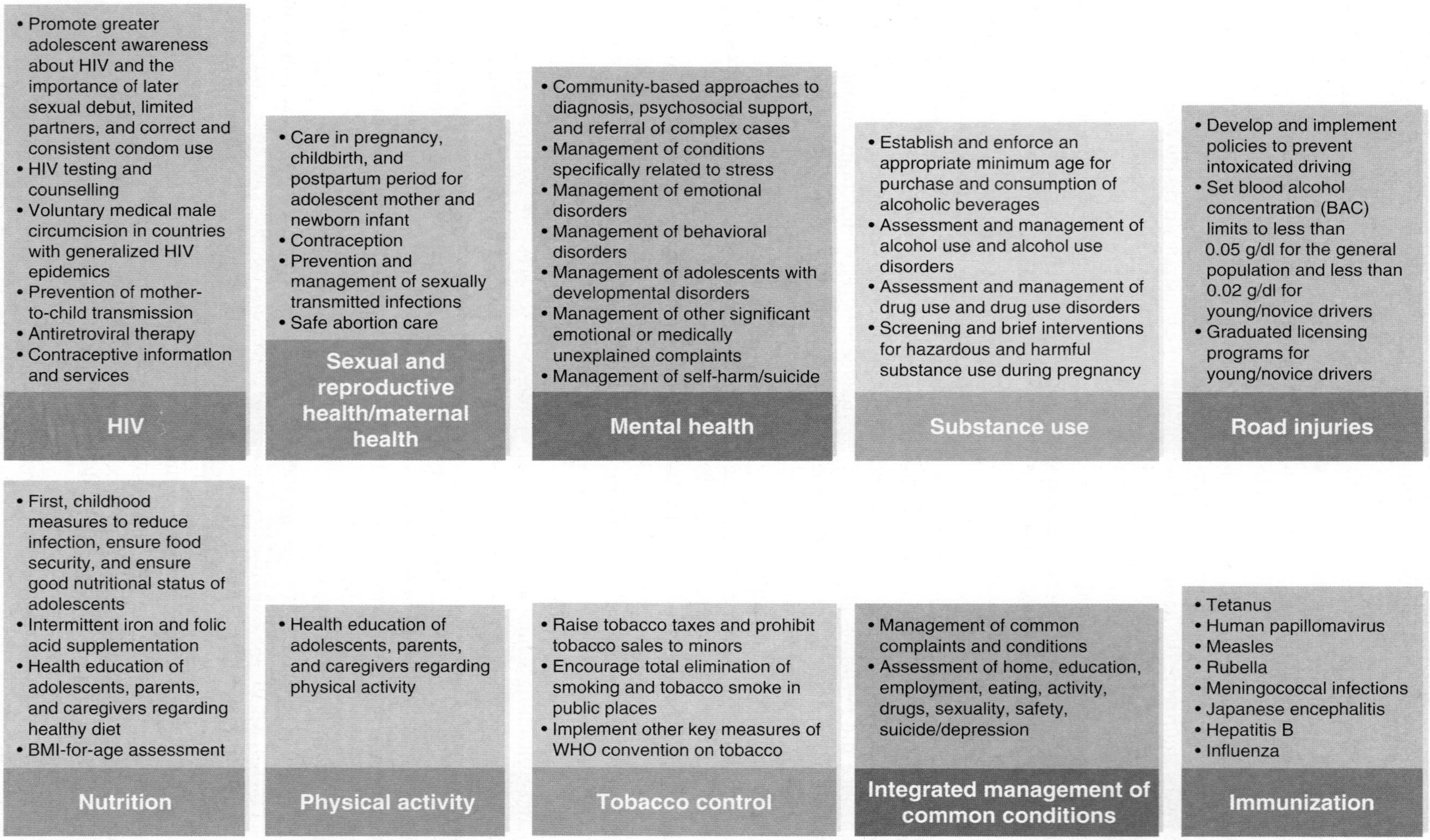

HIV

- Promote greater adolescent awareness about HIV and the importance of later sexual debut, limited partners, and correct and consistent condom use
- HIV testing and counselling
- Voluntary medical male circumcision in countries with generalized HIV epidemics
- Prevention of mother-to-child transmission
- Antiretroviral therapy
- Contraceptive information and services

Sexual and reproductive health/maternal health

- Care in pregnancy, childbirth, and postpartum period for adolescent mother and newborn infant
- Contraception
- Prevention and management of sexually transmitted infections
- Safe abortion care

Mental health

- Community-based approaches to diagnosis, psychosocial support, and referral of complex cases
- Management of conditions specifically related to stress
- Management of emotional disorders
- Management of behavioral disorders
- Management of adolescents with developmental disorders
- Management of other significant emotional or medically unexplained complaints
- Management of self-harm/suicide

Substance use

- Establish and enforce an appropriate minimum age for purchase and consumption of alcoholic beverages
- Assessment and management of alcohol use and alcohol use disorders
- Assessment and management of drug use and drug use disorders
- Screening and brief interventions for hazardous and harmful substance use during pregnancy

Road injuries

- Develop and implement policies to prevent intoxicated driving
- Set blood alcohol concentration (BAC) limits to less than 0.05 g/dl for the general population and less than 0.02 g/dl for young/novice drivers
- Graduated licensing programs for young/novice drivers

Nutrition

- First, childhood measures to reduce infection, ensure food security, and ensure good nutritional status of adolescents
- Intermittent iron and folic acid supplementation
- Health education of adolescents, parents, and caregivers regarding healthy diet
- BMI-for-age assessment

Physical activity

- Health education of adolescents, parents, and caregivers regarding physical activity

Tobacco control

- Raise tobacco taxes and prohibit tobacco sales to minors
- Encourage total elimination of smoking and tobacco smoke in public places
- Implement other key measures of WHO convention on tobacco

Integrated management of common conditions

- Management of common complaints and conditions
- Assessment of home, education, employment, eating, activity, drugs, sexuality, safety, suicide/depression

Immunization

- Tetanus
- Human papillomavirus
- Measles
- Rubella
- Meningococcal infections
- Japanese encephalitis
- Hepatitis B
- Influenza

FIGURE 12-4 Key Health Services and Interventions for Improving Adolescent Health

Data from the author and World Health Organization (WHO). (2014). *Health for the world's adolescents: A second chance in the second decade.* Geneva, Switzerland: Author. Retrieved from http://apps.who.int/adolescent/second-decade/

TABLE 12-7 Recommended Action Bundles for Adolescent and Young Adult Health Problems and Risks

	Community and Family	Schools	Social Marketing	Legal/ Governmental
Undernutrition	Provide micronutrient and protein-energy supplements, deworming, cash transfer programs, and nutrition education	Provide micronutrient supplements and healthy meals at school		Fortify foods with micronutrients such as folate and iron
Overweight and obesity	Create opportunities for physical activity in daily life	Implement multi-component programs involving physical activity and healthy diet education	Promote physical activity	Tax foods high in sugar, salt, or fat Restrict fast-food advertising Mandate nutrition labels on the front of products
Infectious diseases	Provide deworming and bed nets	Require HPV vaccination		
Mental disorders and suicide	Provide gatekeeper training for suicide prevention to adults who interact with adolescents and young adults	Provide school-based mental health services and gatekeeper training	Promote mental health literacy	Restrict access to suicide means
Unintentional injury			Promote knowledge of risks	Enhance traffic control Mandate helmet wearing Implement stepwise driver's licensing
Violence	Promote gender equality, economic empowerment, and parent–child communication	Implement multi-component interventions targeting violent behavior and substance abuse	Promote knowledge of the impact of violence and available services	Implement gun control Legalize homosexuality Protect women from violence and sexual coercion Make 16 years the minimum age for criminal responsibility

(continues)

TABLE 12-7 Recommended Action Bundles for Adolescent and Young Adult Health Problems and Risks *(continued)*

	Community and Family	Schools	Social Marketing	Legal/ Governmental
Sexual and reproductive health	Implement peer education and cash transfer programs incentivizing school attendance	Provide access to quality secondary education, sexuality education, condoms, and modern contraceptives in clean, safe schools	Promote community support for sexual and reproductive health	Establish 18 years as the minimum age for marriage Allow access to contraception for legal minors
Alcohol and illicit drugs	Provide access to needle/syringe exchanges	Implement alcohol-free policies	Restrict advertising of alcohol Create campaigns to build community awareness	Tax alcohol Limit alcohol sales to underage adolescents Implement drunk driving laws
Tobacco	Promote parent-child communication	Implement smoke-free policies	Create anti-tobacco campaigns	Tax tobacco Restrict tobacco advertising Implement smoke-free air laws Limit access to youth

Modified from Patton, G. C., Sawyer, S. M, Santelli, J. S., Ross, D. A., Afifi, R., Allen, N. B., . . . Viner, R. M. (2016). Our future: A *Lancet* commission on adolescent health and wellbeing. *The Lancet*, 387(10036), 2458.

Besides the elements shown in the table, the commission also recommended a number of ways in which mobile technologies could be used for social marketing and health education. The commission also recommended that countries include in their package of universal health coverage services that are sensitive to the needs of adolescents and young adults, evidence-based, and cost-effective. The commission recommended such packages should focus on nutrition and physical activity; TB, malaria, and HIV; reproductive health; violence; mental health; injuries; tobacco and alcohol; and chronic physical disorders. The specific contents of such packages are discussed in detail elsewhere in the text.

▶ Main Messages

The health of adolescents and young adults is critical to the global health agenda. Adolescents and young adults constitute an important part of the population in all countries. In addition, the health of adolescents and young adults is central to preserving the gains made in child health. It is also central to laying a solid foundation for the health of future adults.

A specific focus on the health of adolescents and young adults is essential because adolescents and young adults are neither children nor fully mature adults and because adolescence and young adulthood is a time of important biological and psychological change. Adolescents go through hormonal and other changes, become more influenced by peers and less by family, and may engage in risk-taking behaviors until they are able to exercise more rational control over their impulses and emotions. A number of biological and psychological changes continue through young adulthood.

In addition, adolescents and young adults have a unique burden of disease. Early adolescents, especially in low- and middle-income countries, continue to fall ill and die from preventable or treatable communicable diseases, such as diarrhea, pneumonia, malaria, meningitis, and HIV/AIDS. Older adolescent girls, especially in low-income countries, face serious risks of dying from maternal causes and of contracting HIV. There is also a substantial burden of anemia. Increasingly, however, as the burden of communicable diseases is reduced, more and more adolescents and young adults, in all parts of the world, face a burden of disease dominated by road injuries, depression, interpersonal violence, and suicide. It is also important to note that, side by side with continuing high prevalence of childhood underweight and micronutrient deficiencies, an increasing share of the world's adolescents and young adults have overweight and obesity.

The risk factors for the communicable diseases that affect adolescents and young adults are well-known and include, among other things, poor nutrition; inadequate water, sanitation, and hygiene; and poor coverage of immunization and other health services. Early pregnancy is also an important risk factor for maternal morbidity and mortality. Social determinants of health, such as poverty, abuse, living in rural areas, poor family educational attainment, and gender discrimination, are also key to understanding the burden of disease among adolescents and young adults. Peer relationships, living with conflict or the aftermath of disasters, and having few economic options are also important determinants of the health and well-being of adolescents and young adults and whether they engage in tobacco use, alcohol abuse, unsafe sex, or risky driving or suffer from mental health issues.

The consequences of poor health among adolescents and young adults to individuals, families, and societies are immense. An unhealthy adolescent or young adult is unlikely to have a healthy and productive adulthood. In addition, adolescents and young adults may fall ill with conditions such as mental health, alcohol, or substance abuse disorders, which can go on for many years and will be costly to themselves and to society.

There are a number of measures that can be taken to address the key health issues faced by adolescents and young adults. At the broadest levels of society, it will be important to promote education of good quality to the secondary level for females, as well as males. Investing in water, sanitation, and hygiene will also be fundamental. Economic policies that encourage job creation and productive employment for the large numbers of adolescents and young adults who will enter the job market will also be essential.

Health systems can also take a number of institutional steps to better address the health needs of adolescents and young adults. They need to train their staff to pay attention to the unique burdens of disease and needs of these groups. They need to improve their collection of data that is specific to adolescents and young adults, as well. It will also be important that specific health programs, such as for TB or HIV, focus particular attention on adolescents and young adults, the risk factors for becoming infected with active TB disease or with HIV, and measures that could be taken to reduce the specific risks for these diseases that adolescents and young adults face. Moving to universal health coverage can also help to reduce the barriers that many adolescents and young adults face in accessing health services, as would ensuring that such health services are friendly to these groups.

Other specific interventions could also be made to reduce the burden of disease among adolescents and young adults. Improving licensing requirements for driving, taking a stepwise approach to adolescent driving, and stricter enforcement of drunk driving laws can reduce road traffic injuries among these groups. Keeping girls in school longer, improving knowledge about reproductive health and family planning, and enhancing access to family planning and maternal health services could reduce the burden of reproductive health issues among adolescents and young adults. Taking a community-based approach to mental health issues, with specific attention to adolescents and young adults, psychosocial support, and referral for difficult cases, could help to reduce the high burden of mental health conditions and suicide among adolescents and young adults.

Study Questions

1. Why is specific attention to the health of 10- to 24-year-olds needed?
2. What are the leading burdens of disease among adolescents and young adults globally?
3. How do these burdens vary between sexes and between low-income and high-income countries?
4. How do they vary between early adolescents, older adolescents, and young adults?
5. What are the most important social determinants of the health of adolescents and young adults?
6. What are some of the most important health and social consequences of health issues among adolescents and young adults?

7. What could be done to reduce the burden of reproductive health issues among adolescents and young adults?

8. What could be done to reduce the burden of road injuries among adolescents and young adults?

9. What could be done to reduce the burden of mental health conditions among adolescents and young adults?

10. What are the most critical health, social, and economic costs of the burden of disease among adolescents and young adults?

References

1. Patton, G. C., Sawyer, S. M, Santelli, J. S., Ross, D. A., Afifi, R., Allen, N. B., . . . Viner, R. M. (2016). Our future: A *Lancet* commission on adolescent health and wellbeing. *The Lancet, 387*(10036), 2423–2478.

2. World Health Organization (WHO). (n.d). *Adolescent health.* Retrieved from https://www.who.int/topics/adolescent_health/en/

3. PopulationPyramid.net. (n.d.). World 2017. Retrieved from https://www.populationpyramid.net/

4. Institute of Health Metrics and Evaluation (IHME). (n.d). GBD Compare: Viz Hub. Retrieved from https://vizhub.healthdata.org/gbd-compare/

5. World Health Organization (WHO). (2014). *Health for the world's adolescents: A second chance in the second decade.* Geneva, Switzerland: Author. Retrieved from http://apps.who.int/adolescent/second-decade/

6. Bundy, D.A.P., de Silva, N., Horton, S., Jamison, D.T., & Patton, G.C. (Eds.). (2017). *Disease control priorities: Child and adolescent health and development* (3rd ed., Vol. 8). Washington, DC: The World Bank.

7. Sawyer, S. M., Afifi, R. A., Bearinger, L. H., Blakemore, S. J., Dick, B., Ezeh, A. C., & Patton, G. C. (2012). Adolescence: A foundation for future health. *The Lancet, 379*(9826), 1630–1640.

8. Patton, G. C., Coffey, C., Sawyer, S. M., Viner, R. M., Haller, D. M., Bose, K., . . . Mathers, C. D. (2009). Global patterns of mortality in young people: A systematic analysis of population health data. *The Lancet, 374*(9693), 881–892.

9. Patton, G. C., Coffey, C., Cappa, C., Currie, D., Riley, L., Gore, F., . . . Ferguson, J. (2012). Health of the world's adolescents: A synthesis of internationally comparable data. *The Lancet, 379,* 1665–1675.

10. World Health Organization (WHO). (2007). *Youth and road safety.* Geneva, Switzerland: Author.

11. Viner, R. M., Ozer, E. M., Denny, S., Marmot, M., Resnick, M., Fatusi, A., & Currie, C. (2012). Adolescence and the social determinants of health. *The Lancet, 379,* 1641–1652.

12. World Health Organization (WHO). (2014). *Adolescents: Health risks and solutions* (Fact Sheet No. 345). Retrieved from https://www.who.int/news-room/fact-sheets/detail/adolescents-health-risks-and-solutions

13. World Health Organization. (2018). *Adolescents: Health risks and solutions: Key facts.* Retrieved from https://www.who.int/news-room/fact-sheets/detail/adolescents-health-risks-and-solutions/

14. Bearinger, L. H., Sieving, R. E., Ferguson, J., & Sharma, V. (2007). Global perspectives on the sexual and reproductive health of adolescents: Patterns, prevention, and potential. *The Lancet, 369,* 1220–1231.

15. USAID. (2019). *Tuberculosis in India.* Retrieved from https://www.usaid.gov/what-we-do/global-health/tuberculosis/technical-areas/tuberculosis-india

16. Gore, F. M., Bloem, P. J., Patton, G. C., Ferguson, J., Joseph, V., Coffey, C., . . . & Mathers, C. D. (2011). Global burden of disease in young people aged 10–24 years: A systematic analysis. *The Lancet, 377*(9783), 2093–2102.

17. World Health Organization (WHO). (n.d.). *School and youth health promotion.* Retrieved from http://who.int/school_youth_health/en/

18. Kieling, C., Baker-Henningham, H., Belfer, M., Conti, G., Erte, I., Omigbodun, O., . . . Rahman, A. (2011). Child and adolescent mental health worldwide: Evidence for action. *The Lancet, 378,* 1515–1525.

19. World Health Organization (WHO). (n.d.). *Child and adolescent mental health.* Retrieved from http://www.who.int/mental_health/maternal-child/child_adolescent/en/

20. UNAIDS. (2013). *HIV and AIDS estimates (2013): Malawi.* Retrieved from http://www.unaids.org/en/regionscountries/countries/malawi

21. Misiri, H., Edriss, A., Aalen, O., & Dahl, F. (2012). Estimation of HIV Incidence in Malawi from cross-sectional population based sero-prevalence data. *Journal of International Aids Society, 15*(1), 14.

22. Baird, S. J., Garfein, R. S., McIntosh, C. T., & Özler, B. (2012). Effect of a cash transfer programme for schooling on prevalence of HIV and herpes simplex type 2 in Malawi: A cluster randomised trial. *The Lancet, 379,* 1320–1329.

23. UNAIDS. (2014). *Scaling up cash transfer for HIV prevention among adolescent girls and young women.* Retrieved from http://www.unaids.org/en/resources/presscentre/featurestories/2014/august/20140818cash-transfers

24. Shinde, S., Weiss, H. A., Varghese, B., Khandeoarkar, P., Pereira, B., Sharma, A., . . . Patel, V. (2018). Promoting school climate and health outcomes with the SEHER multi-component secondary school intervention in Bihar, India: A cluster-randomised controlled trial. *The Lancet, 392*(10163), 2465–2477.

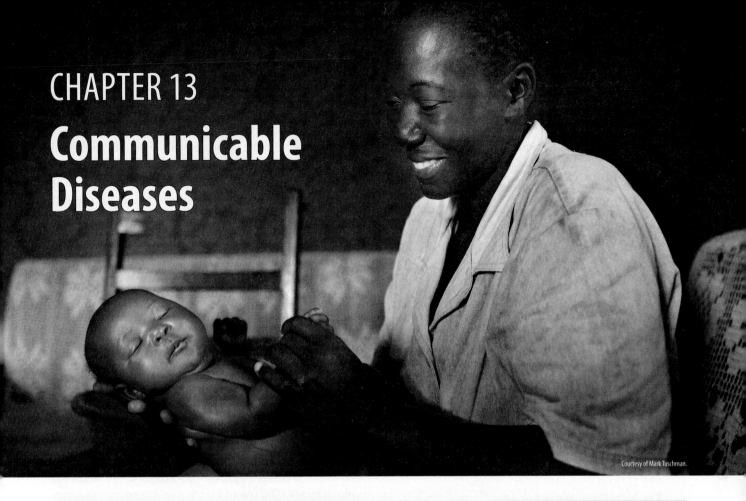

Courtesy of Mark Tuschman.

CHAPTER 13
Communicable Diseases

LEARNING OBJECTIVES

By the end of this chapter, the reader will be able to do the following:

- Review the burden of communicable diseases
- Discuss the determinants of selected communicable diseases, including emerging and re-emerging infectious diseases and antimicrobial resistance
- Understand key concepts concerning the prevention, transmission, and treatment of those diseases
- Review the costs and consequences of communicable diseases of importance
- Outline some of the most important examples of successful interventions against communicable diseases
- Discuss key challenges to the future prevention and control of these diseases

▶ Vignettes

Henrietta was a 35-year-old Kenyan mother of four who lived in Mombasa. Over the last 4 months, Henrietta was barely able to digest her food, had frequent bouts of diarrhea, and had been losing weight. She worried about having AIDS. Henrietta went to a local clinic where she was tested and found to be HIV-positive. She had been infected by her husband, who was a long-distance truck driver.

Maria was 33 years old and lived in the mountains of Peru. For some time, she had not been feeling well. She often had a fever, was coughing a lot, and had night sweats. Maria had tuberculosis (TB) earlier

and worried that this might be TB again. Maria was correct. In fact, this time she had drug-resistant TB, which would be difficult and expensive to treat and might not be curable. When Maria was sick the first time, she started her prescribed 6 months of treatment. However, because she felt much better after the first 2 months of drugs, she did not take the rest of them.

Wole was 4 years old and lived in southwestern Nigeria. He had flulike symptoms, a fever, and a headache. His mother suspected he might have malaria but decided she would see if he got better before taking him to the doctor. In another few days, however, Wole was much sicker and weaker. He was also dizzy and, shortly thereafter, lapsed into a coma. His mother rushed him to the local health center, but he died within a few hours. Unfortunately, Wole had the most virulent form of malaria.

Sanjay was 18 months old and lived in Lucknow, India. His mother was a day laborer and his father was a rickshaw driver. They lived in a hut in a large slum with little access to water and no toilet. Sanjay was below the normal height and weight for his age and looked only 12 months old. Over the past year, Sanjay had six bouts of severe diarrhea.

Sam was a 35-year-old man in Liberia. He had been generally healthy until he fell ill in 2015, while helping to take care of his sick mother. Sam felt very weak, had diarrhea, was vomiting, and had unexplained bleeding. Only a week into the course of his illness did the news reach Sam's village that an outbreak of Ebola hemorrhagic fever was under way in Liberia. Sam's mother succumbed to the disease shortly after health workers visited the village and transported her to a treatment center. Sam also went to the treatment center but was able to survive and is now back in his village.

▶ The Importance of Communicable Diseases

Communicable diseases are immensely important to the global burden of disease. In 2016, they accounted for about 15 percent of all deaths globally and 19 percent of all disability-adjusted life years (DALYs). However, in low-income countries, they accounted for about 40 percent of all deaths and 40 percent of all DALYs.[1] In 2017, it was estimated that tuberculosis (TB) was responsible for about 1.6 million deaths,[2] HIV/AIDS killed about 940,000 people,[3] and malaria accounted for 425,000 deaths.[4] In 2016, diarrhea killed about 525,000 children under 5 years of age.[5] Parasitic infections also account for an enormous burden of disease and disability and some deaths.[1] In addition, the world faces important threats from emerging and re-emerging infectious diseases and from antimicrobial resistance.

Communicable diseases are the most important burden of disease in sub-Saharan Africa, where they account for about 46 percent of deaths and 46 percent of DALYs. They are also especially important in South Asia, where they account for about 20 percent of total deaths and DALYs.[1] These diseases disproportionately affect the poor. Better-off people have the knowledge and income to protect themselves from diseases spread by unsafe water. They do not live in the crowded circumstances that can spread TB, and they

also protect themselves as much as possible against malaria. In addition, they immunize their children against vaccine-preventable diseases at higher rates than poor people do.

Communicable diseases are also of enormous economic consequence. These diseases constrain the physical and mental development of infants and young children and reduce their future economic prospects. The impacts of HIV, TB, malaria, and the neglected tropical diseases on adult productivity are also exceptionally large. In addition, the direct and indirect costs of treatment for an infected person are often a substantial share of their income, causing them to borrow money or sell their already limited assets and forcing them to sink into poverty. High rates of communicable diseases are also impediments to the investment needed to spur economic growth. The appearance of an emerging infectious disease or the re-emergence of a disease can cause billions of dollars in lost income for individuals, communities, and countries.

Much of the burden of communicable diseases is avoidable because many of these diseases can easily be prevented or treated. Vaccines are an extremely cost-effective way to prevent a number of communicable diseases. The use of safe water can reduce the burden of diarrhea and certain parasitic diseases. There are inexpensive, safe, and cost-effective approaches to prevention and treatment for TB, HIV/AIDS, malaria, and many parasitic infections. In addition, the more rational use of antibiotics could reduce the development of antimicrobial resistance, and the global community needs to act more effectively on such resistance and on emerging and re-emerging infectious diseases.

Given their importance and their impact on the poor, the communicable diseases are of immense relevance to the Sustainable Development Goals (SDGs), as noted in **TABLE 13-1**.

This chapter introduces the reader to some of the major communicable diseases and their associated burden of morbidity, disability, and mortality, especially in low- and middle-income countries. It will also outline how selected communicable diseases can be controlled. The chapter then presents a number of case studies on efforts to address communicable diseases. The chapter concludes by reviewing some of the key challenges the world faces in the control of these diseases.

This chapter focuses on emerging and re-emerging infectious diseases and antimicrobial resistance, HIV/AIDS, TB, malaria, and a set of parasitic and bacterial infections often referred to as "neglected tropical diseases." This chapter will not comment on bio-terrorism. This chapter does offer brief comments on diarrhea and pneumonia, which are both covered more extensively in the chapter on child health.

TABLE 13-1 Selected Links Between Communicable Diseases and the SDG Health Targets
Target 3.1 By 2030, reduce the global maternal mortality ratio to less than 70 per 100,000 live births.
HIV/AIDS, TB, and malaria are risks to poor maternal health outcomes. Addressing them effectively will help reduce maternal mortality.
Target 3.2 By 2030, end preventable deaths of newborns and children under 5 years of age, with all countries aiming to reduce neonatal mortality to at least as low as 12 per 1,000 live births and under-5 mortality to at least as low as 25 per 1,000 live births.
A number of communicable diseases are major causes of young child death, including pneumonia, diarrhea, and malaria. Addressing them more effectively is central to any efforts to reduce newborn and under-5 deaths.
Target 3.3 By 2030, end the epidemics of AIDS, tuberculosis, malaria, and neglected tropical diseases and combat hepatitis, waterborne diseases, and other communicable diseases.
This target is directly related to the reduction of communicable diseases.
Target 3.4 By 2030, reduce by one-third premature mortality from noncommunicable diseases through prevention and treatment and promote mental health and well-being.
A number of communicable diseases, including the neglected tropical diseases, are important causes of disability. These disabilities can have a major impact on the mental health of the affected people.
Target 3.7 By 2030, ensure universal access to sexual and reproductive healthcare services, including for family planning, information and education, and the integration of reproductive health into national strategies and programs.
HIV/AIDS remains one of the largest infectious killers. There is also a high prevalence in many communities of other sexually transmitted infections. Both must be addressed as part of sexual and reproductive health services.
Target 3.8 Achieve universal health coverage, including financial risk protection, access to quality essential healthcare services, and access to safe, effective, quality, and affordable essential medicines and vaccines for all.
Universal health coverage that is of good quality reduces out-of-pocket costs to the poor to a minimum. In addition, if it is fairly prioritized and delivered, it can have a major impact on the health services most needed to address communicable diseases.

Modified from United Nations Sustainable Development Goals Knowledge Platform. (n.d.). Sustainable Development Goals. © United Nations. Reprinted with the permission of the United Nations.

This chapter is introductory. Communicable diseases are a very important topic about which an exceptional amount of material has been written. Those interested in gaining a deeper understanding of these diseases are encouraged to read some of the materials cited in this chapter.

▶ Key Terms, Definitions, and Concepts

As you begin to explore communicable diseases in greater detail, there are a number of terms and concepts with which you should be familiar. These are defined in **TABLE 13-2**. It is also important to note that a communicable disease is a disease that is transmitted from an animal to another animal, an animal to a human, a human to another human, or a human to an animal. Transmission can be direct, such as through respiratory means, or indirect through a vector, such as a mosquito in the case of malaria. Most people use the term **communicable disease** in a manner that is synonymous with **infectious disease**. However, others prefer to speak separately about diseases caused by infectious agents, such as TB, and those caused by parasites, such as hookworm. This chapter generally uses the term *communicable disease* to refer to both infectious and parasitic diseases. However, because

TABLE 13-2 Communicable Disease Definitions

Case—An individual with a particular disease.
Case fatality rate—The proportion of persons with a particular condition (cases) who die from that condition.
Control (disease control)—Reducing the incidence and prevalence of a disease to an acceptable level.
Elimination (of disease)—Reducing the incidence of a disease in a specific area to zero.
Emerging infectious disease—A newly discovered disease.
Eradication (of disease)—Termination of all cases of a disease and its transmission globally.
Parasite—An organism that lives in or on another organism and takes its nourishment from that organism.
Re-emerging infectious disease—An existing disease that has increased in incidence or has taken on new forms.

Data from Centers for Disease Control and Prevention (CDC). (n.d.). Epidemiology glossary. Retrieved from https://www.cdc.gov/reproductivehealth/data_stats/glossary.html; Dowdle, W. R. (1999). The principles of disease elimination and eradication. *Morbidity and Mortality Weekly Report, 48*(Suppl. 1), 23–27. Retrieved from http://www.cdc.gov/mmwr/preview/mmwrhtml/su48a7.htm

it is common to refer to "emerging and re-emerging *infectious* diseases," that term will also be used when appropriate.

As we examine the basic concepts concerning communicable diseases, it is also important to know how such diseases can be spread. This is shown in the following list, which includes examples of diseases spread in each manner:

- **Foodborne**: Salmonella, *Escherichia coli, Entamoeba histolytica*
- **Waterborne**: Cholera, rotavirus
- **Sexual or bloodborne**: Hepatitis, HIV
- **Vector-borne**: Malaria, onchocerciasis
- **Inhalation**: Tuberculosis, influenza, meningitis
- **Nontraumatic contact**: Anthrax
- **Traumatic contact**: Rabies

In addition, it is critical to understand the ways in which communicable diseases can be controlled. These are noted in the following list of examples of control measures that may be used against the given diseases. The reader should note, however, that a number of different control measures are taken against many diseases.

- **Vaccination**: Smallpox, polio, measles, diphtheria, pertussis, tetanus, hepatitis B, yellow fever, meningitis, influenza
- **Mass chemotherapy**: Onchocerciasis, hookworm, lymphatic filariasis
- **Vector control**: Malaria, dengue, yellow fever, onchocerciasis, West Nile virus
- **Improved water, sanitation, hygiene**: Diarrheal diseases
- **Improved care seeking, disease recognition**: Diarrheal disease and respiratory disease
- **Case management (treatment) and improved caregiving**: Diarrheal disease, respiratory disease, HIV/AIDS, TB
- **Case surveillance, reporting, and containment**: Avian influenza, meningitis, cholera

- **Behavioral change**: HIV, sexually transmitted infections, Guinea worm, Ebola virus

A final concept of exceptional importance when discussing communicable diseases is the concept of drug resistance. This refers to the extent to which infectious and parasitic agents develop an ability to resist drug treatment.

▶ Note on the Use of Data in This Chapter

It is important to note the data sources for this chapter. Some of the data on the burden of disease comes from the Global Burden of Disease Study 2016.[1] Most other data are taken from the World Health Organization (WHO) and UNAIDS, or *Disease Control Priorities, Third Edition* (DCP3),[6] a recent nine-volume study of disease control priorities for low- and middle-income countries.

▶ The Burden of Communicable Diseases

As noted earlier, in 2016 communicable diseases accounted for about 16 percent of total deaths and about 19 percent of total DALYs globally. However, they were a much larger share of the burden of deaths and disease in low-income countries: in low-income countries they accounted for 40 percent of deaths and 40 percent of DALYs.[1]

TABLE 13-3 summarizes the major causes of death globally by broad age group. Communicable diseases are highlighted.

This table reflects the continuing importance of communicable diseases for all three age groups. However, it also shows that communicable diseases

TABLE 13-3 Leading Causes of Death Globally, by Broad Age Group, 2016, as Percentage of Total Deaths

Under-5		Ages 5–14		Ages 15–49	
Cause	Percentage of Total Deaths (%)	Cause	Percentage of Total Deaths (%)	Cause	Percentage of Total Deaths (%)
Lower respiratory infections	15.3	Road injuries	8.6	HIV/AIDS	19.7
Preterm birth complications	12.1	Typhoid and paratyphoid	7.9	Road injuries	8.8
Neonatal encephalopathy	9.8	Malaria	7.3	Ischemic heart disease	8.4
Diarrheal diseases	9.8	Drowning	7.0	Self-harm	5.9
Other neonatal disorders	6.4	Lower respiratory infections	6.0	Tuberculosis	4.9
Malaria	6.4	Diarrheal diseases	5.9	Stroke	4.8
Congenital heart anomalies	4.0	HIV/AIDS	5.8	Cirrhosis	4.3
Sepsis and other infections	3.7	Congenital defects	3.7	Interpersonal violence	3.9
Protein-energy malnutrition	2.6	Meningitis	3.2	Maternal disorders	2.5
Other congenital birth defects	2.3	Leukemia	3.1	Lower respiratory infections	2.2

Note: Highlighted causes represent communicable causes.
Data from Institute for Health Metrics and Evaluation (IHME). (n.d.). GBD Compare: Viz Hub. Retrieved from https://vizhub.healthdata.org/gbd-compare/

are especially important causes of death for 5- to 14-year-olds.

TABLE 13-4 examines the leading causes of death globally by sex. Communicable diseases are also highlighted in this table.

Globally, for all age groups, we see that the overwhelming majority of deaths are caused by noncommunicable diseases. However, for males, lower respiratory infections and TB remain in the top 10 causes of death, as do lower respiratory infections and diarrhea for females.

TABLE 13-5 examines the leading communicable causes of death by World Bank country income group and globally.

The table brings out a number of points:

- As noted earlier, the burden of communicable causes of death remains greatest in the low-income countries.
- As country incomes rise, the share of deaths associated with communicable causes falls dramatically.
- In high-income countries, only a very small share of total deaths, mostly among the elderly, are caused by communicable diseases.

In addition, the relative importance of specific communicable diseases to the burden of disease varies by region. HIV/AIDS is of particular importance in

TABLE 13-4 Leading Causes of Death Globally, by Sex, 2016, as Percentage of Total Deaths

Males		Females	
Cause	**Percentage of Total Deaths (%)**	**Cause**	**Percentage of Total Deaths (%)**
Ischemic heart disease	16.1	Ischemic heart disease	15.8
Stroke	10.5	Stroke	11.7
COPD	5.9	Alzheimer's disease	6.5
Lower respiratory infections	4.4	COPD	5.5
Lung cancer	4.2	Lower respiratory infections	4.8
Neonatal disorders	3.3	Diarrheal diseases	3.3
Road injuries	3.1	Neonatal disorders	3.0
Cirrhosis	2.9	Diabetes mellitus	2.8
Alzheimer's disease	2.9	Breast cancer	2.4
Tuberculosis	2.5	Lung cancer	2.3

Note: Highlighted causes represent communicable causes.
Data from Institute for Health Metrics and Evaluation (IHME). (n.d.). GBD Compare: Viz Hub. Retrieved from https://vizhub.healthdata.org/gbd-compare/

TABLE 13-5 Deaths from Selected Communicable Diseases, as Percentage of Total Deaths, by World Bank Country Income Group and Globally, 2016

	Globally	Low-income countries	Lower middle-income countries	Upper middle-income countries	High-income countries
Lower Respiratory Infections	4.6	8.6	5.6	2.9	4.0
Diarrheal Diseases	2.3	6.9	5.3	0.3	0.3
Tuberculosis	2.2	5.6	3.8	0.5	0.1
HIV/AIDS	1.9	5.7	2.1	1.6	0.1
Malaria	1.1	6.5	1.4	<0.1	<0.1
Measles	0.2	0.9	0.3	<0.1	<0.1

Data from Institute for Health Metrics and Evaluation (IHME). GBD Compare: Viz Hub. Retrieved from https://vizhub.healthdata.org/gbd-compare/

sub-Saharan Africa, as is malaria. The neglected tropical diseases are also much more important in sub-Saharan Africa than in any other region.

The Costs and Consequences of Communicable Diseases

The economic and social costs of communicable diseases are very high. First, these diseases constrain the health and development of infants and children, often by having an impact on their schooling and on their productivity as adult workers. Second, stigma and discrimination against people with HIV, those with TB, and those with a variety of other debilitating communicable diseases, such as leprosy and lymphatic filariasis, are strong and pervasive. Third, adults who suffer from the diseases discussed in this chapter suffer substantial losses in productivity and income. Fourth, families spend considerable sums of money trying to treat these illnesses. Fifth, high rates of communicable diseases in any country reduce investments in that country's development. Finally, as noted earlier, emerging and re-emerging infectious diseases can have enormous economic consequences, far in excess of their impact on health.

The Leading Burdens of Communicable Diseases

The sections that follow examine emerging and re-emerging infectious diseases and antimicrobial resistance, HIV, TB, malaria, diarrhea, and neglected tropical diseases. The chapter reviews the nature and magnitude of each of these causes, as well as who is affected by them, their risk factors, their social and economic consequences, and what can be done to address these problems in cost-effective ways. The chapter also discusses future challenges in addressing the most important communicable diseases.

Emerging and Re-emerging Infectious Diseases and Antimicrobial Resistance

The Burden of Emerging and Re-emerging Infectious Diseases

Throughout human history, new diseases have appeared periodically, sometimes wreaking substantial damage. The first recorded epidemic of the bubonic plague, for example, was in the 6th century. More recently, new diseases have emerged, such as the Ebola virus in 1976, HIV in the 1980s, severe acute respiratory syndrome (SARS) in the 1990s, and H5N1 influenza, commonly called "bird flu," which first appeared in humans in 2003. These new diseases are referred to as emerging infectious diseases.[7,8] Some examples of emerging infectious diseases are shown in **TABLE 13-6**. It is important to note that some diseases, like those in the table, have infected only a limited number of people, while other diseases that have emerged, such as HIV, have infected tens of millions of people.

Even as new diseases have emerged, some existing diseases have spread more widely in areas in which they had already been present, have spread to places in which they had not appeared before, or have taken on new forms. These diseases are referred to as

TABLE 13-6 Selected Examples of Emerging Infectious Diseases

Year of Outbreak	Disease	Place
1967	Marburg	Germany and Yugoslavia
1976	Ebola	Zaire (Democratic Republic of Congo)
1993	Cryptosporidiosis	Milwaukee, United States
1993	Hantavirus	New Mexico, Arizona, Colorado, and Utah, United States
1996	Variant Creutzfeldt-Jakob disease (vCJD; mad cow disease)	United Kingdom

(continues)

TABLE 13-6 Selected Examples of Emerging Infectious Diseases		*(continued)*
Year of Outbreak	**Disease**	**Place**
1997	H5N1 (avian influenza)	Hong Kong, China
1999	Nipah virus	Malaysia and Singapore
2002	SARS	China
2012	Middle East Respiratory Syndrome (MERS)	Arabian Peninsula
2013	Chikungunya	St. Martin Island, Caribbean
2015	Zika virus	Brazil

Data from Multiple sources: Centers for Disease Control and Prevention (CDC). (2014). Known cases and outbreaks of Marburg hemorrhagic fever, in chronological order. Retrieved from http://www .cdc.gov/vhf/marburg/resources/outbreak-table.html

Centers for Disease Control and Prevention (CDC). (2018). Years of Ebola disease outbreaks. Retrieved from http://www.cdc.gov/vhf/ebola/outbreaks/history/chronology.html

MacKenzie, W., Hoxie, N., Proctor, M., Gradus, M. S., Blair, K. A., Peterson, D. E., . . . Rose, J. B. (2004). A massive outbreak in Milwaukee of cryptosporidium infection transmitted through the public water supply. *New England Journal of Medicine, 331*, 161–197.

Centers for Disease Control and Prevention (CDC). (2012). Hantavirus: History of HPS. Retrieved from http://www.cdc.gov/hantavirus/hps/history.html

Centers for Disease Control and Prevention (CDC). (2002). New variant CJD: Fact Sheet. Retrieved from http://www.cdc.gov/media/pressrel/fs020418.htm

World Health Organization (WHO). (2018). Influenza (Avian and other zoonotic). Retrieved from http://www.who.int/mediacentre/factsheets/avian_influenza/en/

Centers for Disease Control and Prevention (CDC). (2014). Nipah virus (NiV). Retrieved from http://www.cdc.gov/vhf/nipah/

Centers for Disease Control and Prevention (CDC). (2005). Frequently asked questions about SARS. Retrieved from http://www.cdc.gov/sars/about/faq.html

Centers for Disease Control and Prevention (CDC). (2017). Middle East Respiratory Syndrome (MERS). Retrieved from http://www.cdc.gov/coronavirus/MERS/about/index.html

Centers for Disease Control and Prevention (CDC). (2018). Chikungunya virus. Retrieved from https://www.cdc.gov/chikungunya/index.html

Centers for Disease Control and Prevention (CDC). (n.d.). Zika. Retrieved from https://wwwnc.cdc.gov/eid/spotlight/zika

re-emerging infectious diseases.[7,8] In recent years, there have been outbreaks of a number of re-emerging infectious diseases, including West Nile virus in the Western Hemisphere; dengue fever, which spread from South America to the Caribbean and into the United States; cholera in South America; and Ebola in West Africa. Some examples of re-emerging infectious diseases are given in **TABLE 13-7**.

Resistant forms of disease can emerge or re-emerge when bacteria, parasites, and viruses are altered through mutation, natural selection, or the exchange of genetic material among strains and species.[9] The development of resistance is a natural phenomenon; however, it can be sped up by human action, as discussed further later in this chapter. It can also develop and spread faster than would otherwise be the case because of human inaction—the failure to address it in timely and effective ways. It took only a few years after penicillin was introduced, for example, before strains of bacteria that were susceptible to penicillin had become resistant to it. The drug of choice for malaria for many years, chloroquine, can no longer be used in most places because the malaria there is resistant to it. **TABLE 13-8** shows when a sample of resistant strains of bacteria, viruses, and parasites were first detected.

Emerging and re-emerging infectious diseases and antimicrobial resistance are excellent examples of critical health issues that are truly global. They can arise anywhere and at any time. They can spread, sometimes rapidly, within and across countries. Different countries, with the help of various international organizations and networks, have to work together in technically sound ways, and sometimes urgently, if these issues are to be addressed effectively.

In fact, the threat of emerging and re-emerging infectious diseases is continuous and has been called "a perpetual challenge."[7] One study examined 335 events related to emerging and re-emerging infectious diseases that had occurred between 1940 and 2004.[10] This analysis revealed that about 60 percent of these events were related to zoonoses—the spread of infection from animals to humans. The study also indicated that most of those events came from wildlife, and that wildlife were related to an increasing share of emerging and re-emerging infections over time. About 23 percent were

TABLE 13-7 Selected Examples of Re-emerging Infectious Diseases

Year of Outbreak	Disease	Place
1994	Plague	India
1997	Cholera	Peru
1998	Rift Valley fever	Ethiopia
2003	Human monkeypox	Texas, United States
2009	Dengue	Florida, United States
2014	Ebola	West Africa
2015	Zika virus	Brazil
2016	Cholera	Yemen
2018	Ebola	Democratic Republic of the Congo

Data from Multiple sources: Centers for Disease Control and Prevention (CDC). (1994). International notes update: Human plague—India, 1994. *Morbidity and Mortality Weekly Report, 43*(41), 761–762. Retrieved from http://www.cdc.gov/mmwr/preview/mmwrhtml/00032992.htm
World Health Organization (WHO). (1998). 1998—Cholera in Peru. Retrieved from http://www.who.int/csr/don/1998_02_25/en/index.html
Food and Agriculture Organization of the United Nations. (2007, January 4). Flare-up of Rift Valley fever in the Horn of Africa. *FAONewsroom*. Retrieved from http://www.fao.org/newsroom/en /news/2007/1000473/index.html
Centers for Disease Control and Prevention (CDC). (2015). Monkeypox. Retrieved from http://www.cdc.gov/ncidod/monkeypox/qa.htm
Centers for Disease Control and Prevention (CDC). (2010). Locally acquired dengue—Key West, Florida, 2009–2010. Retrieved from http://www.cdc.gov/mmwr/preview/mmwrhtml/mm5919a1.htm
World Health Organization (WHO). (2018). Ebola virus disease fact sheet. Retrieved from http://www.who.int/mediacentre/factsheets/fs103/en/
World Health Organization (WHO). (2018). Zika virus. Retrieved from http://www.who.int/en/news-room/fact-sheets/detail/zika-virus
Centers for Disease Control and Prevention (CDC). (2017). Cholera in Yemen. Retrieved from https://wwwnc.cdc.gov/travel/notices/watch/cholera-yemen
Centers for Disease Control and Prevention (CDC). (2019). 2018 Eastern Democratic Republic of the Congo. Retrieved from https://www.cdc.gov/vhf/ebola/outbreaks/drc/2018-august.html

TABLE 13-8 Selected Examples of Drug Resistance, by Disease

Disease	Resistant Drug	Place	Description
HIV	Any first-line drug	United States	Primary resistance was 24.1% in 2003–2004.
		United Kingdom	Primary resistance was 19.2% in 2003.
Malaria	Chloroquine	Iran	Median failure rate in the presence of *P. falciparum* was 72.5% in 1996–2004.
		Ecuador	Median failure rate in the presence of *P. falciparum* was 85.4% in 1996–2004.
	Sulfadoxine-pyrimethamine	Philippines	Median failure rate in the presence of *P. falciparum* was 42.6% in 1996–2004.
		Myanmar	Median failure rate in the presence of *P. falciparum* was 27.8% in 1996–2004.

(continues)

TABLE 13-8 Selected Examples of Drug Resistance, by Disease (continued)

Disease	Resistant Drug	Place	Description
Multidrug-resistant tuberculosis (MDR-TB)	At least isoniazid and rifampicin	United States	In this outbreak in the early 1990s, 1 in 10 cases of TB was MDR-TB.
		Russia	16.3% of TB cases in Russia were MDR-TB in 2007–2008.
Methicillin-resistant Staphylococcus aureus (MRSA)	Beta-lactams (methicillin and other common antibiotics such as oxacillin, penicillin, and amoxicillin)	Colombia	Over 50% of S. aureus–infected individuals carried resistant strains in 2006.
		Japan	Over 50% of S. aureus–infected individuals carried resistant strains in 2006.
Pneumonia	Penicillin	Israel, Poland, Romania, Spain	Over 25% of S. pneumoniae isolates were resistant in 2002.
		France	Over 53% of S. pneumoniae isolates were resistant in 2002.
	Erythromycin	Vietnam	92% resistance rate in 2001.
		Taiwan	86% resistance rate in 2001.

Data from Nugent, R., Back, E., & Beith, A. (2010). Center for Global Development. *The race against drug resistance.* Retrieved from http://www.cgdev.org/content/publications /detail/1424207
Global Alliance for TB Drug Development. (n.d.). Drug-resistant TB. Retrieved from http://www.tballiance.org/why/mdr-tb.php
World Health Organization (WHO). (2010). Multidrug and extensively drug-resistant TB (M/XDR-TB): 2010 Global Report on Surveillance and Response. Retrieved from http: //www.who.int/tb /features_archive /world_tb_day_2010/en/index.html

related to vector-borne diseases that are spread by arthropods, such as mosquitoes, ticks, or fleas. The Global Outbreak Alert and Response Network (GOARN) verified 578 outbreaks in 132 countries that occurred just between 1998 and 2001.[11] The large share of these diseases that are zoonotic suggests the importance of taking a One Health approach to these diseases, as discussed further in a case study later in the chapter.

The problem of drug resistance is also substantial. It is estimated that in 2017 there were 558,000 cases of TB globally that were resistant to the most effective first-line drug, rifampicin. In addition, about 82 percent of these cases were multidrug resistant.[2] There is also resistance to all of the drugs that treat malaria. A study in Uganda showed that 100 percent of the samples of *Shigella*, a bacterium that causes diarrhea, were resistant to a drug that had been commonly used to treat it.[12] In addition, methicillin-resistant *Staphylococcus aureus*, commonly known as MRSA, which used to be of concern mainly in hospital settings, has now spread to the community in many countries. Indeed,

in 2014 WHO noted that antimicrobial resistance is a serious threat to global public health that threatens the gains of modern medicine and could even lead to a "post-antibiotic era."[13]

The U.S. Institute of Medicine (IOM) carried out important assessments of emerging and re-emerging infectious diseases in 1992 and 2003.[14] The IOM highlighted the most important factors that contribute to the emergence and re-emergence of infectious diseases, which are summarized in **TABLE 13-9**.

It is clear that changes in these factors and changes in their relationship with one another have been linked to the emergence and re-emergence of infectious diseases. Change in the environment and land use, for example, can have a major impact on disease emergence. This could include the well-known example of Lyme disease in the suburbs of the United States, as housing has pushed up against deer populations and deer ticks have spread Lyme disease to humans. The emergence of Ebola virus as populations have pushed up against tropical rain forests also shows the potential

TABLE 13-9 Key Factors Contributing to the Emergence and Re-emergence of Infectious Diseases

Microbial adaption and change
Human susceptibility to infection
Climate and weather
Changing ecosystems
Economic development and land use
Human demographics and behavior
Technology and industry
International travel and commerce
Breakdown of public health measures
Poverty and social inequality
War and famine
Lack of political will
Intent to harm

Data from Smolinski, M. I, Hamburg, M. A., & Lederberg, J. (Eds.). (2004). *Microbial threats to health* (pp. 4–7). Washington, DC: The National Academies Press.

impact of environmental change on the emergence of disease. The increasing amounts of travel and commerce in food and other goods also have the potential to spread communicable diseases more rapidly than ever. Improvements in technology may yield many benefits. Yet, they might also create the conditions for the emergence of disease, such as Legionnaire's disease in the cooling towers of air conditioners.[15]

The factors that contribute to the development of drug resistance are well known. They include the following[16,17]:

- The increasing use of antibiotics in some settings now and in the past
- Poor prescribing and dispensing practices
- Inappropriate use of the drugs by prescribers, dispensers, and patients
- Failure of patients to take appropriate doses of drugs
- The use of counterfeit or poor quality drugs that do not contain the appropriate level of therapeutic ingredients
- Too much use of antibiotics in agriculture, cattle and poultry raising, and fish farming
- Weak health systems, with poor laboratory capacity to diagnose disease and test for drug susceptibility

Some of the factors that might contribute to the more rapid spread of resistant forms of disease include the following[16,18,19]:

- Weak infection control in healthcare settings
- Poor sanitation and hygiene
- A lack of surveillance, leading to late detection of the disease

It is important to highlight that weaknesses in public health measures or breakdowns in public health services can also contribute in a number of ways to the emergence and re-emergence of infectious diseases, including the development and spread of drug resistance. During the Ebola outbreak in West Africa in 2014 and 2015, for example, already weak health systems were even less able to combat other communicable diseases such as malaria. In addition, from the end of World War II until the advent of HIV, there was an increasing sense in high-income countries that "infectious diseases had been conquered."[20] As a consequence, many countries scaled back their attention to such diseases, including TB. This reduction of attention to TB was associated, for example, with a resurgence of TB and drug-resistant TB in a number of settings, such as in New York City in the late 1980s.[20]

The Consequences of Emerging and Re-emerging Infectious Diseases

The costs of emerging and re-emerging diseases have varied considerably but have sometimes been very large, as shown in **TABLE 13-10**. In each of these cases, there were direct costs of caring for those affected, such as the costs of hospitalization. In addition, there were substantial indirect costs. The 1991 cholera epidemic in Peru, for example, led to a decline in people's social activities and their normal expenditures and had a major impact on the local economy. It also led to a substantial decline in tourism in a country in which this sector plays an important role. The plague in India in 1994 led to a significant short-term decline in trade and commerce between India and the rest of the world. The U.K. government had to kill livestock to eliminate the possibility of mad cow disease and to convince a world that would not eat beef from the United Kingdom that this beef would be safe in the future. SARS led to a worldwide fear of a pandemic and to major reductions in trade, travel, and commerce between parts of Asia and the rest of the world. SARS also had an impact on the economy of Canada, after travelers received a warning from WHO about the risk of SARS in that country.[8] The World Bank estimated that the Ebola outbreak in 2014 in West Africa could cause the economies of Guinea, Liberia, and Sierra Leone to grow by 2.1 percent, 3.4 percent, and 3.3 percent less, respectively, than they would have grown in the absence of Ebola.[21] One later estimate suggested that the combined economic and social costs of the outbreak were about $53 billion, an enormous amount for such small economies.[22]

TABLE 13-10 Selected Examples of the Economic Costs of Emerging and Re-emerging Infectious Diseases

Disease	Country/Region	Year(s)	Cost
Cholera epidemic	Peru	1991	$771 million
Plague	India	1994	$1.7 billion
Mad cow disease	United Kingdom	1990–1998	$30 billion
Anthrax	United States	2001	$1 billion
SARS	Asia	2003	$30 billion

Data from World Health Organization (WHO). (2007). *Infectious diseases across borders: The international health regulations*. Geneva, Switzerland: Author.

It is important to note that these costs are not in proportion to deaths from these events. Between 1990 and 1998, for example, only 41 people died in the United Kingdom of mad cow disease.[8] Although SARS generated great fears, only 774 deaths were caused by this disease.[23] By the time the Ebola outbreak in West Africa had ended, it had infected 28,600 people in Guinea, Liberia, and Sierra Leone and had killed 11,325 people.[24] It had also had extensive social and economic impacts. Clearly, a substantial number of deaths *are* associated with some outbreaks, especially the West Africa Ebola outbreak. Yet, in many regards, the economic costs of these events appear to be related to the fear of possible spread rather than the actual morbidity and mortality caused by the disease.

The costs and consequences of drug resistance are also very high. A recent WHO report suggested, for example, that the median cost among 30 countries of treating multidrug-resistant TB was almost six times as high as the cost of treating drug-susceptible TB.[25(p135)] The Centers for Disease Control and Prevention (CDC) estimated that the costs of treating a patient with drug-resistant TB in the United States, which has the highest healthcare costs in the world, was $513,000, almost 30 times greater than the cost of treating a drug-susceptible case.[26] The lowest cost of curing a patient of malaria with artemisinin-based combination therapy (ACT) is about 10 times the cost of curing a patient with chloroquine.[27] The cost of treating someone for certain infections with amoxicillin/clavulanic acid can be 25 to 60 times more expensive than treating them with penicillin. In addition, people are sicker longer and sometimes die from resistant strains of disease as health providers try to find drugs to which these diseases are susceptible. Moreover, the use of some drugs actually encourages the development of resistance to other drugs, making it harder to treat some conditions.[16]

Addressing Emerging and Re-emerging Infectious Diseases

In some respects, the development of emerging and re-emerging infectious diseases, including antimicrobial resistance, is inevitable, given that it partially arises as a result of natural processes. On the other hand, we do have control over some of the factors that drive the development of these diseases. In principle, for example, population pressure on the environment could be reduced and land use planning could limit destruction of animal habitats. In practice, however, these approaches will require substantial change in the way people live and will not occur unless incentives are in place and reasonable alternatives exist. There are also many ways we can more appropriately use drugs. The use of drugs can also be decreased when they are not needed.[10,28]

Thus, even as people work both within and across countries to change some of the structural factors that drive the emergence and re-emergence of infectious diseases, they can take more immediate actions to reduce these threats and the threat of antimicrobial resistance. Some measures to address these problems will have to be taken within nations, but others will require international action.

The foundation for strengthening the capacity to address emerging and re-emerging infectious diseases has to focus on "highly sensitive national surveillance systems, public health laboratories that can rapidly detect outbreaks caused by emerging and re-emerging infections, and mechanisms that permit timely containment."[8] This must also be coupled with the willingness of countries to share information about disease outbreaks in a timely manner with other countries. There is also a need for global coordination of these efforts.

Disease surveillance is based on GOARN, a network of existing disease surveillance networks established in 2000.[29] Those who participate in it include an array of technical institutions, networks, and organizations that can contribute information to the global network, such as United Nations agencies, the International Federation of Red Cross and Red Crescent Societies, and Doctors Without Borders. WHO coordinates the network, building on the resources of its participants.

WHO published an updated version of the International Health Regulations (IHR) in 2005.[29] The IHR laid out a framework that is intended to guide national and global efforts at strengthening surveillance capacity and the national and global capacity to respond to outbreaks. They make provisions for generating and reviewing information about disease outbreaks from a variety of sources, including both official sources and information from nonstate actors. This approach is meant to broaden the potential sources of information about outbreaks and overcome risks that would be posed by states that do not want to share information in a timely manner about disease outbreaks within their own country.

National action and global cooperation on disease surveillance and response were tested during an outbreak of H1N1 swine flu in Mexico in 2009, which was thought to pose a serious risk of becoming a global pandemic. In this case, the Mexican government did report the outbreak to WHO in a timely manner, there was a rapid global response coordinated by WHO, and a vaccine was developed quickly against this virus. However, when a pandemic did not come about, there was some criticism of WHO for exaggerating the risks that this outbreak posed.[30] Nonetheless, it appears that the response of Mexico in this case was considerably more helpful to the world than the long delay that China had in notifying the world about its SARS outbreak in 2003.

National and global capacity was also tested during the 2014 and 2015 Ebola outbreak in West Africa. In this case, Guinea, Liberia, and Sierra Leone were unable to respond adequately, given the weak governance and health systems in those countries. In addition, the international community appeared to respond very slowly and long after assistance should have first been provided. The reasons for this will continue to be examined, but the poor international response appears to have stemmed at least partly from budget and staff cuts to the appropriate units of WHO in Geneva and weaknesses in the Africa office of WHO.[31]

In 2014, in fact, the global community established a new program for cooperation to help address emerging and re-emerging infectious diseases more effectively, the Global Health Security Agenda. This organization aims to raise awareness about the threats of emerging and re-emerging diseases. It also aims to help countries strengthen their capacity to prevent, detect, and respond to these diseases. Thus far, 64 countries are participating in this program.[32]

In many ways, global efforts to address drug resistance have been inadequate. There has been some progress in addressing resistance on a disease-by-disease basis, such as efforts to better diagnose, track, and treat drug-resistant TB or drug-resistant malaria. There have also been countries, particularly in Europe, that have sought to reduce the use of antibiotics in both humans and animals. Nonetheless, the world has continued to fail to establish a well-coordinated mechanism that can work across countries and diseases to address, in a coherent, timely, and effective manner, the factors that drive the development of drug resistance.[16] Some believe that this is a critical failure that places the world at grave risk of additional threats from resistant forms of disease and a real risk of running out of antibiotics and other drugs that can effectively address such diseases.

The Center for Global Development in Washington, DC, convened a Drug Resistance Working Group from 2007 to 2010. The final report of the group made a number of recommendations about how the world might more forcefully move against drug resistance. These are shown in **TABLE 13-11**.

WHO prepared a major report on antimicrobial resistance that was published in 2012.[33] WHO proposed that, to better combat antimicrobial resistance, countries should adopt a policy package that would include the following elements[34]:

- A comprehensive national plan that would be financed, that would engage civil society, and for which the government would be accountable
- Improved surveillance and laboratory capacity
- Uninterrupted access to essential medicines of assured quality
- The regulation and promotion of rational use of medicines, including in animal husbandry

TABLE 13-11 Key Recommendations from the Center for Global Development Drug Resistance Working Group on Addressing Drug Resistance

- Improve surveillance by collecting and sharing resistance information across networks of laboratories.
- Establish an expert technical working group to develop, maintain, and monitor global standards for postmarketing drug quality and ensure that publicly funded drug procurement requires adherence to this standard.
- Create a new partnership of associations of medicine providers, regulators, and others involved in the drug supply chain to promote quality-assured provision of drugs, with accreditation of suppliers and better information to consumers.
- Strengthen national drug regulatory authorities in low- and middle-income countries.
- Catalyze research and development of resistance-fighting technologies by creating a web-based marketplace for the sharing of research in this area.

Data from Nugent, R., Beck, E., & Beith, A. (2010). *The race against drug resistance*. Washington, DC: Center for Global Development.

- Improved infection control
- The fostering of innovation in the fight against resistance

The Lancet also established an infectious disease commission, which issued in 2013 a major study of antimicrobial resistance. The commission suggested a plan of action against drug resistance that included the following[35]:

- Studies of the economic burdens of drug resistance
- A global surveillance system for resistance
- Better regulation and stricter monitoring of prescribing practices for antibiotics
- Enhanced education of the public of the dangers of overprescribing antibiotics
- The phaseout of the use of antibiotics for animal husbandry
- The development of new models for research and development on antibiotics
- Improved governance of antibiotics, both nationally and globally

Most recently, in 2015, WHO published a Global Action Plan on Antimicrobial Resistance.[36] The plan aims to raise awareness of the problem, strengthen the evidence base for action, reduce the incidence of infection, optimize the use of antimicrobials in human and animal health, and develop the economic case for action against antimicrobial resistance. The plan lays out a range of actions that can be taken by member states of WHO, the WHO secretariat, and international partners. The 2018 WHO surveillance report on antibiotic use, however, reports continuing insufficient progress in meeting some of the key the aims of the plan.[37]

Future Challenges

An important question concerns the extent to which diseases are emerging and re-emerging more rapidly than before, given the pace of changes in our environment and the increasing globalization of travel, trade, and transport. A detailed analysis of this question concluded that between 1940 and 2004, the number of occurrences of emerging and re-emerging infectious diseases did increase over time and peaked in the 1980s, probably in association with the spread of HIV.[7,10] However, a recent study by the World Economic Forum suggested that local outbreaks that are highly disruptive are occurring more frequently and could cost the global economy as much as 0.7 percent of global GDP annually.[38]

Indeed, the factors that contribute to the emergence and re-emergence of infectious diseases are becoming more prominent in some places. Infectious disease specialists predict that in the face of rapidly evolving and adapting pathogens, continued population growth, popular encroachment into areas with forests and wildlife, and climate change, new diseases will emerge and already known diseases will re-emerge at an increasing pace.[39,40]

In addition, these tendencies will be exacerbated by poverty, environmental degradation, war, or the lack of effective public health interventions. Public health specialists also believe that the world must be vigilant about the possibility that a major pandemic could arise from a newly emerging or re-emerging infectious disease. This could be the case, for example, with H5N1 influenza if that virus developed the ability to spread more efficiently from human to human.[10,20,28]

When considering measures to address emerging and re-emerging infectious diseases, it is critical to remember that, for diseases that spread from human to human, there may be only a limited window for action after an outbreak begins if a pandemic is to be averted.[8] There is also a growing concern about the potential impact of the recent economic and political trends in the United States and Europe on the ability or willingness of governments to fund critical public health services. This is despite the fact that the potential economic consequences of possible disease outbreaks should make them more willing, rather than less willing, to address such threats during times that are already economically distressed.

The development of drug resistance is also accelerating and spreading to places where it has not been prevalent before.[17] This stems partly from the growing use of antibiotics in low- and middle-income countries, as some of them have witnessed significant economic growth and increasing levels of education. It also reflects, however, that this increasing use is taking place in environments in which the other drivers of resistance have not yet been managed effectively.[16]

Of course, once drug-resistant forms of bacteria, viruses, or parasites do develop, they can spread more easily than ever, given the extent to which people travel, for example.[19] In addition, the behaviors in which people engage can also have an important bearing on the spread of resistant forms of microbes, such as people's failure to adhere to drug regimens or their use of poor quality drugs.

The problem of drug resistance is also compounded by the limited number of new anti-infective drugs that are under development and the speed with which even new drugs become subject to resistance.[16] In addition, there has been insufficient research and development for drugs to combat some of the most important burdens of disease for the poor in low- and middle-income countries, including those for which there is increasing resistance. Until recently, for example, almost all of the existing TB drugs were at least 40 years old. WHO, among others, has recently sought to encourage investment in new antibiotics by establishing a working group on "high priority pathogens." This group suggested that special attention be given to developing antibiotics to fight multidrug-resistant TB, **gram-negative bacteria**, and the agents responsible for resistant strains of salmonella, campylobacter, gonorrhea, and *H. pylori*.[41]

A final note should be added about **pandemic preparedness**, which refers to the ability to effectively deal with a global outbreak of disease. The 1918 flu epidemic infected over 500 million people worldwide and killed more than 50 million people.[42] There have also been additional pandemic influenza outbreaks

since then, in 1957–1958, 1968, and 2009, without the dramatic impact on morbidity and mortality of the 1918 pandemic.[43] WHO has suggested that the likelihood of another influenza pandemic is one of the 10 greatest health threats facing the global community.[44]

An important question, therefore, is the extent to which individual countries and the global community as a whole are "ready" to identify and respond to the emergence of a pandemic influenza, or other pandemic pathogen. On the one hand, important measures have been taken to carry out this work. These include the promulgation of the International Health Regulations, referred to earlier, as well as the development of global mechanisms to carry out surveillance and reporting and ensure adequate supplies globally of diagnostics, vaccines, and therapeutics. A number of countries have also taken measures to be prepared to address the development of a pandemic. On the other hand, there appears to be widespread agreement among those who have studied pandemic preparedness carefully that there are major gaps in such preparedness and that many countries and the world as a whole are *not* adequately prepared to detect, prevent, or respond to a major global emergency.[38,45,46]

HIV/AIDS

The Burden of HIV/AIDS

Rarely has a single pathogen had a greater impact on the human condition than HIV. Some of the basic facts about HIV/AIDS are presented in **TABLE 13-12**. HIV is a virus that can be spread through several ways:

- Unprotected sex, primarily vaginal and anal intercourse
- Mother-to-child transmission, during birth, or through breastfeeding
- Blood, including by transfusion, needle sharing, or accidental needle stick
- Transplantation of infected tissue or organs

Being an uncircumcised male increases the risk of acquiring HIV. Females are also at greater biological and social risk than males of being infected with HIV. Having a sexually transmitted disease also increases the risk of HIV infection.

The efficiency with which the virus is transmitted varies. The virus is spread most efficiently from exposure to infected blood products and through the sharing of infected needles. There is a 90 percent probability of being infected by a transfusion of blood from an HIV-positive person.[47] The efficiency of transmission is also relatively high from sharing needles with an HIV-infected person. Sexual transmission depends

TABLE 13-12 HIV/AIDS Basic Facts: 2017

Number of people living with HIV/AIDS: 36.9 million

Number of new HIV infections: 1.8 million

Prevalence among adults ages 15–49: 0.8%

Children under 15 newly infected with HIV: 180,000

Global distribution of new infections:
   Eastern and southern Africa: 19.6 million
   Asia and the Pacific: 5.2 million
   Western and central Africa: 6.1 million
   Latin America: 1.8 million
   The Caribbean: 310,000
   Middle East and North Africa: 220,000
   Eastern Europe and central Asia: 1.4 million
   Western and central Europe and North America: 2.2 million

Number of HIV-related deaths: 940,000

Number of HIV-positive people being treated with antiretroviral therapy (ART): 21.7 million

Proportion of all adults living with HIV receiving ART: 59%

Proportion of all children living with HIV receiving ART: 52%

Proportion of pregnant women living with HIV who have access to ART: 80%

Fast Track Targets for 2020:
- Fewer than 500,000 people newly infected with HIV per year globally—a 75% reduction across all populations compared with 2010, with particular emphasis on men who have sex with men, transgender people, sex workers, people who inject drugs, prisoners, and adolescent girls and young women in certain high-burden settings.
- Ensure 90% of people living with HIV know their HIV status, 90% of people who know their HIV status are receiving antiretroviral therapy, and 90% of people on treatment have a suppressed viral load.
- Everyone, everywhere, living a life free from HIV-related discrimination. Achieve and sustain the elimination of new HIV infections among children.

Data from UNAIDS. (2015, June). *Understanding Fast-Track: Accelerating action to end the AIDS epidemic by 2030.* Geneva, Switzerland: Author. Retrieved from http://www.unaids.org/sites/default/files/media_asset/201506_JC2743_Understanding_FastTrack_en.pdf; UNAIDS. (2018). Global HIV & AIDS statistics: 2018 fact sheet. Retrieved from http://www.unaids.org/en/resources/fact-sheet

on the type of sexual act and whether the HIV-positive person is male or female. Male-to-female transmission is higher than female-to-male transmission. The risk of unprotected receptive anal intercourse is about 30 times greater than it is for receptive or insertive vaginal intercourse.[47]

HIV attacks the human immune system. The time from becoming infected until one is diagnosed with AIDS varies. However, without treatment for HIV, about half of those infected will be diagnosed with AIDS in 10 years. The extent to which the virus can be transmitted is high during the initial period of infection and also increases as the immune system weakens. It is also heightened in the presence of other sexually transmitted infections.[48]

As the immune system of an HIV-positive person deteriorates, that person, if untreated, will suffer from a variety of what are called opportunistic infections, because they take advantage of the person's compromised immunity. As their disease reaches a fairly advanced state, HIV-positive people who are not on antiretroviral therapy may fall ill with TB, herpes infections, a variety of cancers, and an array of significant communicable diseases such as toxoplasmosis and cryptococcal meningitis, which has become a major killer of those infected with HIV.[49]

The main routes of transmission of HIV vary by location. In the first phases of the epidemic in high-income countries and in Brazil, HIV was largely spread through unprotected sex among men who have sex with men. In sub-Saharan Africa, the disease has been spread overwhelmingly through unprotected sex between men and women, especially among those engaging in high-risk behaviors, such as sex workers and their clients and men engaging in sex with multiple female partners. In China, one center of the HIV epidemic was in a group of people who received transfusions from blood that had been infected with the blood of HIV-positive people. From there, it spread largely through sex between men and women but also through injecting drug use. In Russia and much of the former Soviet Union, the epidemic is driven by injecting drug users who are HIV-positive and who share needles. The epidemic is spreading from them to other groups largely through unprotected sex.

When HIV first appears in a population, it is generally concentrated in certain key populations, such as sex workers, men who have sex with men, and injecting drug users. These groups were earlier referred to as "groups engaging in high-risk behaviors," "high-risk groups," or "most at risk populations." If the virus is controlled in these groups, then the spread to the general population can be limited. However, if it is not controlled, then the epidemic becomes more widespread in the general population and prevalence can be quite high. The Cambodian epidemic was concentrated largely among sex workers and their clients. South Africa and Zimbabwe, by contrast, have epidemics that have broadly spread in the population.

It is estimated that about 77 million people have been infected with HIV since the start of the epidemic, and about 35 million people have died AIDS-related deaths since then. It was estimated that about 37 million people worldwide were infected with the HIV virus in 2017, of whom about 35 million were adults and 1.8 million were children under 15 years of age. AIDS-related deaths have declined by 51 percent since the peak of the epidemic. Still, about 940,000 million people suffered AIDS-related deaths in 2017.[47]

It is also estimated that about 1.8 million people were newly infected with HIV in 2017, of which about 1.62 million were adults and 180,000 were children under 15 years of age. In sub-Saharan Africa, 75 percent of new infections in people aged 15 to 24 years are in women, and women in sub-Saharan Africa are twice as likely as men to be living with HIV.[47]

The prevalence of HIV varies considerably by region and by country. The prevalence rate of HIV by country is shown in **FIGURE 13-1**.

The region with the highest prevalence rate of HIV/AIDS is sub-Saharan Africa, where about 4.7 percent of the adults 15 to 49 years of age were estimated to be HIV-positive in 2017. The Caribbean is also significantly impacted by HIV, with a prevalence

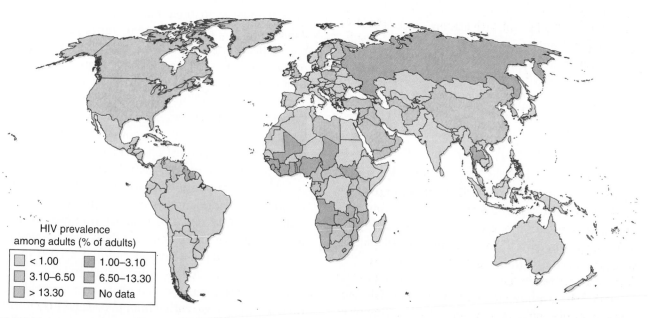

HIV prevalence among adults (% of adults)

- < 1.00
- 1.00–3.10
- 3.10–6.50
- 6.50–13.30
- > 13.30
- No data

FIGURE 13-1 HIV Prevalence by Country, 2017

Data from The World Bank (n.d.). Data: Prevalence of HIV, total (% of population ages 15–49). Retrieved from https://data.worldbank.org/indicator/SH.DYN.AIDS.ZS?view=map

rate of about 1.6 percent. The rate in Europe and Central Asia was about 0.7 percent.[50]

Eswatini, formerly known as Swaziland, had the highest HIV/AIDS prevalence rate in 2017, at 27.4 percent. The next highest rates were found in Lesotho, 23.8 percent; Botswana, at 22.8 percent; and South Africa, at 18.8 percent. Only three other countries have rates of prevalence over 10 percent, including Mozambique, Zambia, and Zimbabwe.[50]

Most WHO regions have seen a decline in the number of new cases of HIV diagnosed relative to the number diagnosed in 2000. However, the European, Eastern Mediterranean, and Western Pacific have seen increases in the number of new diagnoses, compared to 2000. The Eastern Mediterranean region is the only WHO region that has seen an increase in deaths in 2017, compared to the number of AIDS-related deaths in 2000.[51]

Thirty-seven percent of new HIV infections in adults over 15 years of age in 2017 were among those ages 15 to 24. Of those, about 58 percent were in females and 42 percent in males. About 180,000 of those newly infected were among those 0 to 14 years of age, as noted earlier. This is a substantial decline from the 420,000 children 0 to 14 years of age who were newly infected in 2000 and 2001.[52] This decline reflects the progress made globally in reducing maternal-to-child transmission.

The Global Burden of Disease Study 2016 indicated that HIV/AIDS was the 14th leading cause of death for all age groups globally, but the leading cause globally for those aged 15 to 49 years. It was the second leading cause in sub-Saharan Africa among all age groups, but the leading cause for those 15 to 49 years. HIV/AIDS was the 11th leading cause of DALYs globally for all age groups and the third leading cause for sub-Saharan Africa. For the 15- to 49-year-old age group, HIV/AIDS was the second leading cause of DALYs globally and the leading cause in sub-Saharan Africa.[1]

HIV Treatment

There has been enormous progress globally in providing antiretroviral therapy to those who are HIV-positive. Earlier WHO guidelines helped countries to ration drugs that were expensive and inadequate in number. Those guidelines recommended placing people on antiretroviral therapy only when their **CD 4 cell count** fell below a certain number, revised to 500 in 2013.[53] Today, however, there is a universal commitment to placing people on antiretroviral therapy as soon as they are diagnosed, which is known to produce the best possible outcomes. In addition, there is

a global commitment to the following goals for those who are HIV-positive:

- 90 percent of those with HIV are aware of their status.
- 90 percent of those who have been diagnosed are placed on antiretroviral therapy.
- 90 percent of those on therapy have an undetectable **viral load**.[54]

Meeting these targets is central to the global plan to reduce new HIV infections to 500,000 in 2020 and 200,000 in 2030.[54] UNAIDS estimated that in 2017, 75 percent of HIV-positive people knew their status, 79 percent of them were on antiretroviral therapy, and 81 percent of them had a suppressed viral load.[52]

The Costs and Consequences of HIV

HIV has significant social and economic consequences, especially in high-prevalence countries in sub-Saharan Africa, which go beyond its impact on morbidity and mortality. HIV affects family cohesion, business, trade, labor, the armed forces, agricultural production, education systems, governance, public services, and even national security.

In the absence of treatment, a person infected with HIV will eventually become sicker, progress to full-blown AIDS, and suffer from a variety of opportunistic infections, as noted previously. As this happens, the person becomes less able to work, loses part or all of his or her income, and becomes dependent on others for care. The caretaker may also lose his or her income.

This cycle has caused enormous economic losses to individuals and their families, especially in sub-Saharan Africa. A study done in Tanzania, for example, indicated that men with AIDS lost an average of 297 days of work over an 18-month period, and women lost an average of 429 days of work over that same period, which implies that these women were essentially unable to attend to any of their normal tasks.[55] A study in Thailand showed that families that suffered from AIDS lost an average of 48 percent of their income as a result of their illness.[56]

Another important consequence of HIV is the creation of a large number of orphans, defined as an individual 15 years old or younger who has lost one or both parents to the disease. UNICEF estimated in 2015 that about 13.4 million children aged 0 to 17 years of age were "AIDS orphans."[57] Despite efforts by many families to care for their relatives, many orphans do not have anyone with whom to live and may resort to living on the street, where they are at risk of falling into commercial sex or crime.

Like a number of other communicable diseases, HIV is a highly stigmatized condition. HIV, however, has a special stigma because people in many societies believe that people acquire HIV by engaging in behaviors that society does not sanction, such as men having sex with men, commercial sex work, or injecting drug use. Understanding the notion of stigma and discrimination against people with HIV/AIDS is central to understanding the epidemic.

In fact, over the course of the epidemic, stigmatization of HIV/AIDS in many societies has led to an unwillingness to allow people with HIV to attend schools or be employed, get health care, live in certain places, or even live with their families. Stigma has also been a major constraint to people getting tested or treated for HIV. It has also complicated prevention efforts in some settings by driving underground some of the very people it is important to reach, such as sex workers and injecting drug users.

There has been enormous progress in making antiretroviral therapy widely available and at much cheaper prices. Today, the annual cost of therapy for first-line drugs is below $100 for low-income countries.[58] Although these costs are dramatically lower than before, the lowest-income countries that are providing antiretroviral therapy to people living with HIV spend less per capita on health each year than the costs of HIV treatment.[59] Thus, it will be difficult for low-income countries with high HIV prevalence to support the costs of such treatment without considerable and sustained external assistance.[60]

Many studies have been done on the potential impact of HIV on the economic growth of different countries. Some of these have helped convince governments that failure to address HIV early could result in lower economic growth of their country. Overall, the early studies suggested that HIV would have a large impact on the economic growth of high-prevalence countries in Africa, largely because HIV tends to strike people in their most productive years.[55] The higher the prevalence and the more families use their savings to help pay for the costs of illness, the more likely HIV will have a negative impact on the growth of per capita income.[61] Although these arguments make sense intuitively, there are very few recent studies that have tried to examine how rates of economic growth for different countries would have changed if they had lower rates of prevalence of HIV/AIDS.

Addressing the Burden of HIV/AIDS

Despite considerable efforts, there is not yet either a preventive or therapeutic vaccine for HIV. In the absence of such a vaccine, halting the spread of HIV will have to focus on the prevention of new infections.

Several countries had earlier prevention efforts that were considered successful, such as Cambodia, Thailand, and Uganda. A case study of Thailand appears later in this chapter. Studies of the success of HIV/AIDS programs suggest that such successes have consistently been associated with a number of factors related to strong political leadership, commitment, and open communications[48]:

- Sustained political leadership at the highest levels
- Involvement of a broad range of civil society efforts to address HIV/AIDS, including opinion leaders and religious leaders
- Broad-based programs to change social norms in the population
- Open communication about HIV/AIDS and related sexual matters
- Programs to reduce stigma and discrimination

In addition, we also know that to be successful, efforts to address HIV/AIDS need to include the following[47]:

- Good epidemic surveillance
- Information, education, and communication
- Voluntary counseling and testing
- Condom promotion
- Screening and treatment for sexually transmitted infections
- Prevention of mother-to-child transmission through antiretroviral treatment and avoiding pregnancy
- Voluntary male medical circumcision
- Interventions that target populations that transmit the virus from high-risk to low-risk populations
- Prevention of bloodborne transmission through blood safety, harm reduction for injecting drug users, and universal precautions in healthcare settings

In addition, these efforts should be linked with pre-exposure prophylaxis in selected populations. They should also be linked with efforts, as noted earlier, to ensure by 2020 the following[62]:

- 90 percent of the people with HIV will know their HIV status.
- 90 percent of those with HIV will be receiving antiretroviral therapy.
- 90 percent of those being treated will have suppressed viral loads.

At the same time, countries need to continue to address stigma and discrimination against HIV-affected people.

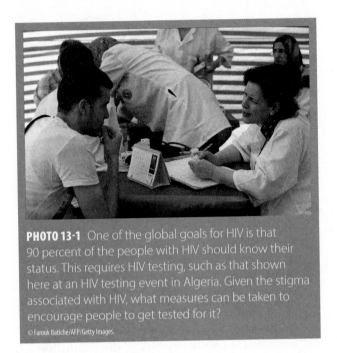

PHOTO 13-1 One of the global goals for HIV is that 90 percent of the people with HIV should know their status. This requires HIV testing, such as that shown here at an HIV testing event in Algeria. Given the stigma associated with HIV, what measures can be taken to encourage people to get tested for it?
© Farouk Batiche/AFP/Getty Images.

Additional comments follow on some of the interventions noted previously.

First, the approach to prevention will need to vary with the nature of the epidemic. In low-level epidemics, some of the focus can be on changing the behaviors of key populations. The approach to prevention in a more generalized epidemic, however, will need to be broader.[49] Unfortunately, many countries have failed to align their investments in addressing HIV with the nature of their epidemics. In Asia, for example, 90 percent of the funds spent on youth were initially spent on low-risk youth, who made up only 5 percent of the new infections.[63]

Second, there is an increasing understanding that prevention efforts have to include a combination of approaches, what is called "combination prevention,"[64] with different weight given to different activities, depending on the nature of the epidemic. These efforts will have to combine three different types of approaches: biomedical, behavioral, and structural. **Biomedical** refers to approaches such as male medical circumcision, the treatment of other sexually transmitted infections, and antiretroviral therapy. **Behavioral** refers to efforts to change people's behavior so they have less risk of becoming infected with HIV. **Structural** refers to societal elements that may predispose a person to the risk of HIV. In this case, for example, adolescent girls who are poor may engage in "transactional sex" in exchange for financial help, in order to support themselves, their schooling, or their families. Yet, if mechanisms can be put in place that can assist the girls in raising the funds needed for these matters, one might be able to reduce transactional

sex, and thereby reduce the number of those infected with HIV.

Education and behavior change efforts must focus on increasing correct knowledge of HIV, increasing the demand for HIV testing, later sexual debut, fewer sexual partners, and correct and consistent condom usage when engaging in high-risk sex. These activities are especially important in key populations, including sex workers and their clients and men who have sex with men.

These behavior change interventions need to be accompanied by efforts at harm reduction for injecting drug users. These are efforts to encourage the use of clean needles among injecting drug users, through needle exchange programs. They also include opioid substitution therapy to try to wean people who use heroin off the drug.

There has also been increasing attention paid to trying to stem mother-to-child transmission of HIV. The most cost-effective measure to reduce mother-to-child transmission of HIV is to avoid unwanted pregnancies of HIV-positive women through contraception. Providing antiretroviral therapy to pregnant women infected with HIV is also cost-effective.[65] If done properly, it can essentially eliminate mother-to-child transmission, whereas in the absence of such treatment, about one-third of HIV-positive pregnant women will give birth to a baby who is HIV-positive.[66]

There is evidence that circumcised males are 40 percent to 60 percent less likely to be infected with HIV than uncircumcised males.[67] A number of voluntary medical male circumcision efforts are now under way as a component of HIV/AIDS prevention activities. Kenya has made important progress in this area, and it will be important to learn from this and other experiences about the most cost-effective approaches to scaling up voluntary male medical circumcision in different settings.[68]

Ensuring that the blood supply is safe and free of the HIV virus, among other infectious agents, is cost-effective and must be a high priority in all settings.

As noted earlier, there has been substantial progress in low- and middle-income countries in placing HIV-infected people on antiretroviral therapy. This is important not only to ensure better health of the HIV-affected person but also to suppress their viral load so that they do not transmit HIV to others. Once patients are under treatment, it is exceptionally important that they take all of their drugs exactly as prescribed in order to avoid developing resistance and to stay as healthy as possible. If the drugs are discontinued because of interrupted supply, poor compliance by the patient, or poor performance of the health system, resistance may develop and the patient may require more expensive second-line drugs. Those infected with drug-resistant strains of HIV can also infect other people with those strains.

Overall, effective HIV/AIDS therapy depends on individuals accessing counseling and testing, a definitive HIV test, a clinical diagnosis of the patient, a laboratory assessment of the individual's immune status with a viral load test, patient adherence to their drug regimen, sound patient nutrition, and sound and continuous monitoring and evaluation of the patient.

A 2015 *Lancet* commission carried out a comprehensive review of the epidemic and what could be done to advance the meeting of global targets on HIV. In addition to the points previously noted, the commission highlighted the need to do the following[69]:

- Put more focus on prevention
- Take measures to address human rights concerns that relate to HIV and that can reduce stigma and discrimination
- Fully fund measures needed to address HIV
- Improve data, transparency, and accountability for HIV efforts
- Invest in needed research and development
- Promote more inclusive governance of HIV and global health efforts

DCP3 recently outlined an "essential package" of actions on a range of communicable diseases. **TABLE 13-13** portrays what DCP3 has recommended for an essential package for HIV/AIDS for low- and middle-income countries.

Critical Challenges in HIV/AIDS

A number of critical challenges constrain the fight against HIV/AIDS. First has been the difficulty of finding an HIV vaccine. Given the fact that there are about 1.6 million new infections a year, it is important to continue the search for a vaccine.[70] The search for a safe and effective **microbicide** must also continue.[71]

Second, although there has been a reduction in HIV incidence globally, the number of new infections annually suggests that it is essential that greater attention be paid to the prevention of such infections. More countries need to focus on prevention, with the political leadership and commitment that has been linked to the HIV success stories to date. We also need to ensure that countries invest in the most cost-effective approaches to combination prevention in their setting. As long as pregnant women continue to be infected, it is important to continue to scale up prevention of mother-to-child transmission. Greater attention must

also be paid to the reduction of stigma among the most stigmatized groups, including men who have sex with men and injecting drug users.

The efforts to offer universal antiretroviral treatment for those eligible will continue. However, this work will confront weak health systems and a lack of trained health workers as it expands further. Successful early treatment of HIV reduces the patient's viral load to an imperceptible level, stems the transmission of HIV, and reduces the likelihood that the patient will contract a number of opportunistic infections, such as TB. Thus, it will be important to diagnose people as early as possible after they are infected, place them on treatment as early in their infection as possible, and ensure that their treatment is effective. This is part of a strategy that is increasingly thought of as treatment as prevention and part of the 90-90-90 goals noted earlier.[62]

Financing treatment, especially in low-income, high-prevalence countries in which there continues to be a substantial number of new infections, will be very difficult and require sustained external support for many years. This highlights the need to continue at every level to reduce the price of antiretroviral therapy as far as possible both for first-line and second-line treatment regimens.

Improving the management of TB and HIV co-infection will also be essential. This is discussed further in the section on TB that follows.

Tuberculosis

The Burden of Tuberculosis

Some of the basic facts concerning TB are noted in **TABLE 13-14**.

Most tuberculosis is caused by the bacteria *Mycobacterium tuberculosis*, which is spread through aerosol droplets. People breathe in the TB bacteria that is transmitted from other people who are ill with tuberculosis disease. Tuberculosis can affect all organs of the body, but in about 80 percent of cases the infection is in the lungs.[2,72]

However, zoonotic TB is another form of tuberculosis that affects humans. It is caused by *Mycobacterium bovis*, which is generally found in cattle (bovine TB) but can also be found in other animals. Most commonly, it is transmitted from infected food products, such as unpasteurized dairy products. This form of TB is often extrapulmonary and may be difficult to diagnose. This type of TB is also naturally resistant to one of the first-line drugs for *Mycobacterium tuberculosis*, making it harder to treat than that bacterium.[73] Most comments below refer to *Mycobacterium tuberculosis*

TABLE 13-13 Essential HIV/AIDS Intervention Package, by Delivery Platform

Intervention type	Delivery Platforms				
	Nationwide policies and regulations	Community health post or pharmacy	Primary health center	First-level hospital	Second- and third-level hospitals
Prevention					
Legal and human rights	Laws and policies to protect and reduce stigma for key populations	Gender-based violence counseling and rape-response referral (medical and justice)			
Structural interventions	Universal access to HIV testing, with immediate linkage to care and treatment and intensified outreach to populations at higher risk of infection				
	Universal access to drug substitution therapy for addiction				
	Brothels: Condoms required				
	Needle exchange encouraged				
Direct (biological) prevention			Pre-exposure prophylaxis for discordant couples		
			Male circumcision service provision		
			Prevention of mother-to-child transmission (Option B+: a three-drug ART regimen for HIV-positive pregnant and postpartum mothers)		
Behavioral interventions: Prevention		HIV education and counseling for pregnant women, sex workers, injection drug users (IDUs), gay, bisexual, and transgender (GBT) males, and HIV+ persons and their partners			

Category			
Social marketing: Information, education, and communication	Promotion of condoms, voluntary male medical circumcision, and testing at national facility	Access to needle exchange for injection drug users	
		Condom distribution	
		Partner notification	
Treatment			
Treatment	Policies and guidelines to support all steps of HIV care continuum, including expanded testing through diverse strategies, linkage to care, ART initiation with support for adherence and retention, and performance and efficiency optimization through data-driven management, task shifting, and decentralization, as appropriate for level of epidemic	Community-based HIV testing and counseling (for example, through mobile units or venue-based testing	Provider-initiated counseling and HIV testing (as well as TB and sexually transmitted infections [STI] testing) for all in contact with healthcare system in high-prevalence settings, including prenatal care
		Household HIV testing and counseling in high-prevalence settings	ART initiation
		Referral and navigation of HIV+ individuals to HIV care sites to ensure linkage	Support for adherence and retention
			Laboratory viral load monitoring
Behavioral and structural interventions: Care		Adherence support including adherence clubs, community-based ART groups, text reminders, and other means	Case manager
		Nutrition, transportation, and other reimbursement	

Adapted from Holmes, K. K., Bertozzi, S., Bloom, B. R., Jha, P., Gelband, H., DeMaria, L. M., & Horton, S. (2017). Major infectious diseases: Key messages from *Disease Control Priorities*. In *Disease control priorities* (Vol. 6). Washington, DC: The World Bank.

TABLE 13-14 TB Basic Facts: 2017

Number of new TB cases: 10 million

Number of new TB cases among people living with HIV: 465,000

Number of TB deaths: 1.6 million

Number of new cases resistant to rifampicin (the most effective first-line drug): 558,000

Proportion of rifampicin-resistant TB cases that were also multidrug resistant: 82%

Incidence rate by WHO region (per 100,000 population): African Region (237), Region of the Americas (28), Eastern Mediterranean Region (113), European Region (30), South-East Asia Region (226), Western Pacific Region (94), Global (133)

Eight countries accounted for 66% of all cases: India, China, Indonesia, the Philippines, Pakistan, Nigeria, Bangladesh, and South Africa

Targets of the End TB Strategy: By 2035, reduce the number of TB deaths by 95% compared to 2015 levels and reduce the TB incidence rate by 90% (to 20 TB cases per 100,000 population)

Modified from World Health Organization (WHO). (2018). *Global tuberculosis report 2018*. Retrieved from https://www.who.int/tb/publications/global_report/en/

but some comments on the burden of zoonotic TB will also be provided.

To get TB (*Mycobacterium tuberculosis*), one has to be exposed to someone with the disease. The likelihood of exposure is greater if you are living with people with active pulmonary TB, especially in crowded circumstances, such as slum dwellings or prisons. Homeless people are also more susceptible to becoming ill with TB. Indeed, TB is generally thought of as a "disease of poverty" and one that has very strong links with the social determinants of health, including low income, low levels of education, a poor living environment, and food insecurity.

An untreated person with active pulmonary TB can infect 10 to 15 people annually. About two-thirds of those with active TB disease will die of the disease if not treated properly. Pulmonary TB can be spread from person to person, but people with TB in other organs (extrapulmonary TB) generally do not spread TB. Active TB disease is characterized by a persistent cough for more than 3 weeks, decreased appetite, general weakness, and profuse night sweats.[2,72]

Not everyone infected with TB bacteria becomes sick with it. Rather, TB remains latent in the bodies of about 90 percent of those infected, and they will not develop active TB disease. People with latent TB do not spread TB to others. About one-third of the world's population is thought to be infected with TB.

It is estimated that the infection will break down to cause active TB in about 10 percent of those people, especially if the person is immune-compromised.[2] This could occur because of malnutrition, HIV infection, use of immune-suppressing drugs, illness such as diabetes, or some cancers. Smoking and alcohol use are also risk factors for TB.[2,74]

The estimated effect of some of these conditions on the risk of a person with latent TB developing active TB disease is noted here[75]:

- *HIV:* People who are HIV-positive are 26 to 31 times more likely to get TB than people not affected by HIV.
- *Diabetes:* Diabetes triples the risk of having active TB disease.
- *Undernutrition:* Undernutrition increases the risk of getting active TB disease, and TB can lead to undernutrition.
- *Tobacco smoking:* Tobacco smoking increases the risk of getting active TB by 2 to 3 times.
- *Alcohol:* Alcohol use also increases the risk of TB by 2 times.

The relationship between TB and HIV is a very important public health issue, as noted above. In addition to greatly increasing the risk of developing active TB disease, HIV is also associated with a higher proportion of TB that is not pulmonary, compared to TB that is not linked to HIV.[2]

WHO now recommends that initial diagnostic testing for anyone suspected of having TB be done with Xpert™ MTB/RIF. This test is also recommended for diagnosing suspected TB meningitis and TB of the lymph nodes. This test uses molecular techniques and can diagnose both TB and resistance to one of the first-line drugs for treatment, rifampicin, in less than 2 hours. Xpert MTB/RIF is more sensitive and more specific than sputum smear microscopy, which has been used traditionally for diagnosis of pulmonary TB and is still used in places that have not yet adopted the Xpert MTB/RIF tool.[76] Diagnosing TB in HIV-positive people and children may require other clinical diagnostic processes, as does extrapulmonary TB, that are not discussed here.[72,77,78]

WHO estimated that there were about 10 million new cases of active TB disease in 2017. Of these, about 5.8 million were in men, 3.2 million were in women, and 1 million were in children.[25] Exposure and susceptibility are linked to males getting active TB disease more than females. However, there is variability in relative burden by sex in different age groups and in different settings.[79] Thus, it is critical to note that TB is also a leading killer of women. About 900,000, or 9 percent of the new cases of active TB, were in people co-infected with HIV.

There were an estimated 147,000 cases of zoonotic TB in 2016.[73]

In addition, WHO estimated that about 560,000 of the new cases of active TB disease were infected with drug-resistant TB, of which 82 percent were multidrug resistant.[25] WHO defines different types of resistance in TB as follows[80]:

- *Mono-resistance:* Resistance to one first-line anti-TB drug only
- *Rifampicin resistance (RR):* Resistance to rifampicin detected using phenotypic or genotypic methods, with or without resistance to other anti-TB drugs. It includes any resistance to rifampicin, in the form of mono-resistance, poly-resistance, MDR, or XDR
- *Poly-resistance:* Resistance to more than one first-line anti-TB drug, other than both isoniazid and rifampicin
- *Multidrug resistance (MDR):* Resistance to at least both isoniazid and rifampicin
- *Extensive drug resistance (XDR):* Resistance to any fluoroquinolone, and at least one of three second-line injectable drugs (capreomycin, kanamycin, and amikacin), in addition to multidrug resistance

In fact, there has been an increase in TB infections that are resistant to one or more TB drugs.[77]

An underlying cause for the development of resistant forms of TB is the failure to complete TB treatment, as was the case for Maria in one of the opening vignettes. However, it is also possible to be infected with drug-resistant TB directly from another person. Drug-resistant strains are found in many countries and are difficult and expensive to treat. Drug resistance is especially important in countries in which drug regulation and TB programs are weak or have fallen into disarray, such as Eastern Europe, and the greatest burdens of drug-resistant TB today are in Eastern Europe, China, and India.[77] In 2006, a number of cases of XDR-TB were found in South Africa among HIV patients, and 52 of 53 patients died within 25 days, despite being on HIV treatment. This caused considerable alarm in the public health community.[81]

The incidence rate of TB varies considerably across countries and regions. In high-income countries the incidence rate is generally below 10 per 100,000 population. By contrast, the highest burden countries have rates between 150 and 400 per 100,000.[25] A few severely affected countries have rates above 500 per 100,000 people, including 513 in the Democratic People's Republic of Korea (North Korea), 513 in the Philippines, 554 in Mozambique, 665 in Lesotho, and 567 in South Africa. The high rates in African countries generally reflect their high rates of HIV. By WHO region, Africa has the highest TB incidence rate, with 237 per 100,000 population, and the Americas have the lowest rate, with 28. TB incidence globally has fallen, but slowly, at a rate of about 2 percent per year. India, China, and Russia accounted for about half of all of the drug-resistant cases in the world.[25]

TB is estimated to have been the cause of about 1.6 million deaths in 2017. 1.3 million of these were among HIV-negative people and 300,000 among people with HIV infection. The number of deaths of HIV-negative people with TB has fallen by almost 30 percent since 2000. The number of deaths from TB among HIV-positive people has fallen by 44 percent since 2000, largely reflecting increasing access to antiretroviral therapy among those with HIV infection.[25] About 12,500 deaths occurred in 2016 from zoonotic TB.[73]

In the 2017 study of the global burden of disease, TB was the 13th most important cause of death worldwide for all age groups and both sexes but it was the 7th leading cause in sub-Saharan Africa. However, for those 15 to 49 years of age in sub-Saharan Africa, TB was the second leading cause of death. When we consider DALYs for the 15- to 49-year-old age group, TB was the second leading cause in sub-Saharan Africa and the 9th leading cause globally. Although TB kills substantially more men than women, TB is the 6th leading cause of death globally among women ages 15 to 49, and for men, TB is the 7th leading cause of death globally in this age group.[1]

The Costs and Consequences of TB

The cost of TB to families, communities, and countries is very high, given the large number of people who are sick with TB, the relatively long course of the illness, and the losses people face when they do have TB. A study of TB in India suggested that those sick with TB lost about 3 months of wages, spent an amount equal to about one-quarter of national income per capita on care and treatment, and took on debts to pay for this care that were equal to about 10 percent of per capita income.[82] A similar study in Bangladesh indicated that those sick with TB lost 4 months of wages.[83] A Thai study showed that TB patients spent more than 15 percent of their annual wages on TB, 12 percent of them took out bank loans to help make up for the costs of their illness, and 16 percent sold part of their property to finance the costs of dealing with their illness.[84] This study also found that TB patients lost about 60 percent of their individual annual income and 40 percent of household income due to TB and that falling ill with TB could be financially catastrophic to many families.[84]

There are also significant social costs associated with TB. Because of the stigma associated with TB, females who fall ill with TB in some parts of the world may be shunned by their families. In one Indian study, 15 percent of the women with TB faced familial rejection.[85] In another Indian study, 8 percent faced rejection.[81]

A study of the macroeconomic impact of TB suggested that the economic growth of a country is inversely correlated with the rate of TB. Every increase of 10 percent in the incidence of TB was associated with a 0.2 percent to 0.4 percent reduction in economic growth.[86] A study of the economic costs of TB in the Philippines indicated that the annual economic loss due to morbidity and premature mortality from TB was equal to almost $150 million. In addition, the cost to the Philippines of treating all of the expected cases of TB would be between $8 million and $29 million.[87]

Addressing the Burden of TB

A vaccine for TB called Bacillus Calmette–Guérin (BCG) is a standard part of the Expanded Program of Immunization for Children. The vaccine reduces severe TB in children, but because children are not important transmitters of TB and due to variable efficacy of the vaccine in different settings, the vaccine

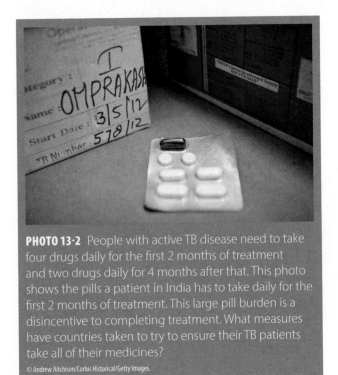

PHOTO 13-2 People with active TB disease need to take four drugs daily for the first 2 months of treatment and two drugs daily for 4 months after that. This photo shows the pills a patient in India has to take daily for the first 2 months of treatment. This large pill burden is a disincentive to completing treatment. What measures have countries taken to try to ensure their TB patients take all of their medicines?
© Andrew Aitchison/Corbis Historical/Getty Images.

has had little impact on the overall incidence or prevalence of TB.[88] Rather, the control of TB depends on effective treatment of active tuberculosis. In many respects, implementing a poor TB program is worse than having no TB program at all because a poor quality TB program can give rise to drug-resistant TB by enabling the use of drugs without quality of care. Poor quality TB care also led to death in patients who should have been treated successfully.

WHO recommends a 6-month regimen for drug-susceptible disease that includes four drugs—isoniazid, rifampicin, pyrazinamide, and ethambutol—for the first 2 months and then isoniazid and rifampicin for the following 4 months.[89]

Once an active case of TB is identified, appropriate drugs of good quality are required in adequate supply for 6 months. It is recommended that drugs be used that are fixed-dose combinations of the required drugs and that they be taken daily. Patient adherence with the TB regimen is required for effective therapy. This should be encouraged through a "patient-centered approach" that encourages health education and counseling and consideration of the most appropriate options for drug administration. This could include material and communications support for the patient. It could also include at-home, community-based, or facility-based treatment and supervision of drug taking by a trained lay provider or health worker. There is also a growing use of digital technologies for encouraging drug adherence, such as video monitoring of drug taking.[90] Globally, 82 percent of people diagnosed with drug-susceptible TB were treated successfully and cured of TB.[25]

Treating active drug-susceptible TB through an organized quality-assured care program is highly cost-effective, with fairly recent studies showing the cost ranging from $5 to $50 per DALY averted in most regions. The cost of treating a TB case, in fact, is below $200 in several countries.[25] BCG is cost-effective in reducing severe cases of childhood TB in high-prevalence settings.[88]

The Management of TB/HIV Co-infection

As noted in the section on HIV/AIDS, TB is an opportunistic infection of HIV. As the immune system of an HIV-positive person declines, TB is one of the diseases that can develop. This is especially so in populations where many people have latent TB. In addition, TB has been the leading cause of death of adults who are HIV-positive and not on antiretroviral therapy, although cryptococcal meningitis may now be responsible for more deaths of HIV-positive people in Africa than TB.

WHO recommends a number of measures to prevent and manage TB and HIV co-infection[91]:

- Intensified case finding to ensure that all of those who are HIV-positive are tested for TB and all of those with TB are tested for HIV
- Giving isoniazid, an antibiotic, to people with HIV to help prevent them from getting TB
- Enhancing infection control in healthcare settings so that TB does not spread among those who are infected with HIV

There are still substantial gaps in many countries in managing TB/HIV co-infection in conjunction with these guidelines. More than half of the people who are co-infected with HIV and TB, for example, did not get TB care. In addition, only about half of the high-burden countries reported offering preventive therapy with isoniazid to HIV-positive people.[91]

TABLE 13-15 portrays the DCP3 recommended essential package for TB.

Challenges in TB Prevention and Care

WHO has developed the End TB Strategy, building on two previous global TB strategies from 1995 to 2015. This strategy seeks to end the global TB epidemic by 2035, with a 95 percent reduction in TB deaths and a drop in incidence to 10 per 100,000 people. It also calls for the elimination of catastrophic costs for TB-affected families by 2020.

The strategy is based on expanding TB prevention and care through a focus on high-impact interventions in a patient-centered way, working with a wider array of public and private partners, pursuing policy shifts associated with universal health coverage, social protection and poverty alleviation, and pursuing basic research, development of new tools, and operational research. The strategy acknowledges the urgent need for better diagnostics and ways of treating latent TB. It also highlights the need for safer and easier drug regimens for active TB disease, as well as a new vaccine, to drive down deaths and incidence much more rapidly.[92]

There has recently been progress in improving TB diagnostics and in developing new and shortened drug regimens for drug-resistant TB. However, significant challenges remain in developing more effective vaccines, inexpensive and rapid diagnostics for all forms of TB, and drug therapy that will lessen the duration of treatment and the number of pills that patients have to take. A related challenge is to ensure that new tools, such as new diagnostics, are put into use, scaled up as rapidly as possible, and coupled with other measures needed to ensure high-quality TB care.

This is essential because there are also major gaps in the quality of care. Some of these gaps relate to the fact that a considerable amount of TB diagnosis and treatment is carried out in the private sector, and often with very poor quality, such as using nonstandard drug regimens, little or no patient follow-up, and excessive diagnostic test charges. However, there are also major quality issues in many national TB programs. In some regions there remains the need to diagnose more of those with TB, and in some regions, particularly Eastern Europe and Central Asia, there is a need to cure a larger share of those who are treated, with low treatment success heavily linked to the large burden of undetected drug-resistant disease. The growing use of Xpert MTB/RIF can be helpful to improving care. However, this can only happen if other parts of the cascade of care are improved in many countries.[93,94]

Improving TB diagnosis and treatment will require that the quality of care be central and that quality be improved at every level of care. It will also require further efforts at linking all providers of TB diagnosis and treatment with national TB control programs. There has been some important progress in this direction, but there remain enormous gaps for public–private partnerships to reach global targets.[77]

There are also still major gaps in the implementation of the WHO guidelines on the collaborative treatment of TB and HIV. Significant improvements are needed in a number of settings to strengthen collaboration between TB and HIV programs so that WHO guidelines can be put more firmly in place in all countries.[77]

TABLE 13-15 Essential Tuberculosis Intervention Package, by Delivery Platform

Intervention Type	Delivery Platform				
	Nationwide policies and regulations	Community health post or pharmacy	Primary health center	First-level hospital	Second- and third-level hospitals
Surveillance and disease detection	Passive case finding Active case finding in high-burden countries	Symptomatic surveillance Active contact tracing of TB-positive patients			
Data collection and patient tracking	Information systems				
Diagnosis and drug sensitivity testing Relapse and reinfection diagnosis	National guidelines promoting the provision of diagnostic labs; diagnostic technology including GeneXpert or culture for drug-susceptible TB; fixed/ mobile X-ray; and training	Symptomatic diagnosis, local sputum smears Referral for diagnosis and drug-susceptible TB tests	Sputum smears Testing of children and household members and HIV+ individuals for case finding in both drug-susceptible and MDR-TB cases Availability of fixed/mobile X-ray for diagnosis	Xpert/RIF or culture for diagnosis of drug-susceptible TB	
Treatment of drug-susceptible TB	WHO guidelines: Four-drug regimen for 2 months, then two-drug regimen for 4 months	Provision and observation of treatment after 1 month at first-level hospital Use of cell-phone SMS to support treatment adherence		Treatment of drug-susceptible TB until transmission is reduced (1 month), then transfer of treatment to community level	
Treatment of drug-resistant TB	WHO guidelines: Multiple-drug regimen after drug-susceptible TB testing for 9 months to 2 years		Provision of appropriate second-line drugs, monitoring INH preventive therapy	Treatment until sputum is negative or GeneXpert is negative, treatment as outpatients after sputum is negative	Specialized treatment for treatment failures, MDR-TB, surgery
Coinfection with HIV		Provider incentives to improve quality of TB care	Referral or provision of HIV treatment as appropriate Information systems to link diagnostic hospital care to outpatient and community care	Separate areas in health facilities for TB to avoid transmission to AIDS patients	

Note: HIV = human immunodeficiency virus; HIV+ = HIV positive; INH = isoniazid; MDR-TB = multidrug-resistant tuberculosis; SMS = short message service (text messaging); TB = tuberculosis; WHO = World Health Organization. Xpert/RIF refers to a new test that simultaneously detects Mycobacterium TB complex (MTBC) and resistance to rifampicin (RIF).

Modified from Holmes, K. K., Bertozzi, S., Bloom, B. R., Jha, P., Gelband, H., DeMaria, L. M., & Horton, S. (2017). Major infectious diseases: Key messages from *Disease Control Priorities*. In *Disease Control Priorities* (Vol. 6). Washington, DC: The World Bank.

The End TB Strategy also emphasizes the importance of embedding TB care in universal health coverage and further linking TB efforts with the strengthening of health systems. This includes the improvement of laboratory services and infection control and further integrating TB care at the primary level, especially through community-based care. The strategy also highlights the importance of promoting more community-based approaches to information and education about TB and the increased involvement of patients, communities, and civil society in TB efforts.[77]

Putting the new strategy in place will require additional financial and technical resources.[78] The fight against TB could face important challenges in finding the needed financial resources in the present global environment.

Malaria

The Burden of Malaria

Some basic facts about malaria are presented in **TABLE 13-16**.

Malaria is caused by parasites in the genus *Plasmodium*, five species of which infect humans: *P. falciparum*, *P. vivax*, *P. ovale*, *P. malariae*, and *P. knowlesi*. These parasite species exist in different proportions in different regions of the world. For example, *P. falciparum* dominates in Africa, *P. vivax* occurs in temperate zones, and *P. ovale* is found in South Asia and tropical Africa.[95] *P. knowlesi* is the least common form and primarily affects macaques. However, it can also infect humans, especially in forested areas of Southeast Asia.[96] Malaria is spread by the bite of the female *Anopheles* mosquito. Essentially, the mosquito carries the parasite from an infected person to an uninfected person.

WHO estimated that in 2017, there were 219 million cases of malaria worldwide. About 92 percent were in Africa, 5 percent in South Asia, and 2 percent in the Eastern Mediterranean. There is also some malaria in Latin America. Fifteen countries in sub-Saharan Africa and India account for 80 percent of the malaria cases worldwide. Five countries have 50 percent of the cases: Nigeria, Democratic Republic of the Congo, Mozambique, India, and Uganda.

There has been dramatic progress in the last decade in reducing the burden of malaria. The global incidence rate has fallen from 72 to 59 per 1,000 from 2010 to 2017. Some regions have also made especially good progress in reducing incidence, such as the WHO South-East Asia region, in which incidence fell from 17 to 7 per 1,000 from 2010 to 2017. In addition, the number of countries moving toward elimination of malaria and that had fewer than 100 cases increased from 15 in 2010 to 26 in 2017. Nonetheless, over the last 3 years there has not been much reduction in the number of cases worldwide.[97]

WHO estimated that there were 435,000 malaria deaths in 2017, down from 607,000 in 2010. Children under 5 years of age are the most vulnerable to malaria, and more than 60 percent of all malaria

TABLE 13-16 Malaria Basic Facts: 2017

Number of malaria cases: 219 million

Global distribution of cases in selected WHO regions: 92% in the African Region, 5% in South-East Asia, and 2% in Eastern Mediterranean Region

Burden of malaria-related deaths: 93% in the African Region, 61% among children under 5 years of age

Proportion of people in Africa sleeping under an insecticide-treated mosquito net: 50%

Estimated proportion of pregnant women in Africa receiving the recommended three or more doses of intermittent preventive treatment in pregnancy for malaria: 22%

Proportion of children under 5 in Africa with a fever given any antimalarial drug: 29%

Number of people protected through indoor residual spraying: 64 million in Africa, 1.5 million in the Americas, 7.5 million in the Eastern Mediterranean, 41 million in South-East Asia, 1.5 million in the Western Pacific Region

Number of countries with fewer than 100 indigenous malaria cases: 26

Data from World Health Organization (WHO). (2018). *World malaria report 2018*. Geneva, Switzerland: Author. Retrieved from https://www.who.int/malaria/publications/world-malaria-report-2018/en/

deaths are among this age group. Pregnant women are also especially vulnerable to malaria. In fact, malaria is the 5th leading cause of death for under-5 children globally and the fourth leading cause of death for under-5 children in sub-Saharan Africa. Malaria is also the 4th leading cause of death for females in sub-Saharan Africa aged 15 to 49 years. Malaria is the 4th leading cause of DALYs for both sexes and all ages in sub-Saharan Africa.[1]

The most important risk factor for malaria is being bitten by mosquitoes that carry the malaria parasite. This risk varies with the feeding habits of various species of mosquitoes, the climate, and the time of year. Some people have a degree of immunity to malaria from having grown up in malarial zones, and the risks of contracting malaria increase if one does not have such immunity.[95]

Pregnant women who contract malaria are at high risk of giving birth to low-birthweight children. Malaria in pregnancy is also associated with spontaneous abortion, stillbirth, premature delivery, and severe anemia in the mother and the baby.[98] An earlier study suggested that 3 to 15 percent of African mothers suffered severe anemia, accounting for 10,000 malaria-related anemia deaths per year. It was further estimated that globally, malaria would cause about 30 percent of low birthweight in newborns and between 75,000 and 200,000 infant deaths per year.[95]

The Costs and Consequences of Malaria

The cost of malaria at the family level is substantial because individuals often have malaria up to five times per year. In one study in Ghana, for example, there were 11 cases of malaria per household, per year, on average.[56] These same studies showed that individuals lost 1 to 5 work days per episode of malaria, that the indirect cost of dealing with their illness was greater than the direct costs of treatment, and that each episode of malaria probably cost an adult about 2 percent of his or her annual income.[56] In many African countries, malaria typically accounts for 30 percent or more of outpatient visits and hospital admissions for children under 5 years of age.[99]

It is estimated that $12 billion is lost annually due to malaria in Africa alone.[99] Roll Back Malaria suggests that the economic cost of malaria in countries with a high malaria burden is a loss of about 1.3 percent of GDP per year. One study suggested that a 10 percent reduction in malaria was associated with a 0.3 percent increase in economic growth. Clearly, malaria in sub-Saharan Africa has been a deterrent to trade, business development, tourism, and foreign investment.[100,101]

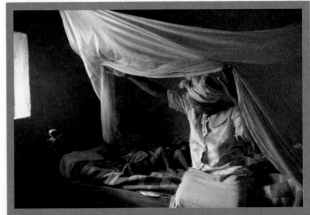

PHOTO 13-3 The increasing and proper use of insecticide-treated bednets has had a major impact on the burden of malaria. Everyone in an endemic zone should sleep under a bednet. Different countries have taken different approaches to promoting their wider use. What approach would you recommend and why? Would you sell them through private channels? Subsidize such sales with vouchers given to pregnant women? Give them away for free at maternal and child health centers?
© Wendy Stone/Corbis Historica/Getty Images.

Addressing the Burden of Malaria

There is widespread agreement on the key interventions required to roll back malaria. These include the following[97]:

- Prompt treatment of those infected, based on confirmed diagnosis
- Intermittent preventive therapy for pregnant women in areas of moderate to high transmission of malaria in Africa
- Intermittent preventive treatment in infants in areas of moderate to high transmission of malaria in Africa
- Seasonal malaria chemoprevention for children under 5 years of age in areas with highly seasonal transmission of malaria in the Sahel region of sub-Saharan Africa
- Long-lasting insecticide-treated bednets for people living in malarial zones
- Indoor residual spraying of the homes of people in malarial zones
- Environmental control measures to reduce mosquito breeding sites

Treatment of malaria should be initiated within 24 hours of diagnosis based on a confirmed diagnosis.[102] Traditionally, diagnoses were supposed to be made through a microscopic examination of a blood smear, but this was often not done. However, a rapid diagnostic test (RDT) was developed to make it easier to test for malaria in low-resource settings, and the use of these kits has become widespread. About 75 percent of the malaria tests in 2017 in Africa were RDTs. In addition, an estimated 245 million RDTs were used by national malaria programs in 2017, mostly in Africa.[97(pxvii)]

Appropriate treatment of malaria is essential to reduce malaria morbidity and mortality. If people with malaria are treated promptly, then mosquitoes that bite them will not carry malaria to another person. Drugs such as chloroquine, Fansidar (sulfadoxine and pyrimethamine), and mefloquine were used earlier as standard treatments for malaria in different settings. However, they faced growing levels of drug resistance.

WHO today, therefore, recommends artemisinin-based combination therapies for treating uncomplicated malaria caused by *P. falciparum* and for treating *P. vivax* infections that are not responsive to chloroquine.[103] From 2010 to 2017, about 2.7 billion treatment courses of ACT were procured, about 60 percent for national malaria programs and the rest for the private sector.[97(pxvii)] WHO also recommends that pregnant women in areas in Africa where malaria is endemic be treated with intermittent preventive therapy as part of antenatal care. WHO recommends that this treatment be given from the second trimester, with doses one month apart and at least three doses before delivery.[103] To protect infants in areas of moderate to high transmission of malaria in Africa, WHO recommends they be given preventive treatment against malaria. This should be given at the time of the second and third rounds of DTP vaccination and the measles vaccination.[103] In the Sahel region of Africa, with highly seasonal transmission of malaria, WHO recommends that all children under 6 years of age be given seasonal monthly treatment against malaria.[103]

The use of long-lasting insecticide-treated bednets (ITNs) is another important pillar of malaria control. Bednets, impregnated with a biologically safe insecticide, are being widely distributed for free and sold by governments, donors, and the private sector. The percentage of people in malaria-endemic areas with access to ITNs has increased from 33 percent in 2010 to 56 percent in 2017.[97(pxvii)]

Spraying the inside of homes, or indoor residual spraying, is also important. Only about 3 percent of the population at risk of malaria globally was covered with such spraying in 2017. This low level and decline from earlier appears to reflect the need to rotate insecticides as mosquitoes become resistant to them and the higher cost of some insecticides.[97(pxvii)] Five insecticides are approved by WHO for indoor residual spraying.[104] Pyrethroids have been the insecticide of choice for spraying, but DDT is also approved for such efforts. Assessments are made to examine resistance to the insecticides and the need to rotate insecticides to slow the development of resistance to them. Particular attention is also being paid to potential environmental risks of the insecticides.[104]

Reducing the number of mosquitoes that carry malaria at the community level relies on effective communication and commitment by local leaders, the identification of breeding sites, and the availability of appropriate larvicides and/or tools to drain potential breeding sites. However, reducing the number of mosquitoes, called source reduction, is particularly difficult in Africa because the vector, *Anopheles gambiae*, is ubiquitous and breeds in all types of standing water.[95]

TABLE 13-17 shows what DCP3 has recommended as an essential package for addressing malaria in low- and middle-income countries.

Challenges in Addressing Malaria

The global goals and targets for the control and prevention of malaria are shown in **FIGURE 13-2**.

It is clear from the data given earlier on the number of cases and on the number of deaths that there has been enormous progress against malaria recently. It is also clear that much of this stems from the concerted efforts of countries and their global partners to ensure better prevention, diagnosis, and treatment of malaria.

Nonetheless, a number of efforts will need to be expanded and improved to meet global goals and, ultimately, to eliminate malaria from an increasing number of countries. Achieving key goals will require, first, the scaling up of key interventions for prevention. This includes trying to ensure 100 percent coverage for people at risk with long-lasting insecticide-treated bednets. Despite enormous progress, today only about 50 percent of the people who should be sleeping under an ITN in Africa are doing so.[97(pxvii)] Progress will have to include not only the dissemination of bednets but also greater efforts at behavior change to ensure that families actually use the nets properly when they have them.

Similar efforts will need to be made in intermittent treatment of pregnant women and infants and seasonal chemoprevention for young children. In 2010, there was almost no intermittent treatment of pregnant women, and in 2017 it was estimated that about 22 percent of pregnant women in 33 African countries received such treatment. While this is important progress, it still means that almost 80 percent of pregnant women are *not* receiving recommended treatment. More than 50 percent of the children in the Sahel

TABLE 13-17 Essential Malaria Intervention Package, by Delivery Platform

Intervention Type	Delivery Platform					
	Population-based health interventions	Community	Health center	First-level hospital	Second- and third-level hospitals

All malaria-endemic countries

Intervention Type	Population-based health interventions	Community	Health center	First-level hospital	Second- and third-level hospitals
Case management: Uncomplicated malaria (or fever)	Prophylaxis for travelers	Diagnosis with RDTs or microscopy, including parasite species Treatment with ACTs (or current first-line combination) for malaria-positive individuals where diagnosis is available Where both RDTs and microscopy are unavailable and malaria is common, presumptive treatment with ACTs for nonsevere suspected malaria; if severe, ACTs plus antibiotics *Plasmodium vivax:* Chloroquine alone or chloroquine plus 14-day course of primaquine (for G6PD-normal individuals) Case investigation, reactive case detection, proactive case detection (including mass screening and treatment)			
Case management: Severe malaria		Single-dose rectal artesunate, then referral to first-level hospital		Parenteral artesunate, then full-course ACTs	
Vector control: ITNs		ITNs available in health centers and antenatal clinics and via social marketing			

Malaria elimination countries

Intervention Type	Population-based health interventions	Community	Health center	First-level hospital	Second- and third-level hospitals
		Mass drug administration to high-risk groups in geographic or demographic clusters Single low-dose primaquine added to first-line treatment			

Malaria-control countries

Intervention Type	Population-based health interventions	Community	Health center	First-level hospital	Second- and third-level hospitals
Vector control: IRS		IRS in selected areas with high transmission and entomologic data on IRS susceptibility			

| Vector control: Larviciding and water management | | Larviciding and water management in specific circumstances where breeding sites can be identified and regularly targeted | | | |
| Mass drug administration | | IPTp, IPTi, and SMC Sahel region | | | |

Note: ACTs = artemisinin-combination therapies; G6PD = glucose-6-phosphate-dehydrogenase; IPTi= intermittent preventive treatment in infants; IPTp= intermittent preventive treatment of pregnant women; IRS = indoor residual spraying; ITN = insecticide-treated net; RDT = rapid diagnostic test; SMC = seasonal malaria chemoprevention

All interventions listed for lower-level platforms can be provided at higher levels. Similarly, each facility level represents a spectrum and diversity of capabilities. The column in which an intervention is listed is the lowest level of the healthcare system in which it would usually be provided.

Modified from Holmes, K. K., Bertozzi, S., Bloom, B. R., Jha, P., Gelband, H., DeMaria, L. M., & Horton, S. (2017). Major infectious diseases: Key messages from *Disease Control Priorities*. In *Disease control priorities* (Vol. 6). Washington, DC: The World Bank.

GTS: global targets for 2030 and milestones for 2020 and 2025

Vision – A world free of malaria

Pillars	
Pillar 1	Ensure universal access to malaria prevention, diagnosis and treatment
Pillar 2	Accelerate efforts towards elimination and attainment of malaria free status
Pillar 3	Transform malaria surveillance into a core intervention

Goals	Milestones		Targets
	2020	**2025**	**2030**
1. Reduce malaria mortality rates globally compared with 2015	At least 40%	At least 75%	At least 90%
2. Reduce malaria case incidence globally compared with 2015	At least 40%	At least 75%	At least 90%
3. Eliminate malaria from countries in which malaria was transmited in 2015	At least 10 countries	At least 20 countries	At least 35 countries
4. Prevent re-establishment of malaria in all countries that are malaria free	Re-establishment prevented	Re-establishment prevented	Re-establishment prevented

GTS: *Global technical strategy for malaria* 2016–2030.

FIGURE 13-2 Targets and Goals for Addressing Malaria

Reproduced from World Health Organization (WHO). (2018). *World malaria report 2018*. Geneva, Switzerland: Author. Retrieved from https://www.who.int/malaria/publications/world-malaria-report-2018/en/

who should receive seasonal chemoprevention are not receiving it either.[97(pxvii)]

There are also substantial gaps in the quality of diagnosis and treatment of malaria, with many cases diagnosed without confirming the presence of malaria by microscopy or a rapid diagnostic test. In addition, many of those who suffer from malaria are not given the right medicine or not given medicine in a timely manner, which can result in death.[105] The latest surveys, for example, show that around 40 percent of children with a fever who should have been checked for malaria received no medical attention. In addition, only about 60 percent who were examined in the public sector were tested for malaria. While progress has been made in ensuring a confirmed diagnosis before treatment, surveys have also suggested that only 74 percent of children treated for malaria had a confirmed diagnosis.[97(pxvii)]

A substantial share of those diagnosed with and treated for malaria seek care in the private sector. The quality of those private services is often inadequate, and people may be given inappropriate or counterfeit drugs. Improving the speed and quality of diagnosis and treatment will require that national malaria programs find effective ways of working with private medical providers in almost all countries in Africa.

Better diagnostics could also be helpful. In addition, the continuous development of new drugs to fight malaria is also critical, given the speed with which malaria has developed resistance to other drugs and the limited number of drugs that now work effectively against malaria. Five countries have now shown resistance to ACT, and there are no new proven drugs available to combat malaria.[106]

There is growing resistance to the insecticides used for indoor residual spraying. It will be extremely important to monitor that resistance. Sixty-one countries have now reported resistance to at least one class of insecticides, and 50 countries have reported resistance to two or more classes.[107]

After many years of effort, there has finally been some progress in the development of a malaria vaccine. The RTS,S/ASO1 (RTS,S) vaccine is the first vaccine to provide partial protection against malaria in young children. In clinical trials done among 15,000 children in seven countries in sub-Saharan Africa, the vaccine prevented about 40 percent of cases over 4 years and about 30 percent of cases of severe malaria. WHO is now coordinating an effort with Ghana, Kenya, and Malawi and their partners to carry out a pilot program that will begin further testing of the vaccine, which requires four doses.[108]

Nonetheless, given the nature of malaria and of resistance to drugs and insecticides, it is crucial that there continue to be important investment in vaccines, drugs, and insecticides that can help to prevent and treat malaria.[97(pxvii)] It will also be important to continue to engage in research and learn what works in cost-effective ways in different settings. Efforts have been under way, for example, to see if relatively small pockets of malaria in countries nearing elimination could be addressed through selective seasonal drug therapy.[109]

Diarrheal Disease

The Burden of Diarrheal Disease

WHO defines diarrhea as "the passage of three or more loose or liquid stools per day (or more frequent passage than is normal for the individual)."[5] Diarrhea is caused by certain bacteria, viruses, and/or parasites that are transmitted by contaminated water or food through the fecal–oral route, such as *Shigella* sp., *Salmonella* sp., *Cholera vibrio*, rotavirus, and *Escherichia coli*. Diarrheal disease agents can be spread by dirty utensils, dirty hands, or flies. Poor recognition of the extent of illness, failed home care, and lack of knowledge about simple therapies increase the severity of diarrhea.[110]

Diarrheal diseases most significantly impact the poor, especially children in low- and middle-income countries. Poor housing, crowding, lack of safe water and sanitation, cohabitation with domestic animals, lack of refrigeration for food storage, and poor personal and community hygiene all contribute to the transmission of diarrheal disease agents. In addition, poor nutrition contributes to poor immunity and increases the frequency and severity of diarrhea. This contributes to a vicious cycle of diarrhea and undernutrition, because diarrhea can cause malnutrition. Diarrhea causes severe dehydration and a loss of body water and can kill infants and young children very quickly.[110]

Diarrheal disease mortality has decreased significantly in the past 30 years. This decline has largely been due to improved nutrition of infants, better disease recognition by families and healthcare providers, improved care seeking, appropriate use of oral rehydration therapy, increasing rates of coverage of the measles vaccine, and the growing use of the rotavirus vaccine.

Nonetheless, the burden of diarrheal disease remains very substantial. Diarrhea is a major cause of death and sickness for children younger than 5 years. WHO estimated in 2016 that there were about 1.7 billion cases of diarrheal disease among children and that diarrhea was responsible for 525,000 deaths of such children.[5] WHO also estimated that children under 3 years of age in low- and middle-income countries suffer on average about three episodes of diarrhea annually, although rates vary worldwide.[5]

Diarrheal diseases are the cause of about 10 percent of all deaths of children under 5 globally, about 12 percent in sub-Saharan Africa, and about 9 percent in South Asia. Diarrheal diseases are the third leading cause of death for under-5 children globally, in sub-Saharan Africa, and in South Asia, behind neonatal disorders and lower respiratory infections.[1]

Addressing the Burden of Diarrhea

There are several major disease prevention strategies for diarrhea. The first is access to safe water and improved sanitation, coupled with better handwashing with soap. Second is the promotion of exclusive breastfeeding for 6 months. This is advantageous to the child because the child receives both maternal antibodies and a nutritious and uncontaminated meal. Mothers benefit from an increased birth interval and a healthier child. This can be coupled with improved complementary feeding, introduced hygienically with breastfeeding after 6 months. Good personal and food hygiene is also central to reducing diarrheal disease, which will, hopefully, follow efforts at health education and hygiene promotion. The next measure is rotavirus immunization.[5] WHO estimated in 2013 that rotavirus was the cause of about 215,000 deaths of children under 5 years of age[5,111]; this was down from 450,000 in 2008, before the vaccine began to be more widely used in low- and middle-income countries.[112]

Measles immunization is also important to reducing diarrheal disease. Data indicate a clear link between measles immunization and reduced incidence and deaths from diarrhea. Ensuring that an increasing share of children have sufficient levels of vitamin A by raising supplementation rates is also important.[113]

A number of case management interventions can significantly reduce the severity and mortality of diarrheal disease. The use of oral rehydration therapy (ORT) is the most cost-effective case management intervention, especially if homemade solutions are administered. Related to this, it was also estimated that zinc supplementation during an acute diarrhea episode lasting 10 to 14 days could reduce the duration of diarrhea by about 25 percent and stool volume by 30 percent. Continuing to feed nutrient nutrient-rich foods is also important. In addition, intravenous fluids may be necessary in the case of severe dehydration or shock. Antibiotics can be given for bloody diarrhea, primarily caused by *Shigella* infection. However, delivering this intervention where it is most needed may depend on careful training of non-physician healthcare personnel because most low-income and many middle-income countries do not have enough physicians living in places where they are most needed.[5,110]

Neglected Tropical Diseases[114]
The Burden of Neglected Tropical Diseases

WHO now lists 22 diseases as neglected tropical diseases (NTDs). Together these diseases affect more than 1 billion people. **TABLE 13-18** is the current list of NTDs.[115]

NTDs are diseases of poverty, affecting nearly everyone in the "bottom billion" of the world's poorest people. NTDs are especially prevalent in subtropical and tropical climates. Women and children who live in unhygienic environments with limited access to clean water and sanitary methods of waste disposal face the biggest threat of NTDs. Pregnant women also face special risks from some NTDs, as discussed later

TABLE 13-18 The Neglected Tropical Diseases
Dengue and severe dengue
Chikungunya
Leishmaniasis
Foodborne trematodiases
Rabies
Yaws
Lymphatic filariasis
Taeniasis/Cysticercosis
Echinococcosis
Chagas disease
Leprosy
Dracunculiasis (guinea-worm disease)
Buruli ulcer
Trypanosomiasis, Human African (sleeping sickness)
Soil-transmitted helminth infections
Onchoceriasis
Schistosomiasis
Vector-borne diseases

Modified from World Health Organization (WHO). (n.d.). *Fact sheets: Neglected tropical diseases*. Retrieved from https://www.who.int/topics/tropical_diseases/factsheets/neglected/en/

in this section. People engaged in farming are particularly susceptible to NTDs because of their close contact with soil, which can harbor many of the parasites and worms that cause NTDs. People who live in Africa and rely on rivers for drinking and bathing are also more likely to be affected by certain NTDs, such as onchocerciasis. Individuals whose labor or domestic chores are centered on freshwater sources are also more likely to contract NTDs.[115] Living in close proximity to livestock and to the vectors of infection also increases risk.[115]

In addition, the burden of the worm diseases concerns not only being infected but also the number of worms in the body. Children of preschool age generally have the greatest number of worms. In addition, the prevalence of intestinal worms in many school-aged children in the most heavily burdened countries is exceptionally high.[115]

Several of these diseases are especially important, given the large number of people at risk of becoming infected, their impact on health and child development, and the manner in which they can be addressed. These include intestinal worms, which are called "soil-transmitted helminths": roundworm (ascariasis), whipworm (trichuriasis), and hookworm. The four other NTDs that will be addressed here include schistosomiasis (snail fever), lymphatic filariasis (elephantiasis), onchocerciasis (river blindness), and blinding trachoma.

NTDs can have a terrible impact on health, impede child growth and development, harm pregnant women, and often cause long-term debilitating illnesses. They cause an extraordinary amount of ill health, disability, and disfigurement. Some deaths are also associated with NTDs, especially from schistosomiasis. Those who suffer from NTDs are frequently shunned by their families and their communities. In addition, people with these diseases are often unable to work productively, leading to enormous economic losses for them, their families, and the nations in which they live.

Many diseases kill more people than NTDs do. However, NTDs can make people sick for long periods of time and cause long-lasting disabilities. In fact, the latest studies suggest that NTDs result in about half as many DALYs annually as are caused by malaria.[1]

Despite their significance, insufficient financial support was provided until recently to address NTDs, compared to the burden of ill health they cause. This was especially regrettable because significant progress has been made to control or eliminate some of the NTDs, including Chagas disease, lymphatic filariasis, onchocerciasis, Guinea worm, and leprosy. It is also lamentable because a package of drugs is available that can prevent through mass drug administration six NTDs for about 50 cents per year.[116] Given the exceptional amount of good health that can be gained in the fight against NTDs for such a small amount of money, an important global challenge has been to spread this package as quickly as possible to all of the places where it can be of benefit.

The Consequences of the Neglected Tropical Diseases

NTDs can have debilitating social and economic consequences as well as a major impact on the health and well-being of those infected. On the clinical side, for example, trachoma can lead to redness and swelling of the eye, sensitivity to light, corneal scarring, and eventually permanent blindness. Schistosomiasis is associated with painful and/or bloody urination, bloody diarrhea, enlargement of the liver and/or spleen, and liver cancer; it is also the most deadly of the NTDs. Lymphatic filariasis is well known for the remarkable swelling it can cause in the limbs and genitals. Onchocerciasis leads to skin problems and blindness.

The helminthic infections are generally associated with abdominal pain, loss of appetite, malnutrition, diarrhea, and anemia. In addition, chronic helminthic infection in children can limit their physical and mental development. Pregnant women with hookworm are at high risk of giving birth to low-birthweight babies, of birthing babies who fail to thrive, and of having poor milk production. In addition, pregnant women with anemia, commonly caused by hookworm in low-income countries, are three and a half times more likely to die during childbirth than women who are not anemic. This risk is especially significant, because one-quarter to one-third of pregnant women in sub-Saharan Africa are infected with hookworm.[117] Whipworm also can lead to severe growth restriction in children.

NTDs by themselves not only have enormous effects on individuals but also worsen the effects of other major infectious diseases or make individuals more susceptible to them. Recent studies have shown that many people have one or more NTDs at the same time as they have HIV/AIDS or malaria, which worsens the intensity of those diseases. In addition, helminthic infections may serve as important factors in the transmission of HIV.[118] Genital schistosomiasis in females may develop into lesions that increase susceptibility to becoming infected with HIV.[119] Neglected tropical diseases are also associated with the onset of some chronic noncommunicable diseases, such as the bladder cancer associated with urinary schistosomiasis.[120]

Social stigma is a major consequence of the NTDs. Many of the NTDs cause disability and disfigurement, resulting in individuals being shunned by their families and their communities. When not treated, for example, leprosy can cause terrible skin lesions that have been stigmatized since biblical times. Few health conditions are as stigmatizing as the swelling of limbs and genitalia that can result from lymphatic filariasis. Individuals who are stigmatized are less likely to seek diagnosis and treatment. Social stigma is particularly demoralizing for young women because they are often left unmarried and unable to work, in settings where the social value of a woman has much to do with her marital status.

NTDs also have a major impact on the productivity of individuals and the economic prospects of communities and nations. Children are disproportionately affected by NTDs and often suffer long-term consequences from them. In some areas, hookworm infection in school-age children contributes to drops in school attendance by over 20 percent, and poor school attendance and poor school performance reduce future earnings. In fact, hookworm has been shown to reduce future wage-earning capacity in some affected areas by up to 43 percent.[121]

NTDs adversely affect economic productivity at the individual, family, community, and national levels. NTDs lead to important losses in income that cause some families to sell assets to try to stay financially solvent. In addition, regions severely affected by onchocerciasis often cannot be used effectively for economic activities such as farming, because families that try to live in these areas are at risk of being blinded by the disease. WHO estimates that blindness due to trachoma costs the world between $2.9 and $5.3 billion annually.[122]

Addressing the Neglected Tropical Diseases

In 2012, WHO published a Roadmap for the prevention, treatment, elimination, and eradication of NTDs.[123] The Roadmap included a number of goals and targets for 2015 and 2020. Shortly after the publication of the Roadmap, global partners issued a London Declaration on Neglected Tropical Diseases. These partners agreed on a range of measures to support the Roadmap, including financial support, the support of research and development, the provision of drug access programs, and technical support.[124]

There has been considerable progress in the fight against a number of NTDs, including continuing declines in the incidence of the diseases discussed, as well as a growing number of people treated for them. The following are other examples of progress[125]:

- Guinea worm has been nearly eradicated.
- Morocco and Oman have eliminated trachoma.
- Six countries have eliminated lymphatic filariasis, and a further 18 countries no longer require mass drug administration for this disease.
- Onchocerciasis has been nearly eliminated in the Americas.

Additional comments follow on the specific diseases under discussion.

There are a number of soil-transmitted helminths. However, the main ones that affect humans are roundworm (*Ascaris lumbricoides*), whipworm

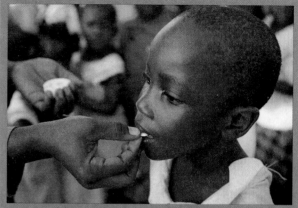

PHOTO 13-4 Preventing the continued spread of some of the "wormy" diseases is based on the mass administration of drugs to populations at risk, as shown here in Uganda. What other measures, both in the short and longer run, should be taken to reduce the risks of soil-transmitted helminths in these communities?
Courtesy of Mark Tuschman.

(*Trichuris trichiura*), and hookworm (*Necator americanus* and *Ancylostoma duodenale*). It is estimated that about 1.5 billion people are infected globally with one or more of these worms. Generally the people most at risk of soil-transmitted helminths are preschool- and school-age children, women of childbearing age, and adults who work in occupations that put them at special risk of infection. In fact, almost 270 million children of preschool age and 570 million school-age children live in regions where these parasites are intensively transmitted. Infections are mostly found in tropical and subtropical regions, with the largest burden being in sub-Saharan Africa, Latin America, China, and East Asia.[126]

The **soil-transmitted helminths** have very similar life cycles. Humans ingest the eggs of the worms. The eggs hatch into larvae, which travel to different parts of the body, depending on the type of worm. The worms might feed on food from the human host or attach themselves to the intestinal lining and live off the blood of the host. Eggs pass from the human host in feces and can then be picked up by others who will get infected.[115]

These parasites can have a number of harmful effects[126]:

- A loss of iron and protein
- A malabsorption of nutrients, including vitamin A
- Anemia
- A loss of appetite, weakness, and malaise
- Abdominal pain, diarrhea, and dysentery
- Impaired physical growth and development

WHO recommends that people who live in areas with a baseline prevalence of soil-transmitted helminths of 20 percent or more should be treated once yearly with albendazole or mebendazole through a program of mass drug administration. WHO recommends twice-yearly treatment for people who live in places with baseline prevalence of 50 percent or more. The drugs are safe, easy to administer by non-health personnel, and have few side effects.[126] The pharmaceutical companies GlaxoSmithKline and Johnson & Johnson donate these drugs to the global NTD program, and WHO provides them for free to any country that needs them.[127]

The global target for addressing soil-transmitted helminths is to eliminate by 2020 morbidity in children that is due to these infections. To achieve this target, 75 percent of all children in endemic areas need to be treated annually as recommended. As of 2016, about 68 percent of children at risk were being treated.[126]

Schistosomiasis is also prevalent in some subtropical environments, and over 90 percent of those at risk live in Africa. Schistosomiasis is caused by a liver fluke. People with schistosomiasis release fluke eggs in their urine or feces. The flukes infect freshwater snails. When humans swim, bathe, or work in water with infected snails, the fluke can penetrate their skin. One form of fluke manifests itself in the intestinal tract (intestinal schistosomiasis) and liver and another in the urinary tract (urogenital schistosomiasis); both can cause severe disease.[115]

Like many of the other NTDs, schistosomiasis is largely prevalent in poorer communities that lack access to safe water and sanitation. People are infected during work that brings them in contact with water that is infested. Young children that play in such water are at particular risk as well. WHO estimates that about 206 million people, in 52 countries, live in areas that require preventive treatment for schistosomiasis.[128]

Schistosomiasis can lead to a number of morbidities. A classic sign of the urogenital disease is blood in the urine. However, it can have much more severe consequences in females, including cervical and vaginal lesions, vaginal bleeding, nodules in the vulva, and pain during sexual intercourse. In some places with high disease endemicity, women have female genital schistosomiasis, which is a risk factor for HIV. Men can also get genital schistosomiasis, which can affect their seminal vesicles, prostate, and other organs. Intestinal schistosomiasis can lead to abdominal pain, diarrhea, blood in the stool, and enlargement of the liver and spleen. Schistosomiasis can also lead to death.[129]

Efforts to reduce the burden of schistosomiasis are based on preventive treatment of people in at-risk areas with prizquantel. This should be complemented by improving access to safe water and sanitation, health education and hygiene, and vector control. Treatment frequency is based on the intensity of infection in school-age children. It could be yearly and has to be repeated for many years. The drug is safe and effective. Some of the needed drug is donated to national programs, and WHO is working with private sector partners to increase the supply of such drugs. In 2016, about 36 percent of all people and 54 percent of school-age children who should have received preventative chemotherapy against schistosomiasis received such treatment.[128]

The cycle of transmission for *lymphatic filariasis* is very different from that for the helminthic infections. In this case, mosquitoes bite infected humans and pick up the larvae, which develop inside the mosquito and migrate to the insect's mouth. When this mosquito bites a human, it transmits the hatched larvae into the skin. Larvae can survive in the lymphatic system for up to 6 years, and when they die, they cause the severe disfigurement associated with lymphatic filariasis.[115]

Some infections are asymptomatic, but still damage the lymph systems and kidneys and alter the immune system. When lymphatic filariasis becomes chronic, it leads to swelling (**lymph edema**), skin/tissue thickening (**elephantiasis**), and scrotal swelling in men (**hydrocele**). It can also involve the breasts. The disease can also lead to bacterial infections of the skin and periodic inflammation of the skin, lymph nodes, and lymphatic tissues, which can be debilitating.[130]

WHO also recommends large-scale preventive chemotherapy through mass drug administration for lymphatic filariasis, with the specific drug regimen depending on the endemicity of onchocerciasis or another parasitic infection, **Loa loa**[130]:

- Albendazole alone is recommended in settings where loaisis (the *Loa loa* parasite) is endemic.
- Ivermectin with albendazole is recommended in areas in which onchocerciasis is endemic.
- Diethylcarbamazine citrate (DEC) plus albendazole is recommended in settings without onchocerciasis.

Some countries have successfully stopped transmission by carrying out preventive chemotherapy by fortifying salt with DEC. In other settings, treatment with two drugs over 4 to 6 years has also been able to interrupt transmission.[130] Two pharmaceutical companies, Merck and Pfizer, have donated drugs for the program against lymphatic filariasis.[127]

In addition to preventive chemotherapy, WHO recommends a package of care to deal with the morbidities associated with lymphatic filariasis:

- Treatment for **adenolymphangitis (ADL)** as it arises
- Guidance in simple measures to manage lymphedema to prevent progression of disease and debilitating, inflammatory episodes of ADL
- Surgery for hydrocele
- Treatment with anti-filarial medicines for infected people

Vector control such as insecticide-treated bednets, indoor residual spraying, and personal protection, as are done for malaria, may also help people avoid infection.[130]

Fourteen countries have eliminated lymphatic filariasis as a public health problem. Seven additional countries no longer have to carry out mass preventive chemotherapy. Overall, in fact, the population requiring such therapy has been reduced by 36 percent since 2000. Nonetheless, there are 52 countries in which some preventive chemotherapy is needed, but not all of them are carrying out such treatment.[130]

The black fly that causes **onchocerciasis**—usually called "river blindness"—carries the larvae from person to person through bites in the skin. These become adult worms, and the females release millions of small larvae into the body, where they can migrate to the skin, eyes, and other organs. The disease manifests itself as a skin and eye disease. In some cases the disease produces severe itching and skin changes. People may also develop eye lesions that cause visual impairment or permanent blindness.[131]

Onchocerciasis is mainly a tropical disease. About 99 percent of those infected are found in 31 countries in sub-Saharan Africa. However, the disease is also found in Brazil, Venezuela, and Yemen. The Global Burden of Disease study estimated that in 2017 that almost 21 million people were infected with this disease, almost 15 million of those infected had skin manifestations, and over 1 million had vision loss caused by the disease.[131]

There are no drugs or vaccines that can prevent onchocerciasis. WHO recommends that countries treat onchocerciasis yearly through mass drug administration for 10 to 15 years with ivermectin. As with lymphatic filariasis, this treatment regimen, however, has to be adjusted in places in which *Loa loa* is endemic, because people with high levels of *Loa loa* may have severe reactions to invermectin. Such treatment through mass drug administration should be what is called "community directed." Treatment should be combined with vector control, as appropriate.[131]

Since 1987, Merck and Pfizer have made a commitment to donate the needed ivermectin for the control of onchocerciasis.[127]

There has been substantial progress in reducing the burden of onchocerciasis. The Onchocerciasis Control Program (OCP) that ran from 1974 to 2002 addressed 40 million infections, prevented 600,000 cases of blindness, and allowed more than 25 million hectares of land to be returned to agricultural use. The African Program for the Control of Onchocerciasis (APOC) ran from 1995 until 2015. APOC treated 119 million people in its last year and important pockets of endemicity in Uganda and South Sudan no longer require treatment. Important progress has also been made in eliminating onchocerciasis in the Americas with twice-yearly treatment with ivermectin. Yet, despite progress, only about 70 percent of the people who should be covered by community-directed treatment with ivermectin are actually receiving treatment.[131]

Trachoma is a disease of the eye that is caused by the bacteria *Chlamydia trachomatis*. It is transmitted when someone comes in contact with discharge from the eyes or nose, usually by touch. However, flies that have been in contact with discharge from the eyes and nose can also spread the disease from person to person.[122]

About 158 million people in 37 countries are thought to live in trachoma-endemic areas. Trachoma is the leading infectious cause of blindness globally. It is responsible for 1.9 million people being visually impaired or blind. Repeated bouts of infection can cause the eyelashes of the infected person to bend down. If untreated, these can rub the surface of the eye, causing considerable discomfort and permanently damaging the eye. The blindness caused by trachoma is irreversible.[122]

Young children are especially susceptible to active trachoma infection, and prevalence declines with age. In highly endemic areas, 60 percent to 90 percent of young children may be affected. Blindness can occur in childhood but is more likely to occur when people are between 30 and 40 years of age. The most important risk factors for trachoma are crowded households, poor hygiene, a lack of water, and poor sanitation. Trachoma is hyperendemic in 37 countries of Africa, Central and South America, Asia, the Middle East, and Australia, with Africa being the most affected region.[122]

In 1997, WHO developed a strategy known as SAFE (Surgery, Antibiotics, Face washing, Environmental change) to combat trachoma worldwide. Surgery is done to treat the blinding stage of the disease. Mass drug administration with azithromycin is done to clear infection. Facial cleanliness is promoted, as is improved access to water and sanitation.[122] The drugs for this program are donated by Pfizer through the International Trachoma Initiative.[127]

The program was particularly effective in Morocco, where the SAFE strategy was the first to be tested at the national level. Through the donation of over $72 million worth of drugs by Pfizer to treat trachoma, as well as interventions to improve environmental hygiene, the prevalence of trachoma declined by an extraordinary 99 percent.[132] Trachoma in Morocco is discussed in one of the following case studies.

In addition, as of 2018, 12 countries had met their elimination goals for trachoma. In 2017, 226,000 people received surgery in Africa alone for trachoma, and 95 million people were treated with antibiotics against the disease. Nonetheless, there remain important gaps in implementing the SAFE program. Despite the fact that the share of those in need of antibiotic treatment rose from 30 percent in 2015 to 52 percent in 2017, almost 50 percent of those needing treatment are not receiving it.[122]

Future Challenges

The successes against NTDs thus far suggest that considerable additional progress can be made, rapidly and at relatively low cost, to combat the exceptional number of cases of NTDs that remain worldwide. However, further progress is likely to require concerted action in a number of areas, including scaling up the treatment package, focusing on deworming, integrating NTD control with other programs and universal health coverage, and developing new technologies to address NTD control.

It is essential to continue to scale up the treatment package referred to earlier in order to address the NTDs discussed here. The basic recommended package of drugs to be used in settings where one or more of these diseases is present is shown in **TABLE 13-19**.

In sub-Saharan Africa, the projected overall cost of the program is about 50 cents per person per year, as noted earlier, which would be a best buy in global health, given its low cost and large impact on public health.

Following the lessons of the onchocerciasis program and others, this package can be implemented rapidly with the help of medicine distributors who are chosen from among members of the affected communities, through community-directed treatment. They are brought into the program through social mobilization activities. These efforts unite key actors from the public and private sectors in a partnership and seek to involve affected communities in the design, implementation, and monitoring of the program.[133] This type of community-directed treatment for onchocerciasis with ivermectin has proven particularly successful in rural Africa.[131] In fact, a study done in 2008 showed that community-directed interventions are much more effective than conventional delivery approaches, which have less community participation, in combating most communicable diseases in sub-Saharan Africa.[133]

Periodic deworming of young children is also a best buy in global health and should be a major focus of attention.[134] Deworming is the single most

TABLE 13-19 Summary NTD Treatment for Selected Endemicity Scenarios

Medicine Set	Endemicity Scenario				Recommended Combination of Medicines
	STH	LF	SCH	ONCHO	Medicines
A	✓	✓	✓	✓	ALB + IVM + PZQ
B	✓	✓		✓	ALB + IVM
C	✓	✓	✓		ALB + DEC + PZQ
D	✓	✓			ALB + DEC
E	✓				ALB/MBD

Note: ALB = albendazole; DEC = diethylcarbamazine; IVM = ivermectin; LF = lymphatic filariasis; MBD = mebendazole; ONCHO = onchocerciasis; PZQ = praziquantel; SCH = schistosomiasis; STH = soil-transmitted helminths
The Rapid Impact Package would also include azithromycin to treat trachoma.
Data from Weaver, S. D. (2008). *The ABCs of NTDs*. Presentation at the USAID Mini-University, September 12, 2008.

cost-effective means to improve school attendance. There is also historical evidence that deworming improves children's cognitive skills and their potential to learn and leads to greater literacy and higher productivity among adults.[135] In addition, recent studies have shown that deworming children may significantly reduce the burden of malaria, because children infected with ascariasis are twice as likely to get severe malaria as children who are not infected.[136]

Moreover, there are considerable opportunities in regions of high prevalence of malaria and HIV/AIDS for effectively integrating NTD treatment programs with existing HIV and malaria control programs. This integration could help to reduce the burden of NTDs and the burden of HIV/AIDS and malaria, while improving the cost-effectiveness of all programs. This is especially important because hookworm and schistosomiasis often worsen the effects of malaria.[137] The distribution of bednets and treatment for NTDs such as onchocerciasis and lymphatic filariasis could also help to control malaria and vice versa. Such a program led to a substantial improvement in the use of bednets in central Nigeria, where insecticide-treated bednet distribution was combined with mass drug administration for treatment of lymphatic filariasis and onchocerciasis.[138]

As we look to the longer run, it is also important to invest in the search for new technologies that could help to address NTDs in more effective and efficient ways. A safe and effective hookworm vaccine, particularly one that would confer lifelong immunity, would eliminate the need to provide medicine for deworming twice a year to all children living in affected areas, which is a substantial undertaking. The development of a vaccine for schistosomiasis is also being carried out by the Institut Pasteur and could also be of great benefit.

It is also critical to develop new drugs to combat the NTDs. The world is now essentially dependent on only four drugs to address the seven NTDs discussed here. There is resistance to some of the drugs, and more extensive use of them could lead to additional resistance. Developing drugs that can combat the NTDs more effectively than the present drugs continues to be a goal of considerable importance.[139]

At the same time as countries seek to prevent and treat NTDs broadly through programs of mass drug administration or treatment of specific diseases, they need to work with communities to address the underlying risks for NTDs. For the NTDs discussed here, these risks overwhelmingly relate to the unsanitary living conditions of the poor. It will remain important for people to better understand the importance of good

hygiene, to have better access to safe water and sanitary disposal of human waste, and to eliminate worm and parasite breeding sites. In the long run, progress in all of these directions will help to reduce the burden of NTDs and sustain such reductions. Unfortunately, however, these developments are not likely to take place quickly. The fastest and most cost-effective route to reducing the burden of NTDs will be to implement the package of prevention and treatment discussed in this chapter as quickly as possible.

▶ Case Studies

The first case discusses the One Health approach, which is fundamental to the control of communicable diseases, some of which are zoonotic in origin. The next case concerns control of HIV/AIDS in Thailand. An additional case addresses a program to control TB in China. This is followed by a case that reviews efforts to control trachoma in Morocco. The last case concerns a recent West African Ebola outbreak.

One Health

Throughout the late 20th and early 21st centuries, many emerging and re-emerging zoonoses have caused epidemics worldwide, including HIV, Ebola, SARS, and Zika. These epidemics have called attention to the need for multiple sectors to address the link between animal and human health. At the same time, there has been an increasing awareness of the role of agriculture, climate change, and other environmental factors in shaping the emergence of these diseases. As population growth, migration patterns, and global warming disrupt the interactions between animals and humans, many anticipate that the rate at which zoonoses emerge will accelerate, perhaps causing an epidemic of catastrophic proportions. The term *One Health* was coined in the early 2000s to describe a growing movement that emphasizes the interrelatedness of human, animal, and environmental health.[140]

One Health is defined by the One Health Commission as:

> a collaborative, multi-sectoral, and transdisciplinary approach, working locally, regionally, nationally, and globally, to achieve optimal health and well-being of all animals, people, plants and their shared environment, recognizing their inextricable interconnections.[141]

Or, put more simply by the One Health Initiative, One Health is:

> a worldwide strategy for expanding interdisciplinary collaborations and communications in all aspects of health care for humans, animals and the environment.[142]

Although One Health has been formally defined in recent years, it is worth noting that health practitioners throughout history—from Hippocrates's day 2,500 years ago to the present—have acknowledged the relationship between animal health, human health, and the environment.[143]

There are several important recent trends in how humans interact with animals and their environment that One Health addresses. First, as the human population expands, more people will live in areas where they are in contact with wildlife, increasing the probability that zoonoses will spread between animals and humans. Second, due to increased deforestation, industrial farming, and carbon emissions, climate change has created many disruptions that can generate new chances for disease transmission. Finally, more trade and travel also means that there are more opportunities for diseases to spread. These recent shifts highlight the need for the One Health approach to bring together individuals from different disciplines to address shifts in how humans and animals interface with each other and their environment.[144]

In practice, the One Health approach has helped to more effectively control, monitor, and mitigate the effects of many different diseases. One example comes from the case of Rift Valley fever virus in East Africa.[145]

Rift Valley fever virus is an infectious disease spread to both humans and livestock through mosquito bites, or by the exchange of blood or tissue between animals and humans. Many outbreaks of Rift Valley fever virus occur during years of heavy rains, when pooled water creates opportunities for infected mosquito eggs to hatch. Although most infections result only in a few days of fever and achy joints, some can become more serious, leading to blindness, hemorrhagic fever, and even death.

In 1997–1998, a serious outbreak of Rift Valley fever occurred in Kenya, Somalia, and Tanzania during a particularly rainy season caused by El Niño weather patterns.[146] The outbreak sickened 90,000 people and killed almost 500. Many livestock also died as a result of the Rift Valley fever outbreak, causing economic hardship for many families.[147] This incident prompted a multifaceted, "One Health" approach to preventing further outbreaks.

First, Assaf Anyamba, a NASA-funded scientist in Kenya, began using satellite images to track vegetation growth: a proxy for the water pooling conditions that allow mosquitos carrying Rift Valley fever virus to proliferate.[148] Based on these images, Anyamba and his team compiled "risk maps" that predicted the areas in which Rift Valley fever virus was most likely to appear. These maps, combined with data on ocean temperatures associated with El Niño rains, predicted an outbreak of Rift Valley fever virus in the fall of 2006. As a result, governments in East Africa were more prepared to address the cases of the disease that broke out in December 2007.[146]

In addition to using weather patterns to predict Rift Valley fever outbreaks, immunizing livestock against Rift Valley fever has also mitigated the spread of the disease. Although there is currently no human vaccine against Rift Valley fever virus, a vaccine against the virus has been developed for the immunization of livestock.[145] By vaccinating animals against Rift Valley fever virus, disease transmission to humans can be reduced, albeit indirectly. Ultimately, the use of One Health strategies in addressing Rift Valley fever virus highlights how collaboration across sectors can create new ways of approaching the prevention and control of infectious diseases.

Despite successes in using a One Health approach, many challenges remain in this field. Critics have called attention to the broadness of the definition of One Health as a barrier to creating a clear agenda for action.[148] Although many organizations and agencies have sought to promote One Health through agreements, resolutions, and declarations, One Health still lacks a formal institutional home, which has resulted in the fragmentation of some One Health efforts.[148] In addition, although One Health is intended to be an interdisciplinary field, the main actors in this field have been veterinary medicine and animal health experts, with less input from experts in other disciplines. In the future, it is important that One Health efforts seek to resolve these challenges to ensure the movement achieves its maximal impact.

Preventing HIV/AIDS and Sexually Transmitted Infections in Thailand[149]

Background

In Thailand in 2002, approximately 1 in every 60 persons were infected with HIV/AIDS and 75,000 children had been orphaned by AIDS. Between 1989 and 1990, HIV among sex workers tripled, from 3.1 percent to 9.3 percent, and a year later reached 15 percent. Over the same period, the proportion of male conscripts already infected with HIV when tested upon entry to the army at age 21 rose sixfold, from 0.5 percent in 1989 to 3 percent in 1991.

The Intervention

In 1989, Dr. Wiwat Rojanapithayakorn, director of a regional office for communicable disease control in Thailand's Ratchaburi province, sought to curb AIDS by making sex in brothels safe, going well beyond the government's approach of raising awareness through mass advertising and education campaigns. Knowing that he could be effective only with political support, he sought the cooperation of the provincial governor. The steep rise in HIV/AIDS persuaded the governor to acquiesce, even though prostitution is illegal in Thailand and the government's intervention could imply that it tolerated or even condoned it.

A program was launched with one straightforward rule for all brothels in Ratchaburi: no condom, no sex. Until then, brothels had been reluctant to insist that their clients use condoms for fear of losing them to other establishments where condoms were not required. However, with condoms mandatory in all brothels, the competitive disincentive to individual workers and brothels was removed. Health officials, with the help of the police, held meetings with brothel owners and sex workers to provide them with information and free condoms. Men seeking treatment for sexually transmitted infections (STIs) were asked to name the brothel they had last visited, and health officials would then visit the establishment to provide more information. This pilot program had dramatic results, bringing down STIs in Ratchaburi within just a few months. In 1991, the National AIDS Committee, chaired by Prime Minister Anand Panyarachun, adopted this 100 percent condom program at the national level.

The Impact

Condom use in brothels nationwide increased from 14 percent in early 1989 to more than 90 percent by June 1992. An estimated 200,000 new infections were averted between 1993 and 2000. New STI cases fell from 200,000 in 1989 to 15,000 in 2001, and the rate of new HIV infections fell fivefold between 1991 and 1993–1995. Such dramatic results have raised questions about their accuracy, as well as about their real causes, but independent studies have found the program to be genuinely effective.

The program did little to encourage the use of condoms in casual but noncommercial sex. Interventions among injecting drug users also did not expand to the national level, and the prevalence of HIV among this group rose as high as 50 percent.

Costs and Benefits

Total government expenditure on the AIDS program remained steady at approximately $375 million from 1998 to 2001, representing 1.9 percent of the health budget. Of this, 65 percent was spent on treatment and care.

Lessons Learned

The success of the program was due, in part, to the sheer scale and level of organization of the sex industry in Thailand, assisting officials in tracing and coopting brothel owners. Thailand also had a good network of STI services within a well-functioning health system, providing treatment and advice, as well as crucial data for decision makers both at the baseline and when the program took effect. Cooperation among health authorities, governors, and the police was critical to success. Strong leadership from the prime minister, backed by significant financial resources, also made swift action possible. Maintaining Thailand's remarkable results in slowing the AIDS epidemic needs continued vigilance. Due to the high cost of treating STIs, the HIV prevention budget declined by two-thirds between 1997 and 2004. Although the Thai experience provides no blueprint for other countries with very different starting conditions, it does demonstrate that targeted strategies and political courage can effect change in deeply entrenched behaviors.

Controlling TB in China[150]
Background

Although China established a national tuberculosis program in 1981, inadequate financial support hindered its success. In 1991, with a $58 million loan from the World Bank, China embarked on the largest effort in TB control in history: the 10-year Infectious and Endemic Disease Control project in 13 of its 31 mainland provinces. The project adopted the DOTS (directly observed therapy, short course) strategy, which was central to the TB control strategy at the time. Individuals demonstrating TB symptoms were referred to county dispensaries, where they received free diagnosis and treatment. Village doctors were given financial incentives for enrolling patients and completing their treatment. Efforts were also made to strengthen the institutions involved with the establishment of a national tuberculosis project office and a tuberculosis control center. Quarterly reports were submitted by each county to the province, the central government, and the National Tuberculosis Project Office, which strengthened monitoring and quality control.

Impact

China achieved a 95 percent cure rate for new cases within 2 years of adopting DOTS, and a remarkable cure rate of 90 percent for those who had previously undergone unsuccessful treatment. The number of people with TB declined by over 37 percent between 1990 and 2000, and 30,000 TB deaths were prevented each year. More than 1.5 million patients were treated, leading to the elimination of 836,000 cases of pulmonary TB.

Costs and Benefits

The program cost $130 million. The World Bank and WHO estimated that successful treatment was achieved at a cost of less than $100 per person. One healthy life was saved for an estimated $15 to $20, with an economic return of $60 for each dollar invested.

Lessons Learned

The success of China's program can be attributed to strong political commitment, leadership, adequate funding, and a sound technical approach delivered through a relatively strong health system. It was found that DOTS could be scaled up rapidly without sacrificing quality. Free diagnosis and treatment served as an effective incentive for patients, and incentives for doctors to diagnose and complete treatment also worked well. However, the overall rate of case detection proved disappointing, mainly due to the inadequate referral of suspected TB cases from hospitals to TB dispensaries; hospitals charging for services had no incentive to refer patients to dispensaries where services were provided for free. In addition, patients at hospitals often abandoned treatment prematurely. Despite the program's success, TB remains a deadly threat in China, and efforts continue to maintain cure rates, as well as to expand TB coverage to the remaining population.

Controlling Trachoma in Morocco[151]

Background

Trachoma is the second leading cause of blindness, after cataracts, and the number one cause of preventable blindness in the world. Although it has been eliminated in North America and Europe, trachoma still afflicted more than 41 million people in 57 countries in 2003, especially in hot, dry regions where access to clean water, sanitation, and health care is limited. In Morocco, trachoma was once widespread, but in the 1970s and 1980s, treatment with antibiotics lowered its incidence in urban areas. A 1992 survey found that 5.4 percent of Moroccans still suffered from trachoma, mainly in five rural provinces in the southeast, where 25,000 people showed a serious decline in vision, 625,000 needed treatment for inflammatory trachoma, and 40,000 urgently required surgery.

The Intervention

Caused by the bacterium *Chlamydia trachomatis*, trachoma is highly contagious, spreading mainly among children through direct contact with eye and nose secretions, infected clothing, and fluid-seeking flies. Transmission of the disease is rapid in overcrowded conditions of poor hygiene and poverty. In endemic areas, prevalence rates in children ages 2 to 5 years can reach 90 percent. Women are infected at a rate two to three times that of men because of their close contact with children. Repeated trachoma infections can lead to a painful in-turning of the eyelash, which can cause blindness.

In 1991, Morocco formed the National Blindness Control Program (NBCP) with several international and other agencies to eliminate trachoma by 2005. Between 1997 and 1999, this program implemented a pilot strategy to treat trachoma, developed by the Edna McConnell Clark Foundation, called SAFE (surgery, antibiotics, face washing, and environmental change). SAFE differed from earlier approaches by emphasizing behavioral and environmental change, in addition to medication. Under this four-part strategy, a quick and inexpensive surgery to prevent blindness was provided for large numbers of patients in small towns and villages. Antibiotics were used to treat infection and prevent scarring. Face washing, especially among children, was promoted through an education campaign. Living conditions and community hygiene were improved by constructing latrines, drilling wells, storing dung away from flies, and providing health education.

In the mid-1990s, Pfizer discovered Zithromax (azithromycin), a one-dose cure to replace the 6-week course of tetracycline that had been used for treatment, ensuring a higher compliance rate. Pfizer donated the drug for Morocco, as well as for a number of other countries, through the International Trachoma Initiative (ITI), a private–public partnership that it forged along with the Clark Foundation.

Impact

Between 1999 and 2003, the SAFE strategy led to a 75 percent decline in trachoma in Morocco. Overall, the prevalence of active disease in children under 10 was reduced by 90 percent since 1997.

Costs and Benefits

The Moroccan government provided most of the financing for the program. ITI supplemented this with several grants, and UNICEF contributed $225,000. Pfizer's donation of tens of millions of dollars' worth of Zithromax (azithromycin) to Morocco and other countries represents one of the largest donations of a patented drug in history.

Lessons Learned

Government commitment to the program was critical to its success, in addition to the array of effective interventions. Four key factors were also listed by ITI: the program was based on solid scientific evidence; it was locally organized and, therefore, responded well to local circumstances; it fit within a broader agenda of health promotion, disease control, and health equity; and treatment was closely linked with prevention and the development of a strong public health infrastructure. ITI and its many partners have helped ensure that Morocco's success with SAFE, like the disease that it has nearly eliminated, is contagious.

The West African Ebola Outbreak of 2014 to 2016

Background

Ebola hemorrhagic fever is caused by the Ebola virus. From its emergence in 1976 until January 2015, Ebola had infected around 25,000 people, all of whom were in Africa, were exposed to someone who acquired the disease in Africa, or were involved in a laboratory accident.[152] As of January 31, 2015, 42.6 percent of those ever infected died of the disease (10,848 deaths).[153,24] However, in some outbreaks the case fatality ratio has been as high as 90 percent. Although there are five types of Ebola virus, only three have been responsible for human outbreaks: *Zaire ebolavirus*, *Sudan ebolavirus*, and *Bundibugyo ebolavirus*.[152]

Ebola is characterized by flulike symptoms, diarrhea, vomiting, and massive hemorrhaging. The incubation period ranges from 2 to 21 days, although symptoms usually begin 8 to 10 days after infection.[154]

The disease is transmitted by exposure to bodily fluids such as blood, saliva, vomit, diarrhea, or semen. However, the disease cannot be transmitted prior to the onset of symptoms. There is no specific cure for Ebola. However, a number of vaccines are under development. One was tried in Guinea in 2015 and another has been used in the 2018/19 outbreak in the Democratic Republic of the Congo.[155,156]

The populations affected have traditionally been medical workers and poor, rural residents of the Democratic Republic of the Congo (DRC), Uganda, South Sudan, the Republic of the Congo (ROC), and Gabon. In previous outbreaks, 10 percent to 25 percent of the cases have been medical workers. Of the 2,348 cases prior to 2014, 41 percent were in the DRC, 25 percent in Uganda, 14 percent in South Sudan, 10 percent in the ROC, and 9 percent in Gabon.[152]

Many believe the main risk factor for initial infection is exposure to sick or dead animals, in particular bats and primates in the forest. Fruit bats are thought to be the natural host of the virus.[157] Once an outbreak has begun, the risk factors for infection include direct contact with symptomatic patients at home or using improper safety procedures in medical facilities.

From 1976 until 2015, there were 35 distinct outbreaks of Ebola. The first outbreak occurred in northwestern DRC, centered around the Yambuku mission. Another large outbreak occurred in the DRC in 1995, infecting 315 individuals and killing 81 percent of those ill.[152] Roughly one-fourth of those infected were healthcare workers.[158] During the first outbreak of Ebola in 1976, 26.7 percent of the cases were infected by accidental needle stick or by reuse of unsanitized needles used on other Ebola patients. Person-to-person transmission accounted for 46.9 percent of the cases. Much of the person-to-person transmission occurs during the process of caring for sick family members or during funeral procedures in which individuals are in close contact with the deceased.[159]

The West African Outbreak of 2014

To date, the 2014 West African outbreak of Ebola is the largest and most complex outbreak ever of the disease. By the end of the outbreak in 2016, there were 28,610 cases and 11,208 deaths.[153] This was the first outbreak of Ebola seen in West Africa and the first to affect major urban centers. The viral strain was *Zaire ebolavirus*, which is very closely related to strains previously seen in the DRC and Gabon.[160]

The outbreak was initially reported in Guinea on March 24, 2014. As of January 31, 2015, Nigeria, Senegal, Spain, the United States, the United Kingdom, Mali, Sierra Leone, and Liberia had also been affected.[24] By early February 2015, however, transmission was ongoing only in Sierra Leone, Liberia, and Guinea. The case fatality rate of around 40 percent was less than in previous outbreaks.

Among other international partners, the primary actors in the outbreak response were the health ministries of the affected countries, the U.S. Centers for Disease Control and Prevention (CDC), WHO, the United Nations (UN), Médecins Sans Frontières (MSF), and UNICEF.

Epidemic Control

Based on previous outbreaks, the best practices for control include community education about safe home care and burial practices, proper hospital safety and sanitation procedures, case management and isolation, laboratory confirmation of cases, and active disease surveillance.

Control efforts for this outbreak were largely consistent with these practices. On August 8, 2014, roughly 8 months after the first case was believed to have occurred and 5 months after the first cases were reported, WHO assigned the Ebola outbreak its highest threat level: public health emergency of international concern.[161] The CDC also deployed staff to all affected countries and Doctors Without Borders (MSF) provided 302 international staff and hired 3,600 local staff at eight Ebola case-management centers.[162] The governments of Sierra Leone, Liberia, and Guinea all instituted travel restrictions and border closures to neighboring countries.

Such efforts had little effect on the outbreak until October 2014, when the overall epidemic hit its peak.[163] The number of cases from then until January 2015 steadily dropped; the week of January 18, 2015, to January 25, 2015, was the first time since June 2014 that the weekly incidence of cases was less than 100.[164] Liberia especially saw a drop in cases, having only 4 during that same week.[163]

The initial failure of control efforts can be attributed to four challenges in this region: poor public health surveillance and border control, lack of medical personnel and supplies, lack of coordination in response, and lack of regional experience and education about the disease. In addition, many believe the international response was late and initially insufficient.

Beginning in 2007, 194 WHO member states instituted the revised International Health Regulations (IHR) in order to coordinate and develop countries'

detection and response capabilities for infectious diseases such as Ebola.[165] However, 80 percent of the ratifying countries, including those affected in this outbreak, had not met their IHR responsibilities by the time of this outbreak.[166] Such inaction on IHR principles affected active case finding and border control. WHO estimated that the actual case count was 2 to 4 times higher than that reported, simply because mobilizing resources for case finding was so challenging.[167] In addition, although border screening and travel bans were enforced, 34 percent of the new cases, as of September 2014, were still occurring in the cross-border region of Sierra Leone, Liberia, and Guinea, indicating a high level of border permeability.[168]

As with previous bouts of Ebola, healthcare staff were particularly affected, making up around 10 percent of the fatalities. Supplies of personal protective equipment and clinic capacity were also grossly inadequate in most areas.[169] Although MSF had eight Ebola treatment centers with a total capacity of 650 beds, the organization reported that it had reached its operational limit numerous times throughout the outbreak. Many individuals thus remained home for care instead of being cared for in a treatment center. UNICEF provided crucial medical resources; however, the procurement of such supplies was hindered by the speed with which they could be produced.[170] In addition, airline travel bans and travel restrictions by countries without ongoing transmission, such as the United States, prevented such supplies from more easily getting into the affected countries. (WHO does not endorse such travel restrictions.)

Furthermore, the lack of education about the disease helped to drive the epidemic. Some families continued to perform burial ceremonies at home; this was responsible for nearly 60 percent of the cases in Guinea.[169] Also, due to a lack of confidence in allopathic medicine and the government, several communities rioted or denied access to healthcare workers. Out of fear of further spread, some violently threatened medical staff and "set free" isolated patients in hospitals.[171]

Meeting Future Challenges

On August 28, 2014, WHO organized its plan for the end of the outbreak in 6 to 9 months in its Ebola Response Roadmap. The tenets of this plan were reiterated in the UN STEPP Strategy from September 2014, which set the primary goals as Stop the outbreak, Treat the infected, Ensure essential services, Preserve stability, and Prevent outbreaks in unaffected countries.[172]

From November 2014 to the end of January 2015, the incidence rate of disease declined. Given this

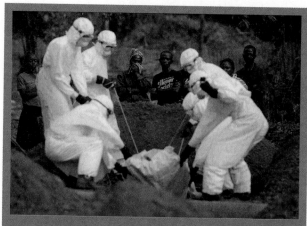

PHOTO 13-5 Addressing an Ebola epidemic requires major changes in people's burial practices, as shown here, in Liberia. What measures need to be taken to build support within affected communities to make needed changes on such culturally sensitive matters?
© John Moore/Getty Images News/Getty Images.

changing epidemiology, which defied most previous estimates of what would occur, on January 21, 2015, the United Nations Office for the Coordination of Humanitarian Affairs released an updated strategy for January to June 2015. This new strategy built upon STEPP. It aimed to reallocate resources in order to prioritize treatment and safe burial practices in areas with high ongoing transmission and to enforce contact tracing in areas with lower risk.[172] After December 17, 2014, MSF also carried out clinical trials for a new drug, favipiravir, from its treatment center in Guéckédou, Guinea. Such a drug, if effective, could have an impact on this and future outbreaks of Ebola.[173]

However, prevention of such a situation in the future is more dependent on ameliorating the fundamental causes of Ebola outbreaks: poor education, poor sanitation, and unsafe burials. As the epidemic waned in Liberia, cases continued in Guinea and Sierra Leone. Future responses will also be aided by a vaccine against Ebola, which was used for the first time in this outbreak.[153] Liberia's early success illustrates the action needed to prevent outbreaks in the future. It is believed that Liberia, which saw a dramatic drop in cases in mid-October 2014, may have benefited from an earlier receipt of foreign resources due to an earlier spike in cases. This enabled the hiring of more safe burial teams and medical staff. Others believe that the concentration of cases in Monrovia, the capital of Liberia, meant that the epidemic affected a more educated population than the outbreaks in Sierra Leone and Guinea, where cases were primarily in rural and less educated populations.[174] The response of the Liberian people to the epidemic revolved around community engagement

and education. Behaviors changed much more rapidly than in Sierra Leone and Guinea, enabling a steep drop in the country's burden of Ebola.

▶ Additional Comments on Future Challenges to the Control of Communicable Diseases

A number of challenges constrain efforts to address the burden of the most important communicable diseases. Some of these relate to the need for countries to cooperate to combat communicable diseases. Some concern the ability of weak health systems in low- and middle-income countries to tackle communicable diseases effectively and efficiently. Others relate to the issues raised by specific diseases.

First, it is imperative to enhance political commitment to the prevention and control of these diseases. Sustained political support at the highest levels is essential if continued progress is to be made against the leading causes of communicable disease. Countries will be successful in acting against these diseases only if they make them a real priority both politically and financially.

It will also be critical that the global community continue to collaborate at high levels to prevent, detect, and respond to communicable diseases, including emerging and re-emerging infectious diseases and antimicrobial resistance. These are in many ways the "perfect" global health issues. No country can carry out this work on its own. Rather, the global community must cooperate politically, technically, and financially to address these issues. The present political environment globally raises some important questions about the continued willingness of some countries to stay involved with these matters at the highest levels. Yet, most people believe that there will be new global outbreaks of disease and the only question is when they will occur.

Many of the underlying causes of communicable diseases in low- and middle-income countries relate to poverty, people's lack of empowerment, people's lack of knowledge of appropriate health behaviors, and a lack of access to basic infrastructure such as safe water, sanitation, and health services. These issues will take many years to address in most low-income countries. Ways must be found in the short and medium term to work with communities to overcome some of these constraints, such as through community-based water supply and sanitation schemes and community-based distribution of drugs for neglected diseases.

Efforts to address communicable diseases must increasingly be embedded in the quest for universal health coverage and in the provision of high-quality primary health care. Yet, it is likely that health systems in many low- and middle-income countries will continue to be weak for many years. This suggests that efforts to address communicable diseases will also have to be based on partnerships with a variety of actors. These include communities, religious groups and other nongovernmental organizations, the private sector, and government. The great successes in the control of communicable diseases to date have all been built upon the foundation of public–private partnerships. The polio eradication effort includes, for example, a remarkable amount of public–private collaboration, as did the campaign against onchocerciasis. It is especially important that these actors work together in the future, in a coherent manner, across an array of diseases and health systems issues and not just on individual diseases. Moreover, only by involving private providers of a variety of types can many diseases, such as TB and malaria, be addressed, because these providers are already so involved in service delivery.

Strengthening the surveillance of disease at the local, national, and global levels is also fundamental to effective disease control. A competent body of public health professionals needs to be responsible for managing surveillance networks. Appropriate laboratory infrastructure must be an essential part of any improved surveillance efforts. Continuous sharing of surveillance information within and across countries is necessary to prepare for special problems, to know when they arise, and to respond to them effectively. Many countries still have substantial gaps in their ability to deal with disease outbreaks, and those gaps need to be closed as rapidly as possible.

The lack of adequately trained and appropriately deployed human resources for health will also remain an issue, especially in low-income countries. There will not be enough personnel, the incentives for their performance will be lacking, and the personnel who do exist may largely be available only in the larger cities for some time to come. Thus, it will be important to have the lowest level of worker possible handle various health services so that scarce higher-level workers can focus on the things they alone can do.

Addressing the need for competent healthcare personnel is one element in the imperative to improve the quality of services at all levels. Poor-quality services can harm people and waste money. Yet, they are pervasive across health systems and across disease control efforts. Quality must become the organizing principle for all public health and clinical services.

Scientific and technical challenges also remain. There has been some progress on diagnostics, but there is still considerable need for improved diagnostics, especially those that are relatively inexpensive, easy to use at the point of care, and can diagnose all forms of a disease, such as TB and malaria. Despite some progress toward a malaria vaccine, there are no effective and licensed vaccines for any of the diseases that are the focus of this chapter, except for rotavirus for some forms of diarrhea. In addition, drug resistance is a constant issue across diseases. This highlights the need for vaccines and for new drugs that can prevent or overcome such resistance and shorten existing courses of treatment for TB.

Another challenge will be the need to develop sustainable models in low- and middle-income countries to provide chronic care of people with HIV/AIDS. Most health service efforts in low-income countries focus on acute care. The treatment of HIV with antiretroviral therapy creates the possibility that people who are HIV-positive can have full and productive lives for many years. However, it also means that countries with very weak health systems that are mostly accustomed to treating acute illnesses will have to develop effective and efficient models for treating some people for many years of their life. Such platforms might be able to serve noncommunicable diseases as well.

Over time, climate change could also create a number of important challenges to the control of communicable diseases. Such change could cause shifts in the spread and manifestation, for example, of vector-borne diseases. It could make other diseases, such as waterborne diseases, more or less prevalent, depending on changes in temperature and precipitation.

Another important issue is how low-income and resource-poor countries, especially those with high burdens of disease, will be able to financially sustain their communicable disease programs. There has been an enormous amount of progress in reducing the burden of NTDs and malaria, and the number of new infections with HIV. There has also been considerable success in getting people with HIV on antiretroviral therapy. Yet, in all of these areas and TB, there are large gaps between the number of people needing services and the number who actually receive them. Enormous gaps in the quality of programs also need to be filled. Improving quality and providing increasing shares of people with appropriate services will raise costs. Many of the low-income countries will require external financial assistance for many years to carry out these programs. Yet, such financing in today's political environment cannot be assured.

Monitoring, evaluation, and operational research are essential tools of public health. If the world is to continue to make progress against the most important communicable diseases, then it is important to enhance the quality of monitoring and evaluation of health investments and to learn increasingly what works, at what cost, and in what ways.

▶ Main Messages

In 2016, communicable diseases accounted for about 40 percent of total deaths and 40 percent of DALYs in low-income countries. These diseases are especially prevalent in sub-Saharan Africa, but they also take a major toll in South Asia. Communicable diseases, such as pneumonia, diarrhea, and malaria, pose especially grave threats for young children in many low- and middle-income countries. Malaria also poses an important risk for women of reproductive age, especially in Africa. TB is now the leading infectious cause of death in the world.

Emerging and re-emerging infectious diseases and antimicrobial resistance represent grave threats to public health in all countries. Emerging and re-emerging infectious diseases have the potential to do great economic damage to individual countries and the international community, vastly in excess of their direct impact on morbidity and mortality. Enhancing global cooperation on disease surveillance and on action against these diseases is essential for the effective prevention, detection, and control of emerging and re-emerging infectious diseases. Substantial efforts will be needed by individual countries and globally to promote more rational use of antibiotics and better quality of antibiotics, if the development of resistant forms of bacteria, viruses, and parasites is to be slowed down.

HIV/AIDS is an especially important burden, but the number of people infected with HIV and HIV-related deaths has been declining. Nonetheless, about 37 million people were estimated to be infected with HIV in 2017. In addition, that same year, there were 1.8 million new HIV infections and 940,000 HIV-related deaths.

The HIV/AIDS epidemic has fueled the burden of TB. In 2017, there were about 10 million new cases of active TB disease in the world and 1.6 million deaths from TB. It is also important to note that

WHO estimates that 560,000 of the new TB cases were infected with drug-resistant TB, and more than 80 percent of them have multidrug-resistant TB.

Malaria killed about 435,000 people in 2017, mostly young children in Africa. It also causes a huge burden of morbidity because cases of malaria are so common, and people may get more than one case a year. Malaria also poses very substantial risks to pregnant women. Diarrhea is an especially important burden of disease for children as well, and in 2016 was responsible for about 525,000 child deaths. A number of parasitic and infectious diseases, referred to as "neglected tropical diseases," pose an exceptional burden of disease, again largely in sub-Saharan Africa and South Asia. More than 1 billion people are infected by one or more of these diseases.

The economic and social consequences of the communicable diseases are very considerable. Diarrhea and worms can cause children to fail to develop properly, delay their entry into and performance in school, and reduce their productivity as adults. HIV/AIDS, TB, and malaria also greatly affect adult productivity. The direct and indirect costs of these diseases to individuals and families are very high and often cause people to borrow money, sell their limited assets, and fall below the poverty line. There is good evidence that high levels of malaria have been an impediment to economic growth in low-income countries in Africa.

The "good news" is that there has been, in many respects, an enormous amount of progress in addressing some communicable diseases. The number of new infections and deaths from HIV and malaria have fallen greatly. Diarrhea causes fewer deaths than ever before in young children. It is also promising that there are affordable, cost-effective interventions or packages of interventions that can further reduce the burden of these diseases. Nonetheless, there is also "less good news": most of the remaining infections are preventable or treatable, and there is still an enormous gap between those needing services and those receiving them. There are also major gaps in the quality of services, including the availability and quality of drugs for some diseases. There is also a need to increasingly embed programs of communicable disease control in efforts to achieve universal health coverage.

Addressing HIV/AIDS will require expanding a range of behavioral, biomedical, and structural investments—called *combination prevention*. These need to be tailored in different countries to the nature of their epidemics. Strong political leadership, focusing on the groups most at risk, and addressing the needs of "bridge populations" are also parts of successful prevention efforts. Testing and counseling and condom promotion need to be enhanced, in connection with efforts to delay sexual debut and reduce the number of sexual partners. It is also important to stem the transmission of HIV from mother to child. Male circumcision programs are being expanded, as is the use of pre-exposure drug therapy for selected groups. An increasing number of people are being treated for HIV worldwide, and efforts are under way to meet 90-90-90 targets by 2020—to ensure that 90 percent of those with HIV know their status, to ensure that 90 percent of them are treated, and to ensure that 90 percent of those treated have suppressed viral loads. Effective treatment reduces transmission and reduces the burden of opportunistic infections, such as TB. The earlier people are put on treatment after becoming infected, the fewer people they will infect with HIV.

The global goal is to eliminate TB as a public health problem by 2035. This will require, among other things, vaccination of children with BCG, expanded efforts at early diagnosis and appropriate early treatment of everyone with TB with quality-assured drugs, and enhanced efforts at managing TB/HIV co-infection. Particular attention must also be paid to treating drug-resistant TB. The aim is to link these efforts with greater involvement of communities, improved regulatory frameworks, and improved efforts to address the social determinants of disease. While important progress has been made with traditional tools of diagnosis and new diagnostic tools are being increasingly used, it will also be important to develop improved diagnostics, a more effective TB vaccine, and more effective and shorter course drug regimens. A central focus must also be on improving the quality of all aspects of national TB programs.

Malaria can be addressed through prompt diagnosis and appropriate treatment, intermittent treatment of pregnant women and young infants, the use of insecticide-treated bednets, and indoor residual spraying. These are now being complemented in selected settings with seasonal chemoprevention for children. Proper treatment on the basis of a confirmed diagnosis is essential to reducing the disease burden and to stemming the development of resistance.

The burden of diarrhea can be reduced through immunization against rotavirus and measles and supplementation with zinc. Oral rehydration therapy is a cost-effective way of managing diarrhea in infants and children. The best approach to diarrhea, of course, would be to try to avoid it through improved hygiene. Better access to safe water and sanitation will also help reduce the burden of diarrhea.

The burden of the NTDs discussed in this chapter can largely be addressed through community-based mass drug administration. This can be complemented by the broader SAFE approach for trachoma and care of morbidities for lymphatic filariasis. Of course, addressing the NTDs in the longer run also requires enhanced hygiene and improved access to safe water and sanitation.

The challenge of addressing the burden of communicable diseases effectively is substantial. They are mostly diseases of poverty that also reflect a lack of access to safe water and sanitation, poor knowledge of appropriate health behaviors, and a lack of health services that are geared to meet the highest-priority needs among the poor. In addition, several of these diseases are highly stigmatized, efforts to control them must be carried out in countries with weak health systems, and considerably more financing is needed for these efforts than has been available. Nonetheless, there has been major, and sometimes exceptional, progress in the last 40 years in addressing a number of these diseases and a number of vaccine-preventable diseases in children. The lessons from those experiences suggest that it is possible to continue making such progress.

Study Questions

1. What are the most important communicable diseases in terms of deaths in low- and middle-income countries? In terms of DALYs?
2. In what regions are the deaths from HIV/AIDS the largest, as a share of total deaths? In what regions is the incidence of malaria the highest?
3. What is driving the HIV epidemic in Russia? In sub-Saharan Africa?
4. In sub-Saharan Africa, what would be the most cost-effective measures to try to prevent further transmission of the HIV virus? What approach would you take to prevention in South Asia, and why would it differ from what you would do in sub-Saharan Africa?
5. What groups are especially at risk for malaria? What steps would you take to try to reduce the burden of malaria?
6. What are the most important steps that need to be taken to reduce the burden of TB?
7. If relatively few people die as a direct result of parasitic diseases, why are they so important?

8. What are the concerns about drug resistance for malaria and TB? How can resistance be kept to a minimum?

9. Why is it important to develop a vaccine for HIV?

10. What are the drivers of antimicrobial resistance? What measures could a country take to try to reduce the development of resistance?

References

1. Institute of Health Metrics and Evaluation (IHME). (n.d.). GBD Compare: Viz Hub. Retrieved from https://vizhub.healthdata.org/gbd-compare/

2. World Health Organization (WHO). (2018). *Tuberculosis: Key facts.* Retrieved from https://www.who.int/en/news-room/fact-sheets/detail/tuberculosis

3. World Health Organization (WHO). (2018). *HIV/AIDS: Key facts.* Retrieved from https://www.who.int/news-room/fact-sheets/detail/hiv-aids

4. World Health Organization (WHO). (2018). *Malaria: Key facts.* Retrieved from https://www.who.int/news-room/fact-sheets/detail/malaria

5. World Health Organization (WHO). (2017). *Diarrhoeal disease: Key facts.* Retrieved from https://www.who.int/news-room/fact-sheets/detail/diarrhoeal-disease

6. Jamison, D. T., R. Nugent, H. Gelband, S. Horton, P. Jha, R. Laxminarayan, & C. N. Mock (Eds.). (2018). *Disease control priorities: Improving health and reducing poverty* (3rd ed.). Washington, DC: World Bank Group.

7. Fauci, A. S. (2005). *2005 Robert H. Ebert memorial lecture. Emerging and re-emerging infectious diseases: The perpetual challenge.* New York, NY: Milbank Memorial Fund.

8. Heymann, D. L. (2005). Emerging and re-emerging infectious diseases from plague and cholera to Ebola and AIDS: A potential for international spread that transcends the defenses of any single country. *Journal of Contingencies and Crisis Management, 13*(1), 29–31.

9. Heymann, D. (2008). Emerging and re-emerging infections. In W. Kirch (Ed.), *Encyclopedia of public health.* New York, NY: Springer.

10. Jones, K. E., Patel, N. G., Levy, M. A., Storeygard, A., Balk, D., Gittleman, J. L., & Daszak, P. (2008). Global trends in emerging infectious diseases. *Nature, 451*(7181), 990–993.

11. Heymann, D. L. (2002). The microbial threat in fragile times: Balancing known and unknown risks. *Bulletin of the World Health Organization, 80*(3), 179.

12. Centers for Disease Control and Prevention (CDC). (1998). Preventing emerging infectious diseases: A strategy for the 21st century. *MMWR Morbidity and Mortality Weekly Report, 47*(No. RR-15), 1–14.

13. World Health Organization (WHO). (2014). *Anti-microbial resistance: Global surveillance report 2014.* Geneva, Switzerland: Author.

14. National Institutes of Health. (2009). *Microbial evolution and co-adaptation: A tribute to the life and scientific legacies of Joshua Lederberg. Workshop summary.* Institute of Medicine Forum on Microbial Threats. Washington, DC: National Academies Press.

15. Cohen, M. L. (2000). Changing patterns of infectious diseases. *Nature, 406*, 762–767.

16. Nugent, R., Beck, E., & Beith, A. (2010). *The race against drug resistance.* Washington, DC: Center for Global Development.

17. Okeke, I. N., Laxminarayan, R., Bhutta, Z. A., Duse, A. G., Jenkins, P., O'Brien, T. F., . . . Klugman, K. P. (2005). Antimicrobial resistance in developing countries. Part I: recent trends and current status. *Lancet Infectious Diseases, 5*(8), 481–493.

18. Okeke, I. N., Klugman, K. P., Bhutta, Z. A., Duse, A. G., Jenkins, P., O'Brien, T. F., . . . Laxminarayan, R. (2005). Antimicrobial resistance in developing countries. Part II: strategies for containment. *Lancet Infectious Diseases, 5*(9), 568–580.

19. Laxminarayan, R., Bhutta, Z. A., Duse, A., Jenkins, P., O'Brien, T., Okeke, I. N., …Klugman, K. P. (2006). Drug resistance. In D. T. Jamison, J. G. Breman, A. R. Measham, et al. (Eds.), *Disease control priorities in developing countries* (2nd ed., pp. 1031–1051). New York, NY: Oxford University Press.

20. Snowden, F. M. (2008). Emerging and re-emerging diseases: A historical perspective. *Immunological Reviews, 225*, 9–26.

21. The World Bank. (2014). *The economic impact of the 2014 Ebola epidemic.* Washington, DC: Author.

22. Huber, C., Finelli, L., & Stevens W. (2018). The economic and social burden of the 2014 Ebola outbreak in West Africa. *Journal of Infectious Diseases, 218*(Suppl. 5), S698–S704.

23. Centers for Disease Control and Prevention (CDC). (n.d.). *Severe acute respiratory infection (SARS): Frequently asked questions about SARS.* Retrieved from http://www.cdc.gov/sars/about/faq.html

24. Centers for Disease Control and Prevention (CDC). (2017). *2014–2016 Ebola outbreak in West Africa.* Retrieved from https://www.cdc.gov/vhf/ebola/history/2014-2016-outbreak/index.html

25. World Health Organization (WHO). (2018). *Global tuberculosis report 2018.* Geneva, Switzerland: Author.

26. Centers for Disease Control and Prevention (CDC). (2017). *Drug-resistant TB.* Retrieved from https://www.cdc.gov/tb/topic/drtb/default.htm

27. Médecins Sans Frontières. (2003). *Q&A: ACT NOW to get malaria treatment that works to Africa.* Retrieved from http://www.msf.org/article/qa-act-now-get-malaria-treatment-works-africa

28. Morens, D. M., Folkers, G. K., & Fauci, A. S. (2008). Emerging infections: A perpetual challenge. *Lancet Infectious Diseases, 8*(11), 710–719.

29. World Health Organization (WHO). (2005). *International health regulations* (2nd ed.). Geneva, Switzerland: Author.

30. Lynn, J. (2010, January 12). WHO to review its handling of H1N1 flu pandemic. *Reuters.* Retrieved from http://www.reuters.com/article/idUSTRE5BL2ZT20100112

31. Salaam-Blyther, T. (2014). *U.S. and international health responses to the Ebola outbreak in West Africa.* Washington, DC: Congressional Research Service.

32. Global Health Security Agenda. (n.d.). *About.* Retrieved from https://www.ghsagenda.org/

33. World Health Organization (WHO). (2012). *The evolving threat of antimicrobial resistance: Options for action*. Geneva, Switzerland: Author.

34. Leung, E., Weil, D. E., Raviglione, M., & Nakatani, H., on behalf of the World Health Organization World Health Day Antimicrobial Resistance Technical Working Group. (2011). The WHO policy package to combat antimicrobial resistance. *Bulletin of the World Health Organization, 89*, 290–292.

35. Laxminarayanan, R., Duse, A., Wattal, C., Zaidi, A. K., Wertheim, H. F. L., Sumpradit, N., . . . Cars, O. (2013). Antibiotic resistance—The need for global solutions. *Lancet Infectious Diseases, 13*(12), 1057–1098. doi: 10.1016/S1473-3099(13)70318-9

36. World Health Organization (WHO). (2015). *Global action plan on antimicrobial resistance*. Geneva, Switzerland: Author.

37. World Health Organization (WHO). (2018). *WHO report on surveillance of antibiotic consumption: 2016–2018 early implementation*. Geneva, Switzerland: Author.

38. World Economic Forum. (2019). *Outbreak readiness and business impact protecting lives and livelihoods across the global economy*. Geneva, Switzerland: Author.

39. Mackey, T. K., & Liang, B. A. (2012). Threats from emerging and re-emerging neglected tropical diseases (NTDs). *Infection Ecology and Epidemiology, 2*. doi: 10.3402/iee.v2i0.18667

40. Dash, A. P., Bhatia, R., Sunyoto, T., & Mourya, D. T. (2013). Emerging and re-emerging arboviral diseases in Southeast Asia. *Journal of Vector Borne Diseases, 50*, 77–84.

41. Tacconelli, E., Carrara, E., Savoldi, A. Harbarth, S., Mendelson, M., Monnet, D. L., . . . Magrini, N. (2018). Discovery, research, and development of new antibiotics: The WHO priority list of antibiotic-resistant bacteria and tuberculosis. *Lancet Infectious Diseases, 18*(3), 318–327.

42. Centers for Disease Control and Prevention (CDC). (2018). *Remembering the 1918 influenza pandemic*. Retrieved from https://www.cdc.gov/features/1918-flu-pandemic/index.html

43. Centers for Disease Control and Prevention (CDC). (2018). *Past pandemics*. Retrieved from https://www.cdc.gov/flu/pandemic-resources/basics/past-pandemics.html

44. World Health Organization (WHO). (2019). *Ten threats to global health in 2019*. Retrieved from https://www.who.int/emergencies/ten-threats-to-global-health-in-2019

45. Quick, J. D., & Fryer, B. (2019). *The end of pandemics: The looming threat to humanity and how to stop it*. New York, NY: St. Martin's Press.

46. Gostin, L. O., & Katz, R. (2016). The international health regulations: The governing framework for global health security. *The Milbank Quarterly, 94*(2), 264–313.

47. UNAIDS. (2018). *Fact sheet: World AIDS day 2018*. Retrieved from http://www.unaids.org/sites/default/files/media_asset/UNAIDS_FactSheet_en.pdf

48. Chin, J. (Ed.). (2000). *Control of communicable diseases manual* (17th ed.). Washington, DC: American Public Health Association.

49. Bertozzi, S., Padian, N. S., Wegbreit, J., DeMaria, L. M., Feldman, B., Gayle, H., . . . Isbell, M. T. (2006). HIV/AIDS prevention and treatment. In D. T. Jamison, J. G. Breman, A. R. Measham, et al. (Eds.), *Disease control priorities in developing countries* (2nd ed., pp. 331–370). New York, NY: Oxford University Press.

50. The World Bank. (n.d.). *Data: Prevalence of HIV, total (% of population 15–49)*. Retrieved from https://data.worldbank.org/indicator/SH.DYN.AIDS.ZS

51. World Health Organization (WHO). (2018). *HIV update: Global epidemic, progress in scale up and policy uptake*. Retrieved from https://www.who.int/hiv/data/en/

52. UNAIDS. (n.d.). *AIDSinfo*. Retrieved from http://aidsinfo.unaids.org/

53. UNAIDS. (2013). *AIDS by the numbers*. Geneva, Switzerland: Author.

54. UNAIDS. (2014). *Fast track: Ending the AIDS epidemic by 2030*. Geneva, Switzerland: Author.

55. Brown, L. R. (1997). *The potential impact of AIDS on population and economic growth rates*. Retrieved from http://ideas.repec.org/p/fpr/2020br/43.html

56. Russell, S. (2004). The economic burden of illness for households in developing countries: A review of studies focusing on malaria, tuberculosis, and human immunodeficiency virus/acquired immunodeficiency syndrome. *American Journal of Tropical Medicine and Hygiene, 71* (2 Suppl.), 147–155.

57. UNICEF. (2016). *For Every Child, End AIDS: Seventh Stocktaking Report, 2016*. New York, NY: Author. Retrieved from https://www.unicef.org/publications/files/Children_and_AIDS_Seventh_Stocktaking_Report_2016_EN.pdf.pdf

58. MSF Treatment Access Campaign. (2018). *Stopping senseless deaths*. Retrieved from https://www.msf.org/sites/msf.org/files/2018-08/HIV_Brief_Stopping_Senseless_Deaths_ENG_2018.pdf

59. The World Bank. (2015). *Data: Health expenditure per capita (current US$)*. Retrieved from http://data.worldbank.org/indicator/SH.XPD.PCAP

60. Resch, S., Ryckman, T., & Hecht, R. (2015). Funding AIDS programmes in the era of shared responsibility: An analysis of domestic spending in 12 low- and middle-income countries. *Lancet Global Health, 3*(1), e52–e61.

61. Ainsworth, M., & Over, M. (1994). AIDS and African development. *World Bank Research Observer, 9*(2), 203–240.

62. UNAIDS. (2014). *90-90-90: An ambitious treatment target to help end the AIDS epidemic*. Geneva, Switzerland: Author.

63. UNAIDS. (2010). *UNAIDS report on the global AIDS epidemic*. Geneva, Switzerland: Author.

64. Kurth, A. E., Celum, C., Baeten, J. M., Vermund, S. H., & Wasserheit, J. N. (2011). Combination HIV prevention: Significance, challenges, and opportunities. *Current HIV/AIDS Reports, 8*(1), 62–72. doi: 10.1007/s11904-010-0063-3

65. World Health Organization (WHO). (n.d.). *Mother-to-child transmission of HIV*. Retrieved from http://www.who.int/hiv/topics/mtct/en/

66. World Health Organization (WHO). (2010). *Guidelines on HIV and infant feeding 2010*. Geneva, Switzerland: Author.

67. Centers for Disease Control and Prevention (CDC). (2008). *Male circumcision and risk for HIV transmission: Implications for the United States*. Retrieved from http://stacks.cdc.gov/view/cdc/13545/

68. Dickson, K. E., Tran, N. T., Samuelson, J. L., Njeuhmeli, E., Cherutich, P., Dick, B., . . . Hankins, C. A. (2011) Voluntary medical male circumcision: A framework analysis of policy and program implementation in Eastern and Southern

Africa. *PLoS Med, 8*(11), e1001133. doi: 10.1371/journal.pmed.1001133

69. Piot, P., Abdool Karim, S. S., Hecht, R., Legido-Quigley, H., Buse, K., Stover, J., . . . Sidibé, M. (2015). Defeating AIDS—advancing global health. *The Lancet, 386*(9989), 171–218.

70. International AIDS Vaccine Initiative. (n.d.). Homepage. Retrieved from http://www.iavi.org/

71. International Partnership on Microbicides. (n.d.). Homepage. Retrieved from http://www.ipmglobal.org/

72. Centers for Disease Control and Prevention (CDC). (2015). *Basic TB facts.* Retrieved from http://www.cdc.gov/tb/topic/basics/

73. World Health Organization (WHO), World Organization for Animal Health (OIE), Food and Agriculture Organization of the United Nations (FAO), & International Union Against Tuberculosis and Lung Disease. (2017). *Zoonotic tuberculosis.* Retrieved from https://www.who.int/tb/areas-of-work/zoonotic-tb/ZoonoticTBfactsheet2017.pdf?ua=1

74. Centers for Disease Control and Prevention (CDC). (n.d.). *Tuberculosis: TB risk factors.* Retrieved from http://www.cdc.gov/tb/topic/basics/risk.htm

75. World Health Organization (WHO). (n.d.). *Tuberculosis (TB): TB comorbidities and risk factors.* Retrieved from https://www.who.int/tb/areas-of-work/treatment/risk-factors/en/

76. World Health Organization (WHO). (n.d.). *Tuberculosis diagnostics: Automated real-time DNA amplification test for rapid and simultaneous detection of TB and rifampicin resistance: Xpert MTB/RIF assay.* Retrieved from https://www.who.int/tb/publications/factsheet_xpert.pdf?ua=1

77. World Health Organization (WHO). (2014). *Global tuberculosis report 2014.* Geneva, Switzerland: Author.

78. World Health Organization. (n. d.) *Tuberculosis. Drug resistant tuberculosis.* Retrieved from https://www.who.int/tb/areas-of-work/drug-resistant-tb/en/

79. World Health Organization (WHO). (n.d.). *Gender, equity, and human rights. Gender and tuberculosis.* Retrieved from https://www.who.int/gender-equity-rights/knowledge/a85584/en/

80. World Health Organization (WHO). (n.d.). *Tuberculosis: TB drug-resistance types.* Retrieved from https://www.who.int/tb/areas-of-work/drug-resistant-tb/types/en/

81. Centers for Disease Control and Prevention (CDC). (n.d.). *Tuberculosis. Fact sheet.* Retrieved from https://www.cdc.gov/tb/publications/factsheets/drtb/xdrtb.htm

82. Chand, N., Singh, T., Khalsa, J. S., Verma, V., & Rathore, J. S. (2004). A study of socio-economic impact of tuberculosis on patients and their family. *Chest, 126*(4), 832S.

83. Croft, R. A., & Croft, R. P. (1998). Expenditure and loss of income incurred by tuberculosis patients before reaching effective treatment in Bangladesh. *International Journal of Tuberculosis and Lung Disease, 2*(3), 252–254.

84. Tanimura, T., Jaramillo, E., Weil, D., Raviglione, M., & Lonnroth, K. (2014). Financial burden for tuberculosis patients in low- and middle-income countries: A systematic review. *European Respiratory Journal, 43*(6), 1763–1775.

85. Rajeswari, R., Balasubramanian, R., Muniyandi, M., Geetharamani, S., Thresa, X., & Venkatesan, P. (1999). Socio-economic impact of tuberculosis on patients and family in India. *International Journal of Tuberculosis and Lung Disease, 3*(10), 869–877.

86. Grimard, F., & Harling, G. (2004). *The impact of tuberculosis on economic growth.* Paper presented at the Northeast Universities Development Consortium Conference, Montréal, Quebec. Retrieved from http://neumann.hec.ca/neudc2004/fp/grimard_franque_aout_27.pdf

87. Peabody, J. W., Shimkhada, R., Tan, C., Jr., & Luck, J. (2005). The burden of disease, economic costs and clinical consequences of tuberculosis in the Philippines. *Health Policy and Planning, 20*(6), 347–353.

88. Dye, C., & Floyd, K. (2006). Tuberculosis. In D. T. Jamison, J. G. Breman, A. R Measham, et al. (Eds.), *Disease control priorities in developing countries* (2nd ed., pp. 289–312). New York, NY: Oxford University Press.

89. World Health Organization (WHO). (2010). *Guidelines for the treatment of tuberculosis* (4th ed.). Geneva, Switzerland: Author.

90. World Health Organization (WHO). (2017). *WHO guidelines for treatment of drug-susceptible TB and patient care.* Retrieved from https://www.who.int/tb/publications/2017/DS_TB_treatmentFactsheet.pdf?ua=1

91. World Health Organization (WHO). (2018). *HIV-associated tuberculosis.* Retrieved from https://www.who.int/tb/areas-of-work/tb-hiv/tbhiv_factsheet.pdf?ua=1

92. World Health Organization (WHO). (2014). *The end TB strategy.* Geneva, Switzerland: Author.

93. Pai, M., & Temesgen, Z. (2019). Quality: The missing ingredient in TB care and control. *Journal of Clinical Tuberculosis Other Mycobacterial Diseases, 14*, 12–13.

94. Pai, M., Schumacher, S.G., & Abimbola, S. (2018). Surrogate endpoints in global health research: still searching for killer apps and silver bullets? *BMJ Global Health, 3*(2), e000755. doi: 10.1136/bmjgh-2018-000755

95. Breman, J. G., Mills, A., Snow, R. W., & Mulligan, J.-A. (2006). Conquering malaria. In D. T. Jamison, J. G. Breman, A. R. Measham, et al. (Eds.), *Disease control priorities in developing countries* (2nd ed., pp. 413–432). New York, NY: Oxford University Press.

96. van Hellemond, J. J., Rutten, M., Koelewijn, R., Zeeman, A.-M., Verweij, J. J., Wismans, P. J., . . . van Genderen, P. J. J. (2009). Human *Plasmodium knowlesi* infection detected by rapid diagnostic tests for malaria. *Emerging Infectious Diseases, 15*(9), 1478–1480.

97. World Health Organization (WHO). (2018). *World malaria report 2018.* Geneva, Switzerland: Author.

98. World Health Organization (WHO). (2017). *Malaria in pregnant women.* Retrieved from http://www.who.int/malaria/areas/high_risk_groups/pregnancy/en/

99. World Health Organization (WHO). (2016). *10 facts on malaria.* Retrieved from https://www.who.int/features/factfiles/malaria/en

100. USAID. (2011). *The president's malaria initiative: Fifth annual report to Congress.* Retrieved from http://www.pmi.gov/docs/default-source/default-document-library/pmi-reports/pmi_annual_report11.pdf

101. Roll Back Malaria Partnership. (n.d.). *Economic costs of malaria.* Retrieved from https://www.malariaconsortium.org/userfiles/file/Malaria%20resources/RBM%20Economic%20costs%20of%20malaria.pdf

102. World Health Organization (WHO). (2018). *Malaria: Overview of malaria treatment.* Retrieved from https://www.who.int/malaria/areas/treatment/overview/en/

103. World Health Organization (WHO). (2015). *Guidelines for the treatment of malaria* (3rd ed.). Geneva, Switzerland: Author.

104. President's Malaria Initiative. (n.d.). *Indoor residual spraying.* Retrieved from http://www.pmi.gov/how-we-work/technical-areas/indoor-residual-spraying

105. World Health Organization (WHO). (2014). *World malaria report 2014.* Geneva, Switzerland: Author.

106. World Health Organization (WHO). (2018). *Q and A on artemisinin resistance.* Retrieved from https://www.who.int/malaria/media/artemisinin_resistance_qa/en/

107. World Health Organization (WHO). (2019). *Malaria: Insecticide resistance.* Retrieved from https://www.who.int/malaria/areas/vector_control/insecticide_resistance/en/

108. World Health Organization (WHO). (2019). *Q and A on the malaria vaccine implementation program (MVIP).* Retrieved from https://www.who.int/malaria/media/malaria-vaccine-implementation-qa/en/

109. World Health Organization (WHO). (2012). *WHO policy recommendation: Seasonal malaria chemoprevention (SMC) for* Plasmodium falciparum *malaria control in highly seasonal transmission areas of the Sahel sub-region in Africa.* Geneva, Switzerland: Author.

110. Keusch, G. T., Fontaine, O., Bhargava, A., & Boschi-Pinto, C. (2006). Diarrheal diseases. In D. T. Jamison, J. G. Breman, A. R. Measham, et al. (Eds.), *Disease control priorities in developing countries* (2nd ed., pp. 371–388), New York, NY: Oxford University Press.

111. World Health Organization (WHO). (2018). *Immunization, vaccines and biological: Rotavirus.* Retrieved from https://www.who.int/immunization/diseases/rotavirus/en/

112. World Health Organization (WHO). (2012). *Estimated rotavirus deaths for children under 5 years of age: 2008, 453,000.* Retrieved from http://www.who.int/immunization/monitoring_surveillance/burden/estimates/rotavirus/en/

113. UNICEF & World Health Organization. (2009). *Diarrhoea: Why children are still dying and what can be done.* New York, NY: Author.

114. This section of the chapter is adapted with permission from Skolnik, R., & Ahmed, A. (2010). *Ending the neglect of neglected tropical diseases.* Washington, DC: Population Reference Bureau.

115. World Health Organization (WHO). (n.d.). *Neglected tropical diseases.* Retrieved from https://www.who.int/neglected_diseases/diseases/en/

116. Centers for Disease Control and Prevention (CDC). (n.d.). *Neglected tropical diseases.* Retrieved from https://www.cdc.gov/globalhealth/ntd/diseases/index.html

117. Brooker, S., Hotez, P. J., & Bundy, D. A. P. (2008). Hookworm-related anemia among pregnant women: A systematic review. *PLoS Neglected Tropical Diseases, 2*(9), e291.

118. Hotez, P. J., Brindley, P. J., Bethony, J. M., King, C. H., Pearce, E. J., & Jacobson, J. (2008). Helminth infections: The great neglected tropical diseases. *Journal of Clinical Investigation, 118*(4), 1311–1321.

119. Kjetland, E. F., Ndhlovu, P. D., Gomo, E., Mduluza, T., Midzi, N., Gwanzura, L., . . . Gundersen, S. G. (2006). Association between genital schistosomiasis and HIV in rural Zimbabwean women. *AIDS, 20*(4), 593–600.

120. Hotez, P. J., & Daar, A. S. (2008). The CNCDs and the NTDs: Blurring the lines dividing noncommunicable and communicable chronic diseases. *PLoS Neglected Tropical Diseases, 2*(10), e312.

121. World Health Organization. (2019) *Soil transmitted helminths. Key facts.* Retrieved from https://www.who.int/en/news-room/fact-sheets/detail/soil-transmitted-helminth-infections

122. World Health Organization. (2018). *Trachoma.* Retrieved from https://www.who.int/en/news-room/fact-sheets/detail/trachoma

123. World Health Organization (WHO). (2012). *Accelerating work to overcome the impact of neglected tropical diseases: A roadmap for implementation.* Geneva, Switzerland: Author.

124. Uniting to Combat Neglected Tropical Diseases. (2012). *London declaration on neglected tropical diseases.* Retrieved from https://unitingtocombatntds.org/london-declaration-neglected-tropical-diseases/

125. World Health Organization (WHO). (2017). *Neglected tropical diseases: Implementing the WHO roadmap on neglected tropical diseases—partners celebrate five years of collaboration.* Retrieved from https://www.who.int/neglected_diseases/news/WHO_Roadmap_five_years_of_collaboration/en/

126. World Health Organization (WHO). (2019). *Soil-transmitted helminth infections.* Retrieved from https://www.who.int/en/news-room/fact-sheets/detail/soil-transmitted-helminth-infections

127. World Health Organization (WHO). (2018). *Essential medicines donated to control, eliminate, and eradicate neglected tropical diseases.* Retrieved from https://www.who.int/neglected_diseases/Medicine-donation-04-july-2018.pdf?ua=1

128. World Health Organization (WHO). (2018). *Schistosomiasis.* Retrieved from https://www.who.int/en/news-room/fact-sheets/detail/schistosomiasis

129. World Health Organization (WHO). (n.d.). *Schistosomiasis: Epidemiological situation.* Retrieved from https://www.who.int/schistosomiasis/epidemiology/en/

130. World Health Organization (WHO). (2018). *Lymphatic filariasis.* Retrieved from https://www.who.int/en/news-room/fact-sheets/detail/lymphatic-filariasis

131. World Health Organization (WHO). (2018). *Onchocerciasis.* Retrieved from https://www.who.int/en/news-room/fact-sheets/detail/onchocerciasis

132. International Trachoma Initiative. (n.d.). *About trachoma.* Retrieved from https://trachoma.org/about-trachoma

133. World Health Organization (WHO). (2008). *Community-directed interventions for major health problems in Africa.* Geneva, Switzerland: Author.

134. Copenhagen Consensus Center. (n.d.). Homepage. Retrieved from http://www.copenhagenconsensus.com/Home.aspx

135. Evidence Action. (n.d.). *Deworm the world initiative: The evidence for deworming.* Retrieved from http://www.evidenceaction.org/dewormtheworld/

136. Hotez, P. J., Molyneux, D. H., Fenwick, A., Ottesen, E., Ehrlich Sachs, S., & Sachs J. D. (2006). Incorporating a rapid-impact package for neglected tropical diseases with programs for HIV/AIDS, tuberculosis, and malaria. *PLoS Medicine, 3*(5), e102. doi: 10.1371/journal.pmed.0030102

137. Hotez, P. J., & Molyneux, D. H. (2008). Tropical anemia: One of Africa's greatest killers and a rationale for linking malaria and neglected tropical disease control to achieve

a common goal. *PLoS Neglected Tropical Diseases, 2*(7), e270.

138. Hopkins, D. R., Eigege, A., Miri, E. S., Gontor, I., Ogah, G., Umaru, J., . . . Richards, F. O. Jr. (2002). Lymphatic filariasis elimination and schistosomiasis control in combination with onchocerciasis control in Nigeria. *American Journal of Tropical Medicine and Hygiene, 67*(3), 266–272.

139. Geraghty, J. (2009). Expanding the biopharmaceutical industry's involvement in fighting neglected diseases. *Health Affairs, 28*(6), 1774–1777.

140. Gibbs, E. P. J. (2014). The evolution of One Health: A decade of progress and challenges for the future. *Veterinary Record, 174*(4), 85–91.

141. One Health Commission. (n.d.). *What is One Health?* Retrieved from https://www.onehealthcommission.org/en/why_one_health/what_is_one_health/

142. One Health Initiative. (n.d.). *About the One Health Initiative*. Retrieved from http://www.onehealthinitiative.com/about.php

143. Mackenzie, J. S., McKinnon, M., & Jeggo, M. (2014). One Health: From concept to practice. In *Confronting emerging zoonoses* (pp. 163–189). Tokyo, Japan: Springer.

144. Centers for Disease Control and Prevention (CDC). (n.d.). *One Health basics*. Retrieved from https://www.cdc.gov/onehealth/basics/index.html

145. World Health Organization. (2018). *Rift Valley fever*. Retrieved from https://www.who.int/news-room/fact-sheets/detail/rift-valley-fever

146. NASA. (2009). *Visible Earth: Predicting Rift Valley fever*. Retrieved from https://visibleearth.nasa.gov/view.php?id=37025

147. Centers for Disease Control and Prevention (CDC). (n.d.). *The story of the Rift Valley fever virus vaccine*. Retrieved from https://www.cdc.gov/onehealth/in-action/rvf-vaccine.html

148. Lee, K., & Brumme, Z. L. (2012). Operationalizing the One Health approach: The global governance challenges. *Health Policy and Planning, 28*(7), 778–785.

149. This case is based on Levine, R. (2007). Preventing HIV/AIDS and sexually transmitted infections in Thailand. In *Millions saved: Case studies in global health* (1st ed.). Burlington, MA: Jones and Bartlett.

150. This case is based on Levine, R. (2007). Controlling tuberculosis in China. In *Millions saved: Case studies in global health* (1st ed.). Burlington, MA: Jones and Bartlett.

151. This case is based on Levine, R. (2007). *Controlling trachoma in Morocco*. In *Millions saved: Case studies in global health* (1st ed.). Burlington, MA: Jones and Bartlett.

152. Centers for Disease Control and Prevention (CDC). (n.d.). *Years of Ebola virus disease outbreak*. Retrieved from http://www.cdc.gov/vhf/ebola/resources/outbreak-table.html

153. World Health Organization (WHO). (2014). *Ebola virus disease*. Retrieved from http://www.who.int/mediacentre/factsheets/fs103/en/

154. Centers for Disease Control and Prevention (CDC). (n.d.). *Ebola: Signs and symptoms*. Retrieved from http://www.cdc.gov/vhf/ebola/symptoms/index.html

155. Centers for Disease Control and Prevention (CDC). (2019). *Ebola Virus Disease*. Retrieved from: https://www.cdc.gov/vhf/ebola/prevention/index.html

156. Stat. (2019). *The data are clear: Ebola vaccine shows 'very impressive' performance in outbreak*. Retrieved from: https://www.statnews.com/2019/04/12/the-data-are-clear-ebola-vaccine-shows-very-impressive-performance-in-outbreak/.

157. Leroy, E., Kumulungui, B., Pourrut, X., Rouquet, P., Hassanin, A., Yaba, P., . . . Swanepoel, R. (2005). Fruit bats as reservoirs of Ebola virus. *Nature, 438*, 575–576.

158. Centers for Disease Control and Prevention (CDC). (2014). *Infection control for viral haemorrhagic fevers in the African health care setting*. Retrieved from http://www.cdc.gov/vhf/abroad/vhf-manual.html

159. Breman, J. G., Piot, P., Johnson, K. M., White, M. K., Mbuyi, M., Sureau, P., Heymann, D. L., ...Ngvete, K. (1978). The epidemiology of Ebola haemorrhagic fever in Zaire, 1976. In S. R. Pattyn (Ed.), *Ebola virus haemorrhagic fever* (pp. 103–124). Amsterdam, The Netherlands: Elsevier/North-Holland. Retrieved from http://www.itg.be/internet/ebola/pdf/EbolaVirusHaemorragicFever-SPattyn.pdf

160. Baize, S., Pannetier, D., Oestereich, L., Rieger, T., Koivogui, L., Magassouba, N., . . . Günther, S. (2014). Emergence of Zaire Ebola virus disease in Guinea—Preliminary report. *New England Journal of Medicine, 371*(15). Retrieved from http://www.nejm.org/doi/pdf/10.1056/NEJMoa1404505

161. World Health Organization (WHO). (2014, August 8). *Statement on the meeting of the International Health Regulations Emergency Committee regarding the 2014 Ebola outbreak in West Africa*. Retrieved from http://www.who.int/mediacentre/news/statements/2014/ebola-20140808/en/

162. Médecins Sans Frontières. (n.d.). *Ebola*. Retrieved from http://www.doctorswithoutborders.org/our-work/medical-issues/ebola

163. Centers for Disease Control and Prevention (CDC). (2019), *Case Counts* Retrieved from https://www.cdc.gov/vhf/ebola/history/2014-2016-outbreak/case-counts.html

164. World Health Organization (WHO). (2015, January 28). *Ebola situation report—28 January 2015*. Retrieved from http://apps.who.int/ebola/en/ebola-situation-report/situation-reports/ebola-situation-report-28-january-2015

165. World Health Organization (WHO). (2008). *International health regulations (2005)* (2nd ed.). Retrieved from http://www.who.int/ihr/9789241596664/en/

166. Levine, M. (2014, July 17). WHO can't fully deal with Ebola outbreak, health official warns. *The Los Angeles Times*. Retrieved from http://www.latimes.com/world/africa/la-fg-who-ebola-20140718-story.html

167. World Health Organization (WHO). (2014). *Ebola response roadmap*. Retrieved from http://apps.who.int/iris/bitstream/10665/131596/1/EbolaResponseRoadmap.pdf?ua=1

168. European Centre for Disease Prevention and Control. (2014). *Rapid risk assessment: Outbreak of Ebola virus disease in West Africa. Fourth update*. Retrieved from http://ecdc.europa.eu/en/publications/Publications/Ebola-virus-disease-west-africa-risk-assessment-27-08-2014.pdf

169. World Health Organization (WHO). (2014, August 12). *WHO Director-General briefs Geneva UN missions on the Ebola outbreak*. Retrieved from http://www.who.int/dg/speeches/2014/ebola-briefing/en/

170. UNICEF. (2014). *Ebola virus disease: Personal protective equipment and other Ebola-related supply update*. Retrieved from http://www.unicef.org/supply/index_75984.html

171. Nossiter, A. (2014, July 27). Fear of Ebola breeds a terror of physicians. *New York Times*. Retrieved from http://www .nytimes.com/2014/07/28/world/africa/ebola-epidemic -west-africa-guinea.html?_r=0

172. United Nations Office for the Coordination of Humanitarian Affairs. (2015). *Ebola outbreak: Updated overview of needs and requirements for January–June 2015*. Retrieved from http://reliefweb.int/sites/reliefweb.int/files/resources /updated_overview_of_needs_and_requirements_for _january-june_2015_0.pdf

173. Médecins Sans Frontières. (2014, December 29). *Clinical trial for potential Ebola treatment starts in MSF clinic in Guinea*. Retrieved from http://www.doctorswithoutborders .org/article/clinical-trial-potential-ebola-treatment-starts -msf-clinic-guinea

174. Onishi, N. (2015, January 31). As Ebola ebbs in Africa, focus turns from death to life. *New York Times*. Retrieved from http://www.nytimes.com/2015/02/01/world/as-ebola-ebbs -in-africa-focus-turns-from-death-to-life.html?emc=edit _th_20150201&nl=todaysheadlines&nlid=67361508

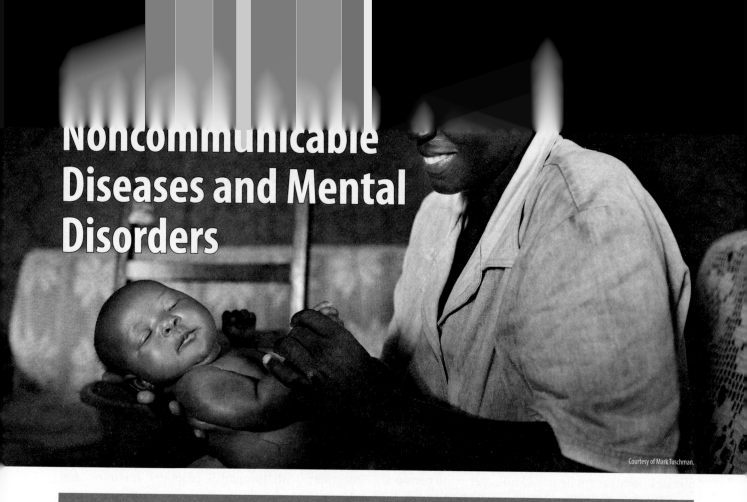

Noncommunicable Diseases and Mental Disorders

Courtesy of Mark Tuschman.

LEARNING OBJECTIVES

By the end of this chapter, the reader will be able to do the following:

- Describe the burden of noncommunicable diseases and mental disorders worldwide
- Discuss the most important risk factors for the burden of these conditions
- Outline the costs and consequences of selected noncommunicable diseases and mental disorders
- Review measures that can be taken to address the burden of these conditions in cost-effective and fair ways
- Describe some successful cases dealing with noncommunicable diseases and mental disorders in low- and middle-income countries

▶ Vignettes

Roberto was 45 years old and lived in Bogota, Colombia. He had a government desk job and had been affected by overweight for most of his adult life. He got little exercise. He had read about increasing rates of diabetes in Colombia but still thought this was largely a disease of people in rich countries. Last year, Roberto started feeling thirsty all the time, had dry mouth, and felt weak after exertion. He went to his doctor and was diagnosed with type 2 diabetes.

Shalini was 35 years old and lived in Sri Lanka. She had grown up in a village, had worked hard on her family's small farm, and had been healthy for all of her adult life. She had two children and had not had any problems during either pregnancy. During a recent visit to the local health center, however, the doctor discovered that Shalini had high blood pressure. The doctor talked with Shalini about changing her diet and also prescribed medication for her. The medicine she needs is not expensive but, unfortunately, Shalini has to take this medicine for the remainder of her life.

Alexei was 47 years old and lived in Moscow, Russia. Alexei had been smoking one pack of cigarettes a day since he was 16 years old. He heard on television and on the radio about the bad effects that cigarettes have on health. Urged by his children to stop smoking, he tried unsuccessfully on several occasions to quit. Over the last few months, Alexei developed a continuous cough and was often short of breath. Alexei had lung cancer.

Lai Ying was a factory worker who lived in Guandong Province, China. Until recently she had been a happy and healthy young woman. Lately, however, Lai Ying had felt very unhappy, did not feel like getting out of bed in the morning, did not want to go to work, and had no energy when she was at work. Lai Ying's family noticed that she was not eating properly and that she was not herself. However, they thought she was having a difficult time at work or with a boyfriend and that she would soon be fine. After some months of this behavior, Lai Ying consumed an overdose of sleeping pills and died by suicide.

Key Definitions

Communicable diseases are illnesses caused by an infectious agent that spreads from a person or an animal to another person or animal. Like noncommunicable diseases, they can be very disabling, can seriously impair the ability of people to engage in day-to-day activities, and often lead to death if they are not treated appropriately. However, noncommunicable diseases (NCDs) are, in some respects, the opposite of most communicable diseases. They cannot be spread from person to person by an infectious agent, even if they might be associated with one. In addition, they tend to last a long time.

In practice, however, the definition of noncommunicable diseases is not as clear as it might seem. First, the terms chronic disease and degenerative disease are often used interchangeably with noncommunicable disease. However, some would say that these are also imperfect terms because some communicable diseases, such as HIV/AIDS, can become "chronic" conditions when those affected receive appropriate treatment. Second, a number of noncommunicable diseases, such as some cancers, have infectious causes. Third, although mental health disorders are included, in principle, in noncommunicable diseases, they are excluded from many discussions of NCDs.

In this text, however, for the sake of simplicity and to conform to the generally used terminology, we shall consistently use the term noncommunicable disease. This will include all causes that are included in the Global Burden of Disease Study 2016 (GBD 2016) under the category of noncommunicable diseases, including mental disorders.[1]

This chapter will focus on selected noncommunicable diseases of importance. This includes cardiovascular disease, cancers, chronic obstructive pulmonary disease, vision and hearing loss, and mental health disorders. Including mental disorders in the chapter title is intended to signal the coverage of the chapter and the importance of mental health.

You are already familiar with most of the terms used in this chapter; however, a few key terms with which you may be less familiar are defined in **TABLE 14-1**.

The Importance of Noncommunicable Diseases

Noncommunicable diseases are of immense and growing importance worldwide. In fact, the burden of these conditions is greater than the burden of communicable diseases in low- and middle-income countries, as well as in high-income countries. Only in sub-Saharan Africa is the burden of communicable diseases higher than that of noncommunicable diseases.[1] This contradicts some people's continuing perception that low-income countries do not face a significant burden of noncommunicable disease and that these diseases are problems only for affluent countries.

Moreover, the burden of noncommunicable diseases will increase in low- and middle-income countries as they develop economically, become more integrated with the global economy, urbanize, and age. Among the most important of the noncommunicable health conditions that low- and middle-income countries face are ischemic heart disease, stroke, chronic obstructive pulmonary disease, diabetes, cancers, musculoskeletal disorders, and mental health disorders.[1] The risk factors for several noncommunicable diseases relate in significant ways to lifestyle, much of which is modifiable. This chapter discusses, for example, the importance of diet, physical activity, tobacco use, and alcohol use for the onset and during the course of certain noncommunicable diseases. By engaging in appropriate health behaviors, it is possible for most people to considerably reduce the risk of getting heart disease, stroke, COPD, some cancers, or diabetes.

Some noncommunicable diseases can be prevented at relatively low cost, but these diseases are often very expensive to treat. It is possible, for example, to significantly reduce the chances of getting lung cancer by making a modest investment in smoking cessation therapy and by quitting smoking. By contrast, the cost of treating lung cancer through drugs and surgery is considerably more expensive.

TABLE 14-2 indicates some of the most important links between noncommunicable diseases and the Sustainable Development Goals (SDGs). The table highlights the importance of noncommunicable diseases in all countries, including low- and middle-income countries.

TABLE 14-1 Key Terms

Blood glucose—Blood sugar, the main source of energy for the body.

Body mass index (BMI)—Body weight in kilograms divided by height in meters squared (kg/m^2).

Cancer—One of a large variety of diseases characterized by uncontrolled growth of cells.

Cardiovascular disease—A disease of the heart or blood vessels. This term encompasses both ischemic heart disease and stroke.

Cholesterol—A fatlike substance that is made by the body and is found naturally in animal-based foods such as meat, fish, poultry, and eggs.

Diabetes—An illness caused by poor control by the body of blood sugar.

Hypertension—High blood pressure, with a reading of 140/90 or greater.

Ischemic heart disease—A disturbance of the heart function due to inadequate supply of oxygen to the heart muscle.

Obesity—A BMI equal to or greater than 30.

Overweight—A BMI equal to or greater than 25 but less than 30.

Stroke—Sudden loss of function of the brain due to clotting or hemorrhaging.

Data from Texas Heart Institute (n.d.). Cardiovascular glossary. Retrieved from https://www.texasheart.org/heart-health/heart-information-center/topics/a-z/; National Institutes of Health. (n.d.). Obesity, physical activity, and weight-control glossary. Retrieved from http://win.niddk.nih.gov/publications/glossary.htm; World Health Organization (WHO). (n.d.). Obesity and overweight. Retrieved from http://www.who.int/mediacentre/factsheets/fs311/en/

The chapter first examines the burden of noncommunicable diseases and the risk factors for those diseases. Following that, it comments on some of the most important costs and consequences of those diseases. It then reviews what steps can be taken to address the burden of these diseases in cost-effective ways and discusses several examples of successful efforts to prevent and deal with noncommunicable diseases. The chapter concludes with comments on some of the future challenges that must be addressed if the burden of noncommunicable diseases is to be reduced.

▶ A Note on Data

This chapter includes data on both deaths and disability-adjusted life years (DALYs) for the most important noncommunicable diseases. An important part of the data in the chapter, therefore, is based on the Global Burden of Disease Study 2016 and its related publications and website.[1] Much of the other data used in this chapter comes from the World Health Organization (WHO). The chapter also uses data from a number of studies of specific diseases, especially from *Disease Control Priorities, Third Edition* (DCP3).[2]

▶ The Burden of Noncommunicable Diseases

Cardiovascular Disease

Ischemic heart disease caused almost 10 million deaths in 2016 and is the leading specific cause of death globally for all age groups and both sexes. Stroke was the second leading cause of death globally among all age groups and for both sexes in 2016 and was responsible for more than 6 million deaths. Together, ischemic heart disease and stroke, generally referred to in burden-of-disease studies as cardiovascular disease (CVD), made up almost 27 percent of all deaths globally in 2016.[1]

Ischemic heart disease is the fifth leading cause of death in low-income countries. However, it is the leading cause of death for both sexes and all ages in lower middle-, upper middle-, and high-income countries. Stroke is the second leading cause of death in lower middle- and upper middle-income countries but is the third leading cause in high-income countries and the eighth leading cause in low-income countries.[1]

TABLE 14-2 Selected Links Between Noncommunicable Diseases and the SDG Health Targets

Target 3.1 By 2030, reduce the global maternal mortality ratio to less than 70 per 100,000 live births.

This is directly linked to the health and well-being of women. Yet, an increasing share of women have obesity and suffer from hypertension and diabetes, all of which are risk factors for poor maternal and fetal outcomes.

Target 3.2 By 2030, end preventable deaths of newborns and children under 5 years of age, with all countries aiming to reduce neonatal mortality to at least as low as 12 per 1,000 live births and under-5 mortality to at least as low as 25 per 1,000 live births.

Good birth outcomes and child survival depend to an important extent on healthy mothers. The growing prevalence of hypertension, obesity, and diabetes among women of reproductive age are risk factors for child survival, as are tobacco smoking, substance abuse, alcohol abuse, and mental disorders.

Target 3.3 By 2030, end the epidemics of AIDS, tuberculosis, malaria, and neglected tropical diseases and combat hepatitis, waterborne diseases, and other communicable diseases.

Diabetes triples the risk for tuberculosis and worsens its clinical course. The growing number of people with diabetes and the growing rates of diabetes in many settings pose a serious threat for the spread of tuberculosis.

Target 3.4 By 2030, reduce by one-third premature mortality from noncommunicable diseases through prevention and treatment and promote mental health and well-being.

This target directly concerns NCDs.

Target 3.5 Strengthen the prevention and treatment of substance abuse, including narcotic drug abuse and harmful use of alcohol.

Substance abuse disorders are a major, and often growing, cause of morbidity, disability and death in many countries. In some, they are leading to a decline in life expectancy. Harmful use of alcohol is a major risk factor for a range of non-communicable diseases.

Target 3.6 By 2020, halve the number of global deaths and injuries from road traffic accidents.

Excess alcohol consumption is a major risk factor for road traffic injuries.

Target 3.8 Achieve universal health coverage, including financial risk protection, access to quality essential healthcare services, and access to safe, effective, quality, and affordable essential medicines and vaccines for all.

Universal health coverage that is of good quality reduces out-of-pocket costs to the poor to a minimum and, if fairly prioritized and delivered, can have a major impact on delivering the health services most needed to help prevent and address NCDs.

United Nations Sustainable Development Goals Knowledge Platform. (n.d.). Sustainable Development Goals. © United Nations. Reprinted with the permission of the United Nations.

Ischemic heart disease is the largest cause of death among all age groups for both sexes in all World Bank regions, except in East Asia and the Pacific, where stroke is a more common cause of death, and in sub-Saharan Africa, where communicable diseases still predominate and where ischemic heart disease is the seventh leading cause of death. Stroke is the leading cause of death in East Asia and the Pacific. It is the second leading cause of death in Europe and Central Asia, Latin America and the Caribbean, and the Middle East and North Africa. It is the third leading cause of death in South Asia, fourth in North America, and eighth in sub-Saharan Africa.[1]

Together, ischemic heart disease and stroke made up about 44 percent of all deaths in Europe and Central Asia in 2016 and about 37 percent of all deaths in East Asia and the Pacific. However, they were associated with only about 12 percent of the total deaths in sub-Saharan Africa.[1] CVD rates are higher in Eastern

Europe than in Western Europe, although the rates of CVD are falling in some Eastern European countries. The highest rates of CVD are in the former Soviet Union, where they earlier contributed to declines in life expectancy.[3]

Ischemic heart disease was the 2nd leading cause of DALYs and stroke was the 3rd leading cause of DALYs among all age groups and both sexes in 2016. For low-income countries, ischemic heart disease was the 9th leading cause of DALYs and stroke was the 11th leading cause of DALYs. However, in the lower middle-income countries and upper middle-income countries, stroke was the leading cause and ischemic heart disease was the 2nd leading cause. In the high-income countries, ischemic heart disease was the leading cause of DALYs and stroke was the 3rd leading cause.[1]

Given limited access to prevention programs or appropriate treatment, deaths from CVD generally occur earlier in life in low- and middle-income countries than in high-income countries. In India, for example, CVD occurs in people at younger ages more often than in high-income countries. Whereas in high-income countries only about 22 percent of CVD deaths occur in people under 70 years of age, in India, about 50 percent of the CVD deaths occur in people under 70.[4]

To help get a better understanding of the importance of CVD to the burden of disease, **TABLE 14-3** shows the burden of deaths and DALYs by World Bank regions that are associated with ischemic heart disease and stroke, compared to some of the other leading causes of deaths and DALYs. **TABLE 14-4** does the same by World Bank country income group.

Some of the risk factors for cardiovascular disease are modifiable while others are not. Men have a higher risk of heart disease than women who are premenopausal, but postmenopausal women have the same risk of cardiovascular disease as men. In addition, men and women have similar risks of stroke. The medical history of one's family is also significant. If a male relative had coronary heart disease before 55 years of age or a female relative before 65 years of age, then one has a higher risk of heart disease. Ancestry is also relevant, as people of African or Asian descent have higher risks than other groups. Aging also increases risk, with the risk of a stroke doubling every 10 years after age 55.[5]

Other risk factors are modifiable, meaning one can change them by changing behavior. These include hypertension, which is the biggest risk factor for stroke and a major risk factor for heart disease. Tobacco use is also a major risk factor for CVD, with higher risks for women and those who started smoking early and smoke a lot. High levels of cholesterol, which are linked to a diet high in saturated fats and the lack of physical activity, are also risks. The lack of physical activity is a risk for obesity that in turn is a risk for diabetes, which doubles one's risk of CVD. Excess alcohol consumption is also associated with heart disease.[5]

Social factors can be important risks for CVD. There is good evidence that higher risks of CVD are associated, for example, with poverty, stress, and being isolated socially. Depression is also an important risk factor for CVD.[5]

Diabetes

There are several types of diabetes. The two most common are called type 1 and type 2 diabetes. Type 1 diabetes is thought to be an autoimmune disorder that attacks and destroys the cells in the pancreas that produce insulin. Without insulin, the body is not able to use glucose (blood sugar) for energy. To treat the disease, a person must inject insulin, follow a diet plan, exercise daily, and test blood sugar several times a day.[6]

Type 1 diabetes usually begins before the age of 30. This type of diabetes was previously known as insulin-dependent diabetes mellitus or juvenile diabetes.[6] Type 2 diabetes was previously known as noninsulin-dependent diabetes mellitus or adult-onset diabetes. Type 2 diabetes is the most common form of diabetes mellitus, present in about 90 percent to 95 percent of all people with diabetes. People with type 2 diabetes are able to produce insulin; however, they either do not make enough insulin or their bodies do not efficiently use the insulin they do make.[6]

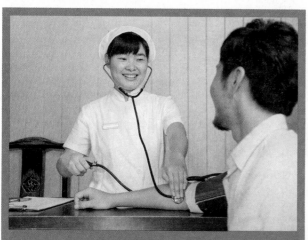

PHOTO 14-1 A Chinese healthcare provider is shown here taking her patient's blood pressure. Hypertension is a major risk factor for noncommunicable diseases. Better prevention and management of hypertension is central to improving health in many countries. In resource-poor settings, how could one make a start at improving the prevention, diagnosis, and management of hypertension?
© XiXinXing/Getty Images.

TABLE 14-3 Deaths and DALYs from Select Noncommunicable and Communicable Causes, by World Bank Region, 2016, as a Percentage of Total Deaths and DALYs

Region	Ischemic Heart Disease	Stroke	Diabetes	COPD	Mental Disorders	Cancer	TB	HIV/AIDS	Malaria
East Asia and Pacific									
Deaths	15%	18%	2%	7%	N/A*	23%	1%	< 1%	< 1%
DALYs	7%	10%	3%	5%	6%	15%	1%	< 1%	< 1%
Europe and Central Asia									
Deaths	25%	12%	2%	4%	N/A*	23%	< 1%	< 1%	< 1%
DALYs	12%	6%	3%	3%	6%	15%	< 1%	< 1%	< 1%
Latin America and the Caribbean									
Deaths	14%	8%	5%	4%	N/A*	18%	< 1%	1%	< 1%
DALYs	6%	4%	4%	2%	6%	10%	< 1%	1%	< 1%
Middle East and North Africa									
Deaths	26%	10%	3%	2%	N/A*	12%	< 1%	< 1%	< 1%
DALYs	10%	4%	3%	2%	7%	6%	< 1%	< 1%	< 1%
South Asia									
Deaths	15%	8%	3%	8%	N/A*	10%	4%	< 1%	< 1%
DALYs	7%	4%	2%	4%	4%	6%	3%	< 1%	< 1%
Sub-Saharan Africa									
Deaths	5%	4%	2%	1%	N/A*	7%	5%	10%	7%
DALYs	2%	2%	1%	< 1%	3%	3%	3%	9%	8%
North America									
Deaths	19%	6%	2%	6%	N/A*	25%	< 1%	< 1%	0%
DALYs	8%	4%	4%	5%	7%	15%	< 1%	< 1%	0%

*Standard global data on deaths due to mental disorders do not exist.
Data from Institute of Health Metrics and Evaluation (IHME). (n.d.). GBD Compare: Viz Hub. Retrieved from https://vizhub.healthdata.org/gbd-compare/

TABLE 14-4 Deaths and DALYs from Select Noncommunicable and Communicable Causes, by World Bank Country Income Level, 2016, as a Percentage of Total Deaths and DALYs

Income Level	Ischemic Heart Disease	Stroke	Diabetes	COPD	Mental Disorders	Cancer	TB	HIV/AIDS	Malaria
Low-income countries									
Deaths	6%	5%	2%	2%	N/A*	7%	6%	6%	7%
DALYs	2%	2%	1%	1%	3%	4%	4%	5%	7%
Lower middle-income countries									
Deaths	16%	9%	3%	6%	N/A*	10%	4%	2%	1%
DALYs	7%	4%	2%	3%	4%	6%	3%	2%	2%
Upper middle-income countries									
Deaths	18%	16%	2%	6%	N/A*	21%	< 1%	2%	< 1%
DALYs	8%	9%	3%	4%	6%	14%	< 1%	2%	< 1%
High-income countries									
Deaths	17%	8%	2%	5%	N/A*	27%	< 1%	< 1%	< 1%
DALYs	7%	4%	3%	4%	7%	17%	< 1%	< 1%	< 1%

*Standard global data on deaths due to mental disorders do not exist.
Data from Institute of Health Metrics and Evaluation (IHME). (n.d.). GBD Compare: Viz Hub. Retrieved from https://vizhub.healthdata.org/gbd-compare/

There is also a third type of diabetes, generally referred to as **gestational diabetes**. A high blood glucose level—hyperglycemia—that is diagnosed first in pregnancy is referred to as **hyperglycemia in pregnancy** or **gestational diabetes mellitus (GDM)**. Hormonal production by the placenta can lead to diminished action of insulin, called **insulin resistance**, and lead to GDM. Other risk factors for GDM include older age, obesity, excessive weight gain during pregnancy, a family history of diabetes, or having had a stillbirth or giving birth to a child with congenital anomalies. GDM usually resolves when the pregnancy is over. However, having had GDM is a risk factor for GDM in subsequent pregnancies and for having type 2 diabetes. GDM in the mother also increases her baby's lifetime risk of obesity and diabetes.[7(p20)] The International Diabetes Federation (IDF) estimates that about 16 percent of pregnancies are associated with GDM.[7(p40)]

IDF estimated that 425 million people aged 20 to 79 years had diabetes in 2017.[7] The corresponding prevalence in this age group is 8.8 percent. The prevalence in men was 9.1 percent and in women was 8.4 percent.[7(p40)] Rates of diabetes rise as people age. IDF also estimates that there were 1.1 million children and adolescents aged 0 to 19 years in the world who suffered from type 1 diabetes in 2017, with more than 130,000 new cases a year in this age group. **FIGURE 14-1** shows IDF estimates of the prevalence rates of diabetes in 2017 by IDF region. **FIGURE 14-2** indicates the number of people estimated to have diabetes in 2017 by IDF region, as well as the number projected to have diabetes in 2045. This shows a significant increase in the number of people likely to be affected by diabetes between 2017 and 2045 in the lowest-income IDF regions, Africa and Southeast Asia. This increase will have important implications for people's health and the costs of health care in the affected countries.

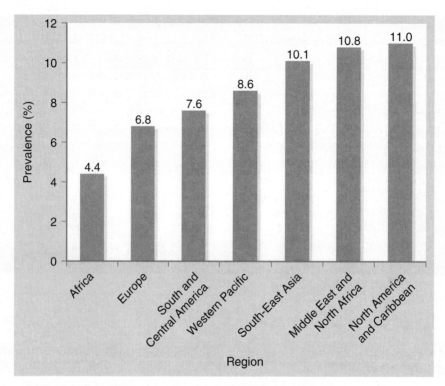

FIGURE 14-1 Prevalence of Diabetes in People 20–79 Years Old by IDF Region, 2017

Data from International Diabetes Federation. (2017). *IDF diabetes atlas* (8th ed.). Retrieved from http://www.diabetesatlas.org/IDF_Diabetes_Atlas_8e_interactive_EN/

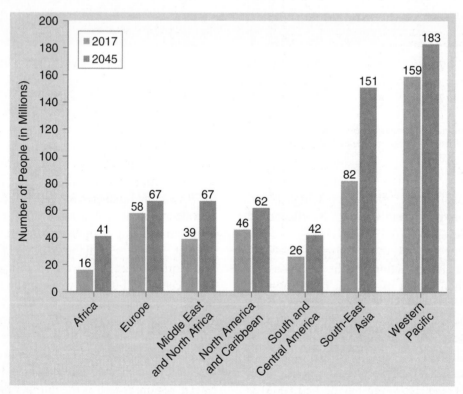

FIGURE 14-2 Number of People 20-79 Years Old with Diabetes by IDF Region, in Millions, 2017 and 2045

Data from International Diabetes Federation. (2017). *IDF diabetes atlas* (8th ed.). Retrieved from http://www.diabetesatlas.org/IDF_Diabetes_Atlas_8e_interactive_EN/

As shown in Figure 14-1, the prevalence of diabetes varies across International Diabetes Federation regions, from a high of 11 percent of the population in North America and the Caribbean to a low of 4.4 percent in Africa. It is also very important to note that many people with diabetes are undiagnosed. IDF estimates that even in high-income countries, only about 63 percent of those with diabetes are actually diagnosed and that in low-income countries, only about 23 percent of those affected are diagnosed.[7(p48)] The prevalence of diabetes also varies by country. The highest rates are found in the island nations of the Western Pacific, where around a quarter to a third of all adults 20 to 79 years of age have diabetes.[7]

The Global Burden of Disease Study estimated that diabetes was the 9th leading cause of death worldwide in 2016 among all age groups and both sexes and that about 1.3 million people died of diabetes in 2016. Diabetes was the 14th leading cause of death in low-income countries, the 9th leading cause in lower middle-income countries, the 11th leading cause of death in upper middle-income countries, and the 11th leading cause in high-income countries.[1] About 80 percent of all deaths from diabetes occur in low- and middle-income countries.[1]

Diabetes has a number of important and costly complications. Among the most common are eye problems that can cause blindness, kidney problems, and circulatory problems that can result in amputation of the lower extremities, stroke, and coronary heart disease. About two-thirds of people with diabetes have some disability, compared to less than one-third of people without diabetes.[8]

The risk factors for type 1 diabetes are still being studied. However, type 1 diabetes is associated with a family history of diabetes. In addition, environmental factors, increased weight and height development, increased maternal age at birth, and exposure to some viral infections have also been linked to developing type 1 diabetes.[9] Type 2 diabetes is also associated with a family history of diabetes. In addition, it is associated with diet and physical inactivity, obesity, insulin resistance, ancestry, and increasing age.[9,10] In high-income countries, less-educated and lower-income individuals have higher rates of diabetes than better-educated and wealthier people.[11]

Chronic Obstructive Pulmonary Disease

Chronic obstructive pulmonary disease (COPD) is a term used to refer to chronic lung diseases that cause limitations in lung airflow. The most common symptoms are shortness of breath, excessive sputum production, and a chronic cough. COPD is a life-threatening disease; it can progress to death.[12]

The main risk factors for COPD are as follows[12,13]:

- Tobacco smoking
- Household air pollution
- Ambient particulate matter pollution
- Occupational exposures to dust, chemicals, fumes, and other irritants
- Frequent lower respiratory infections as a child

Exposure to household air pollution as a child can also be a risk factor for developing COPD later in life.[13] COPD cannot be cured. However, treatments can alleviate symptoms, reduce disability, and prolong life.

Males and females now have roughly equal risk of being affected by COPD.[12] In 2016, it was estimated that there were about 250 million cases of COPD worldwide.[13] In that same year, about 5.6 percent of all deaths, or about 3.1 million deaths in the world, were associated with COPD.[1] About 90 percent of all of

Nutrition Facts

Serving Size 3 oz. (85g)
Serving Per Container 2

Amount Per Serving

Calories 200	Calories from Fat 120

	% Daily Value*
Total Fat 15g	**20 %**
Saturated Fat 5g	**28 %**
Trans Fat 3g	
Cholesterol 30mg	**10 %**
Sodium 650mg	**28 %**
Total Carbohydrate 30g	**10 %**
Dietary Fiber 0g	**0 %**
Sugars 5g	
Protein 5g	

Vitamin A 5%	•	Vitamin C 2%
Calcium 15%	•	Iron 5%

*Percent Daily Values are based on a 2,000 calorie diet. Your Daily Values may be higher or lower depending on your calorie needs.

	Calories	2,000	2,500
Total Fat	Less than	65g	80g
Sat Fat	Less than	20g	25g
Cholesterol	Less than	300mg	300mg
Sodium	Less than	2,400mg	2,400mg
Total Carbohydrate		300mg	375mg
Dietary Fiber		25g	30g

PHOTO 14-2 The number of people who have overweight and obesity continues to grow throughout the world. Yet there have been few successful efforts at addressing this problem at scale. Still, there is good evidence that food labeling, as shown here, can alter the choices people make about what and how much to eat. Can better food labeling make a difference in people's diets in low- and lower middle-income countries?
© mustafahacalaki/Getty Images.

those deaths were in low- and middle-income countries, reflecting their disproportionate exposure to the risks of COPD.[12,13]

In 2016, COPD was the 3rd leading cause of death globally and the 6th leading cause of DALYs globally. COPD was the 11th leading cause of death in low-income countries, the 4th leading cause in lower middle-income countries, the 3rd in upper middle-income countries, and the 4th in the high-income countries.[1]

Cancer

Cancer poses a unique challenge because there are many forms of cancer and each may have different characteristics concerning who it affects, its risk factors, and how it can be prevented and treated.

All forms of cancer were associated with almost 16 percent of all deaths in 2016, or about 9.5 million deaths. This would make cancers the second leading cause of death after cardiovascular disease. However, all forms of cancer combined led to more deaths than either ischemic heart disease or stroke when considered separately.[1] About 70 percent of all cancer deaths occur in low- and middle-income countries.[14]

Globally, all forms of cancer made up 9.2 percent of all DALYs in 2016. This was the second leading cause of DALYs after CVD. However, as with deaths, all forms of cancer when taken together led to more DALYs than either ischemic heart disease or stroke.[1]

WHO has estimated that the following are the most commonly occurring cancers worldwide[14]:

- Lung (2.09 million cases)
- Breast (2.09 million cases)
- Colorectal (1.80 million cases)
- Prostate (1.28 million cases)
- Skin cancer (non-melanoma) (1.04 million cases)
- Stomach (1.03 million cases)

WHO has also estimated that the most common causes of cancer deaths are the following[14]:

- Lung (1.76 million deaths)
- Colorectal (862,000 deaths)
- Stomach (783,000 deaths)
- Liver (782,000 deaths)
- Breast (627,000 deaths)

As noted earlier, there are a number of different types of cancer, and their prevalence varies across regions. **FIGURE 14-3** shows data on the leading types of cancer by WHO region.

The distribution of deaths caused by different types of cancers in each region is shown in **FIGURE 14-4**.

In the simplest of terms, there are a number of points that are striking about Figure 14-3:

- Liver cancers are uniquely important in Africa.
- Cervical cancer is a much larger share of all cancers in Africa than elsewhere.
- Stomach cancers are uniquely important in the WHO Western Pacific region.
- Bladder cancers are a larger share of the total cancers in Europe than elsewhere.

There are also a number of points that are striking about Figure 14-4:

- Cervical cancer deaths as a share of all cancer deaths are much more important in Africa than in any other WHO region.
- Deaths from cervical cancer are not among the top five leading causes of cancer deaths in several regions.
- Lung cancer deaths are not an important share of total cancer deaths in Africa.
- Bladder cancer deaths are the leading cause of cancer death only in Europe.
- Stomach and esophageal cancer deaths are an important share of cancer deaths only in the Western Pacific.

The global burden of cancer has continued to grow as more people in more places continue to live longer and the burden of communicable diseases decreases in these populations. Although cancer is common everywhere, the types of cancer most prevalent in a region can depend on environmental factors and the standard of living.[15] Generally, worldwide trends show that in low- and middle-income countries, the economic and societal shift toward lifestyles typical of high-income countries leads to a rising burden of cancers associated with reproductive, dietary, and hormonal risk factors. As income levels increase, cancers for which sedentary behavior or high fat consumption is a risk factor tend to increase as a proportion of all cancers.[16] Increases in breast cancer in low-income countries will be largely due to changes in reproductive practices, with women choosing to have fewer children, have their first pregnancy later in life, and breastfeed for a shorter period.[17]

Although cancer incidence has been increasing in most regions of the world, there are obvious differences and inequalities between low- and high-income countries in incidence and mortality rates. Incidence rates remain highest in higher-income regions due to longer average life spans, but mortality is relatively much higher in lower- and middle-income countries, likely due to a lack of early detection and access to treatment facilities. For example, breast

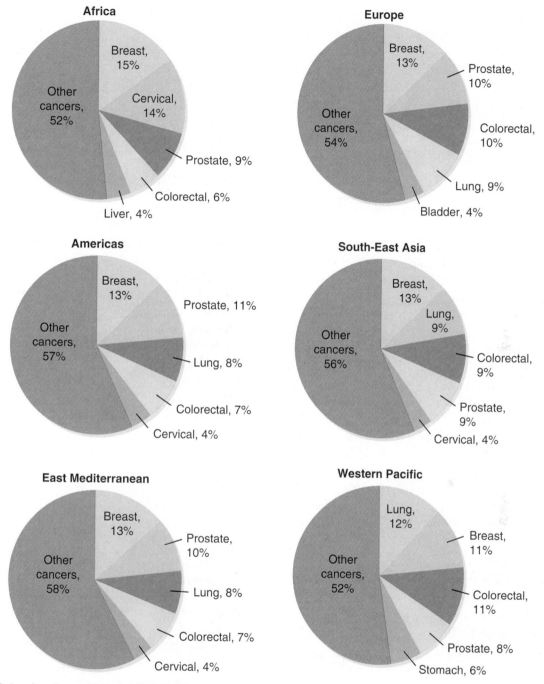

FIGURE 14-3 Leading Types of Cancer by WHO Region, as a Percentage of Total, 2018

Data from International Agency for Research on Cancer. (2018). GLOBOCAN 2018: Cancer today. Retrieved from https://gco.iarc.fr/today/explore

cancer incidence has reached more than 90 new cases per 100,000 women annually in Western Europe, a high-income region, compared with 30 per 100,000 in Eastern Africa, a low-income region. However, breast cancer mortality rates in these two regions are almost identical, at about 15 per 100,000.[16]

Moreover, many low- and middle-income countries face a double burden of cancer due to cancers caused by infectious agents combined with cancers associated with behavioral risks. The situation in high-income countries is more nuanced, depending on the country. Incidence for some cancer types, including prostate, colorectal, and female breast cancer, is increasing in several countries.[17] Decreasing mortality trends in high-income countries can largely be attributed to decreases in risk factors, such as changing smoking habits, especially in men, plus better screening and early detection, and improved treatment.[18]

In both low- and high-income countries, both men and women are affected by cancer. Certain cancers have higher incidence rates in women, like breast cancer, while others affect men and women equally.

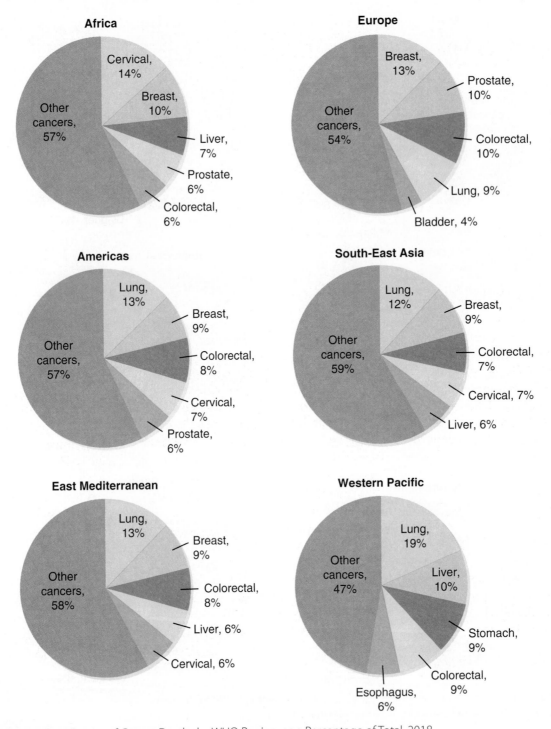

FIGURE 14-4 Leading Causes of Cancer Deaths by WHO Region, as a Percentage of Total, 2018

Data from International Agency for Research on Cancer. (2018). GLOBOCAN 2018: Cancer today. Retrieved from https://gco.iarc.fr/today/explore

Certain cancers, such as cervical cancer or prostate cancer, are specific to women or men. Although men and women of all ages are at risk for developing cancer, this risk increases with age. Cancer has a higher incidence in older individuals above 65 years due to more prolonged exposure to environmental risk factors and the accumulation of genetic changes. Moreover, the incidence of cancer tends to be higher in urban regions because of the differences in lifestyle and increased risk of exposure to carcinogens.[19]

There are many risk factors for cancer, and they vary by the type of cancer, as noted in **TABLE 14-5**. Some cancers are associated with tobacco use, such as lung and esophageal cancers. Tobacco use is one of the greatest risk factors for cancer in general. Tobacco is most directly linked to lung cancer, but using tobacco can also indirectly increase the risk of other cancers such as prostate and breast cancers. Alcohol is associated with liver, upper digestive tract, breast, and colorectal cancers, whereas diets high in red and

TABLE 14-5 Leading Risk Factors by Cancer Type

Cancer	Leading Risk Factors
Breast	Genetic predisposition, radiation exposure, alcohol, obesity (postmenopausal)
Cervical	HPV
Colorectal	Diets high in red meat and low in fiber; alcohol (men)
Liver	Hepatitis B virus, hepatitis C virus, schistosomiasis, alcohol
Lung	Tobacco use, asbestos exposure, air pollution
Pancreatic	Alcohol, obesity
Skin	UVA/UVB exposure

Data from World Health Organization (WHO). (2014). Cancer prevention. Retrieved from http://www.who.int/cancer/prevention/en/

processed meats and low in fiber have been associated with colorectal cancer. Obesity is a risk factor for breast (postmenopausal), colorectal, endometrial, kidney, esophageal, and pancreatic cancers. Similarly, low physical activity can be a major risk factor for colon, breast, and endometrial cancers.[17]

As noted, other cancers are associated with infectious agents. Liver cancer, for example, is associated with the hepatitis B virus, cervical cancer is associated with the human papillomavirus (HPV), and stomach cancer is associated with the bacteria *Helicobacter pylori*. Liver cancer is also associated with schistosomiasis, a parasitic worm that is also called "bilharzia," which infects more than 200 million people worldwide.[20] There are also numerous environmental and occupational carcinogens, such as asbestos, which was the cause of lung cancer in many roofing workers in the United States, for example.

Mental Disorders

Parallel with its definition of health, the World Health Organization defines mental health as "a state of well-being in which every individual realizes his or her own potential, can cope with the normal stresses of life, can work productively and fruitfully, and is able to make a contribution to her or his community."[21]

One of the major categories of noncommunicable diseases in the *Global Burden of Disease Study 2016* is "mental disorders." This includes depressive disorders, anxiety disorders, bipolar disorder, and schizophrenia. The category also includes conduct disorders, autism spectrum disorders, eating disorders, attention deficit hyperactivity disorder, and idiopathic developmental disability disorder. In earlier studies of the burden of

disease, alcohol and drug use disorders were included in mental disorders, but they are now categorized separately as "substance use disorders."[1] In addition, some of the writing on mental disorders globally discusses neurological and substance abuse disorders and self-harm. This chapter does contain comments on alcohol use and a case study on dementia. However, self-harm is treated in the chapter on adolescents and young adults and the chapter on injuries. In addition, this chapter does not discuss mental health issues in complex emergencies, which are discussed in the chapter on such emergencies.

Four mental disorders contribute the largest share to the burden of mental disorders and are the main focus of comments on mental disorders in this chapter. These are unipolar depressive disorders, which will be referred to here as depression; schizophrenia; anxiety disorders; and bipolar affective disorder. These conditions are defined briefly in **TABLE 14-6**.

Mental disorders have generally been thought to be associated overwhelmingly with disability, rather than with deaths. However, a recent study for the first time estimated the number of deaths associated with mental disorders. It suggested that more than 2.2 million deaths may have been associated in 2010 with depression, 1.3 million with bipolar disorder, and about 110,000 with autism spectrum disorder. The deaths from depression would be linked with suicide and comorbid conditions such as cardiovascular disease and infectious conditions. Those associated with bipolar disorder would be linked with comorbid causes such as cardiovascular disease, plus intentional injuries and suicide. Those associated with autism spectrum disorder would be linked with accidents, respiratory diseases, intellectual disability, epilepsy, and seizures.[22(p3)]

TABLE 14-6 Key Mental Health Terms and Definitions

Bipolar disorder—A serious mood disorder characterized by swings of mania and depression.
Depression—A mental state characterized by feelings of sadness, loneliness, despair, low self-esteem, and self-reproach.
Panic disorders—An anxiety disorder characterized by attacks of acute intense anxiety.
Schizophrenia—A mental illness, the main symptoms of which are hallucinations, delusions, and changes in outlook and personality.

Data from Ohio Psychological Association. *Psychological Glossary*; The Royal College of Psychiatrists. *Diagnoses or Conditions*; American Psychological Association. (n.d.). *APA Dictionary of Psychology*. Retrieved from https://dictionary.apa.org/.

Estimates of the Global Burden of Disease Study 2016 indicate that mental disorders contributed 4.8 percent of the total DALYs globally. This is more, for example, than the DALYs associated with unintentional injuries, chronic respiratory diseases, or HIV and sexually transmitted diseases. Depression alone is estimated to have been associated with 1.7 percent of the DALYs globally for both sexes and all age groups.[1]

The Global Burden of Disease Study 2016 suggests that there is a significant difference between the burden of mental disorders in females and males. Globally, they are associated with 5.6 percent of DALYs for females and 4.1 percent for males. The 2016 study also suggests that DALYs associated with mental disorders as a share of total DALYs for both sexes and all age groups rise as country income levels rise. Mental disorders are associated with 2.7 percent of DALYs in low-income countries, 4.1 percent in lower middle-income countries, 5.8 percent in upper middle-income countries, and 7.1 percent in high-income countries.[1]

It is also essential to examine how the burden of disease from mental disorders varies by age group. Mental disorders are the largest cause of DALYs for the 15- to 49-year-old age group, globally and in high-income, upper middle-income, and low-income countries. Only cardiovascular disorders cause more DALYs than mental disorders in this age group in lower middle-income countries. In fact, looking at specific causes for this age group globally, major depressive disorder is the 7th leading cause of DALYs and anxiety disorder is the 14th. Mental disorders (including suicide) take a particular toll on older adolescents aged 15 to 19 years. Major depressive disorders are the 4th leading cause of DALYs in this age group and anxiety disorders are the 9th leading cause of DALYs in this age group globally for both sexes.[1]

One reason for the large disability burden of these conditions is the substantial number of people who suffer mental disorders. Other reasons are that mental disorders often start at relatively young ages, they go on for a long time, they are often not cured, and they, therefore, produce large amounts of disability.

The determinants of mental disorders are complex, not very well understood, and appear to be both genetic and nongenetic. The recent *Lancet* Commission on Global Mental Health and Sustainable Development suggests that the causes of mental disorders relate to "the complex interplay of psychosocial, environmental, biological, and genetic factors across the life course, but in particular during the sensitive developmental periods of childhood and adolescence."[23(p4)]

Studies have also suggested that a number of social determinants have an especially important impact on mental health[22(p3)]:

- Demographic factors: age, gender, and ethnicity
- Socioeconomic status: low income, unemployment, income inequality, low education, and low social support
- Neighborhood factors: inadequate housing, overcrowding, neighborhood violence
- Environmental events: natural disasters, war, conflict, climate change, and migration
- Social change associated with changes in income, urbanization, and environmental degradation

It is also clear that there is a "vicious cycle" between social determinants and mental disorders, because having a mental disorder can cause disability, constrain one's ability to function and earn income, and further immiserate the affected person.[22(p3)]

WHO suggests that:

Determinants of mental health and mental disorders include not only individual attributes such as the ability to manage one's thoughts, emotions, behaviors and interactions with others, but also social, cultural, economic, political and environmental factors such as national policies, social protection, standards of living, working conditions, and community support.

Stress, genetics, nutrition, perinatal infections and exposure to environmental hazards are also contributing factors to mental disorders.[24]

Vision and Hearing Loss

Vision Loss

Vision loss is a major cause of disability. In addition, the aging of populations globally and continued improvements in life expectancy will increase the importance of vision loss as a burden of disease. These factors will also shift the types of problems that cause visual impairment toward those suffered by older populations.

The latest estimates suggest that almost 190 million people in the world suffer mild vision impairment.[25] It has also been estimated that there were almost 217 million people in the world in 2015 who suffered moderate to severe impairment of their vision. The major reasons for moderate to severe impairment were the following[26]:

- Refractive errors such as near- and farsightedness and astigmatism: 53 percent
- Cataract: 24 percent
- Age-related macular degeneration: 4 percent
- Glaucoma: 1 percent

The same study suggested that about 36 million people suffered from blindness in 2015. The following were the major reasons for blindness[26]:

- Cataract: 35 percent
- Uncorrected refractive errors: 21 percent
- Glaucoma: less than 1 percent

Besides the causes noted, blindness can also be caused by, among other things, glaucoma, vitamin A deficiency, and rubella. Some blindness also has parasitic and infectious causes, such as trachoma and onchocerciasis, although the number of people who are blind because of these causes has declined as progress has been made against these diseases.[27] Diabetes-related eye disease can also cause blindness. Over 80 percent of vision loss can be prevented or cured.[25]

The main risk factors for visual impairment are poverty, gender, age, and a lack of access to health services. Cigarette smoking is also a risk factor for cataracts and glaucoma.[28]

The causes of vision loss and blindness also vary by age and country income group. In young children, the leading cause of blindness in low-income countries is congenital cataracts, whereas in high-income countries it is eye problems associated with prematurity. In adults in low-income countries, a substantial burden of vision loss and blindness is associated with conditions that could be treated but are not, such as refractive errors and cataracts. In high-income countries, adult vision loss is much more often associated with macular degeneration.[25]

WHO has estimated that about 90 percent of those who suffer visual impairment live in low- and middle-income countries. About 65 percent of those who suffer visual impairment are over 50 years of age. About 19 million children also suffer such impairment, and 12 million have refractive errors that could be corrected with appropriate services.[27]

Females are more likely than males to suffer blindness and visual impairment from diabetic retinopathy and cataracts. Males are more likely to suffer visual impairment and blindness due to glaucoma and corneal opacity than females.[26]

The Global Burden of Disease Study 2016 suggests that visual impairment and blindness were responsible for about 1.2 percent of all DALYs in 2016, for both sexes and all ages. This was more than the burden for any individual cancer, except lung cancer, and about the same as the DALYs associated with anxiety disorder. The study also indicated that visual impairment and blindness were responsible for 0.6 percent of DALYs in low-income countries, 1.3 percent in lower middle-income countries, 1.4 percent in upper middle-income countries, and 0.8 percent in high-income countries.[1]

Hearing Loss

WHO estimates that about 432 million adults and 34 million children worldwide have disabling hearing loss. This means that more than 5 percent of the world's population suffers disabling hearing loss.[29] About 80 percent of them had adult-onset hearing loss and about 20 percent had childhood-onset hearing loss.[30] About one-third of people over 65 years of age are affected by disabling hearing loss.[30] More males have suffered hearing loss than females, probably as a result of exposure to noise.[30]

The 2016 Global Burden of Disease Study indicated that 1.3 percent of DALYs globally, for all ages and both sexes, could be attributed to hearing loss. This was greater than the burden globally of vision loss and more than any of the individual mental health disorders, except depression. The proportion of DALYs from hearing loss varied by country income group[1]:

- Low-income: 0.6 percent
- Lower middle-income: 1.0 percent
- Upper middle-income: 1.8 percent
- High-income: 2.1 percent

There are a range of factors in lower-income countries that affect hearing loss. These countries are also less able to treat hearing loss than higher-income countries. However, population aging is probably the most significant factor that will propel an increase in the number of people globally who suffer hearing loss.

Childhood-onset hearing loss is primarily related to congenital conditions, infection of the ear, or complications of other diseases, such as meningitis. Adult-onset hearing loss is largely related to exposure to noise and chemicals, as well as to aging. Poverty, poor hygiene, a failure to get vaccinated, and other causes that contribute to children getting infections are also risk factors for hearing loss.[28] Some medicines and recreational exposures can also cause hearing loss.[29]

Tobacco Use

Tobacco is such an important risk factor for cardiovascular disease, COPD, cancer, and diabetes that it bears specific mention of its own. Globally and for all ages and both sexes, tobacco is the third leading attributable risk factor for death. Tobacco is also the third leading risk factor for death in high-income and upper middle-income countries, the fourth in lower middle-income countries, and the eighth in low-income countries. Tobacco is the fourth leading risk factor globally for DALYs.[1]

It is estimated that about 7 million deaths annually are associated with the use of tobacco. More than 80 percent of these deaths are the result of direct tobacco use, and almost all of the remainder are due to the effects of secondhand smoke.[1,31] It is also estimated that 1 in 5 males over the age of 30 and 1 in 20 females over the age of 30 who die worldwide die of tobacco-related causes.[32,33] Ultimately, one-half to two-thirds of those who smoke will die of causes related to tobacco.[32] In addition, half of all tobacco-related deaths occur among people ages 35 to 69.[32] The most common tobacco-related deaths are from CVD; diseases of the respiratory system, such as emphysema; and cancers. Tobacco use can also increase the risk of getting tuberculosis (TB) or dying from it, as well as substantially increase the risk of developing diabetes.[33]

Most tobacco is used through smoking either cigarettes or *bidis*, which are hand-rolled cigarettes used largely in South Asia. It is estimated that about 1.1 billion people smoke worldwide.[31] Of countries that participated in a review of tobacco prevalence by WHO, Russia had the highest rate of smoking prevalence at about 39 percent of all adults. Indonesia was the second highest with 34.8 percent of adults smoking. The lowest rate of the countries surveyed was in Nigeria, with 3.9 percent prevalence.[33]

In all regions of the world, men smoke more than women do (see **TABLE 14-7**). This is most pronounced in low-income countries, in which relatively small shares of women smoke. Prevalence for men was estimated

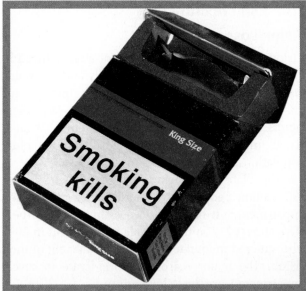

PHOTO 14-3 Reducing tobacco consumption is the single most important investment in reducing the burden of noncommunicable diseases. There is a well-known and evidence-based package of interventions to accomplish this. Especially in low- and lower middle-income countries, what forces impede the implementation of this package?
© Gannet77/E+/Getty Images.

earlier to vary from 18 percent in sub-Saharan Africa to 49 percent in East Asia and the Pacific. The rates for women were estimated to vary from 2 percent in a number of regions, including the Middle East and North Africa, South Asia, and sub-Saharan Africa, to 9 percent in Latin America and the Caribbean.[32] The highest rate of smoking prevalence among males is 76 percent in Indonesia.[34] The highest rate of smoking among women was 44 percent in Montenegro.[35]

The extent to which people take up smoking varies not only by sex but also by socioeconomic status and level of educational attainment. The higher the socioeconomic status and the higher the level of education, the less likely a person is to smoke. Most people who smoke start when they are teenagers. In addition, it is important to note that tobacco is physically addictive and that once one starts to smoke, it is difficult to stop.[36]

In some countries, such as Canada, Poland, Thailand, the United Kingdom, the United States, and Uruguay, the use of tobacco has been declining. However, usage is increasing among men in low- and middle-income countries and among women in all regions. Unless steps are taken to stop the spread of tobacco use, we are likely to see continued growth in CVD, COPD, and cancers related to smoking. CVD, COPD, and cancers related to smoking are often avoidable, and the overwhelming majority will occur in today's low- and middle-income countries.[33]

TABLE 14-7 Smoking Prevalence by Sex, by World Bank Regions and Country Income Groups, 2016

Region	Females	Males
East Asia and Pacific	3%	49%
Europe and Central Asia	21%	38%
Latin America and Caribbean	9%	21%
Middle East and North Africa	2%	35%
North America	18%	24%
South Asia	2%	25%
Sub-Saharan Africa	2%	18%
Low- and middle-income countries	4%	36%
High-income countries	19%	29%

Note: Data were not available for low-income countries only, so the data for low- and middle-income countries combined were used.

Data from The World Bank. (n.d.). Data: Smoking prevalence, females (% of adults). Retrieved from https://data.worldbank.org/indicator/SH.PRV.SMOK.FE; The World Bank. (n.d.). Data: Smoking prevalence, males (% of adults). Retrieved from https://data.worldbank.org/indicator/SH.PRV.SMOK.MA

Alcohol

Alcohol is a major public health problem. Alcohol use is associated with 0.7 percent of all DALYs globally. This varies by country income group:

- Low-income: 0.3 percent
- Lower middle-income: 0.5 percent
- Upper middle-income: 1 percent
- High-income: 1 percent

Globally, this is similar to the burden of breast and colorectal cancers. In addition, alcohol use disorders are the 9th leading attributable risk factor for deaths globally, the 9th leading risk factor in low- and middle-income countries, and the 6th leading risk factor in high-income countries. In 2016, alcohol was the 9th leading attributable risk factor for deaths and the 8th leading attributable risk factor for DALYs globally, for both sexes and all ages. This ranking did not vary much by country income group. However, there is substantial difference in ranking for males compared to females. It was the 5th leading risk factor for DALYs for males globally, but the 13th for females. There is also a substantial difference across regions in the importance of alcohol. It was the 6th leading attributable risk factor in Europe and Central Asia but the 15th in the Middle East and North Africa.[1]

High-risk drinking is defined as drinking 20 grams or more per day of pure alcohol for a woman and 40 grams a day for a man.[37] This is equal to about one-quarter of a bottle of wine for a woman and one-half a bottle of wine for a man. High-risk drinking may also be defined to include the total amount that is consumed, the frequency with which it is consumed, and the extent to which one engages in binge drinking.

High-risk drinking has a negative effect on people's health in a number of ways. Among other things, it increases the risks for hypertension, liver damage, pancreatic damage, hormonal problems, and heart disease.[37] In addition, alcohol intoxication is associated with accidents, injuries, accidental death, and a variety of social problems, including the first sexual encounters of teenagers, unprotected sex, and intimate partner violence. It is also possible to become dependent on alcohol, which has a number of negative psychological and physical consequences. Moreover, fetal alcohol syndrome is associated with low birthweight babies who are at risk of developmental disabilities.

The prevalence of high-risk drinking varies by region. It has been estimated that men in Europe and Central Asia have the highest prevalence of high-risk drinking: about 21 percent between ages 45 to 59. People in the Middle East and North Africa have the lowest prevalence, which is reported to be very low. South Asia also has a very low prevalence of high-risk drinking.[37] The prevalence rate of high-risk drinking also varies by age, with fewer people engaging in high-risk drinking after age 60 than at younger ages. In each region, high-risk drinking is higher among men than women, except in South Asia.[37]

There is very little evidence on the determinants of high-risk drinking, especially in low-income settings. Studies done in high-income countries suggest that lower socioeconomic status and lower educational attainment are risk factors for drinking to the level of intoxication.[37]

▶ The Costs and Consequences of Noncommunicable Diseases, Mental Health Disorders, Tobacco Use, and Alcohol Use

Overview

The economic costs of noncommunicable diseases are substantial and are growing, given the increasing burden of cardiovascular disease and diabetes, as well as a number of other conditions, such as vision and hearing loss. These costs include the direct costs of treating noncommunicable diseases, which by their nature often require many years of treatment. They also include indirect costs that result from lost productivity. These are also very substantial, given that noncommunicable diseases often start at relatively younger ages, often cause substantial disability, and can persist for many years.

In addition, many actors in the global health arena previously carried out their work as if high-income countries faced the burden and costs of noncommunicable diseases and low- and middle-income countries faced only the burden and costs of communicable diseases. However, in light of the increasing amount of noncommunicable diseases in low- and middle-income countries, it is clear that these countries do not have the luxury of facing *either* communicable *or* noncommunicable diseases. Rather, even low-income countries now *simultaneously* face the burden and costs of communicable diseases, noncommunicable diseases, and injuries. Some additional comments follow on the costs and consequences of noncommunicable diseases.

A study conducted in 2007 estimated the economic costs of selected noncommunicable diseases in 23 low- and middle-income countries. In those countries, the selected diseases make up 80 percent of the noncommunicable disease burden. This study noted that men in low- and middle-income countries are 56 percent more likely to die at the same age of

such causes than men in high-income countries, and women are 86 percent more likely to die at the same age than women in high-income countries of these causes. The study further concluded that these countries would lose $84 billion in economic production between 2006 and 2015 alone as a result of the large and growing burden of noncommunicable diseases.[38]

The World Economic Forum commissioned a study in 2011 on noncommunicable diseases in low- and middle-income countries. That study concluded that the cumulative output lost due to these conditions in low- and middle-income countries over the next 2 decades would be $47 trillion. The study also suggested that low- and middle-income countries would bear an increasing share of the costs of these diseases in the future.[39]

A more recent study examined the costs of noncommunicable diseases in China and India from 2012 to 2030. This study concluded that China would face costs of $27.8 trillion and India, $6.2 trillion. These costs would largely be driven in both countries by the costs of CVD, mental health, and respiratory diseases. The costs in China would be substantially greater than in India largely because of the much larger share of the population in China that would be older and because China is further along the epidemiological transition than India.[40]

Another study done recently suggested that, especially for populations without insurance, as many as 60 percent of the families affected by NCDs faced catastrophic out-of-pocket healthcare expenditures.[41] A study done on the costs of NCDs in the Eastern Caribbean island states found that patients suffering from noncommunicable diseases spent on average 36 percent of their annual household income on care for the management and treatment of these diseases.[42]

WHO has also estimated that implementing a package of "best buys" to address NCDs, which is discussed later, could generate $350 billion in additional economic activity between 2018 and 2030.[43]

Cardiovascular Disease

Only a small number of studies have been done on the direct and indirect costs of CVD in low- and middle-income countries. A study conducted in South Africa suggested that the direct costs of treating cardiovascular disease were about 25 percent of all healthcare expenditures, which was equal to between 2 percent and 3 percent of the gross domestic product (GDP) in that country.[44] The indirect costs of cardiovascular disease on the economy are likely to be substantial, given the relatively low age at which such diseases affect people in many countries.

Chronic Obstructive Pulmonary Disease

There is a limited amount of data on the costs of COPD in low- and middle-income countries. However, a small number of studies have been done on those costs in high-income countries. One study in Canada and Sweden, with data from the last decade, suggested that the annual indirect plus direct costs of COPD varied by severity of the illness and ranged, as noted here, from the least to the most severe illness[45]:

- Canada: $2,462 to $5,520
- Sweden: $696 to $20,260

These numbers suggest that the trajectory for treating COPD as populations age will be a challenging one, especially in resource-poor countries.

Diabetes

It is estimated that the direct costs of treating diabetes vary between 2.5 percent and 15 percent of health expenditures in different countries, depending on the prevalence of disease and the extent and costs of the treatment available.[9] Given the level of development of different low- and middle-income regions, it is likely that the Latin America and Caribbean region has the highest expenditure on diabetes per capita and sub-Saharan Africa the lowest such expenditures.[9]

Moreover, the International Diabetes Federation has estimated that expenditure by people with diabetes on this condition has risen from $232 billion in 2006 to $727 billion in 2017.[7(p51)] Given the increasing numbers of people with diabetes, these numbers should be expected to increase. In addition, the 10 countries spending the most on diabetes care spend from $5,700 a year per affected person to almost $12,000.[7(p52)] The International Diabetes Federation also estimates that countries in the different IDF regions are already spending between 6 percent and almost 17 percent of their annual healthcare expenditures on diabetes.[7(p54)]

The indirect costs of diabetes in low- and middle-income countries are substantial, partly reflecting the fact that many people in those countries live with diabetes without proper treatment and, therefore, suffer from disability and related losses in productivity. In fact, the direct and indirect costs of diabetes are likely to grow in all regions as the number of people with diabetes increases, as noted earlier.

Mental Disorders

There are relatively few reliable data on the direct and indirect costs of mental disorders. In addition, the studies that have been done largely refer to high-income countries. Nonetheless, they are indicative of the large and usually unappreciated costs of mental illness in all countries. A study done in the United States estimated that the direct and indirect costs of mental illness were equal to about 2.5 percent of gross national product (GNP), and a similar study done in Europe estimated that the costs of mental illness there were between 3 percent and 4 percent of GNP.[46] Studies done in Canada, the United Kingdom, and the United States showed that about half of the total costs of mental illness were direct costs and about half were indirect costs. These indirect costs are so substantial for mental illness that one study done in the United States estimated almost 60 percent of the productivity losses that come from illness, accidents, or injuries are linked with mental illness.[46] Studies done in the United States and the United Kingdom showed, in addition, that workers suffering from depression lost 40 to 45 days of work in a year as a result of their illness.[46]

The most comprehensive study done on the costs of noncommunicable diseases suggested that annual economic losses due to mental, neurological, and substance abuse disorders combined was about $8.5 trillion per year. The study also suggested that such costs are rising.[39] *The Lancet* Commission on Global Mental Health and Sustainable Development estimates that the economic losses to the global economy from mental health disorders will be about $16 trillion from 2010 to 2030.[23(p8)]

Hearing and Vision Loss

Unfortunately, very little information is available about the economic costs of vision and hearing loss, especially in low- and middle-income countries. This is despite the large number of DALYs attributed to them now and the growing number of DALYs that will be associated with them as populations age.

Some of the limited information that is available refers to the United States. A study done in 1995, for example, suggested that the economic cost to the United States from vision loss was almost $40 billion annually, of which about 60 percent was direct costs and 40 percent indirect costs.[47] Another study, published in 2006, estimated that the annual economic loss from major vision disorders in the United States was about $35 billion, of which about $16 billion was direct medical costs, about $11 billion other direct costs, and about $8 billion in productivity losses.[48]

A study of tea pickers in India confirmed the important economic consequences to individuals of vision loss, as well as the low cost of preventing some of those losses. This study sought to identify the economic impact of offering eyeglasses to treat presbyopia, the age-related decline in near vision, on individuals who picked tea and on the tea company for which they worked. Those tea pickers who were given eyeglasses were able to substantially increase the amount they picked per day, which increased their income and the income of the company. Compliance with the intervention was high, as was the benefit-to-cost ratio of the intervention. At the end of the study, those in the control group also received eyeglasses.[49]

A comprehensive review of the existing literature on hearing loss in low- and middle-income countries was published in 2010. It did not indicate either country or global estimates of the economic costs of hearing loss; however, it did indicate some of the costs that would be associated with hearing loss, for which economic costs could be calculated[50]:

- Constraints to the formal education of children with hearing loss, with its attendant consequences on their employment and earning prospects
- The number of school days missed by children with disabilities
- The costs of additional medical visits associated with children with disabilities
- The high cost of education for students with hearing loss
- The difficulties faced by adults with hearing loss in finding and keeping employment
- Income levels for people with hearing loss, which can be 45 percent of the levels of people without hearing loss, even in high-income countries

Tobacco Use

Calculating the costs of smoking to an economy can be very complicated.[51] The simplest way to do so is to calculate gross costs, which include all the costs associated with smoking-related diseases. Studies on the costs of smoking have largely focused on the costs of smoking in high-income countries. These studies suggested that the gross costs of smoking to various high-income economies range from 0.1 percent to 1.1 percent of GDP and that the costs to low- and middle-income countries might be just as high.[51]

However, a recent report by the National Cancer Institute of the United States, in collaboration with WHO, cited a study that concluded that the total economic costs of smoking to the world economy in 2012 were $1.4 trillion, or 1.8 percent of the world's GDP. The direct healthcare costs of smoking in 2012 were $422 billion, or about 5.7 percent of all healthcare expenditures that year.[52]

The prevalence rates of smoking are increasing among women everywhere and among men in low-income countries. We should expect, therefore, that the economic costs of smoking in those countries will increase for some time. In fact, it is estimated that 70 million people died of smoking-related causes between 1950 and 2000 and that, if present trends in tobacco use continue, an additional 150 million people will die of smoking-related causes between 2000 and 2025. Of course, the economic costs of this will be great.[53]

Alcohol Use Disorders

For the economic costs of alcohol use disorders, as for many other issues, there are relatively few data for low- and middle-income countries. Excessive alcohol use, as discussed earlier, is linked with health problems of the drinker. In addition, it is linked with violence and injuries caused by the drinker, such as when driving while intoxicated. When calculating the economic costs of excessive alcohol drinking, therefore, one has to take account of the costs of health care for the user and for others whose injuries or health conditions were caused by the user. The indirect costs of excessive alcohol drinking will include the productivity losses of the drinker and people hurt by the drinker because of excessive drinking.

The limited studies that have been done on the costs of alcohol abuse can only be considered indicative because they did not follow any standard methodology. However, they all reveal substantial costs of alcohol abuse, as a share of GDP[54]:

- Canada: 1.1 percent
- France: 1.4 percent
- Italy: 5.6 percent
- New Zealand: 4.0 percent
- South Africa: 2.0 percent

A 2009 study examined the economic costs attributable to alcohol in four high-income countries and two middle-income countries. The costs were greater than 1 percent of GDP in all countries. The highest costs were found in the United States, at 2.7 percent of GDP, and South Korea, at 3.3 percent of GDP.[55] In another estimate, the United States Centers for Disease Control and Prevention (CDC) estimated that excessive alcohol consumption costs the United States $290 billion annually.[56]

▶ Addressing the Burden of Noncommunicable Diseases

The global community has focused much more attention on NCDs in the last decade than ever before. The

United Nations, for example, convened a high-level meeting on noncommunicable diseases in September 2011. This meeting resulted in an international political commitment to trying to reduce the burden of NCDs by 25 percent by the year 2025.[57] This meeting highlighted the idea that all countries, including today's low- and middle-income countries, must take measures now to reduce the burden of noncommunicable diseases. This includes efforts that can reduce the burden of NCDs for those already afflicted by them, as well as efforts to prevent the burden of NCDs from growing.

The final declaration of the meeting indicated a number of steps that countries could take to address their burden of NCDs[58]:

- Focusing on prevention and the main risk factors of tobacco, alcohol, dietary risks, and the lack of physical activity
- Engaging all government parties in the battle against NCDs
- Increasing funding to address NCDs

The declaration further noted that countries should focus on the following actions[58]:

- Take multisectoral, cost-effective approaches to addressing NCDs
- Speed action on the measures indicated in the Framework Convention on Tobacco
- Implement WHO-recommended approaches to diet, physical activity, alcohol, and the marketing of unhealthy foods to children
- Promote cost-effective measures to reduce salt, sugar, and saturated fats in foods and eliminate trans fats in food
- Promote vaccination against the infectious causes of NCDs, including the vaccines against hepatitis B and HPV

The declaration from the meeting also highlighted a number of measures that should be taken to strengthen the ability of health systems to monitor NCDs and to act on them effectively, such as enhancing universal health coverage and improving access to affordable medicines.[58]

As a follow-up to the high-level meeting, the World Health Assembly, the governing body of WHO, endorsed in May 2013 the Global NCD Action Plan 2013–2020. The action plan includes a number of voluntary global targets as noted in **TABLE 14-8**. The action plan also contains a number of indicators for each of the targets.

The Global NCD Action Plan also lays out a series of evidence-based, cost-effective measures that are "best

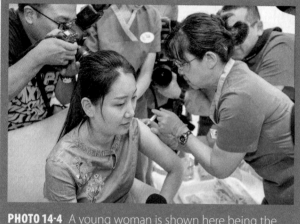

PHOTO 14-4 A young woman is shown here being the first in rural areas of China to get a vaccine against 9 strains of HPV. This vaccine and the one against hepatitis B are, in effect, "cancer vaccines." While there has been good progress in increasing their uptake, additional progress is needed. What measures can be taken globally and locally to increase the use of these vaccines, especially in low- and middle-income countries?
© China News Service/Visual China Group/Getty Images.

buys" in addressing the burden of some of the most important NCDs, other than mental disorders. The most significant of these measures are shown in **TABLE 14-9**.

More recently, a WHO report of a high-level commission on NCDs recommended a number of updated best buys for the control of NCDs that focused on CVD, COPD, and diabetes. These are shown in **TABLE 14-10**.

The DCP3 has recently suggested that countries adopt what it calls "essential packages" of interventions to prevent and address CVD, COPD, and diabetes in low- and middle-income countries. **TABLE 14-11** summarizes the DCP3 recommendations. The package recommended by DCP3 goes somewhat beyond the best buys suggested by WHO. One important advance of the DCP3 report was that it organized recommended interventions by platforms for their delivery. Table 14-11 shows the package that DCP3 has recommended and where such interventions could be delivered.

▶ Additional Comments on Addressing Key Risk Factors for CVD, COPD, and Diabetes

Some additional comments follow on steps that countries can take to address some of the key risk factors for CVD, COPD, and diabetes—tobacco, alcohol, hypertension, high cholesterol, and obesity.

TABLE 14-8 Global NCD Action Plan Voluntary Global Targets

Framework Element	Target
Mortality and morbidity	
Premature mortality from noncommunicable disease	A 25% relative reduction in the overall mortality from cardiovascular diseases, cancer, diabetes, or chronic respiratory diseases
Behavioral risk factors	
Harmful use of alcohol	At least 10% relative reduction in the harmful use of alcohol, as appropriate, within the national context
Physical inactivity	A 10% relative reduction in prevalence of insufficient physical activity
Salt/sodium intake	A 30% relative reduction in mean population intake of salt/sodium
Tobacco use	A 30% relative reduction in prevalence of current tobacco use in persons aged 15+ years
Biological risk factors	
Raised blood pressure	A 25% relative reduction in the prevalence of raised blood pressure or contain the prevalence of raised blood pressure, according to national circumstances
Diabetes and obesity	Halt the rise in diabetes and obesity
National systems response	
Drug therapy to prevent heart attacks and strokes	At least 50% of eligible people receive drug therapy and counseling (including glycemic control) to prevent heart attacks and strokes
Essential noncommunicable disease medicines and basic technologies to treat major noncommunicable diseases	An 80% availability of the affordable basic technologies and essential medicines, including generics, required to treat major noncommunicable diseases in both public and private facilities

Reproduced from World Health Organization (WHO). (2013). *Global action plan for the prevention and control of noncommunicable diseases, 2013–2020*. Geneva, Switzerland: Author.

Tobacco Use

The Framework Convention on Tobacco, agreed upon in 2003, outlines the measures that countries have agreed to undertake to reduce both the demand for and the supply of tobacco.[59] WHO then elaborated on these measures by outlining the MPOWER program for tobacco control, which consists of six elements[60]:

- Monitor tobacco use and prevention policies
- Protect people from tobacco smoke
- Offer help to quit tobacco use
- Warn about the dangers of tobacco use
- Enforce bans on tobacco advertising, promotion, and sponsorship
- Raise taxes on tobacco

The following comments elaborate on these points. Evidence suggests a number of steps can be taken to reduce the use of tobacco. Almost all countries tax cigarettes; however, low- and middle-income countries

TABLE 14-9 Selected Policy Measures in the Global NCD Action Plan

Objective	Selected Policy Measure
Tobacco use	Reduce affordability of tobacco products by increasing tobacco excise taxes Create by law completely smoke-free environments in all indoor workplaces, public places, and public transport Warn people of the dangers of tobacco and tobacco smoke through effective health warnings and mass media campaigns Ban all forms of tobacco advertising, promotion, and sponsorship
Harmful use of alcohol	Regulating commercial and public availability of alcohol Restricting or banning alcohol advertising and promotions Using pricing policies such as excise tax increases on alcoholic beverages
Physical inactivity and unhealthy diet	Reduce salt intake Replace trans fats with unsaturated fats Implement public awareness programs on diet and physical activity
Cardiovascular disease and diabetes	Drug therapy (including glycemic control for diabetes mellitus and control of hypertension using a total risk approach) and counseling to individuals who had a heart attack or stroke and to persons with high risk (greater than 30%) of a fatal and nonfatal cardiovascular event in the next 10 years Acetylsalicylic acid for acute myocardial infarction
Cancer	Prevention of liver cancer through hepatitis B immunization Prevention of cervical cancer through screening (visual inspection with acetic acid or Pap smear if cost-effective), linked with timely treatment of precancerous lesions

Reproduced from World Health Organization (WHO). (2013). *Global action plan for the prevention and control of noncommunicable diseases, 2013–2020.* Geneva, Switzerland: Author.

tend to tax cigarettes at lower rates than do high-income countries. Public demand for cigarettes is sensitive to price, and the lower the country income level, the more price increases will affect demand. Studies conducted in low- and middle-income countries indicate that a 10 percent increase in cigarette taxes can lead to an 8 percent reduction in the demand for cigarettes. Under these circumstances, taxing cigarettes would be an effective policy for reducing cigarette consumption.[32] Smuggling is a significant issue when countries raise tobacco taxes. However, there is evidence that 10 percent greater expenditure on efforts to reduce smuggling can lower smuggling by 5 percent and tobacco consumption by 2 percent.[33]

For countries where there is weak government enforcement of laws, it will be more difficult to enforce restrictions on smoking; however, an increasing number of countries are undertaking these measures. Studies suggest that countries that can enforce legal restrictions can reduce the number of cigarettes smoked between 5 percent and 25 percent and can reduce smoking uptake by about 25 percent.[32] The effectiveness of these actions is likely to be enhanced

in settings in which there are also strong social norms against smoking.

There is also evidence from high-income countries that consumption of cigarettes can be reduced by about 6 percent through a total ban on cigarette advertising, which is another step that low- and middle-income countries should consider.[32] Countries should also provide the public with information about the negative effects of smoking tobacco. There is evidence from high-income countries that such efforts led to short-term reduction in cigarette consumption of between 4 percent and 9 percent and long-term declines of between 15 percent and 30 percent.[32]

High-income settings that have had the biggest impact on reducing tobacco consumption have undertaken comprehensive tobacco control programs that generally included efforts to prevent young people from starting smoking, encouraging all smokers to quit smoking, reducing exposure to passive smoking, and eliminating disparities in smoking among different population groups by helping those most at risk to reduce tobacco consumption.[32] It remains critically important to stop people from taking up smoking;

TABLE 14-10 WHO Best Buys for the Prevention and Control of Noncommunicable Diseases

Goal	Strategy
Reduce tobacco use	<ul><li>Increase excise taxes and prices on tobacco products</li><li>Implement standardized health warnings on tobacco packaging</li><li>Enforce bans on tobacco advertising</li><li>Eliminate exposure to secondhand smoking in all indoor work places, public places, and public transport</li><li>Educate the public about the harms of tobacco through mass media campaigns</li></ul>
Reduce the harmful use of alcohol	<ul><li>Increase excise taxes on alcoholic beverages</li><li>Implement restrictions on alcohol advertising</li><li>Implement restrictions on the physical availability of alcohol via reduced hours of sale</li></ul>
Reduce unhealthy diet	<ul><li>Reduce the amount of salt used in food production and set target levels for the amount of salt in foods</li><li>Provide lower-sodium options in hospitals, schools, workplaces, and other public institutions</li><li>Implement a mass media campaign to reduce salt intake</li><li>Implement front-of-package labels for sodium content on food products</li></ul>
Reduce physical inactivity	<ul><li>Implement awareness campaigns and community-based programs to increase levels of physical activity</li></ul>
Manage cardiovascular disease and diabetes	<ul><li>Provide drug therapy and counseling to people who have had a stroke or heart attack or at risk of having one</li></ul>
Manage cancer	<ul><li>Vaccinate 9- to 13-year-old girls against HPV</li><li>Screen women aged 30 to 49 years for cervical cancer</li></ul>

Adapted from World Health Organization (WHO). (2018). *Time to deliver: Report of the WHO Independent High-Level Commission on Noncommunicable Diseases* (p. 33). Retrieved from https://www.who.int/ncds/management/time-to-deliver/en/

however, in order to reduce tobacco-related deaths in the near future, it is essential to reduce consumption among those already smoking. Preventing young people from taking up smoking will have an impact on tobacco-related deaths only in the more distant future. There is evidence that brief counseling sessions by medical providers can double quit rates to about 4 percent to 8 percent. Medications that aid quitting tobacco smoking can triple the rates of quitting to 8 percent to 12 percent.[33]

Alcohol

Despite the high burden of disease and economic costs that are related to excessive drinking of alcoholic beverages, very few countries have embarked on coherent efforts to reduce alcohol consumption. Those that have done so generally focused their attention on policy and legislative actions, such as taxation, laws on

drunk driving, and restricting alcohol sales to selected places, times, and age limits. Controlled advertising and tightened law enforcement, such as through more widespread breath testing of drivers, have also been imposed. Another successful part of such programs was to encourage counseling by healthcare providers through "brief interventions with individual high risk drinkers."[37(p893)]

Just as is the case for cigarette taxation, increased taxation on alcohol will likely lead to a decrease in the purchase and consumption of alcohol. Whereas in the case of tobacco increased taxation can lead to the smuggling of untaxed cigarettes, in the case of alcohol increased taxation can lead to a rise in the consumption of illicit alcohol. This is an issue that countries must take into account when considering raising taxes on alcohol.

In selected high-income countries, studies suggest that reducing the number of hours during

TABLE 14-11 Essential Interventions for the Prevention or Management of Risk Factors and Selected NCDs

All Cardiovascular and Respiratory Disease Conditions

Condition	Type of intervention		Personal health services, by delivery platform				
	Fiscal interventions	Intersectoral interventions	Public health interventions	Community based	Primary health center	First-level hospital	Referral and specialized hospitals
All conditions	Large excise taxes on tobacco products Product taxes on sugar-sweetened beverages	Improving the built environment to encourage physical activity School-based programs to improve nutrition and encourage physical activity Regulations on advertising and labeling tobacco products Actions to reduce salt content in manufactured food products Ban on trans fatty acids	Nutritional supplementation for women of reproductive age Use of mass media concerning harms of specific unhealthy foods and tobacco products	Use of community health workers for CVRD screening, improving adherence, and referral to primary health centers	Screening for hypertension for all adults Screening for diabetes in all high-risk adults	Tobacco cessation counseling and use of nicotine replacement therapy	
Specific Diseases							
Ischemic heart disease, stroke, and peripheral artery disease					Long-term management with aspirin, beta-blockers, ACEi, and statins to reduce risk of further events Use of aspirin in all cases of suspected myocardial infarction	Use of unfractionated heparin, aspirin, and generic thrombolytics in acute coronary events	Use of percutaneous coronary intervention for acute myocardial infarction

(continues)

TABLE 14-11 Essential Interventions for the Prevention or Management of Risk Factors and Selected NCDs *(continued)*

Condition	Type of intervention		Personal health services, by delivery platform				
	Fiscal interventions	Intersectoral interventions	Public health interventions	Community based	Primary health center	First-level hospital	Referral and specialized hospitals
Specific Diseases							
Heart failure					Medical management with diuretics, beta-blockers, ACEi, and mineralocorticoid antagonists	Medical management of acute heart failure	
Diabetes				Diabetes self-management education	Prevention of long-term complications through blood pressure, lipid, and glucose management		Retinopathy screening via telemedicine, followed by treatment using laser photocoagulation
Respiratory disease				Self-management for obstructive lung disease to promote early recognition and treatment Exercise-based pulmonary rehabilitation for patients with obstructive lung disease	Annual flu vaccination and five-yearly pneumococcal vaccine for patients with underlying lung disease Low-dose inhaled corticosteroids and bronchodilators for asthma and for selected patients with COPD	Management of acute exacerbations of asthma and COPD using systemic steroids, inhaled beta-agonists, and, if indicated, oral antibiotics and oxygen therapy	Management of acute ventilatory failure due to acute exacerbations of asthma and COPD

Note: ACEi = angiotensin-converting enzyme inhibitors; ARB = angiotensin receptor blocker; COPD = chronic obstructive pulmonary disease; CVRD = cardiovascular, respiratory, or related disorder

Adapted from Prabhakaran, D., Anand, S., Watkins, D., Gaziano, T., Wu, Y., Mbanya, J. C., & Nugent, R. (2018). Cardiovascular, respiratory, and related disorders: key messages from Disease Control Priorities. *The Lancet, 391*(10126), 1224–1236.

which alcohol can be sold can lead to a 1.5 percent to 3 percent decrease in high-risk drinking and a 1.5 percent to 4 percent decrease in alcohol-related traffic deaths.[37] Government authorities have to assess the extent to which such measures could be implemented effectively, especially in low- and middle-income countries with weak governance, as well as the extent to which such measures might also drive people to seek illicit alcohol.

Bans on alcohol advertising can be put into effect, as discussed for tobacco; however, it appears that such bans have had relatively little effect on the consumption of alcohol.[37] In healthcare settings in a number of countries, efforts have been made to engage high-risk drinkers in brief but specific education and counseling about the risks of excessive drinking. Even when taking relapses into account, it appears that such counseling is effective in reducing excessive consumption by 14 percent to 18 percent, compared to no treatment at all.[37] Although this approach might be effective in middle-income countries, it is unlikely to be effective in many low-income countries, given the scarcity of effective health services, the lack of health providers, and the already excessive demands on their weak health systems.

A study that was part of a broader major review of alcohol and health suggested that countries should take a stepwise approach to reducing alcohol consumption. Such an approach would allow countries to implement an increasing number of and levels of policies on alcohol as their capacity to legislate and enforce such approaches grew. The study recommended, at a minimum, that all countries make alcohol more expensive through excise taxes; reduce availability through regulation, licensing, and controlled sales to minors; check sobriety of drivers; and engage in the brief treatment approach noted above. As countries move to the next level of addressing alcohol abuse, they can, for example, ban sales and drinking in public places, regulate discounts on alcohol, and do random breath testing. At the last level, countries could set high minimum prices for alcohol, ban all forms of product marketing and restrict the design of packaging, and provide mandatory treatment for drunk driving, as well as treatment options for alcoholism.[61]

High Blood Pressure, High Cholesterol, and Obesity

The majority of risks associated with cardiovascular disease relate to a combination of high blood pressure, high cholesterol, high body mass index, low intake of fruits and vegetables, physical inactivity, and tobacco and alcohol use. The single most important risk factor for type 2 diabetes is obesity. This section comments on measures that can be taken to improve diet and to reduce obesity.

To reduce the burden of CVD and diabetes, healthy eating and maintaining a healthy weight are key. Generally, this requires eating more fruits and vegetables and decreasing the intake of salt and foods that are high in saturated fats and trans fats. It also entails limiting the intake of sugar and replacing refined grains with whole grains. People with overweight generally need to consume fewer calories each day and need to become more active physically.[62] Tax policies can be used to subsidize healthier foods and tax those that are less healthy.

The lack of regular physical activity, in fact, is associated, among other things, with CVD, stroke, type 2 diabetes, and colon and breast cancer. Urbanization, motorization, and television watching all reduce physical activity. Countries can use public policies to try to limit the role of automobiles, promote walking and biking, and design communities in ways that encourage healthy lifestyles. In Singapore and London, for example, taxes are levied on cars that enter the center of the city to reduce the use of vehicles and their attendant traffic and pollution. Many cities promote the use of bicycles and have bicycle lanes, as one can see in a number of European cities, such as Amsterdam. By contrast, other places have features that may encourage the use of automobiles over other types of transport. Some communities in the United States, for example, have limited or no sidewalks, little public transport, and services that are very spread out, all of which provide an incentive for people to use automobiles to get from place to place, rather than to walk or bike.[62]

One way to promote healthier diets is through population-based health education. Large-scale education efforts of this type, often through the mass media, have had mixed results because it is difficult to successfully promote the reduction of obesity on a large scale.[44] Generally, mass programs are more effective when they are combined with direct communication with individuals.

Few efforts to undertake population-based education measures have been studied. However, a study on a project to reduce salt intake among men in one part of China found a reduction in both hypertension and obesity after 5 years. In another effort, the government of Mauritius encouraged the population to switch from cooking with palm oil, which is high in saturated fat, to soybean oil, which has less saturated fat. Over a 5-year period, the intake of saturated fat decreased and the total cholesterol intake levels in the population fell.[44] Regulations and legislation on labeling food products and the reduction of unhealthy ingredients in commercial food products can also contribute to reducing obesity. New York City, for example, banned the use of trans fats in its restaurants.

Studies suggest the following goals for large-scale health education efforts if they are to succeed in changing what people eat[44]:

■ Have a realistic time frame that takes account of the time it takes to change deeply ingrained behaviors

■ Be carried out by a respected organization and headed by a competent manager, with clear responsibility

■ Encourage different organizations and agencies to work together to maximize the reach of the program and ensure that messages get disseminated in appropriate ways

■ Involve the food industry and enhance food labeling

Even as countries undertake the steps noted, they will still need to treat those who already have CVD or who have some of the key risk factors for CVD, including hypertension. Most low-income countries and some middle-income countries do not have the level of health system or the financial resources needed to carry out sophisticated medical procedures. In such settings, however, an important reduction in risks and in the burden of disease can be realized through preventive interventions, such as getting people with high cholesterol and hypertension to take inexpensive medicines to lower blood pressure and cholesterol.[44]

▶ Additional Comments on Addressing Diabetes, Cancer, Mental Health, and Vision and Hearing Loss

Given the growing importance of diabetes, the increasing amount of vision and hearing loss to be expected in aging populations, and the relative neglect historically of mental health issues, the following section offers additional comments on these topics. The section also includes additional comments on cancer, given that many lower-income countries are paying additional attention to preventing certain cancers and treating others.

Further Addressing Diabetes

Avoiding overweight and obesity is the single most important way to prevent type 2 diabetes. Although large-scale efforts to reduce obesity have generally not been very successful, a pilot project that used intensive personal counseling to promote weight loss through healthier eating and more physical activity was successfully carried out in China, Finland, Sweden, and the United States. The average weight loss after almost 3 years of participation in this study was about 10 pounds more than in the control group. In addition, the study group had a 58 percent lower rate of type 2 diabetes than the control group.[11]

Treatment for people with diabetes is needed in all countries. Treating people with type 1 diabetes with insulin is a cost-effective investment, although difficult to afford or manage in the poorest countries, especially for people living outside of the main cities. For all people with diabetes, it is cost-effective to control hypertension because the combination of the two diseases can produce major vascular complications. People with diabetes are also subject to foot problems from circulation difficulties associated with their diabetes, so appropriate foot care is another cost-effective investment. The cost of not doing this can be ulcers and eventual amputation of the foot.[6] Those countries with greater resources and a health system that can deliver additional interventions can also consider other cost-effective measures for treating diabetes, including vaccination against influenza and pneumococcal infections, diagnosis and treatment of retinal problems associated with diabetes, and treating hypertension with ACE inhibitors to prevent kidney problems from getting worse.[11]

Cancer

DCP3 recently recommended a package of interventions that are cost-effective and that low-resource countries should be able to carry out effectively to reduce the burden of cancers.[63] This package is shown in **TABLE 14-12**.

Tobacco control is overwhelmingly the first priority for preventing cancer, as noted earlier. Countries should also try to reduce the burden of cancer by vaccinating against infectious agents that are associated with cancers, such as hepatitis B and HPV. An increasing number of countries are adding the hepatitis B vaccine and the HPV vaccine to their national immunization programs. This is especially important in countries where a relatively large share of the population carries hepatitis B. However, additional progress is needed in ensuring that the first dose of the hepatitis B vaccine is given at birth to reduce mother-to-child transmission.[63]

The prevention and treatment of cancer face many challenges due to the fact that each type of cancer has

TABLE 14-12 Essential Cancer Intervention Package

Cancer type	Platform for intervention delivery			
	Nationwide policies, regulation, or community information	Primary health clinic or mobile outreach	First-level hospital	Specialized cancer center/unit
All cancers	Education on tobacco hazards, HPV and HBV vaccination, and importance of seeking early treatment for common cancers Palliative care, including, at a minimum, opioids for pain relief			
Selected tobacco-related cancers (oral, lung, and esophagus)	Taxation of tobacco products Warning labels or packaging Bans on public smoking, advertising, and promotion	Cessation advice and services, mostly without pharmacological therapies		
Breast cancer				Treat early-stage cancer with the intention to cure it
Cervical cancer	School-based HPV vaccination	Opportunistic screening (visual inspection or HPV DNA testing) Treat precancerous lesions	Treat precancerous lesions	Treat early-stage cancer
Colorectal cancer			Emergency surgery for obstruction	Treat early-stage cancer with the intention to cure it
Liver cancer		Hepatitis B vaccination (including birth dose)		
Childhood cancers				Treat selected early-stage cancer in pediatric cancer units/hospitals

Note: HBV = hepatitis B virus; HPV = human papillomavirus

Adapted from Gelband, H., Jha, P., Sankaranarayanan, R., Gauvreau, C. & Horton, S. (2017). Summary. In H. Gelband, P. Jha, R. Sankaranarayanan, et al. (Eds.), *Disease control priorities* (3rd ed., Vol. 3, p. 9). Washington, DC: The World Bank.

its own risk factors and the most appropriate form of treatment depends on the type of cancer and the level of resources available. Prevention is the most cost-effective method to reduce the economic burden of cancer because cancer treatment can require very advanced and expensive interventions over a long period of time. The importance of prevention and early detection in low- and middle-income countries is highlighted by the fact that the stage of cancer at the time of detection in these countries is, on average, substantially further advanced than in wealthier countries. In some countries, in fact, as much as 80 percent of cancers may already be incurable when first diagnosed. Patients in low- and middle-income countries also tend to have additional health conditions that make their recovery from cancer less likely than patients in high-income countries.[15]

Although screening is possible for a number of cancers, DCP3 has suggested that only opportunistic screening for cervical cancer is generally cost-effective and manageable in low-income settings. However, that study also suggested that screening for some other cancers, such as oral cancers in places with a high prevalence rate of such cancers, might also be warranted.[63]

To be effective, cancer treatment programs in most low-income countries and many middle-income countries will require considerable strengthening of a range of health services:

- Laboratory services
- Pathology
- Surgery
- Chemotherapy
- Radiotherapy

In addition, substantial training of health providers will be needed. It will also be very important that cancer treatment be of appropriate quality. This means, among other things, that all of the inputs needed to treat a particular cancer must be in place and must be delivered appropriately if desired cure rates are to be achieved.[63] Collective global effort could be very important for helping countries to reduce the costs of and improve procurement of cancer-related drugs, including drugs for palliative care. Collective efforts could also help countries address the key constraints to providing appropriate detection and treatment of cancer that are noted here.[64]

Even considering the present limitations on cancer treatment in a number of settings, DCP3 has suggested that it is cost-effective in low-resource settings to treat precancerous lesions of the cervix and to treat early stage cervical, breast, and colorectal cancers. DCP3 also suggests that low-resource countries should seek to treat those childhood cancers that have high cure rates, a recommendation that goes beyond those of WHO.[63]

Another aspect of cancer treatment is palliative care. There exists a substantial need to limit suffering and discomfort for the many individuals who will die from cancer each year. Unfortunately, low- and middle-income countries generally have only limited access to palliative care. This is despite the fact that two-thirds of cancer patients will suffer from moderate to severe pain and the majority of them will have no access to pain relief. Palliative care comprises both medical interventions and psychosocial support, but oral morphine is underused on a global level and there is a shortage of qualified counselors and therapists for such care.[65]

In addition to preventive measures, improved early detection methods are also critical to reducing the global burden of cancer. The world must continue to devise low-cost, effective screening tests for detecting cancer in low-resource settings. For example, cervical cancer screening is traditionally done via a Papanicolaou (Pap) smear in higher-income countries. However, Pap smear programs can be unfeasible where there is little infrastructure, so a direct visualization method, using visual inspection of the cervix with acetic acid, was developed that allows for testing and treatment of precancerous lesions in a single visit.[15]

Mental Health

There has been little progress until relatively recently in most low-income countries and many middle-income countries in addressing mental disorders. Unfortunately, despite the enormous and growing importance of mental disorders, there is generally an inadequate understanding of the importance of mental health, a lack of funds for mental health, a shortage of people who understand mental health issues, and stigma around mental disorders.

In addition, the more limited the resources of a country, the wider the gaps are likely to be between what is needed to address mental disorders and what is available to do so. In fact, estimates suggest that in low- and middle-income countries, only between 15 percent to 24 percent of people in need of mental health services receive them; even in high-income countries, it is estimated that only 35 percent to 50 percent of the people in need of mental health services receive them.[66] There is also an exceptional lack of human resources in most low- and middle-income countries to help address mental disorders. High-income countries have 170 times the number of psychiatrists and 70 times the number of nurses per capita as in low-income countries.[21]

Moreover, a significant amount of the mental health care in low- and middle-income countries is offered in large psychiatric hospitals that consume an overwhelming share of the mental health budget in those countries. Yet, a range of mental disorders can be prevented and treated effectively outside such settings. In fact, the evidence is growing that for $3 to $4 per person per year, countries could provide more community-based approaches to care that would offer drug therapy combined with psychosocial support for bipolar disorder, depression, and schizophrenia, as well as drug therapy for panic disorder.[67,68]

It is also clear that low- and middle-income countries have scarce financial resources and a limited number of mental health professionals. Thus, they are very unlikely to be able to take an approach to mental health that is medically oriented and depends on psychiatrists and psychiatric nurses, as is the case in most high-income countries. Rather, approaches that are cost-effective, scalable, and sustainable will have to depend on the community and on family-based efforts.

In this light, and with increasing attention to mental disorders, in 2013 WHO published the *Mental Health Action Plan, 2013–2020*.[66] This plan takes a comprehensive view of both needed actions and the various actors who must be involved in improving action on mental disorders, from stakeholders to government to the global community. Some of the key recommended actions in the plan are noted here:

- Countries should have national plans for mental health that are consistent with international human rights instruments.
- Countries should have updated their laws on mental health, and those laws should also be consistent with international human rights instruments.
- Services for people with severe mental disorders should be increased by 20 percent by 2020.
- Countries should implement multisectoral promotion and prevention programs for mental health.
- Steps should be taken to reduce suicides by 10 percent by 2020.
- Countries should take steps to improve their collection of and reporting on key mental health indicators.

The plan also recommended that countries should do the following:

- Involve a broader range of stakeholders in their work on mental health and involve those affected by mental disorders in the planning, implementation, and monitoring of mental health programs
- Shift services away from long-stay mental hospitals and toward non-specialized community-based approaches, evidence-based approaches, and community support
- Provide integrated and responsive care that brings together promotion, prevention, care, and support
- Reduce disparities by paying particular attention to groups most in need[66]

As noted earlier, *The Lancet* Commission on Global Mental Health and Sustainable Development issued a comprehensive report in late 2018.[23] The Commission strongly recommended dealing with mental health as an issue of sustainable development and of human rights, if progress in this field is to be enhanced. It also recommended that it be addressed as an essential component of universal health coverage.

TABLE 14-13 outlines the specific interventions the Commission recommended for addressing mental disorders in low-, medium-, and high-resource settings. It is important to remember as one considers this table that the services suggested for high-income countries are a long-run goal for all countries. Clearly, countries will need to take a stepwise approach to achieving such comprehensive services.

The Commission also put forward a number of other suggestions that could be important to health services beyond mental health[23]:

- Moving care away from hospitals and toward the community
- Involving patients and family members in planning and providing care
- Using multidisciplinary teams to provide social interventions alongside clinical and pharmacological interventions
- Focusing on comorbidities, while dealing with mental health conditions

There have been few mental health success stories in low- and middle-income countries. Uganda was one low-income country that sought before most others to improve mental health services through a model of community-based care that was truly integrated into the national health system. There have also been some instructive efforts to provide community-based care for schizophrenia in India. This has been coupled with shifting of tasks to community-based health workers, given the absence of trained mental health professionals in much of India. In addition, although Chile is now considered a high-income country, it will be important to follow the progress of mental health services for depression in Chile, which has become a model for a national effort to address depression.[67] A community-based intervention in Zimbabwe called the Friendship Bench has tackled common mental disorders by training lay health workers to deliver problem-solving therapy over the course of 6 weeks on benches outside of public clinics.[23] This is an example of a success story in which a program utilizing community members has been scaled up in many districts across the country. Another evidence-based intervention delivered through community health workers originated in Rawalpindi, Pakistan. The

TABLE 14-13 Mental Health Service Components Relevant to Low-Resource, Medium-Resource, and High-Resource Settings

	Community (provided across relevant sectors)	Primary Health Care (provided by general primary care workers)	Secondary Health Care (provided in general hospitals)	Tertiary Health Care (provided by mental health specialist services)
Low-resource settings	■ Basic opportunities for occupation/employment and social inclusion ■ Basic community interventions to promote understanding of mental health ■ Interventions to reduce stigma and promote help-seeking ■ Range of community-level suicide prevention programs (e.g., reduce access to pesticides) ■ Early childhood and parenting intervention programs ■ Basic school-based mental health programs ■ Promotion of self-care interventions ■ Integration of mental health into community-based rehabilitation and community-based inclusive development programs ■ Home-based care to promote treatment adherence ■ Activating social networks	■ Case identification ■ Basic evidence-based psychosocial interventions ■ Basic evidence-based pharmacological interventions ■ Basic referral pathways to secondary care	■ Training, support, and supervision of primary care staff ■ Outpatient clinics ■ Acute inpatient care in general hospitals ■ Basic referral pathways to tertiary care	■ Improve quality of care in psychiatric hospitals ■ Initiate move of mental health inpatient services from psychiatric hospitals to general hospitals ■ Initiate closure of long-stay institutions and develop alternatives in community settings ■ Establish means of licensing all practitioners treating people with mental disorders, including non-formal care facilities ■ Range of evidence-based psychological treatments ■ Ensure compliance with relevant human rights conventions ■ Initiate consultation-liaison services in collaboration with other medical departments and improve physical health care of people in mental health services
Medium-resource settings	Services as provided in low-resource settings and: ■ Coordinated opportunities for occupation/employment and social inclusion ■ Coordinated community interventions to promote understanding of mental health ■ Coordinated interventions to reduce stigma and promote help-seeking	Services as provided in low-resource settings and: ■ Equitable geographical coverage of mental health care integrated in primary care ■ Coordinated, collaborative care across service delivery platforms	Services as provided in low-resource settings and: ■ Multidisciplinary mobile community mental health teams for people with severe mental disorders	Services as provided in low-resource settings and: ■ Consolidate move of mental health inpatient services from psychiatric hospitals to general hospitals ■ Basic range of targeted specialized services (e.g., for children and young people, older adults, forensic settings)

High-resource settings					
Services as provided in low-resource settings and: ■ Intensive opportunities for occupation/employment and social inclusion ■ Intensive community interventions to promote understanding of mental health ■ Intensive interventions to reduce stigma and promote help-seeking ■ Full range of independent and supported accommodation for people with long-term mental disorders ■ Range of evidence-based services in community platforms (e.g., in schools, colleges, and workplaces) ■ Intensive drug and alcohol use prevention programs ■ Intensive childhood and parenting intervention programs (e.g., life-skills training) ■ Intensive community-level suicide prevention programs (e.g., hotlines, media training, reduce access to means of self-harm)	Services as provided in low-resource settings and: ■ Full geographic coverage of mental health care integrated in primary care ■ Collaborative care model with specialists supporting primary care practitioners	Services as provided in low-resource settings and: ■ Full range of evidence-based psychosocial interventions delivered by trained experts ■ Full range of evidence-based pharmacological interventions available	Services as provided in low-resource settings and: ■ Complete move of mental health inpatient services from psychiatric hospitals to general hospitals ■ Full range of targeted specialist services (e.g., for early intervention for psychoses, for children and young people, older adults, addictions, and forensic settings)	■ City-wide and district-wide coordination of integrated mental healthcare plans ■ Attention to mental health in policy across all sectors ■ Range of independent and supported accommodation for people with long-term mental disorders ■ Drug and alcohol use prevention programs ■ Range of services for homeless people with mental or substance use disorders ■ Community-based rehabilitation for people with psychosocial disabilities	■ Comprehensive mental health training for general healthcare staff ■ Integration of mental health care with other secondary health care (e.g., maternal and child health, HIV) ■ Consolidate consultation-liaison services

Reproduced from Patel, V., Saxena, S., Lund, C., Thornicroft, G., Baingana, F., Bolton, P., ... Unützer, J. (2018). *The Lancet* commission on global mental health and sustainable development. *Lancet Commissions, 392*(10157), 1553–1598. Retrieved from http://dx.doi.org/10.1016/S0140-6736(18)31612-X

Thinking Healthy Program (THP) has since been implemented in other parts of Pakistan and has been adopted by WHO's Mental Health Gap Action Program. THP has reduced rates of perinatal depression among mothers by using cognitive and behavioral therapy to improve mental well-being and social support. This is an example of a successful intervention in a low-resource setting that has been integrated with existing maternal and child health programs to facilitate scaling up.[23]

Vision Loss

In 2013, the World Health Assembly approved a global action plan for universal eye health. The plan has three objectives: generate evidence to enhance understanding and commitment; develop coherent national policies, plans, and programs on eye health; and enhance multisectoral collaboration and partnerships to improve eye health.[69]

The plan sets a target of reducing preventable blindness globally by 2019, from the 2010 baseline. The plan encourages countries to establish comprehensive eye care programs that are well integrated into their health systems and that focus on cost-effective interventions to address refractive errors and the burden of unoperated cataracts. The plan also encourages countries to continue to work across sectors to help address the infectious and parasitic causes of blindness, as well as the growing threat of blindness related to diabetes. Eye care is an area in which there has been considerable success with task shifting, and the plan also comments on the training of personnel for eye care, including allied healthcare personnel.[69] This could include, for eye care, for example, ophthalmic assistants who are trained to do cataract surgeries, especially in places where there are an insufficient number of ophthalmologists.

Hearing Loss

Despite the substantial burden of disease and economic costs related to hearing loss, the world has not yet adopted any coherent plan or targets to address this problem. WHO suggests, however, that about half of all cases of hearing loss can be addressed by primary prevention:

- Immunizing children against childhood diseases, including measles, meningitis, rubella, and mumps
- Immunizing adolescent girls and women of reproductive age against rubella before pregnancy

- Screening for and treating syphilis and other infections in pregnant women
- Improving antenatal and perinatal care, including promotion of safe childbirth
- Avoiding the use of ototoxic drugs, unless prescribed and monitored by a qualified physician
- Referring babies with high risk factors (such as those with a family history of deafness or those born with low birthweight, birth asphyxia, jaundice, or meningitis) for early assessment of hearing, prompt diagnosis, and appropriate management, as required
- Reducing exposure (both occupational and recreational) to loud noises by creating awareness, using personal protective devices, and developing and implementing suitable legislation

WHO also suggests that attention be paid to early diagnosis and appropriate medical or surgical intervention for middle ear infections that can lead to hearing loss.[30]

For that part of hearing loss that cannot be addressed through primary prevention, or for which it is too late, WHO also recommends that countries focus on early detection of hearing loss, accompanied by appropriate management of the problem. In principle, screening and diagnosis can be done in preschools, schools, and the community. However, WHO acknowledges that both diagnosis and appropriate management of hearing loss requires greater attention and resources in most low- and middle-income settings. WHO estimates, for example, that only about 1 in 40 people in low- and middle-income countries who need a hearing aid have one. In addition, the resources available in these settings for speech therapy, training in sign language, cochlear implants, and related efforts are limited.[30]

▶ Case Studies

Three case studies follow. The first brief deals with mental health, specifically on the growing costs of dementia. Few countries and few actors in global health have paid much attention to oral health, so the second study deals with that topic. The third study examines Poland's efforts to reduce tobacco consumption.

Dementia

Dementia is a syndrome—usually of a chronic or progressive nature—in which there is deterioration in cognitive function beyond what might be expected from normal aging.[70] The number of people living with dementia in 2013 was estimated to be about 44 million.[71]

Dementia mainly affects older people, and the likelihood of developing dementia after age 65 roughly doubles every 5 years. However, there is a growing awareness of cases with an onset before the age of 65.[72] The most important risk factors for dementia are age, family history, and heredity. Other risk factors include alcohol use, atherosclerosis, obesity, smoking, diabetes, and high cholesterol. Some evidence suggests an association between decreased blood flow conditions and the onset of vascular dementia.[73]

Dementia is a global problem on the rise. The number of people living with dementia is predicted to reach 115 million by 2050. Population aging is the main driver of projected increases in the prevalence of dementia. Low- and middle-income countries going through the demographic transition are predicted to see the largest increase in prevalence, and it is projected that by 2050, 71 percent of dementia patients will live in today's low- and middle-income countries, an increase from 68 percent in 2013. The largest increases are projected in East Asia and sub-Saharan Africa.[71]

The social and economic costs of dementia are great. In 2010, the total global societal cost of dementia was estimated to be $604 billion annually. This corresponded to 1 percent of worldwide GDP. The total cost of dementia as a proportion of GDP varied from 0.24 percent in low-income countries to 1.24 percent in high-income countries.[70] Costs of informal care provided by families and friends accounted for about 42 percent of worldwide total costs associated with dementia and the direct costs of care provided by professionals accounted for 42 percent of costs, as well. Direct medical care costs were much lower and were about 16 percent of worldwide total costs.[72] People with dementia and their families face a significant financial impact from the cost of providing health and social care and from the reduction or loss of income.[74]

Little is known on how to treat dementia, and there is no cure. However, there are many prospective treatments in clinical trials. In the absence of a cure or a treatment to reverse any cognitive loss, emphasis is put on supporting and comforting dementia patients and their families. A high proportion of people with dementia need some care, ranging from support with activities of daily living to full personal care and round-the-clock supervision.

In some high-income countries, between one-third and one-half of all people with dementia live in resource- and cost-intensive residential or nursing home care facilities.[71] In the Netherlands, care facilities have reached a new level. Self-contained villages for those experiencing late-stage dementia allow patients to enhance their quality of life by living in a surrogate environment. These villages are set up to allow residents to go about their daily lives of going to the grocery store, shopping, or restaurants safely because everyone working in the village, from the storekeeper to the neighbors, is trained to be a dementia caregiver.[75] It is known that with appropriate care and support, dementia patients can live many years after the onset of symptoms and can maintain a good quality of life.[74]

Special challenges arise in meeting the needs of dementia patients in low- and middle- income countries. In these settings, there are few social protection programs for the elderly and sick and also fewer overall services for their support and care.[71] In low-resource settings, it is recognized that primary care physicians or community-based workers will be the primary case managers, compared to specialists in more developed settings. With this in mind, primary care physicians and community-based personnel must be properly trained to handle dementia cases in these settings with a focus on continuing care and support rather than curative interventions.[76]

There is an urgent need to develop cost-effective packages for medical and social care that meet the needs of people with dementia and their caregivers across the course of the illness and a need to develop evidence-based prevention strategies. Only by investing now in research and cost-effective approaches to care can future societal costs be anticipated and managed.[71] Moreover, universal social support through pensions and insurance schemes could provide protection to this vulnerable group.[74] Governments and health and social care systems need to be adequately prepared for the future and must seek ways now to improve the lives of the growing number of people with dementia and their caregivers.[72]

Oral Health

The Burden of Disease

Seven oral diseases and conditions account for most of the oral disease burden globally:

- Dental caries (tooth decay)
- Periodontal (gum) diseases
- Oral cancers
- Oral manifestations of HIV
- Oro-dental trauma
- Cleft lip and palate
- Noma

Yet, these diseases and conditions are either largely preventable or can be treated in their early stages.[77]

Oral diseases were estimated by GBD 2016 to have affected at least 3.58 billion people worldwide in 2016. Caries of the permanent teeth were the most prevalent of all conditions assessed.[78] It was also estimated that 2.4 billion people suffered from caries of permanent teeth and that almost 500 million children suffered from caries of primary teeth.[77]

In fact, "oral disorders," as they are called in GBD 2016, are among the most common of the noncommunicable diseases. Oral diseases were the 15th leading cause of years of life lived with disability (YLD) globally, for all ages and both sexes, in 2016. The ranking of such disorders by country income group in 2016 was as follows[1]:

- Low-income: 23rd
- Lower middle-income: 24th
- Upper middle-income: 14th
- High-income: 13th

This ranking reflects, among other things, the interaction among changing diets, access to oral health services, and population aging. In fact, oral disorders were the 11th leading cause of YLD globally for people 50 to 69 years of age and over 70 years of age.[1] Yet, despite the enormous amount of disability related to oral disorders, such disorders have never been part of mainstream discussions of global health.

Dental caries and periodontal disease are two prominent but often neglected burdens of disease in low- and middle-income countries.[79] Dental caries, commonly known as tooth decay or cavities, are present in 90 percent of the global population,[80] including an estimated 60 percent to 90 percent of all school-aged children worldwide.[79] Caries result when naturally occurring oral bacteria break down foods, particularly those containing sugars and starches, into acidic by-products. These acids combine with saliva and food remnants to form plaque, a substance that builds up and adheres to teeth.[81] Without removal, the plaque acids will either degrade the enamel of teeth and create cavities or turn into tartar, which can be removed only with a professional dental cleaning.[82]

Together, plaque and tartar cause gingivitis, or inflammation of the gums. When left untreated, gingivitis advances to periodontitis, a disease characterized by inflammation around the teeth and also gums that retract from teeth to form spaces that are prone to oral infection.[82] Once infection occurs, the body's immune system responds with bacterial toxins that break down the bone and connective tissue, resulting in tooth loss.[80,82] Severe forms of periodontal disease

affect 5 percent to 15 percent of most populations,[80] including about 2 percent of youth worldwide who suffer from juvenile or early-onset aggressive periodontitis.[79] In addition, dental caries and periodontal disease can lead to tooth loss, including the loss of all natural teeth. This is a very important cause of years of life lived with disability in countries with a large share of older people in their population.

Moreover, many people fail to understand or underestimate the importance of oral health to child health. Both dental caries and periodontal disease contribute to childhood morbidity and have a negative impact on their quality of life.[80] Research suggests that the discomfort associated with biting and chewing for children who suffer from problems of oral health contributes to school absenteeism. It has been estimated, for example, that 50 million school hours are lost annually due to oral health issues.[83] Malnutrition prevalence rates also increase if children are too pained to eat.[80] A child's psychosocial well-being and ability to smile and speak may also be impaired.[77]

Another oral health disease of importance is noma. This condition originates as an untreated gingival inflammation, which then evolves into a gangrenous lesion that causes necrosis of the lips, chin, and facial tissues.[77,84] Noma has generally been reported in children ages 2 to 6 who reside in low-income communities with poor sanitation in sub-Saharan Africa.[79,84] However, it has also been reported in Asia and Latin America. The progression of noma can be halted when it is detected at an early stage and treated appropriately. Such treatment would include good hygiene, antibiotics, and nutritional rehabilitation. Yet, it has been estimated that 90 percent of children who are exposed to this illness die as a result of receiving no medical care,[79] and survivors in those settings must often cope with severe facial disfigurement.[85]

Risk Factors for Dental Caries, Periodontal Disease, and Noma

There are a number of risk factors for dental caries, periodontal disease, and noma in low- and middle-income countries. These include low education levels, low socioeconomic status, poor oral hygiene practices, alcohol and tobacco use, and excessive intake of dietary sugars.[79,86] These often occur in settings with limited access to safe water and modern sanitary facilities, insufficient community infrastructure, and the presence of cultural beliefs that do not support preventive oral health efforts.[88] Diabetes is also thought to be linked with periodontitis in reciprocal ways.

Current epidemiological data indicate that the oral health burden for children is most prominent in the Americas and has least affected Africa.[79] However, the prevalence of these diseases is expected to rise in low- and middle-income countries due to increased sugar consumption that accompanies economic growth and globalization of the food industry.[79] Illustratively, Dr. Karen Sokal-Gutierrez, a pediatrician working with the Children's Oral Health Nutrition Project in Latin America and Asia, has noted an "explosion in the availability of soda, chips and other junk food."[87] These products are low-priced and contain large amounts of sugars and starches. Unfortunately, children are often exposed to these products without nutrition education to inform them of the potential negative health effects of consuming such food.[87] The result is a pandemic of tooth decay, and Dr. Sokal-Gutierrez estimates that between one-third and one-half of the children she works with in El Salvador, Ecuador, Nepal, Peru, and Vietnam have baby teeth that are black, rotten, and decayed.[87]

Barriers to Treatment and Prevention

In addition to risk factors, there are several barriers to treatment that are prominent in resource-poor countries. In these countries, almost all tooth decay goes untreated.[88] The dental healthcare workforce in these countries is insufficient to satisfy service needs or demands.[80] In high-income countries such as the United States and Germany, for example, the dentist-to-patient ratio is 1 per 1,000 population. In low- and middle-income countries, the ratio decreases to 1 per 50,000 population. In some extreme cases in sub-Saharan Africa, the figure is as low as 1 dentist per 900,000 population. To further exacerbate this crisis, dentists in low-resource settings tend to practice in urban settings, neglecting rural populations, as families in these areas are more likely to be of low socioeconomic status and unable to afford dental care.[80]

Another barrier to treatment is the high cost of dental services. In high-income countries, oral diseases rank as the fourth most expensive health condition to treat,[79] yet insurance coverage for oral health is insufficient, even in many high-income countries. For instance, in the United States, about 130 million Americans lack dental coverage under their insurance plan. This includes 22 percent of children ages 1 to 17. Estimates suggest that, in low-income countries, the cost of treating dental caries in children alone would exceed the total current budget for child health activities.[79]

Some prevention efforts are also hindered by the limited infrastructure in many low- and middle-income countries, as well as constrained family incomes. There is strong evidence that long-term, low exposure to fluoride reduces the prevalence of dental caries in children.[87] Dispersing fluoride treatment in salt and public water systems has proven to be an effective prevention method in many countries.[89] However, successful implementation is largely contingent on the capacity of infrastructure of the affected population, and most low- and middle-income countries lack the resources to accomplish this.[80] With the world population now over 7 billion, estimates from the British Fluoridation Society's most recent global report suggest that only about 435 million people have access to fluoridated water sources. Moreover, even on a household level in the lowest-income countries, fluoridated toothpaste can exceed a family's budget. In the United Kingdom, for example, only 0.02 percent of a household's annual expenditure is accounted for by toothpaste; in Zambia this percentage rises to 4 percent of annual household expenses.[90]

Addressing Oral Health Issues

Interventions focused on cost-effective prevention methods that combine social policy and individual action will have the most impact in low- and middle-income countries.[87] It will be important to include oral health within the scope of comprehensive chronic disease prevention programs.[88] Oral diseases share many risk factors with the four most prominent chronic conditions—CVD, diabetes, cancer, and COPD. Using a shared risk factor approach has the potential to address several health issues simultaneously, benefiting resource-poor countries by reducing the required amount of physical and financial resources.[79] Government programs supporting subsidy and taxation relief of fluoridated toothpaste can also help to address financial barriers.[80] The U.S. Centers for Disease Control and Prevention suggests that every dollar spent on community-based fluoridation interventions saves $38 on dental treatment.[91]

Emphasis also needs to be placed on strengthening oral health education and promotional methods in community settings.[92] With an estimated 1 billion children attending primary and secondary schools globally, public schools are an optimal venue for health promotion and education among this population.[82] Oral health education reinforced in this environment can foster productive health attitudes and good oral health habits early in life. Pilot studies conducted in the United States and Ireland have shown that school-based interventions improve knowledge related to oral cleanliness and gingival health among school-age children.[91,93] The World Health Organization also strongly supports similar efforts on a global scale.[82]

The Challenge of Curbing Tobacco Use in Poland[94]

Background

More than three-quarters of the world's smokers live in low- and middle-income countries, where smoking is on the rise. In the late 1970s, Poland had the highest rate of smoking in the world, with the average Pole smoking 3,500 cigarettes a year and nearly three-quarters of Polish men smoking daily. The impact on the nation's health was staggering. In 1990, the probability of a 15-year-old boy in Poland reaching his 60th birthday was lower than in most countries, including China and India. Lung cancer rates were among the highest in the world. But because tobacco production, run by the state, provided a significant source of revenue, the government did not fully disclose to the population the negative consequences of smoking. The fall of communism further exacerbated smoking because tobacco, the first industry to be privatized, was taken over by powerful multinational corporations who flooded the market with international brands, spent vast sums on advertising, and kept prices so low that cigarettes cost less than a loaf of bread.

The Intervention

As the tobacco epidemic escalated, Poland's scientific community laid the foundation of the anti-tobacco movement. Research in the 1980s by the Marie Sklodowska-Curie Memorial Cancer Centre and Institute of Oncology contributed to the first Polish report on smoking, highlighting the link between tobacco and the country's alarming rise in cancer. A series of international workshops and scientific conferences in Poland further strengthened these findings. Civil society was experiencing a renewal at the time, with the formation of anti-tobacco groups such as the Polish Anti-Tobacco Society, which began to interact with international bodies, such as WHO and the International Union Against Cancer. In addition, the Health Promotion Foundation was established to lead public efforts on health issues and anti-tobacco education efforts.

With the fall of the Berlin Wall, the media became free to cover health topics and played an important role in disseminating information, raising awareness about the dangers of smoking, and shaping public opinion. When tobacco control legislation was introduced in 1991, a heated public debate ensued between health advocates and the powerful tobacco lobby, increasingly viewed by the public as a contest between David and Goliath. In 1995, groundbreaking legislation was finally passed, requiring sweeping measures such as large health warnings on cigarette packs and bans on smoking in enclosed workspaces and health centers, on electronic media advertising, and on tobacco sales to minors. A 30 percent increase in taxes levied on cigarettes was subsequently passed in 1999 and 2000, and advertising was completely banned. In parallel, the Health Promotion Foundation also launched extensive health education and consumer awareness efforts. These included an annual "Great Polish Smoke-Out" competition to encourage smokers to quit, with incentives like winning a weeklong stay in Rome and a chance to meet the Polish-born Pope John Paul II. Since the first smoke-out in 1991, more than 2.5 million Poles have permanently snuffed out their cigarettes because of the campaign.

The Impact

Cigarette consumption dropped 10 percent between 1990 and 1998, and the number of smokers declined from 14 million in the 1980s to under 10 million by the end of the 1990s. The reduction in smoking led to 10,000 fewer deaths each year, a 30 percent decline in lung cancer among men ages 20 to 44, a nearly 7 percent decline in CVD, and a reduction in infant mortality and low birthweight. Life expectancy in the 1990s increased by 4 years.

Lessons Learned

Poland's experience shows that once smoking is seen for what it is—the leading cause of preventable deaths among adults worldwide—governments do act. Working in concert with civil society and using state-of-the-art communication strategies, the Polish government succeeded in countering the powerful economic influence of the tobacco industry and inducing major shifts in smoking, an addictive behavior that was also then an ingrained social norm. Poland's sweeping legislative measures came to serve as a model for other countries. The experience of South Africa provides an interesting parallel: once the African National Congress came to power in 1994, the antismoking movement gained a powerful ally in Nelson Mandela and his first health minister, ultimately leading to the passage of strict tobacco control legislation and dramatic price control measures that increased the real value of cigarette taxes by 215 percent. As a result, cigarette consumption fell by more than 30 percent, from 1.9 billion packs in 1991 to 1.3 billion packs in 2002. As a South African researcher noted, "You need the right combination of science, evidence, and politics to succeed. If you have one without the other, you don't see action." For a more detailed discussion of the Polish efforts, see *Case Studies in Global Health: Millions Saved.*

► Future Challenges of Preventing and Addressing NCDs and Mental Disorders

The world must face a number of challenges if it is to reduce the burden of noncommunicable diseases in low- and middle-income countries. First, the number of people with new cases of noncommunicable diseases will grow in low- and middle-income countries as a result of the aging of the population, urbanization, globalization, and lifestyle changes. In addition, because noncommunicable diseases are chronic, the number of people with these diseases will also rise. The increasing number of people who will be at risk of and living with chronic diseases in low- and middle-income countries will pose a huge challenge to the health of these countries, their health systems, and their national finances.

Related to this, a number of low-income countries will have to deal with the challenge of addressing increasing amounts of noncommunicable disease simultaneously with having to address substantial burdens of communicable diseases and injury. This will severely tax the managerial, technical, and financial capacity of many low- and middle-income countries. It will also require greater attention by low-income countries to noncommunicable diseases and to improved surveillance of these diseases. Low- and middle-income countries will need to strengthen primary care and integrate the prevention and control of noncommunicable diseases into it.

In addition, it will be important to spread as rapidly as possible to low- and middle-income countries the lessons that high-income countries have already learned about how to address noncommunicable diseases in cost-effective ways. It will also be critical to generate much greater evidence about what works in low- and middle-income countries. This body of evidence, especially for low-cost interventions that have a high payback, needs to be disseminated in low- and middle-income countries as rapidly as possible. Ongoing mechanisms need to be established to ensure that cost-effective diagnostics and drugs get used as early as possible after their development in low- and middle-income countries and not just in high-income countries.

Even as they continue to learn from the experience of the high-income countries, the low- and middle-income countries need to take the measures that are known to prevent noncommunicable diseases, as discussed earlier in the chapter. However, many countries have limited administrative capacity, insufficient financial resources, and major gaps in human resources for health. Thus, lessons will also need to be generated and disseminated on the operational efforts needed to put effective NCD programs in place in low-resource settings. In addition, such countries will almost certainly need to take a stepwise approach to strengthening their NCD programs, starting with those efforts that will have the highest return.

Most low- and lower middle-income countries have little experience in dealing with NCDs in a major way. In addition, many of these countries have health systems with major structural weaknesses that are not ready to address NCD prevention and control more broadly, effectively, or efficiently. Thus, many countries will have to substantially strengthen their health systems if they are to meet the challenges of a growing burden of NCDs. They will also have to strengthen their ability to act across agencies to tackle measures such as taxation policies that are needed to reduce the consumption of tobacco, alcohol, and sugar.

A major goal of public health policy is to try to help people live longer lives that are as healthy as possible. The epidemiologic and demographic changes that are occurring globally suggest this goal can be achieved only if countries take measures now to prevent as much noncommunicable disease as possible. To achieve this aim, countries need to increasingly prepare their health systems to deal with the prevention and treatment of noncommunicable diseases in cost-effective and efficient ways. The failure to address these aims effectively will result in older but unhealthy populations, whose needs for care and cost of care will overwhelm the health systems of a number of countries.[95]

TABLE 14-14 portrays a number of measures that low- and middle-income countries could take to strengthen their health systems to address CVD, COPD, and diabetes. It is also clear that some of these measures can be extrapolated to what is needed for health systems to better address mental health disorders. Of course, in addition to the specific measures noted in the table, moving as rapidly as possible toward universal health coverage will allow for more services to be provided to a larger share of the population, with less financial risk than they face now. As countries do this, achieving services of appropriate quality will also be essential.

► Main Messages

Noncommunicable diseases constitute the largest burden of disease worldwide. In all regions of the world, except sub-Saharan Africa, the burden of these

TABLE 14-14 Recommendations for Health Systems Improvements that Enable Implementation of the Recommended Interventions

Policy	Platform
Improve access to the following essential medications: aspirin, beta-blockers, diuretics, ACEi or ARBs, statins, mineralocorticoid agents, nonanalog insulin, bronchodilators, and inhaled corticosteroids	Policy, public health
Develop a category of trained (nonphysician) health worker	Policy, intersectoral
Offer public emergency medical transport services	Policy, intersectoral
Create standardized care pathways for first-level hospitals to manage acute episodes for myocardial infarction, stroke, critical limb ischemia, heart failure, acute kidney injury, chronic obstructive pulmonary disease, or asthma exacerbation	Policy, public health
Issue national targets for secondary prevention to enable primary health centers to manage CVRD effectively	Policy, public health

Note: ACEi = angiotensin-converting enzyme inhibitors; ARB = angiotensin receptor blocker; CVRD = cardiovascular, respiratory, and related disorders.
Reproduced from Jamison, D.T., Gelband, H., Horton, S., Jha, P., Laxminarayan, R., Mock, C.N., & Nugent, R. (Eds.). (2018). *Disease control priorities* (3rd ed.). Washington, DC: The World Bank.

diseases is greater than the burden of communicable diseases and other Group I causes, including maternal, perinatal, and nutritional conditions. Cardiovascular disease is the single largest cause of death worldwide. Diabetes, some forms of cancer, and mental disorders are also major causes of disability and death from noncommunicable diseases. In fact, about 14 percent of the DALYs in 2016 were attributable to CVD, almost 9 percent to cancer, about 5 percent to the four mental disorders discussed earlier, about 3 percent to COPD, and almost 3 percent to diabetes.[1] Moreover, economic development, globalization, urbanization, and aging will encourage the growth of noncommunicable diseases globally as a share of the total burden of disease.

The leading risk factors for cardiovascular disease are hypertension, obesity, high cholesterol, and tobacco use. Tobacco use is also the leading risk factor for COPD. A lack of physical activity contributes to CVD and obesity, and the main risk factor for diabetes is obesity. Some cancers are associated with an infectious agent, such as hepatitis B, *H. pylori*, or the human papillomavirus. Other cancers are linked with tobacco use. The nongenetic risk factors that are associated with mental disorders are not well understood. However, the recent *Lancet* Commission on Global Mental

Health and Sustainable Development suggested that mental health disorders relate to a "complex interplay of psychosocial, environmental, biological, and genetic factors across the life course, but in particular during the sensitive developmental periods of childhood and adolescence."[23(p4)]

The costs of noncommunicable diseases and the use of tobacco and alcohol abuse are substantial. They have a considerable impact on people in their productive years of life. In addition, mental disorders and diabetes are associated with very large amounts of disability. The costs of trying to prevent the burden of noncommunicable diseases include efforts to promote healthier lifestyles, including a healthy diet, maintaining an appropriate weight, and increasing physical activity, while trying to reduce obesity, cigarette smoking, and excessive drinking. The costs of treating noncommunicable diseases can be high, both because of the high cost of some medical treatments for specific episodes of illness and the need to treat some diseases and conditions for many years. Mental disorders, for example, frequently start early in life and often continue throughout life. Nonetheless, some medicines used for hypertension and high cholesterol, for example, are highly cost-effective in dealing with CVD, even in low- and middle-income settings, as are some medicines and treatment for mental health disorders.

The single most important step that low- and middle-income countries can take now to reduce the burden of noncommunicable diseases is to reduce the consumption of tobacco. There is good evidence from high-income and some lower- and middle-income countries that taxing cigarettes more heavily, banning smoking from public places, and trying to educate the population about the impact of tobacco on health can all contribute to reducing tobacco consumption.

Reducing the burden of noncommunicable diseases will also require that alcohol-related harm be reduced, which can be done in cost-effective ways by taking measures analogous to those taken for dealing with tobacco. In addition, it is critical that obesity be reduced through healthier diets, consumption of fewer calories, increased intake of fruits and green leafy vegetables, and more physical activity. Tax policies can also be used to subsidize healthy foods and tax unhealthy foods. Other measures to reduce obesity can be complemented with food labeling legislation and legislation to encourage the use of healthier ingredients in food products. The intake of salt must also be reduced.

Low-resource countries will need to embed approaches to mental health in their communities and at the family level. This can be coupled with better training of primary healthcare staff at all levels to deal with mental health, improved access to low-cost drugs, and enhanced financing by deconcentrating the budgets so that they are not disproportionately allocated to large psychiatric hospitals.

A number of countries are making important progress in addressing vision loss by reducing the loss from infectious and parasitic causes and taking steps to address unoperated cataracts. To meet the global goals of reducing preventable blindness, countries will need to take additional measures to establish more comprehensive eye care programs at all levels of their healthcare systems.

There are substantial gaps in attention to hearing loss. However, about 50 percent of all hearing loss can be addressed through primary prevention, including better maternal nutrition and care, enhanced vaccination, and reduction in syphilis. Increasing the attention of resource-poor health systems to the remaining burden of hearing loss will require increases in financial, human, and health system resources with greater attention to early screening and appropriate management.

Study Questions

1. How important are noncommunicable diseases to the global burden of disease?
2. Why are noncommunicable diseases less important to the burden of disease in sub-Saharan Africa than in other regions?
3. What are the leading risk factors for cardiovascular disease?
4. What are the most important cancers that affect low-income countries?
5. What are the most important risk factors for cancers?
6. What factors are causing the epidemic of diabetes that is occurring worldwide?
7. Why are mental disorders so important to the burden of disease?
8. What measures have proven effective in reducing the use of tobacco?
9. What evidence is developing about community-based mental health programs?
10. What measures have been effective in reducing the abuse of alcohol?

References

1. Institute of Health Metrics and Evaluation (IHME). (n.d.). GBD Compare: Viz Hub. Retrieved from https://vizhub .healthdata.org/gbd-compare/
2. Jamison, D.T., Gelband, H., Horton, S., Jha, P., Laxminarayan, R., Mock, C.N., & Nugent, R. (Eds.). (2018). *Disease control priorities* (3rd ed.). Washington, DC: The World Bank.
3. Nichols, M., Townsend, N., Luengo-Fernandez, R., Leal, J., Gray, A., Scarborough, P., & Rayner, M. (2012). *European cardiovascular disease statistics 2012*. Brussels, Belgium: European Heart Network; Sophia Antipolis, France: European Society of Cardiology.
4. Gaziano, T. A., Srinath Reddy, K., Paccaud, F., Horton, S., & Chaturvedi, V. (2006). Cardiovascular disease. In D. T. Jamison, J. G. Breman, A. R. Measham, et al. (Eds.), *Disease control priorities in developing countries* (2nd ed., pp. 645–662). Washington, DC: The World Bank.
5. World Heart Federation. (2015). *Cardiovascular disease risk factors*. Retrieved from http://www.world-heart-federation .org/cardiovascular-health/cardiovascular-disease -risk-factors/
6. National Institutes of Health (NIH). (n.d.). *Obesity, physical activity, and weight control glossary*. Retrieved from http:// win.niddk.nih.gov/publications/glossary.htm

7. International Diabetes Federation. (2017). *IDF diabetes atlas* (8th ed.). Retrieved from http://www.diabetesatlas.org/IDF_Diabetes_Atlas_8e_interactive_EN/

8. Ryerson, B., Tierney, E. F., Thompson, T. J., Engelgau, M. M., Wang, J., Gregg, E. W., & Geiss, L. S. (2003). Excess physical limitations among adults with diabetes in the U.S. population, 1997–1999. *Diabetes Care, 26*(1), 206–210.

9. International Diabetes Federation. (2013). *IDF diabetes atlas* (6th ed.). Brussels, Belgium: Author.

10. Haffner, S. M. (1998). Epidemiology of type 2 diabetes: Risk factors. *Diabetes Care, 21*(Suppl. 3), C3–6.

11. Venkat Narayan, K., Zhang, P., Kanaya, A. M., Williams, D. E., Engelgau, M. M., Imperatore, G. & Ramachandran, A. (2006). Diabetes: The pandemic and potential solutions. In D. T. Jamison, J. G. Breman, A. R. Measham, et al. (Eds.), *Disease control priorities in developing countries* (2nd ed., pp. 591–603). Washington, DC: The World Bank.

12. World Health Organization (WHO). (n.d.). *Chronic obstructive pulmonary disease (COPD).* Retrieved from https://www.who.int/respiratory/copd/en/

13. World Health Organization (WHO). (2017). *Chronic obstructive pulmonary disease (COPD): Key facts.* Retrieved from https://www.who.int/en/news-room/fact-sheets/detail/chronic-obstructive-pulmonary-disease-(copd)

14. World Health Organization (WHO). (2018). *Cancer: Key facts.* Retrieved from https://www.who.int/en/news-room/fact-sheets/detail/cancer

15. Sloan, F. A., & Gelband, H. (Eds.). (2007). *Cancer control opportunities in low- and middle-income countries.* Washington, DC: National Academies Press.

16. International Agency for Research on Cancer. (2013). *Latest world global cancer statistics* (Press Release No. 233). Lyon, France: Author.

17. Veneis, P., & Wild, C. P. (2013, December 16). Global cancer patterns: Causes and prevention. *The Lancet.* Retrieved from https://www.thelancet.com/journals/lancet/article/PIIS0140-6736(13)62224-2/fulltext

18. Torre, L.A., Seigel, R.L., Ward, E.M. & Jemal, A. Global Cancer Incidence and Mortality Rates and Trends—An Update. *Cancer Epidemiol Biomarkers Prev.* 2016; 2016 (25) (1) 16-27; DOI:10.1158/1055-9965.EPI-15-0578.

19. Magrath, I. (2010). Cancer in low and middle-income countries. In M. Carballo (Ed.), *Health G20: A briefing on health issues or G20 leaders* (pp. 58–68). Sutton, United Kingdom: Probrook.

20. Centers for Disease Control and Prevention (CDC). (2012). *Parasites: Schistosomiasis.* Retrieved from http://www.cdc.gov/parasites/schistosomiasis/index.html

21. World Health Organization (WHO). (2014). *Mental health: A state of well-being.* Retrieved from https://www.who.int/features/factfiles/mental_health/en/

22. Patel, V., Chisholm, D., Dua, T., Laxminarayan, R., & Medina-Mora, M. E. (2015). Mental, neurological, and substance use disorders. In D. T. Jamison, H. Gelband, S. Horton et al. (Eds.), *Disease control priorities* (3rd ed., Vol. 4). Washington, DC: World Bank.

23. Patel, V., Saxena, S., Lund, C., Thornicroft, G., Baingana, F., Bolton, P., . . . UnÜtzer, J. (2018). *The Lancet* Commission on Global Mental Health and Sustainable Development. *Lancet Commissions, 392*(10157), 1553–1598. Retrieved from http://dx.doi.org/10.1016/S0140-6736(18)31612-X

24. World Health Organization (WHO). (2018). *Mental disorders: Key facts.* Retrieved from https://www.who.int/en/news-room/fact-sheets/detail/mental-disorders

25. World Health Organization (WHO). (2018). *Blindness and vision impairment: Key facts.* Retrieved from https://www.who.int/en/news-room/fact-sheets/detail/blindness-and-visual-impairment

26. Flaxman, S. R., Bourne, R. R.A., Resnikoff, S., Ackland, P., Braithwaite, T., Cicinelli, M. V., . . . Taylor, H. R. (2017). Global causes of blindness and distance vision impairment 1990–2020: A systematic review and meta-analysis. *The Lancet Global Health, 5*(12), e1221–1234.

27. World Health Organization (WHO). (2014). *Visual impairment and blindness* (Fact Sheet No. 282). Retrieved from http://www.who.int/mediacentre/factsheets/fs282/en/

28. Cook, J., Frick, K. D., Baltussen, R., Resnikoff, S., Smith, A., Mecaskey, J., & Kilima, P. (2006). Loss of vision and hearing. In D. T. Jamison, J. G. Breman, A. R. Measham, et al. (Eds.), *Disease control priorities in developing countries* (2nd ed., pp. 953–962). Washington, DC: The World Bank

29. World Health Organization (WHO). (2018). Deafness and hearing loss: Key facts. Retrieved from https://www.who.int/en/news-room/fact-sheets/detail/deafness-and-hearing-loss

30. World Health Organization (WHO). (2012). WHO global estimates on prevalence of hearing loss. Retrieved from https://www.who.int/pbd/deafness/WHO_GE_HL.pdf

31. World Health Organization (WHO). (2018). Tobacco: Key facts. Retrieved from https://www.who.int/en/news-room/fact-sheets/detail/tobacco

32. Jha, P., Chaloupka, F. J., Moore, J., Gajalakshmi, V., Gupta, P., Peck, R.,... Zatonski, W. (2006). Tobacco addiction. In D. T. Jamison, J. G. Breman, A. R. Measham, et al. (Eds.), *Disease control priorities in developing countries* (2nd ed., pp. 869–885). Washington, DC: The World Bank.

33. Jha, P., MacLennan, M., Yurekli, A., Ramasundarahettige, C., Palipudi, K. , et. al. (2015). Global hazards of tobacco and the benefits of smoking cessation and tobacco tax. In D. T. Jamison, H. Gelband, S. Horton, et al. (Eds.), *Disease control priorities* (3rd ed., Vol. 3). Washington, DC: The World Bank.

34. The World Bank. (n.d) Data: Smoking prevalence males, (% of adults). Retrieved from https://data.worldbank.org/indicator/SH.PRV.SMOK.MA

35. The World Bank. (n.d) Data: Smoking prevalence, females (% of adults). Retrieved from https://data.worldbank.org/indicator/SH.PRV.SMOK.FE

36. Jamison, D. T., Breman, J. G., Measham, A. R., Alleyne, G., Claeson, M., Evans, D. B., . . . Musgrove, P. (Eds.). (2006). *Priorities in health.* Washington, DC: The World Bank.

37. Rehm, J., Chisholm, D., Room, R., & Lopez, A. D. (2006). Alcohol. In D. T. Jamison, J. G. Breman, A. R. Measham, et al. (Eds.), *Disease control priorities in developing countries* (2nd ed., pp. 887–906). Washington, DC: The World Bank.

38. Abegunde, D. O., Mathers, C. D., Adam, T., Ortegon, M., & Strong, K. (2007). The burden and costs of chronic diseases in low-income and middle-income countries. *The Lancet, 370*(9603), 1929–1938.

39. Bloom, D. E., Cafiero, E. T., Jané-Llopis, E., Abrahams-Gessel, S., Bloom, L.R., Fathima, S., . . . Weinstein, C. (2011). *The global economic burden of noncommunicable diseases.* Geneva, Switzerland: World Economic Forum.

40. Bloom, D. E., Cafiero, E. T., McGovern, M. E., Prettner, K., Anderson Stanciole, J. W., Bakkila, S., . . . Weinstein, C. (2013). *The economic impact of non-communicable disease in China and India: Estimates, projections, and comparisons* (NBER Working Paper No. 19335). Cambridge, MA: National Bureau of Economic Research.

41. Jan, S., Laba, T-L., Essue, B. M., Gheorghe, A., Muhunthan, J., Engelgau, M., . . . Atun, R. (2018). Action to address the household economic burden of non-communicable diseases. *The Lancet, 391*(10134), 2047–2058.

42. The World Bank. (2012). *The growing burden of non-communicable diseases in the Eastern Caribbean.* Washington, DC: Author. Retrieved from http://documents.worldbank .org/curated/en/2012/01/15978036/growing-burden-non -communicable-diseases-eastern-caribbean

43. World Health Organization (WHO). (2018). *Saving lives, spending less: A strategic response to noncommunicable diseases.* Geneva, Switzerland: Author.

44. Rodgers, A., Lawes, C. M., Gaziano, T. A., & Vos, T. (2006). The growing burden of risk from high blood pressure, cholesterol, and bodyweight. In D. T. Jamison, J. G. Breman, A. R. Measham, et al. (Eds.), *Disease control priorities in developing countries* (2nd ed., pp. 859–868). Washington, DC: The World Bank.

45. S. Ehteshami-Afshar, S., FitzGerald, J. M., Doyle-Waters, M. M., & Sadatsafavi, M. (2016). The global economic burden of asthma and chronic obstructive pulmonary disease. *International Journal of Tuberculosis and Lung Disease, 20*(1), 11–23. doi: 10.5588/ijtld.15.0472

46. World Health Organization (WHO). (2003). *Investing in mental health.* Geneva, Switzerland: Author.

47. National Institutes of Health. (2010). *Healthy people 2010: Vision and hearing loss* (Working Paper 28). Retrieved from http://www.healthypeople.gov/2010/Document/pdf /Volume2/28Vision.pdf

48. Rein, D. B., Zhang, P., Wirth, K. E., Lee, P. P., Hoerger, T. J., McCall, N., . . . Saaddine, J. (2006). The economic burden of major adult visual disorders in the United States. *Archives of Ophthalmology, 124*(12), 1754–1760.

49. Reddy, P. A., Congdon, N. MacKenzie, G., Gogate, P., Wen, Q., Jan, C., . . . Ali, R. (2018). Effect of providing near glasses on productivity among rural Indian tea workers with presbyopia (PROSPER): A randomised trial. *Lancet Global Health, 6*(9), e1019–e1027.

50. Tucci, D. L., Merson, M. H., & Wilson, B. S. (2010). A summary of the literature on global hearing impairment: current status and priorities for action. *Otology & Neurotology, 31*(1), 31–41.

51. Lightwood, J., Collins, D., Lapsley, H., & Novotny, T. E. (2000). Estimating the costs of tobacco use. In P. Jha & F. J. Chaloupka (Eds.), *Tobacco control in developing countries* (pp. 63–104). London, United Kingdom: Oxford University Press.

52. U.S. National Cancer Institute and World Health Organization. (2016). *The economics of tobacco and tobacco control.* National Cancer Institute Tobacco Control Monograph 21. NIH Publication No. 16-CA-8029A. Bethesda, MD: U.S. Department of Health and Human Services, National Institutes of Health, National Cancer Institute; and Geneva, Switzerland: World Health Organization.

53. Chaloupka, F. J., Tauras, J. A., & Grossman, M. (2007). The economics of addiction. In P. Jha & F. J. Chaloupka (Eds.), *Tobacco control in developing countries* (pp. 107–130). London, United Kingdom: Oxford University Press.

54. World Health Organization (WHO). (2004). *Global status report on alcohol 2004.* Geneva, Switzerland: Author.

55. Rehm, J., Mathers, C., Popova, S., Thavorncharoensap, M., Teerawattananon, Y., & Patra, J. (2009). Global burden of disease and injury and economic cost attributable to alcohol use disorders. *The Lancet, 373*(9682), 2223–2233.

56. Centers for Disease Control and Prevention (CDC). (n.d.). *Excessive drinking is draining the US economy.* Retrieved from https://www.cdc.gov/features/costsofdrinking/index .html

57. United Nations. (2011). *2011 high-level meeting on the prevention and control of non-communicable diseases.* Retrieved from http://www.un.org/en/ga/ncdmeeting2011/

58. NCD Alliance. (2011). *Political declaration of the high-level meeting on the prevention and control of non-communicable diseases (NCDs): Key points.* Retrieved from http://www .ncdalliance.org/sites/default/files/rfiles/Key%20Points %20of%20Political%20Declaration.pdf

59. Conference of the Parties to the WHO FCTC. (2003). *WHO framework convention on tobacco control.* Geneva, Switzerland: World Health Organization.

60. World Health Organization (WHO). (2013). *Tobacco free initiative.* Retrieved from http://www.who.int/tobacco /mpower/en/

61. Casswell, S., & Thamarangsi, T. (2009). Reducing harm from alcohol: A call to action. *The Lancet, 373*(9682), 2247–2257.

62. Willett, W. C., Koplan, J. P., Nugent, R., Dusenbury, C., Puska, P., & Gaziano, T. A. (2006). Prevention of chronic disease by means of diet and lifestyle changes. In D. T. Jamison, J. G. Breman, A. R. Measham, et al. (Eds.), *Disease control priorities in developing countries* (2nd ed., pp. 833–850). Washington, DC: The World Bank.

63. Gelband, H., Jha, P., Sankaranarayanan, R. & Horton, S. (2015). Cancer. In D. T. Jamison, H. Gelband, S. Horton, et al. (Eds.), *Disease control priorities* (3rd ed., Vol. 3). Washington, DC: The World Bank.

64. Collective global effort will also be very important for helping countries to reduce the costs of and improve procurement of cancer-related drugs, including for palliative care. Collective efforts could also help countries address the key constraints with laboratories they now face to providing appropriate detection and treatment of cancer, as noted.

65. Horton, S., & Gauvreau, C. Cancer in low- and middle-income countries: An economic overview. In D. T. Jamison, H. Gelband, S. Horton, et al. (Eds.), *Disease control priorities* (3rd ed., Vol. 3). Washington, DC: The World Bank.

66. World Health Organization (WHO). (2013). *Mental health action plan, 2013–2020.* Geneva, Switzerland: Author.

67. Patel, V., Araya, R., Chatterjee, S., Chisholm, D., Cohen, A., De Silva, M., . . . van Ommeren, M. (2007). Treatment and prevention of mental disorders in low-income and middle-income countries. *The Lancet, 370*(9591), 991–1005.

68. Lancet Mental Health Group. (2007). Scale up services for mental disorders: A call to action. *The Lancet, 370*(9594), 1241–1252.

69. World Health Organization (WHO). (2013). *Universal eye health: A global action plan 2014–2019.* Geneva, Switzerland: Author.

70. World Health Organization (WHO). (2014). *Dementia (Fact Sheet No. 362)*. Retrieved from http://www.who.int/mediacentre/factsheets/fs362/en/

71. Alzheimer's Disease International. (2013). *Policy brief for heads of government: The global impact of dementia 2013–2050*. London, United Kingdom: Author.

72. Alzheimer's Disease International. (2010). *World Alzheimer report 2010: The global impact of dementia*. London, United Kingdom: Author.

73. Mayo Clinic Staff. (2014). *Dementia: Risk factors*. Retrieved from http://www.mayoclinic.org/diseases-conditions/dementia/basics/risk-factors/con-20034399

74. Alzheimer's Disease International & World Health Organization. (2012). *Dementia: A public health priority*. London, United Kingdom: Author.

75. Moisse, K. (2012, April 10). Alzheimer's disease: Dutch village doubles as nursing home. *ABC News*. Retrieved from http://abcnews.go.com/Health/AlzheimersCommunity/alzheimers-disease-dutch-village-dubbed-truman-show-dementia/story?id=16103780

76. Prince, M. J., Acosta, D., Castro-Costa, E., Jackson, J., & Shaji, K. S. (2009). Packages of care for dementia in low- and middle-income countries. *PLoS Med*, 6(11), e1000176. doi: 10.1371/journal.pmed.1000176

77. World Health Organization (WHO). (2018). *Oral health: Key facts*. Retrieved from https://www.who.int/news-room/fact-sheets/detail/oral-health

78. Institute of Health Metrics and Evaluation (IHME). (2013). *The global burden of disease: Generating evidence, guiding policy*. Seattle, WA: Author.

79. World Health Organization (WHO). (2014). *What is the burden of oral disease?* Retrieved from http://www.who.int/oral_health/disease_burden/global/en/

80. The Lancet. (2009). Oral health: Prevention is key. *The Lancet*, 373(9657), 1. doi: 10.1016/S0140-6736(08)61933-9

81. MedlinePlus. (2014). *Dental cavities*. Retrieved from http://www.nlm.nih.gov/medlineplus/ency/article/001055.htm

82. National Institute of Dental and Craniofacial Research. (2014). *Periodontal (gum) disease: Causes, symptoms, and treatments*. Retrieved from http://www.nidcr.nih.gov/oralhealth/topics/gumdiseases/periodontalgumdisease.htm

83. Kwan, S., Petersen, P., Pine, C., & Borutta, A. (2005). Health-promoting schools: An opportunity for oral health promotion. *Bulletin of the World Health Organization*, 83, 677–685.

84. Enwonwu, C. O., Falkler, W. A., & Phillips, R. S. (2006). Noma (cancrum oris). *The Lancet*, 368(9530), 147–156. doi: 10.1016/S0140-6736(06)69004-1

85. World Health Organization (WHO). (2014). *Noma*. Retrieved from http://www.who.int/topics/noma/en/

86. Peterson, P. (2004). Challenges to improvement of oral health in the 21st century—The approach of the WHO Global Oral Health Programme. *International Dental Journal*, 54 (Suppl. 6), 329–343.

87. Evert, J., Drain, P. K., & Hall, T. (2014). Vignette: Dr. Karen Sokal-Gutierrez and the Children's Oral Health Nutrition Project. In *Developing global health programming: A guidebook for medical and professional schools* (pp. 219–220). San Francisco, CA: Global health Education Collaborations Press.

88. Benzian, H., Hobdell, M., & Mackay, J. (2011). Putting teeth into chronic diseases. *The Lancet*, 377(9764), 464. doi: 10.1016/S0140-6736(11)60154-2

89. McDonagh, M. S., Whiting, P. F., Wilson, P. M., Sutton, . J., Chestnutt, I., Cooper, J., . . . Kleijnen, J. (2000). Systematic review of water fluoridation. *BMJ*, 321(7265), 855–859.

90. Goldman, A. S., Yee, R., Holmgren, C. J., & Benzian, H. (2008). Global affordability of fluoride toothpaste. *Globalization and Health*, 4(1), 7. doi: 10.1186/1744-8603-4-7

91. Gauba, A., Bal, I., Jain, A., & Mittal, H. (2013). School based oral health promotional intervention: Effect on knowledge, practices and clinical oral health related parameters. *Contemporary Clinical Dentistry*, 4(4), 493. doi: 10.4103/0976-237X

92. Children's Dental Health Project. (2013). *Cost effectiveness of preventive dental services*. Retrieved from https://www.cdhp.org/resources/163-cost-effectiveness-of-preventive-dental-services

93. Friel, S. (2002). Impact evaluation of an oral health intervention amongst primary school children in Ireland. *Health Promotion International*, 17(2), 119–126. doi:10.1093/heapro/17.2.119

94. Levine, R. (2007). Curbing tobacco use in Poland. In *Millions saved: Case studies in global health* (1st ed.). Burlington, MA: Jones and Bartlett.

95. Adeyi, O., Smith, O., & Robles, S. (2007). *Public policy and the challenge of chronic noncommunicable diseases*. Washington, DC: The World Bank.

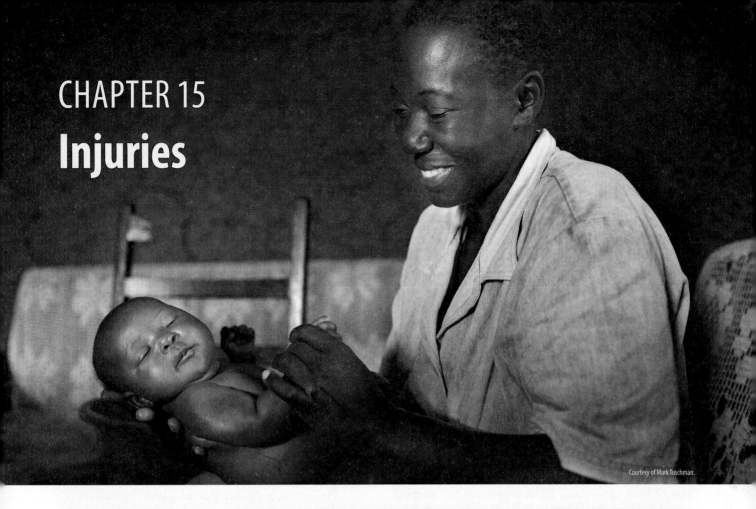

CHAPTER 15
Injuries

Courtesy of Mark Tuschman.

LEARNING OBJECTIVES

By the end of this chapter, the reader will be able to do the following:

- Define the most important types of injuries
- Describe the burden of disease related to those injuries
- Discuss how that burden varies by age, sex, region, country income group, and type of injury
- Outline the costs and consequences of those injuries
- Review measures that can be taken to address key injury issues in cost-effective, feasible, sustainable, and fair ways
- Describe some successful cases of preventing and addressing injuries at large scale

▶ Vignettes

Rodrigo was 25 years old. He was driving his 15-year-old car from Lima, Peru, to a small town in the mountains, where he planned to visit his grandmother. Rodrigo had received only a small amount of driver training. His car was very old, had never been inspected for safety, and had worn tires and poor brakes. The road was very mountainous, did not have good lane markings or signs, and had few safety barriers. As the sun was setting, another car came rapidly around a mountain bend, headed right toward Rodrigo's car. He tried to avoid the car but he swerved, slid down the side of the mountain, and was killed in the crash.

Mary was 12 years old and lived in a farming community in northern Tanzania. People in her village used fertilizer and pesticide in their agricultural work. They cooked with kerosene stoves. One day, after coming home from school, Mary was thirsty and saw some of her favorite soft drink near the area in which her mother cooked. Mary reached for the drink and began to consume it quickly. As she did so, she realized that her mother was storing in the soft drink bottle the kerosene that she used for cooking. Mary lived far from health services, got very sick that evening, and died of kerosene poisoning before she could receive proper medical treatment.

Paitoon was a 75-year-old physician in Bangkok, Thailand. He was still practicing medicine but was becoming frail. He fancied himself to be a young man and enjoyed fixing things around his house. While standing on a stool to repair a broken light, Paitoon

451

fell. Like many people his age who suffer falls, Paitoon broke his hip. Paitoon was hospitalized, had surgery, and could not attend to his patients for several months while he recovered.

Asma was a 26-year-old woman in Lahore, Pakistan. She lived in a very small house with a tiny cooking area. While preparing dinner one evening, the sleeve of Asma's clothing dipped into the cooking fire. Before her family could help her, Asma was engulfed in flames. She died the next day from burns.

▶ The Importance of Injuries

Injuries are exceptionally important and are among the leading causes of deaths and disability-adjusted life years (DALYs) worldwide. In 2016, about 8.4 percent of total deaths worldwide, equal to about 4.6 million deaths, were due to injuries. This is fewer than the number who died of ischemic heart disease or stroke that year. However, it is more than the number of people who died of chronic obstructive pulmonary disease or lower respiratory infections in 2016. In addition, it is more than twice as many as the number of people who died that year of lung cancer and about four times the number who died from HIV/AIDS. Injuries also represent about 11 percent of total DALYs globally and addressing them is an important SDG goal (**FIGURE 15-1**)[1].

This chapter is about injuries. It first reviews definitions that are commonly used when discussing injuries. The chapter then reviews the burden of disease from these injuries and how that burden varies by type of injury, sex, age, region of the world, and country income group. Although the chapter does include some data on conflicts and interpersonal

violence, the chapter focuses on what the *Global Burden of Disease Study* calls "unintentional injuries" and "transport injuries" (which are further broken down into "road injuries" and "other transport injuries"). It looks at the costs and consequences of those injuries and select measures that can be taken to reduce their burden in cost-effective ways. The chapter concludes with a case of successful prevention of transport-related injuries. Additional information on self-harm is given in the chapter on adolescent health and in the section on mental health in the chapter on noncommunicable diseases. Additional information on the impact of conflicts on health is in the chapter on complex humanitarian emergencies.

▶ Key Definitions

As we begin this chapter, it is important to define key terms and to outline more precisely the focus of the chapter.

For the purposes of this chapter, we can define an **injury** as follows:

> The result of an act that damages, harms, or hurts; unintentional or intentional damage to the body resulting from acute exposure to thermal, mechanical, electrical, or chemical energy or from the absence of such essentials as heat or oxygen.[2]

Some injuries, such as being shot by someone with the intention of harming you, are **intentional injuries**.

The *Global Burden of Disease Study 2016* includes a number of causes in the category of "injuries"[1]:

- Road injury
- Other transport injury
- Poisonings
- Falls
- Fires, heat, and hot substances
- Drowning
- Exposure to mechanical forces
- Adverse effects of medical treatment
- Animal contact
- Self-harm
- Interpersonal violence
- Conflict and terrorism
- Foreign body
- Environmental heat and cold exposure
- Other unintentional injuries not classified elsewhere

Unintentional injuries are "that subset of injuries for which there is no evidence of predetermined intent."[3] When this text refers to unintentional injuries, it refers to everything on the previous list except self-harm,

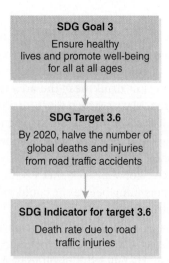

FIGURE 15-1 The Sustainable Development Goals and Injuries

SDG Goal 3
Ensure healthy lives and promote well-being for all at all ages

SDG Target 3.6
By 2020, halve the number of global deaths and injuries from road traffic accidents

SDG Indicator for target 3.6
Death rate due to road traffic injuries

Data from United Nations Sustainable Development Goals Knowledge Platform. (n.d.). Sustainable Development Goals. © United Nations. Reprinted with the permission of the United Nations.

interpersonal violence, and conflict and terrorism. As noted above, the *Global Burden of Disease Study* separates "transport injuries" from "unintentional injuries." This chapter *will* include "transport injuries" in its discussion of "unintentional injuries." However, it will refer specifically to transport injuries, including road injuries and other transport injuries, as appropriate.

This chapter pays particular attention to the largest causes of unintentional injury globally, including road injuries, and what might be done to address them:

- Road injury
- Poisonings
- Falls
- Fires
- Drownings

The Burden of Injuries

TABLE 15-1 shows the share of deaths by region that can be attributed to injuries (Group III causes) and how that compares with deaths from Group I and Group II causes.

TABLE 15-2 examines deaths from injuries by country income group, compared to deaths in

TABLE 15-1 Deaths from Injuries Compared to Total Deaths from Group I and Group II Causes, by World Bank Region, 2016

Region	Deaths from Group I Causes (Percentage of All Deaths)	Deaths from Group II Causes (Percentage of All Deaths)	Deaths from Group III Causes (Percentage of All Deaths)
East Asia & Pacific	8%	84%	8%
Europe & Central Asia	4%	90%	6%
Latin America & the Caribbean	12%	77%	11%
Middle East & North Africa	11%	74%	15%
North America	5%	89%	6%
South Asia	27%	63%	10%
Sub-Saharan Africa	59%	33%	7%

Note: Group I = communicable, maternal, neonatal, and nutritional disorders; Group II = noncommunicable diseases; Group III = injuries.
Institute of Health Metrics and Evaluation (IHME). (n.d.). GBD Compare: Viz Hub. Retrieved from https://vizhub.healthdata.org/gbd-compare

TABLE 15-2 Deaths from Injuries Compared to Total Deaths from Group I and Group II Causes, by World Bank Country Income Group, 2016

Income Group	Deaths from Group I Causes (Percentage of All Deaths)	Deaths from Group II Causes (Percentage of All Deaths)	Deaths from Group III Causes (Percentage of All Deaths)
High-Income Countries	5%	89%	6%
Upper Middle-Income Countries	7%	84%	9%
Lower Middle-Income Countries	29%	62%	9%
Low-Income Countries	54%	38%	8%

Note: Group I = communicable, maternal, neonatal, and nutritional disorders; Group II = noncommunicable diseases; Group III = injuries.
Institute of Health Metrics and Evaluation (IHME). (n.d.). GBD Compare: Viz Hub. Retrieved from https://vizhub.healthdata.org/gbd-compare/

those country income groups from Group I and Group II causes.

When examining deaths by region, injury deaths vary from 6 percent of all deaths in Europe and Central Asia, and North America to 15 percent in the Middle East and North Africa. When looking at injury deaths by country income group, we see that they range from 6 percent in high-income countries to 9 percent in lower middle- and upper middle-income countries. Both ranges largely reflect the level of motorization of a region, its ability to ensure safe transport, and its

ability to effectively address injuries, especially road transport injuries, when they do occur.

TABLE 15-3 shows DALYs from injuries by region, compared to Group I and Group II causes. **TABLE 15-4** shows DALYs from injuries by country income group, compared to Group I and II causes.

DALYs from injuries, as a percentage of all DALYs, vary from 7 percent in sub-Saharan Africa to 17 percent in the Middle East and North Africa. When looking at injury-related DALYs by country income group, we can see they vary from 8 percent of total DALYs in

TABLE 15-3 DALYs from Injuries Compared to Total DALYs from Group I and Group II Causes, by World Bank Region, 2016

Region	DALYs from Group I Causes (Percentage of All DALYs)	DALYs from Group II Causes (Percentage of All DALYs)	DALYs from Group III Causes (Percentage of All DALYs)
East Asia & Pacific	11%	78%	11%
Europe & Central Asia	7%	83%	11%
Latin America & the Caribbean	15%	71%	15%
Middle East & North Africa	17%	66%	17%
North America	5%	85%	10%
South Asia	33%	55%	12%
Sub-Saharan Africa	64%	29%	7%

Note: Group I = communicable, maternal, neonatal, and nutritional disorders; Group II = noncommunicable diseases; Group III = injuries.
Institute of Health Metrics and Evaluation (IHME). (n.d.). GBD Compare: Viz Hub. Retrieved from https://vizhub.healthdata.org/gbd-compare/

TABLE 15-4 DALYs from Injuries Compared to Total DALYs from Group I and Group II Causes, by World Bank Country Income Group, 2016

Income Group	DALYs from Group I Causes (Percentage of All DALYs)	DALYs from Group II Causes (Percentage of All DALYs)	DALYs from Group III Causes (Percentage of All DALYs)
High-Income Countries	5%	86%	10%
Upper Middle-Income Countries	11%	77%	13%
Lower Middle-Income Countries	36%	53%	11%
Low-Income Countries	61%	32%	8%

Note: Group I = communicable, maternal, neonatal, and nutritional disorders; Group II = noncommunicable diseases; Group III = injuries.
Institute of Health Metrics and Evaluation (IHME). (n.d.). GBD Compare: Viz Hub. Retrieved from https://vizhub.healthdata.org/gbd-compare/

low-income countries to 13 percent in upper middle-income countries.

Injury-related deaths as a share of total deaths are the same as injury-related DALYs only in the low-income countries. In all other country income groups, injury-related DALYs as a share of total DALYs are larger than injury-related deaths as a share of total deaths. These patterns in the data almost certainly reflect the same factors noted earlier, plus the ability of the higher-income countries to address injuries medically. This will save lives but may also lead to people living with injury-related disabilities.

It is important to understand the significance of injuries to the burden of disease in different regions, different country income groups, and different settings globally. We also need to note their importance in low-income and lower middle-income countries. The data on the burden of injuries highlights the fact that low-income and lower middle-income countries simultaneously face the burdens of communicable diseases, noncommunicable diseases, and injuries. This has important implications for the approach these countries must take to improving the health of their people and the potential costs of such efforts.

As shown in **TABLE 15-5** and **TABLE 15-6**, the leading categorized cause of injury-related deaths and DALYs varies by country income group.

In three of the four country income groups, road injuries are the leading cause of injury-related death. However, in high-income countries, both self-harm and falls are larger causes of injury-related death than transport injuries. This likely reflects greater safety in road transport in those countries and the ability of the health system to manage road injuries.

The data on DALYs are similar in many ways to the data on deaths. However, in high-income countries, falls are the leading cause of injury-related DALYs. This probably reflects the aging of high-income populations and the fact that self-harm often leads to death. In addition, transport injuries in lower middle-income countries are a much higher share of total DALYs than of total deaths. This may reflect the extensive motorization of those countries and the substantial number of related injuries. **TABLE 15-7** examines deaths from injuries by sex for different country income groups.

Table 15-7 highlights a number of points:

- Substantially more males than females die of injuries in all country income groups.
- This is true for all country income groups for almost all of the categories of injuries in the table.

- Males are around three times more likely than females, in all country income groups, to die from road injuries.
- The only category in the table for which more females die than males is from fires in lower middle-income countries.
- In low-income and high-income countries, the ratio of female-to-male deaths from fire is also higher than the ratio of deaths from any other injuries.

TABLE 15-8 provides data on the importance of injury-related deaths by broad age group.

Table 15-8 indicates clearly the exceptional importance of deaths from injuries for relatively younger age groups. Above 5 years of age, most children, adolescents, and young adults in low- and middle-income countries will succumb much less than at younger ages to pneumonia, diarrhea, and malaria, and injuries will rise as a share of their total deaths. By contrast, the 50- to 69-year-old age group are generally less subject to road injury deaths and are at the age when deaths from other causes are the most important.

Of course, deaths are only part of the injury story. Although the number of deaths is significant, the number of people who suffer disability annually from an injury is much greater than those who actually die from an injury. As an example, a study of fatal and nonfatal injuries in two states in the United States reported 13,052 deaths from injury but also identified over 2 million injuries for which medical care was sought over the course of the study.[4] In other words, for every person who died from an injury, there were approximately 153 people who were injured seriously enough to seek the help of a health professional. Moreover, this figure does not include those injuries for which people did not seek medical help, whether due to the minor nature of the problem, lack of access to care, a lack of health insurance, or other unknown reasons.

A similar study done with children in the United States showed that for each child under 19 years of age who was fatally injured, 45 children required hospitalization and another 1,300 children sought care in emergency rooms. This study also did not indicate how many injuries were treated at home.[5]

It is apparent that when disability due to injuries is taken into consideration, as well as mortality, the scope of the problem presented by such injuries is magnified. Moreover, these figures likely underestimate the total impact of injuries around the world. The true burden is likely to be much higher than that based on simple reporting of injuries, especially for low- and middle-income countries. Indeed, some

TABLE 15-5 Leading Causes of Death from Injuries, by World Bank Country Income Group, 2016

High-Income Countries

Rank	Cause	Percentage of Total Deaths from Injuries
1	Self-harm	29%
2	Falls	23%
3	Road injuries	21%
4	Interpersonal violence	5%
5	Foreign body	5%

Upper Middle-Income Countries

Rank	Cause	Percentage of Total Deaths from Injuries
1	Road injuries	34%
2	Self-harm	16%
3	Interpersonal violence	12%
4	Falls	12%
5	Drowning	6%

Lower Middle-Income Countries

Rank	Cause	Percentage of Total Deaths from Injuries
1	Road injuries	28%
2	Self-harm	17%
3	Falls	16%
4	Drowning	7%
5	Interpersonal violence	6%

Low-Income Countries

Rank	Cause	Percentage of Total Deaths from Injuries
1	Road injuries	27%
2	Self-harm	11%
3	Falls	10%
4	Interpersonal violence	9%
5	Drowning	9%

Institute of Health Metrics and Evaluation (IHME). (n.d.). GBD Compare: Viz Hub. Retrieved from https://vizhub.healthdata.org/gbd-compare/

TABLE 15-6 Leading Causes of DALYs from Injuries, by World Bank Country Income Group, 2016

High-Income Countries

Rank	Cause	Percentage of Total DALYs from Injuries
1	Falls	25%
2	Road injuries	24%
3	Self-harm	22%
4	Interpersonal violence	6%
5	Mechanical forces	6%

Upper Middle-Income Countries

Rank	Cause	Percentage of Total DALYs from Injuries
1	Road injuries	33%
2	Interpersonal violence	13%
3	Falls	13%
4	Self-harm	12%
5	Drowning	6%

Lower Middle-Income Countries

Rank	Cause	Percentage of Total DALYs from Injuries
1	Road injuries	37%
2	Self-harm	21%
3	Falls	18%
4	Drowning	10%
5	Interpersonal violence	10%

Low-Income Countries

Rank	Cause	Percentage of Total DALYs from Injuries
1	Road injuries	24%
2	Falls	10%
3	Interpersonal violence	10%
4	Drowning	9%
5	Conflict and terror	9%

Institute of Health Metrics and Evaluation (IHME). (n.d.). GBD Compare: Viz Hub. Retrieved from https://vizhub.healthdata.org/gbd-compare/

TABLE 15-7 Distribution of Deaths from Selected Injuries, Males and Females, by World Bank Country Income Group, 2016 (in Thousands)

| | High-Income Countries | | |
| | Total Deaths from Injuries | | |
	Males	Females	Total
Drownings	15	6	21
Falls	69	66	135
Fires	9	8	17
Forces of nature	0	0	0
Poisonings	2	1	3
Road injuries	92	35	127
Other	23	15	38
Total	210	131	341
	Upper Middle-Income Countries		
	Total Deaths from Injuries		
	Males	Females	Total
Drownings	78	27	105
Falls	125	64	189
Fires	22	13	35
Forces of nature	2	1	3
Poisonings	15	9	24
Road injuries	428	129	557
Other	70	25	95
Total	740	268	1008

	Lower Middle-Income Countries		
	Total Deaths from Injuries		
	Males	**Females**	**Total**
Drownings	96	44	140
Falls	167	144	311
Fires	24	33	57
Forces of nature	1	1	2
Poisonings	12	6	18
Road injuries	423	123	546
Other	110	79	189
Total	833	430	1263
	Low-Income Countries		
	Total Deaths from Injuries		
	Males	**Females**	**Total**
Drownings	27	11	38
Falls	23	20	43
Fires	12	11	23
Forces of nature	1	1	2
Poisonings	6	4	10
Road injuries	81	31	112
Other	32	18	50
Total	182	96	278

Note: The classification "Other" includes injuries due to animal contact, mechanical forces, and adverse effects of medicine.
Institute of Health Metrics and Evaluation (IHME). (n.d.). GBD Compare: Viz Hub. Retrieved from https://vizhub.healthdata.org/gbd-compare/

TABLE 15-8 Deaths Due to Injuries as a Share of Total Deaths, by Selected Age Group, Globally, 2016

Age (Years)	Percentage of Deaths Due to Injuries
5–14	28%
15–49	27%
50–69	7%

Institute of Health Metrics and Evaluation (IHME). (n.d.). GBD Compare: Viz Hub. Retrieved from https://vizhub.healthdata.org/gbd-compare/

authorities have questioned the reliability of disability data from lower-income settings where mechanisms to accurately collect and report injury data are lacking and where many injured persons do not seek or do not have access to medical care.[6-8]

When considering transport injuries, it is especially important to note that in some settings nearly 50 percent of the victims of road traffic accidents are pedestrians. In addition, a larger share of the transport injury victims are pedestrians in low- and middle-income countries than in high-income countries.[9]

Injury in Children, Adolescents, and Young Adults

Discussion thus far has centered primarily on data concerning all age groups combined. However, children throughout the world sustain an alarming number of injuries with high levels of attendant death and disability. The overwhelming majority of childhood injury deaths occur in the low- and middle-income countries.[1]

TABLE 15-9 examines in greater detail the four leading causes of injury-related deaths for children, younger adolescents, older adolescents, and young adults. It also shows the share of total deaths in each age group related to injuries.

The following are the most important messages from Table 15-9:

- Road injuries are the most important cause of injury-related deaths for these age groups. However, drowning is also important, especially in the younger age groups.
- As children age into adolescents and young adults, self-harm and interpersonal violence become very important causes of death.

Risk Factors for Injuries

Numerous reasons are thought to underlie the high prevalence of injuries in young children, especially in low- and middle-income countries. A partial list of factors includes developmental immaturity relative to the dangers these children face within their environments, the influence of poverty on families' ability to provide adult supervision and child care, and exposure to workplaces with unsafe, hazardous, and developmentally inappropriate machinery.[10-12] In support of this last point, a study in the

TABLE 15-9 Leading Causes of Injury-Related Deaths for Children, Younger Adolescents, Older Adolescents, and Young Adults, Globally, 2016

| Rank | Children Ages 5–9 | Younger Adolescents Ages 10–14 | Older Adolescents Ages 15–19 | Young Adults Ages 20–24 |
	Cause	Cause	Cause	Cause
1	Road injuries	Road injuries	Road injuries	Road injuries
2	Drowning	Drowning	Self-harm	Self-harm
3	Conflict & terror	Conflict & terror	Interpersonal violence	Interpersonal violence
4	Falls	Self-harm	Drowning	Conflict & terror
5	Mechanical forces	Interpersonal violence	Conflict & terror	Drowning

Institute of Health Metrics and Evaluation (IHME). (n.d.). GBD Compare: Viz Hub. Retrieved from https://vizhub.healthdata.org/gbd-compare

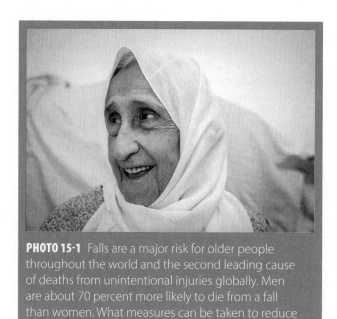

PHOTO 15-1 Falls are a major risk for older people throughout the world and the second leading cause of deaths from unintentional injuries globally. Men are about 70 percent more likely to die from a fall than women. What measures can be taken to reduce injuries and deaths from falls, especially in low-resource settings?
© Jasmin Merdan/Moment/Getty Images.

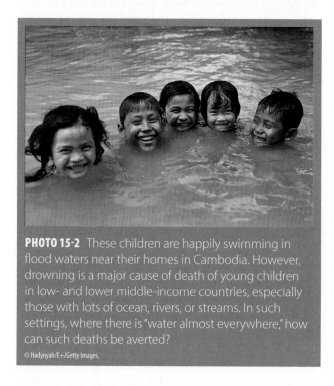

PHOTO 15-2 These children are happily swimming in flood waters near their homes in Cambodia. However, drowning is a major cause of death of young children in low- and lower middle-income countries, especially those with lots of ocean, rivers, or streams. In such settings, where there is "water almost everywhere," how can such deaths be averted?
© Hadynyah/E+/Getty Images.

within their environments and thus encounter more risks and complex situations, which challenge their reasoning and ability to react.

The risk factors for falls for young people in low- and middle-income countries appear to be associated with physical activity and also may vary with socio-economic status.[3] By contrast, the risk factors for injury from falls for older people are mostly related to age and overall physical condition.[3]

Low income, poor housing, and living in a crowded area are all risk factors for burns. Rural dwellers also suffer higher rates of burns than urban people. Children are more likely to suffer burns than any other age group.[3]

The risk factors for drowning in low- and middle-income countries are consistent with what we would expect. Young children are the most likely age group to drown, and males are more likely to drown than females. Most drownings occur during activities in which children regularly engage that take place near water. This is unlike in high-income countries, where most drownings are associated with recreational activities. Data suggest that children from poorer and larger families drown more frequently than other children.[3]

Studies done on poisoning in low- and middle-income countries have shed some light on risk factors. Poisoning tends to be correlated with using non-standard containers for poisonous goods and storing them within the reach of young children. Lower-income parents who are unable to spend time super-vising their children sufficiently around poisons are also more likely to experience the death of their child by poisoning than better-off parents.[3]

There are several well-known risk factors for road traffic injuries in low- and middle-income countries that are different from those in high-income countries. First is the increasing use of motor vehicles in low- and middle-income coun-tries. Second, in many countries, two-wheeled vehi-cles, which are especially unsafe, are very common. Third, most low- and middle-income countries pay insufficient attention to road planning, design, engi-neering, signage, or traffic management. Fourth, enforcement of speed limits is lax in many low- and middle-income countries; studies done on road traf-fic accidents show that about half of all such acci-dents are associated with excessive speed. It is also true in low- and middle-income countries that vehi-cles are less safe than in high-income countries, that many vehicles will not have safety belts or airbags, and that infant seats for cars are barely known or used. Motorcycle helmets are also used much less than in high-income countries.[3]

Philippines found that 60 percent of working chil-dren were exposed to unsafe conditions, and 40 percent of those children had suffered a serious workplace injury.[13]

It might be assumed that as children grow older, they become less susceptible to injury. However, the reality is that as children grow older and are better able to maneuver in their environment, the incidence of injuries does not decrease. More developmentally mature young persons tend to roam more widely

▶ The Costs and Consequences of Injuries

The costs associated with unintentional injuries worldwide are considerable. The economic burden due to such injury includes direct costs such as medical care, hospitalization, rehabilitation, and funeral fees, as well as indirect costs such as lost wages, sick leave from work, disability payments, insurance payouts, and costs associated with family care. These costs may be catastrophic for people within certain socioeconomic strata or those without access to sufficient health insurance. In this case, costs are frequently borne by government or private social services. In all cases, however, injuries represent a significant drain on personal and societal resources.

The World Health Organization (WHO) estimated in 2006 that the direct costs due to road traffic injuries alone were about $500 billion annually, with the share borne by the low- and middle-income countries estimated at $65–$100 billion. WHO also estimated that those costs were 1 percent to 2 percent of the GNP of low- and middle-income countries. At the regional level, Asia had the highest direct costs attributable to road traffic injuries, at $24.5 billion. Africa, the least affected region by cost, still bore a significant burden, with an estimated $3.7 billion annually in total costs.[14,15]

Few studies have been done on the costs of road traffic injuries for individual countries. However, a study on Iran concluded that the total cost of road traffic injuries in Iran between 2009 and 2010 was just over 2 percent of GDP.[16] A study of similar costs over 3 years in Jordan suggested they were between 2.2 percent and 2.5 percent of GDP in each of the years studied.[17] A 2014 study conducted for the United Nations indicated that the economic costs of road traffic accidents was between 2 percent and 4 percent for different countries in Asia.[18] The U.S. Centers for Disease Control and Prevention (CDC) suggests that in 2015 the medical and other costs associated in the United States with road traffic injuries was about $63 billion, which would have been about 0.35 percent of total GDP in the United States that year.[19]

The consequences of unintentional injury are not limited to financial costs. There are significant social consequences for individuals and families that may be associated with such injury. Numerous studies have documented the long-term physical and psychosocial consequences of unintentional injuries. Persisting problems with pain, fatigue, memory, and psychosocial functioning are common among victims of trauma.[20-22] Moreover, these social consequences may be relatively independent of injury severity and reflect the influence of other noninjury variables.[23] The psychosocial consequences for families of child injury victims may be significant, with difficulties relating to finances, changes in work status required to care for injured children, and altered family dynamics.[24]

▶ Addressing Key Injury Issues

TABLE 15-10 summarizes some of the key policy measures that countries can take to address the main burdens of unintentional injuries. The comments that follow elaborate on some of those points.

One of the key issues in addressing the burden of unintentional injuries is to raise awareness about how to apply rigorous methods of prevention and control to these injury problems. In fact, even among the high-income countries, the prioritization of such injuries as a significant health problem and the application of scientific methods of injury prevention and control are relatively recent phenomena.[7,25] Many public policymakers and public health actors in low- and middle-income countries may not yet appreciate the importance of unintentional injuries to the burden of disease or understand what can be done to prevent unintentional injuries.

In order to design effective prevention and control activities for unintentional injuries, formal surveillance systems are fundamental to obtain reliable information as to numbers and patterns of injury. Minimal standards for codifying injury morbidity and mortality should be implemented in all countries. In this light, WHO published guidelines for collecting, coding, and reporting injury data, which have been specifically developed for use in low-resource settings and do not require the use of technology-intensive data management systems or specialized training.[26,27]

In addition, it will be important to develop local capacity to analyze injury data and design injury prevention and mitigation programs. Injury prevention and control activities from one setting cannot be grafted onto another setting. Rather, planners with an intimate understanding of local knowledge, attitudes, beliefs, and practices are required to design effective interventions for injury prevention in specific settings.

The theoretical foundation of many injury prevention and control efforts is called Haddon's matrix, and it is widely used in efforts to understand and address injury issues. Haddon's matrix models the interaction of host, vector, and environment in an injury event. It is dynamic and models the events prior to, during, and after an injury.[25]

The example of road traffic injuries provides a useful learning tool for thinking about injuries using

TABLE 15-10 Essential Health Policies to Prevent Injuries

Fiscal and Intersectoral Policies

Domain of Action	Taxes and Subsidies	Infrastructure, Built Environment, and Product Design	Regulation	Information, Education, and Communication
Road Safety				
Overall	Subsidized public transportation	Mass transport infrastructure and land use (bus rapid transit, rail)	Adoption and enforcement of harmonized motor vehicle standards	
Pedestrian safety		Increased visibility, areas for pedestrians separate from fast motorized traffic		Increased supervision of children walking to school
Motorcycle safety		Exclusive motorcycle lanes	Mandatory use of daytime running lights for motorcycles; Mandatory motorcycle helmet laws	
Bicycle safety		Increased visibility, lanes for cyclists separate from fast motorized traffic		Social marketing to promote helmet use by child bicyclists
Child passenger safety			Legislation for and enforcement of child restraints (including seats)	
Speed control		Traffic-calming infrastructure (for example, speed bumps), especially at dangerous road segments	Setting and enforcement of speed limits appropriate to function of roads	
Driving under the influence of alcohol			Setting and enforcement of blood alcohol concentration limits	
Seat belt use			Mandatory seat belt use laws for all occupants	Social marketing to promote seat belt use

(continues)

TABLE 15-10 Essential Health Policies to Prevent Injuries

(continued)

Domain of Action	Taxes and Subsidies	Infrastructure, Built Environment, and Product Design	Regulation	Information, Education, and Communication
Other Unintentional Injury				
Drowning			Legislation and enforcement of use of personal flotation devices for recreational and other high-risk boaters	Parental or other adult supervision (for example, use of crèches) in high-risk areas Swimming lessons for children
Burns		Safer stove design		
Poisoning		Child-resistant containers		Information, education, and communication for safe storage of hazardous substances

Data from Mock, C. N., Smith, K. R., Kobusingye, O., Nugent, R., Abdalla, S., Ahuja, R. B., . . . Watkins, D. A. (2017). Injury prevention and environmental health: Key messages from *Disease Control Priorities*, third edition. In D. T. Jamison, J. G. Breman, A. R. Measham, et al. (Eds.), *Disease control priorities in the developing world* (3rd ed., Vol. 07, pp. 1–24). Washington, DC: The World Bank.

Haddon's matrix and how they can be prevented. The roadway (environment), automobile (vector), and human driver and behavior (host) interact in the moments leading up to a collision, during the collision, and in the moments after the collision.

Measures to prevent unintentional injuries have usually focused on education, enforcement, and engineering in the context of Haddon's matrix. Recent efforts to reduce road traffic injuries have emphasized safer roads, safer vehicles, and safer systems. They have also paid increasing attention to land use and transport planning.[3] A study of the cost-effectiveness of approaches to reducing road traffic injuries in sub-Saharan Africa and South-East Asia suggested that combined approaches to enforcement, such as enforcing speed limits, drunk driving laws, and motorcycle helmet laws, would likely be the most cost-effective approach but that the specifics of the effort would need to be tailored to the local context.[28] In addition, one important report reminded low- and middle-income countries of the importance of investing in a multidisciplinary approach to road safety as they increase motorization to avoid problems of road traffic accidents later.[29]

Roads can be made safer from the engineering point of view by paying particular attention to building safety into road designs, improving high-risk intersections and routes, providing separate lanes or areas for slow-moving vehicles and pedestrians, improving barriers and median strips, and enhancing lighting. Ghana was able to reduce road traffic injuries by installing speed bumps at selected places.[3] In countries in which there are many types of vehicles, it would also help to separate those that can travel at high speed from those, like two-wheeled motorized rickshaws, that can only travel slowly and that are unsafe in many ways.[3]

Vehicles can be made safer by engineering safety features into them, such as crash protection zones, headrests, seat belts, and daytime running lights. For example, including daytime running lights on motorcycles in China did reduce injuries.[3] People can be encouraged to use vehicles in safer ways through enforcement of speed limits, restricting the driving of those consuming alcohol, limiting the hours allowed for commercial driving, and enforcing the use of bicycle and motorcycle helmets.[3] Although there is considerable corruption in the police forces of many countries, enforcement of driving laws has helped in a number of settings to reduce road traffic injuries by up to 34 percent.[3] The introduction of mandatory seat belt and child restraint laws has been associated in high-income countries with a reduction in deaths and injuries by 25 percent.[3]

Few low- and middle-income countries have taken measures to deal with poisonings. However, South Africa carried out a program in which childproof containers were given to families for free. This program was associated with a cost-effective reduction in child poisonings and deaths.[30] It appears that to reduce poisonings in low- and middle-income countries, it is important to educate families to store poisons away from other household goods and out of the reach of children, to store them in appropriate and marked containers, and to enforce rules that prohibit the sale of poisons in unmarked and inappropriate containers.[3]

It is not easy to prevent falls among older people. It appears, however, that steps that have been taken in high-income countries to address such falls have included working with the elderly to improve their balance and modifying their home environment to reduce risks.[3] In low-income and many middle-income countries, it may be that the only cost-effective measure that could be taken to reduce falls among the elderly would be to provide community-based education to families about the risks of falls to their elderly relatives and about measures that are appropriate in that cultural context to reducing those risks.

Few efforts at reducing childhood injuries from falls have taken place in a systematic way in low- or middle-income countries. Here, too, it may be that the most reasonable step initially is community-based education to families about the risks of falling and what can be done to reduce those risks. Of course, if schools do have play equipment, it will be valuable to design that equipment in a way that reduces falls and injuries from such falls.

There is also little evidence from low- and middle-income countries about what might be done in cost-effective ways to reduce drownings. Perhaps on this front, as well, one has to start with community-based information efforts about increased parental and older sibling supervision and with obvious measures, such as covering wells.[3] A community-based pilot program was carried out in Bangladesh to determine if communities would accept door barriers and playpens as means for protecting children from the risk of being unsupervised around water and drowning. Families provided with a playpen were almost seven times more likely to use it than were the families provided with a door barrier. Further study, however, is needed to determine if such an approach will translate into fewer deaths by drowning of young children.[31]

Not unexpectedly, there is also very little data on effective measures to reduce burns in low- and middle-income countries, despite their importance both generally and specifically for women. Separate from the special circumstances of "dowry deaths," it appears that, for this, too, community-based efforts at behavior change must be the starting point for improved action.[3]

▶ Emergency Medical Services

Unintentional injuries will remain an important component of the burden of disease for some time in almost all countries. In addition, that burden may grow in both absolute and relative importance as countries witness economic growth, urbanization, and increasing motorization of transport. Thus, even low-income countries should now examine investments in low-cost but effective ways of improving emergency medical services.

One important measure would be to arrange for emergency transport. This could take the form of special vehicles made for low-income or rural communities, or it could be arranged in advance with owners of available transport. A bicycle ambulance was established in Malawi for the transport of obstetric emergencies, and it turned out to be used more frequently for other medical emergencies and dealing with accident victims.[32] In addition, one could train members of the community who frequently come in contact with road accidents, such as truck drivers, to provide first aid and transport to accident victims. This was done with some important successes, for example, in Ghana.[33]

Low-income countries could also begin to invest in better training of healthcare personnel who work in emergency services. They could also invest in emergency transport services based out of selected locations known to the public so that the emergency transport could be hailed quickly, even in environments in which most people would not have a telephone.[34]

▶ Case Study

A case study follows concerning the successful efforts in Vietnam to reduce injury and death by ensuring the use of motorcycle helmets.

Vietnam Motorcycle Helmets: Saving Lives Through Helmet Laws in Vietnam[35]

Introduction

Vietnam is home to some of the most dangerous road traffic in the world. In part, this is a result of rapid economic growth in the 1990s, which enabled many families to purchase motorcycles instead of the bicycles they used earlier. By 2014, motorcycles accounted for nearly 95 percent of all vehicles on Vietnamese roads.

However, without proper infrastructure to support this influx of motorized vehicles, roads in Vietnam became notoriously perilous.

In 2007, road traffic accidents were the leading cause of death for working-age Vietnamese individuals. High rates of road traffic accidents had economic consequences, too: in 2003, road accidents cost Vietnam at least $900 million each year, or 2.7 percent of the gross domestic product of the country.

Helmets have been shown to reduce the risk of injury and death by 40 percent and 70 percent, respectively, during a motorcycle accident. However, despite the effectiveness of helmets in preventing injuries and deaths, less than one-third of Vietnamese motorcyclists were wearing helmets in the early 2000s. This was in part attributed to lax enforcement of mandatory helmet use laws, as well as the small penalties associated with helmet violations.

The Intervention

An opportunity to address road traffic accidents and deaths in Vietnam arose in 2002, when new leadership arrived in the National Traffic Safety Committee (NTSC) of the Vietnamese government. Buy Huynh, the incoming director of the NTSC, strongly supported helmet legislation. Several other initiatives to improve use of motorcycle helmets also coincided with legal and political approaches to addressing road traffic safety.

In 2007, legislation called "Resolution 32" was introduced in parliament. This law made helmets mandatory for all motorcyclists and passengers, beginning on "Helmet Day" in December 2007. The price for riding without a helmet was a hefty VND10,000–VND200,000 ($6–$12)—or one-third of the average monthly income. Police were trained in how to identify offenders, and ticketed nearly 680,000 riders for noncompliance in the first year that the law was implemented. Around this time, political leaders also began to take ownership for preventing motorcycle accidents by signing pledges to wear helmets, or even taking on local leadership of NTSC chapters.

Beyond legislation, a campaign was started to educate and motivate the public to use helmets. Concerts, billboards, and TV commercials were all used as venues to promote helmet wearing and inform the public about the penalties for not doing so.

Impact

Resolution 32 and the initiatives surrounding its implementation had a demonstrated influence on helmet use, road traffic head injuries, and road traffic deaths. A study conducted by the Hanoi School of Public Health with support from WHO found

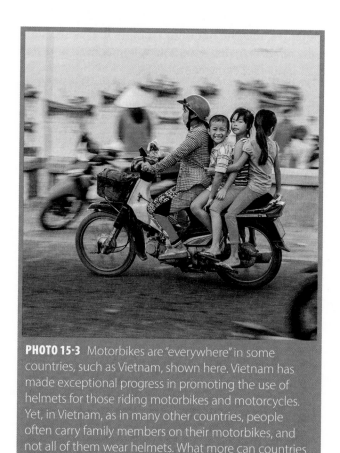

PHOTO 15-3 Motorbikes are "everywhere" in some countries, such as Vietnam, shown here. Vietnam has made exceptional progress in promoting the use of helmets for those riding motorbikes and motorcycles. Yet, in Vietnam, as in many other countries, people often carry family members on their motorbikes, and not all of them wear helmets. What more can countries like Vietnam do to ensure that all riders wear helmets, all the time?
© Hadynyah/E+/Getty Images.

that helmet compliance rose from 40 percent in 2007 (before Helmet Day) to 93 percent in 2009. There was also a 16 percent decline in road traffic head injuries and an 18 percent decline in risk of road traffic death. In addition, an assessment by the Asia Injury Prevention Foundation suggested that 20,609 deaths and 412,175 serious injuries were prevented from 2008 to 2013 as a result of the law.

Cost

Traffic-related head injuries are costly: one study found that the medical costs for severe brain injuries in Vietnam were approximately $2,370. The high cost of medical treatment can threaten the economic stability of individuals who suffer head injuries. Two-thirds of traffic accident victims in Vietnam take on debt in order to pay for treatment.

The available evidence also suggests that mandatory laws that are appropriately enforced are among the most cost-effective interventions to address the burden of road traffic accidents. Considering the impact on health outcomes and the cost of implementing the law, it has been estimated that the complete implementation of Resolution 32 cost $1,249 per

DALY averted, which would be cost-effective according to WHO thresholds.

Lessons Learned

The Vietnam helmet law benefited from strong political leadership, thorough enforcement, and harsh penalties for violators, as well as a culturally appropriate approach to motivating behavior change. With enthusiastic support from Buy Huynh and others, there was momentum to pass Resolution 32, and local leaders became more involved with NTSC chapters in their region.

Once the law was passed, implementing a large fine for violation, as well as consistent enforcement of that fine, ensured that the law strongly incentivized helmet use. The fact that conformity is valued in Vietnamese society also made the public awareness efforts surrounding Resolution 32 an effective approach to promoting helmet compliance. By organizing a campaign to educate the public on the law and promote helmet use, as well as by instituting Helmet Day, the government promoted the law in a visible way that created, in essence, a new social norm.

Effective implementation of the helmet law did not come without challenges. The original law did not cover individuals younger than 16, and many motorcyclists would wear helmets without attaching the chinstrap. Many young people purchased flimsy helmets that did not provide adequate protection. Over time, however, incremental policy changes closed many of these loopholes. Nonetheless, in 2011, helmet quality still suffered, with less than 20 percent of helmets passing safety tests.

Despite room for improvement, the Vietnam helmet law demonstrates that legal approaches to behavior change can be effective. However, passing a law alone is insufficient to motivate this change. To be successful, legislation must be accompanied by enforcement, sufficient penalties, and public awareness initiatives. As other countries—such as Uganda and Tanzania—follow the example of Vietnam, it is critical that they address the context in which helmet law mandates are implemented.

▶ Future Challenges

One key challenge for the future will be to ensure that low- and middle-income countries show the political commitment needed to reduce the burden of injuries. This burden is too large a source of deaths and disabilities to ignore, even in the face of continuing communicable diseases and a growing burden of noncommunicable diseases.

There is increasing information about what works in cost-effective ways to reduce the burden of injury in high-income countries, and this can serve as a starting point for adapting this learning to other settings. It will be important for selected low- and middle-income countries to carry out pilot schemes in preventing injury, especially from road traffic accidents, and then to expand them more broadly as they learn how to make them work effectively in different settings.

As low- and middle-income countries develop economically and become more urbanized and motorized, it will be valuable for them to engineer safety into their newer investments in road transportation. It will also be important to increase efforts to provide information and education to the public about key areas of injury prevention. Governance is weak in many countries. Nonetheless, such countries can take measures in a phased manner to enforce laws concerning road safety that can have a high return with little effort, such as encouraging the use of motorcycle helmets, and enforcing drunk driving laws and speed limits. As governance improves and people have more knowledge of road safety and trust that enforcement of laws will be honest, the government can enforce additional regulations affecting road safety. The challenge of reducing injuries from falls, burns, and drowning will depend almost completely on informing and educating the public in a community-based manner.

▶ Main Messages

Injuries are an important cause of deaths and DALYs in all regions of the world. In 2016, about 4.6 million people died of injuries worldwide. This was more than 8 percent of total deaths. In addition, these injuries are major causes of disability, with many people being disabled by injuries, even if they do not die from them.

Moreover, the rate of deaths from injuries is substantially higher in low- and middle-income countries than in high-income countries.

The leading cause of both deaths and DALYs attributable to injuries is road traffic accidents. This is followed by deaths from falls, drowning, poisoning, and fires. About three times as many men die in road traffic accidents as women. The number of deaths from road traffic accidents as a share of total deaths is particularly high in the Middle East and North Africa region, compared to other regions. Injuries are an important source of deaths for young children.

The risk factors for road traffic injuries revolve around education, enforcement, and engineering. The risk factors of other leading causes of unintentional injuries relate largely to lower socioeconomic status, inadequate supervision of children, lack of safe storage of poisons, and household cooking arrangements that pay insufficient attention to fire hazards in areas that tend to be crowded and hazardous.

Although there have been few studies of the economic costs of injuries in low- and middle-income countries, estimates of such costs for road traffic accidents alone suggest that they range from 2 percent to 4 percent of GNP.[16-18] The social costs of dealing with the disabilities caused by accidents can also be very high.

There is increasing evidence from a range of countries of measures that can be taken to improve vehicle operator safety, build safety into vehicles, make plans for land use and traffic, and enforce key traffic rules. These measures can be implemented in a phased manner in low- and middle-income countries and adapted to local settings. Reducing the burden of road traffic injuries and other injuries will require enhancing community-based approaches to providing information about how the community can reduce risk factors for such injuries.

Study Questions

1. How important are injuries to the global burden of disease?
2. What injuries cause the most deaths?
3. How does the rate of death from road traffic accidents vary by region, and why?
4. What are the most important injuries that affect children?
5. Do men and women suffer from injuries at the same rates? Why or why not?
6. What are the risk factors for road traffic accidents?
7. What are the risk factors for drownings?
8. What are the key risk factors for burning, and how do they vary by region?
9. What is Haddon's matrix, and how would you apply it to analyze accidents?
10. What are the most cost-effective steps that low- and middle-income countries can take to reduce the burden of road traffic accidents on health?

References

1. Institute of Health Metrics and Evaluation (IHME). (n.d.). GBD Compare: Viz Hub. Retrieved from https://vizhub.healthdata.org/gbd-compare/

2. National Highway Traffic Safety Administration. *Trauma system agenda for the future: Glossary.* Retrieved from http://www.nhtsa.dot.gov/people/injury/ems/emstraumasystem03/glossary.htm

3. Norton, R., Hyder, A. A., Bishai, D., & Peden, M. (2006). Unintentional injuries. In D. T. Jamison, J. G. Breman, A. R. Measham, et al. (Eds.), *Disease control priorities in developing countries* (2nd ed., pp. 737–753). New York, NY: Oxford University Press.

4. Wadman, M., Muelleman, R., Coto, J., & Kellermann, A. L. (2003). The pyramid of injury: Using ecodes to accurately describe the burden of injury. *Annals of Emergency Medicine, 42,* 468–478.

5. UNICEF. (2008). *World report on child injury prevention.* Geneva, Switzerland: World Health Organization.

6. Bangdiwala, S., Anzola-Perez, E., Rommer, C., Schmidt, B., Valdez-Lazo, F., Toro, J., & D'Suze, C. (1990). The incidence of injuries in young people: I. Methodology and results of a collaborative study in Brazil, Chile, Cuba, and Venezuela. *International Journal of Epidemiology, 19,* 115–124.

7. Bartlett, S. (2002). The problem of children's injuries in low-income countries: A review. *Health Policy and Planning, 17*(1), 1–13.

8. Mohan, D. (1997). Injuries in less industrialized countries: What do we know? *Injury Prevention, 3,* 241–242.

9. World Health Organization & Indian Institute of Technology Delhi. (2006). *Road traffic injury prevention.* Geneva, Switzerland: World Health Organization.

10. Jordan, J., & Valdez-Lazo, F. (1991). Education on safety and risk. In M. Manciaux & C. Romer (Eds.), *Accidents in childhood and adolescence: The role of research* (pp. 106–120). Geneva, Switzerland: World Health Organization.

11. Ljungblom, B.-A., & Köhler, L. (1991). Child development and behavior in traffic. In M. Manciaux & C. Romer (Eds.), *Accidents in childhood and adolescence: The role of research* (pp. 97–105). Geneva, Switzerland: World Health Organization.

12. Leflamme, L., & Diderichsen, F. (2000). Social differences in traffic injury risk in childhood and youth—A literature review and a research agenda. *Injury Prevention, 6,* 293–298.

13. International Labour Office. (1996). *Child labour: Targeting the intolerable.* Geneva, Switzerland: International Labour Office.

14. Hoffman, K., Primack, A., Keusch, G., & Hrynkow, S. (2005). Addressing the growing burden of trauma and injury in low- and middle-income countries. *American Journal of Public Health, 95,* 13–17.

15. Jacobs, G., Aaron-Thomas, A., & Astrop, A. (2000). *Estimating global road fatalities.* London, UK: Transport Research Laboratory.

16. Rezaei, S., Arab, M., Matin, B. K., & Sari, A. A. (2014). Extent, consequences and economic burden of road crashes in Iran. *Journal of Injury and Violence Research, 6*(2), 57–63.

17. Ghadi, M., Török, Á., Tánczos, K. (2018). Study of the economic cost of road accidents in Jordan. *Periodica Polytechnica Transportation Engineering, 46*(3), 129–134.

18. Mohan, D. (2014). *Impact of road traffic crashes in Asia: A human and economic assessment.* United Nations Centre for Regional Development. Retrieved from https://www.researchgate.net/publication/274075965_IMPACT_OF_ROAD_TRAFFIC_CRASHES_IN_ASIA_A_HUMAN_AND_ECONOMIC_ASSESSMENT

19. Centers for Disease Control and Prevention. (n.d.). *Motor vehicle safety: Cost data and prevention policies.* Retrieved from https://www.cdc.gov/motorvehiclesafety/costs/index.html

20. Depalma, J., Fedorka, P., & Simko, L. (2003). Quality of life experienced by severely injured trauma survivors. *AACN Clinical Issues, 14*(1), 54–63.

21. van der Sluis, C., Eisma, W., Groothoff, J., & ten Duis, H. (1998). Long-term physical, psychological and social consequences of severe injuries. *Injury, 29*(4), 281–285.

22. Landsman, I., Baum, C., Arnkoff, D., Craig, M. J., Lynch, I., Copes, W. S., & Champion, H. R. (1990). The psychosocial consequences of traumatic injury. *Journal of Behavioral Medicine, 13*(6), 561–581.

23. Mayou, R., & Bryant, B. (2001). Outcome in consecutive emergency department attenders following a road traffic accident. *British Journal of Psychiatry, 179,* 528–534.

24. Osberg, J., Khan, P., Rowe, K., & Brooke, M. (1996). Pediatric trauma: Impact on work and family finances. *Pediatrics, 98*(5), 890–897.

25. Haddon, W. (1999). The changing approach to epidemiology, prevention, and amelioration of trauma: The transition to approaches etiologically rather than descriptively based. *Injury Prevention, 5,* 231–235.

26. Holder, Y., Peden, M., Krug, E., Lund, J., Gururaj, G., & Kobusingye, O. (Eds.). (2001). *Injury surveillance guidelines.* Geneva, Switzerland: World Health Organization.

27. McGee, K., Peden, M., Waxweiler, R., & Sleet, D. (2003). Injury surveillance. *Injury Control and Safety Promotion, 10,* 105–108.

28. Chisholm, D., Naci, H., Hyder, A. A., Tran, N. T., & Peden, M. (2012, March 2). Cost-effectiveness of strategies to combat road traffic injuries in sub-Saharan Africa and South East Asia: Mathematical modelling study. *BMJ, 344*(e612).

29. Global Road Safety Facility The World Bank Group; Institute For Health Metrics and Evaluation, University of Washington. (2014). *Transport for health: The global burden of disease from motorized road transport.* Washington, DC: The World Bank.

30. Krug, A., Ellis, J. B., Hay, I. T., Mokgabudi, N. F., & Robertson, J. (1994). The impact of child-resistant containers on the incidence of paraffin (kerosene) ingestion in children. *South African Medical Journal, 84,* 730–734.

31. Callaghan, J. A., Hyder, A. A., Blum, L. S, Arifeen, S., & Baqui, A. H. (2010). Child supervision practices for drowning prevention in rural Bangladesh: A pilot study of supervision tools. *Journal of Epidemiology and Community Health, 64,* 645–647.

32. Kobusingye, O. C., Hyder, A. A., Bishai, D., Hicks, E. R., Mock, C., & Joshipura, M. (2005). Emergency medical systems in low- and middle-income countries: Recommendations for action. *Bulletin of the World Health Organization, 83*(8), 626–631.

33. Mock, C., Arreola-Risa, C., & Quansah, R. (2003). Strengthening care for injured persons in less developed countries: A case study of Ghana and Mexico. *Injury Control and Safety Promotion, 10*(1–2), 45–51.

34. Kobusingye, O. C., Hyder, A. A., Bishai, D., Joshipura, E. R. H., & Mock, C. (2006). Emergency medical services. In D. T. Jamison, J. G. Breman, A. R. Measham, et al. (Eds.), *Disease control priorities in developing countries* (2nd ed., pp. 1261–1279). New York, NY: Oxford University Press.

35. This case is based on Glassman, A., & Temin, M. (2016). Improving road safety: Vietnam's comprehensive helmet law. In A. Glassman, M. Temin, & the Millions Saved Team and Advisory Group, *Millions saved: New cases of proven success in global health* (pp. 181–189). Washington, DC: Center for Global Development.

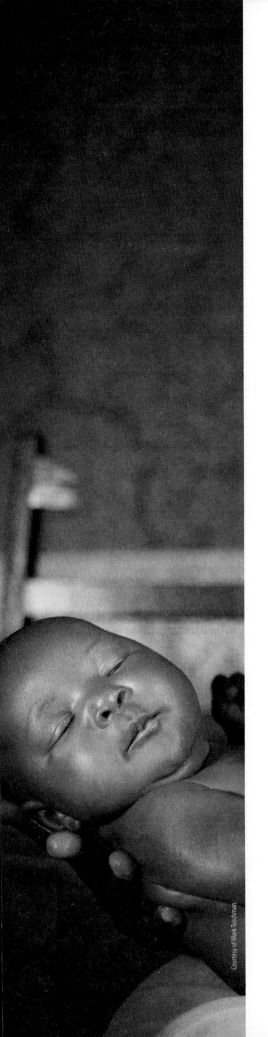

Courtesy of Mark Tuschman.

PART IV

Working Together to Improve Global Health

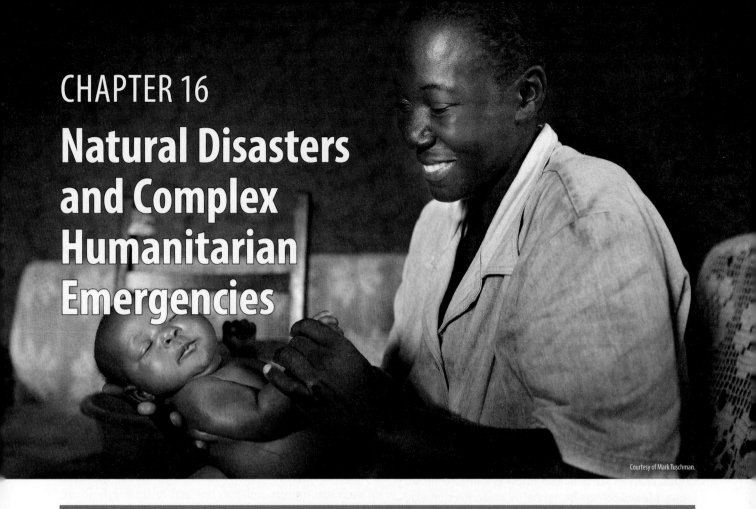

Courtesy of Mark Tuschman.

CHAPTER 16

Natural Disasters and Complex Humanitarian Emergencies

LEARNING OBJECTIVES

By the end of this chapter, the reader will be able to do the following:

- Describe several types of disasters that affect human health
- Discuss the health effects of natural disasters and complex humanitarian emergencies
- Review how those health impacts vary by age, sex, location, and type of disaster
- Describe key measures that can be taken to mitigate the health impacts of natural disasters and complex humanitarian emergencies

▶ Vignettes

Javad lived in the Pakistani province of Kashmir when the earthquake hit. All the buildings in his village were destroyed. Hundreds of people in the village were killed, mostly a result of being buried in the rubble. Many other people were badly injured from rubble falling on them. Their injuries were overwhelmingly orthopedic in nature. As the earthquake destroyed the village, it also destroyed wells, a health center, and roads leading to and from the village. Javad feared that many of those injured would soon die.

Samuel was living in the eastern part of Sierra Leone when the war started. He did all that he could to protect his family, but it was not enough. In the first year of the conflict, as he and his family were getting ready to flee, a band of armed men stormed the village. As Samuel had heard they would do, they used machetes to kill or take limbs off of many village people. They also raped a large number of women. In addition, they kidnapped some of the children in hopes of making them into sex slaves or soldiers.

As the civil war spread in Rwanda, Sarah and her family fled across the border to what was quickly becoming a large refugee camp in Zaire, later called the Democratic Republic of Congo. Although the camp workers did what they could to help the refugees, the circumstances at the camp were not good. There was little shelter, water, or food. In addition, a cholera epidemic spread through the camp not long after Sarah's arrival there. It hit the camp especially hard and led to a large number of deaths. A number of international organizations rushed staff to refugee camps, just across the border from intense fighting. Some of the agencies had many years of experience doing such work and had clear guidelines for their staff concerning relief efforts. Other agencies, however, were not so experienced in this work and their efforts were poorly coordinated. In addition, some of the inexperienced agencies brought food, medicine, and clothing that was not appropriate to the local situation. Over the last decade, however, the international humanitarian response to such emergencies has become, in many respects, more professional, better coordinated, and more effective and efficient.

▶ The Importance of Natural Disasters and Complex Emergencies to Global Health

Complex emergencies and natural disasters have a significant impact on global health. They can lead to increased death, illness, and disability, and the economic costs of their health impacts can also be very large. Measures can be taken in cost-effective ways, however, to reduce the toll of disasters and conflicts and to address the major health problems that relate to them. These measures are most effective when those involved in disaster relief work together according to agreed-upon standards that focus on the most important priorities for action.

This chapter reviews the relationships between natural disasters and health and complex humanitarian emergencies (CHEs) and health. The chapter begins by introducing some key concepts and definitions that relate to these topics. It then reviews the incidence of natural disasters and CHEs and their main health impacts. The chapter then reviews a number of case studies related to natural disasters and CHEs. Lastly, the chapter examines measures that can be taken in cost-effective ways to prevent and address some of the health effects of natural disasters and CHEs.

▶ Key Terms

Understanding the health impacts of natural disasters and CHEs requires an introduction to several terms and concepts that are examined briefly here.

A disaster is "any occurrence that causes damage, ecological destruction, loss of human lives, or deterioration of health and health services on a scale sufficient to warrant an extraordinary response from outside the affected community area."[1] Another way to think of this would be as "an occurrence, either natural or manmade, that causes human suffering and creates human needs that victims cannot alleviate without assistance."[1] Some disasters are natural. These include, for example, the results of floods, volcanoes, and earthquakes. Some, however, are caused by humans, such as the cloud of poisonous gas that rained over the town of Bhopal, India, in 1984 as a result of an industrial accident. Some disasters are rapid onset, such as an earthquake, whereas others are slow onset, such as a drought or famine. Although the long-term effects of these natural and human-made disasters can be substantial, they are often characterized by an initial event and then its aftereffects. Some examples of recent natural disasters that caused a significant loss of life are listed in **TABLE 16-1**.

In response to the large number of civil conflicts that have taken place, the term complex emergency or complex humanitarian emergency (CHE) has been established. A complex emergency can be defined as a "complex, multi-party, intra-state conflict resulting in a humanitarian disaster which might constitute multi-dimensional risks or threats to regional and international security. Frequently within such conflicts, state institutions collapse, law and order break down, banditry and chaos prevail, and portions of the civilian population migrate."[2] CHEs have also been described as "situations affecting large civilian populations which usually involve a combination of factors, including war or civil strife, food shortages, and population displacement, resulting in significant excess mortality."[3(p1012)]

Such emergencies include war and civil conflict. They usually affect large numbers of people and often have severe impacts on the availability of food, water, and shelter. Linked to these phenomena and the displacement of people that often go with them, CHEs usually result in considerable excess mortality, compared to what would be the case without such an emergency.[4] Some examples of CHEs are listed in **TABLE 16-2**.

Complex emergencies create refugees. Under international law, a refugee is a person who is outside his or her country of nationality or habitual residence; has a well-founded fear of persecution because of his or her race, religion, nationality, membership in a particular social group, or political opinion; and is unable or unwilling to avail him- or herself of the protection of that country, or to return there, for fear of persecution. They are a subgroup of the broader category of displaced persons.[5] It is important to note that there are a number of international conventions that define refugees and that accord them rights according to international law, as well. **TABLE 16-3** notes a number of countries with significant refugee populations and the countries they fled. A United Nations Agency,

TABLE 16-1 Selected Natural Disasters, 2008–2017

2008

Cyclone Nargis hit Myanmar, causing a record 138,366 deaths. The government resisted foreign relief efforts, intensifying the morbidity and mortality associated with the cyclone. The cyclone also damaged infrastructure and destroyed the rice and shrimp industries.

2010

A magnitude-7.0 earthquake hit Haiti, killing 222,570 people and leaving approximately a million homeless. The damage to infrastructure was extensive and shut down roads, electric grids, and hospitals.

2011

A magnitude-9.0 earthquake, one of the most powerful ever reported, hit off the coast of Japan. It created tsunami waves over 30 feet high in Japan, and smaller waves throughout the Pacific basin, including Hawaii and the west coast of the United States. In Japan, the tsunami killed approximately 20,000 people and triggered a nuclear disaster at the Fukushima plant.

2012

In November, Typhoon Bopha, a category-5 super typhoon, hit the Philippines with winds up to 175 mph. The typhoon caused 1,900 deaths and extensive damage.

2015

In April, the Gorkha earthquake killed 8,831 people in Nepal. Throughout the summer in France, India, and Pakistan, record heat waves killed over 6,000 people.

2016

In April, an earthquake in Ecuador caused 676 deaths, the highest mortality of any disaster that year. In August, Hurricane Matthew killed 546 people in Haiti while causing damage and flooding throughout the southeastern United States and the Caribbean. Meanwhile, flooding in North Korea caused 538 deaths, and an ongoing drought affected 330 million people in India.

2017

Monsoon rains in South Asia led to flooding and landslides that killed over 1,000 people in India, Nepal, and Bangladesh. The flooding affected 40 million people, shutting down schools and businesses while forcing hundreds of thousands from their homes.

Data from Centre for Research on the Epidemiology of Disasters (CRED). (2017). *Annual disaster statistical review 2016*. Retrieved from https://reliefweb.int/sites/reliefweb.int/files/resources /adsr_2016.pdf. See also *Annual Disaster Statistical Review 2015: The Numbers and Trends*. https://reliefweb.int/sites/reliefweb.int/files/resources/ADSR_2015.pdf, and *Natural Disasters in 2017: Lower Mortality, Higher Cost*. https://reliefweb.int/sites/reliefweb.int/files/resources/CredCrunch50.pdf

the United Nations High Commissioner for Refugees (UNHCR), is responsible for protecting the rights of most refugees, while Palestinians fall under the mandate of a separate agency, the United Nations Relief and Works Agency (UNRWA). Some migrants are also called asylum-seekers. **Asylum-seekers** are those claiming protection outside of their home country, but their request for sanctuary has yet to be processed.[6]

Some of the people who flee or are forced to migrate during a disaster or CHE leave their homes but stay in the country in which they were living. These are called **internally displaced people (IDP)**. Although there is no legal definition of an internally displaced person, they are considered to be "someone who has been forced to leave their home for reasons such as religious or political persecution or war, but

has not crossed an international border."[7] As with the term *refugee*, the term *IDP* is a subset of the more general *displaced person*. **TABLE 16-4** shows selected examples of countries with large numbers of internally displaced persons. It is important to note that the legal status of IDP is not as well defined as that for refugees.[8] It is also important to understand that, unlike refugees, no agency or organization is responsible for IDPs. Rather, their own government is responsible for them but that government is often part of the reason why these people are fleeing.

One of the important indicators of the health impact of a CHE is the **crude mortality rate**. This is the proportion of people who die from a population at risk over a specified period of time.[9] For addressing CHEs, the crude mortality rate is generally expressed

TABLE 16-2   Selected Complex Humanitarian Emergencies of Importance Since 1980

Afghanistan: There are currently 1.3 million internally displaced people (IDP) due to conflict between the Taliban and international forces supporting the government, led by the United States. Many Afghans have also fled the country, including over 2 million in Pakistan and between 2.5 and 3 million in Iran.

Bosnia and Herzegovina: Between 1992 and 1994, war with various parts of the former Yugoslavia led to more than 100,000 deaths and 1.8 million people displaced.

Colombia: Conflict between government and non-state armed groups, primarily the Revolutionary Armed Forces of Colombia (FARC), continued from 1985 until 2016 and displaced 7.7 million people internally.

The Democratic Republic of Congo: Fighting since the mid-1990s between government forces and rebels has displaced millions to neighboring countries and created 4.5 million IDP within Congo.

Ethiopia: A border war with Eritrea from 1998 to 2000 and ongoing fighting between the Ethiopian military and separatist rebel groups have created 1.7 IDP within Ethiopia. Many Ethiopians and Eritreans have fled to nearby countries, as well.

Myanmar: Government offensives against a number of ethnic groups, including the Rohingya, have continued for more than 20 years and produced between 500,000 and 1 million IDP.

Palestine: The establishment of Israel in 1948 is associated with the displacement of over 700,000 Palestinians. Today, 5 million Palestinians are registered as refugees, including descendants of people who fled in 1948. Over 1.5 million Palestinians live in refugee camps in Jordan, Lebanon, Syria, Gaza, and the West Bank.

Rwanda: More than 800,000 people were killed in the 1994 genocide, which also produced more than 2 million refugees who fled to Burundi, what is now the Democratic Republic of Congo, Tanzania, and Uganda.

Somalia: Conflict between al-Shabaab and the Transitional Federal Government allied forces exacerbated previous displacement from famine and civil war. There are currently 2.1 million IDP.

Sudan: A civil war from 1983 to 2005, which included genocide against people in the Darfur region and eventually led to the independence of South Sudan, displaced 5–6 million people. Today, 1.76 people are still internally displaced within South Sudan, and 2.1 million are within Sudan.

Syria: An ongoing civil war since 2011 has displaced 6.8 million within Syria and created 5.6 million refugees.

Yemen: Clashes between rebel groups and government forces have resulted in over 2 million IDP.

Data from Central Intelligence Agency (CIA) and the United Nations Relief and Works Agency (UNRWA). (n.d.). *The world fact book. Field listing: Refugees and internally displaced persons*. Retrieved from https://www.cia.gov/library/publications/the-world-factbook/fields/2194.html; UNRWA. (n.d.). *Palestinian refugees*. Retrieved from https://www.unrwa.org/palestine-refugees

TABLE 16-3 Selected Refugee Populations and Source of Refugees, 2018		
Country	**Number of Refugees**	**Source Countries**
Turkey	3,918,337	Afghanistan, Iraq, Iran, Syria
Jordan	2,920,029	Palestine, Syria, Iraq, Yemen
Iran	2,528,268	Afghanistan, Iraq
Pakistan	2,400,000	Afghanistan
Lebanon	1,452,130	Syria, Palestine
Uganda	1,441,126	Democratic Republic of Congo, Rwanda, Burundi, South Sudan, Somalia

Gaza Strip	1,348,536	Palestine
Bangladesh	915,000	Burma
Ethiopia	912,499	Somalia, South Sudan, Eritrea, Sudan
Sudan	881,819	Eritrea, Chad, Syria, South Sudan
West Bank	809,738	Palestine
Kenya	517,982	Somalia, South Sudan, DRC, Ethiopia, Burundi, Sudan
Syria	454,879	Palestine, Iraq
Chad	448,541	Sudan, Central African Republic, Nigeria
Cameroon	355,146	Central African Republic, Nigeria
China	317,098	North Korea, Vietnam
Egypt	288,117	West Bank and Gaza Strip, Sudan, South Sudan, Somalia, Iraq, Syria, Ethiopia, Eritrea
South Sudan	279,995	Sudan, Democratic Republic of Congo
Yemen	261,771	Somalia, Ethiopia
India	196,514	Tibet/China, Sri Lanka, Burma, Afghanistan
Colombia	182,529	Venezuela
Venezuela	171,920	Colombia
Niger	166,422	Mali, Nigeria
Rwanda	159,644	Democratic Republic of Congo, Burundi
Ecuador	153,895	Colombia, Venezuela
Algeria	100,000	Western Sahara
Malaysia	87,036	Burma
Burundi	71,055	Democratic Republic of the Congo
Austria	70,506	Syria, Afghanistan, Russia, Iraq
Afghanistan	59,737	Pakistan
Angola	36,094	Democratic Republic of Congo
Burkina Faso	24,216	Mali
Nepal	23,313	Tibet/China, Bhutan
Armenia	14,626	Syria (ethnic Armenians)

Data from Central Intelligence Agency (CIA). (n.d.). *The world factbook. Field listing: Refugees and internally displaced persons*. Retrieved from https://www.cia.gov/library/publications/the-world -factbook/fields/2194.html

TABLE 16-4 Internally Displaced People: Selected Countries of Importance, 2018

Country	Number of IDP
Colombia	7,708,465
Syria	6,784,000
Democratic Republic of Congo	4,500,000
Iraq	3,159,380
Somalia	2,100,000
Sudan	2,072,000
Yemen	2,014,026
Nigeria	1,881,198
Afghanistan	1,286,000
Turkey	1,113,000
India	806,000

Data from the Central Intelligence Agency (CIA). (n.d.). *The world factbook. Field listing: Refugees and internally displaced persons.* Retrieved from https://www.cia.gov/library/publications/the-world-factbook/fields/2194.html

per 10,000 population, per day. The extent to which diseases might spread in a refugee camp depends partly on the **attack rate** of a disease, which is "the cumulative incidence of infection in a group observed over a period of time during an epidemic."[9(p8)] Finally, it is important to understand **case fatality rate**, which is "the number of deaths from a specific disease in a given period, per 100 episodes of the disease in the same period."[10]

▶ The Characteristics of Natural Disasters

There are several types of natural disasters. Some of these are related to the weather, including droughts, hurricanes, typhoons, cyclones, and heavy rains. Tsunamis, like the one that occurred in Japan in 2011, can also cause extreme devastation, injuries, and death. In addition, earthquakes and volcanoes can have important impacts on the health of various communities. Despite the exceptional nature of tsunamis and the

deaths associated with them, earthquakes are the natural disasters that generally kill the most people.

It appears that the number of natural disasters is increasing, affecting larger numbers of people and causing more economic losses than earlier but causing proportionately fewer deaths than before. The countries most often hit by natural disasters are China, the United States, India, Indonesia, and the Philippines.[11] However, the biggest relative impact is in low- and middle-income countries: more than 90 percent of the deaths from natural disasters occur in low- and middle-income countries.[12] The relative impact of natural disasters on the poor, of course, is greater than on the better off because the share of poorer people's total assets that are lost in these disasters is greater than that lost by higher-income people. Moreover, the poor are often the most vulnerable to losses from natural disasters because they often live in places at risk of experiencing such disasters or have housing that cannot withstand such shocks.[12] Climate change already appears to be having an impact on the number, type, and severity of natural disasters. It is anticipated that climate change will continue to affect such disasters in the future, as well.

Natural disasters can cause significant harm to infrastructure that is needed for safe water and sanitation, and roads that may be needed to transport people requiring health care. Natural disasters can also damage the health infrastructure itself, such as hospitals, health centers, and health clinics. People can die directly as a result of the natural disaster, such as from falling rubble during an earthquake or drowning during a flood. However, they may also die as an indirect result of the disaster because of epidemics linked to the lack of safe water or sanitation, food, or access to health services.[12] Disasters can also destroy homes and displace communities. Some people affected end up living in camps, which poses a range of health hazards.

▶ The Characteristics of Complex Emergencies

It is estimated that at the end of the 1990s there were about 40 complex emergencies per year in countries in which more than 300 million people live.[8] In 2018 there was record displacement as the number of forced migrants worldwide reached 68.5 million. The number of internally displaced persons increased to 40 million, while the number of refugees increased to 25.4 million.[13] This high displacement was linked to the persistence of many severe complex emergencies.[14]

Although natural disasters have been associated with considerable death and economic loss, the impact of complex emergencies on health over the last decade has been considerably greater than that of natural disasters.

CHEs have a number of features that particularly relate to their health impacts. First, these emergencies often go on for long periods of time. The strife in the Democratic Republic of Congo, for example, has gone on for more than two decades. The latest conflict in Afghanistan began in 2001. In addition, these emergencies are often related to civil wars, as in Sudan, Syria, Somalia, and Yemen. As a result of the nature of the conflict, it is quite common that one or more of the groups that are fighting will not allow humanitarian assistance to be provided to other groups. In fact, humanitarian workers have increasingly been the targets of those who are fighting, despite the fact that they should have protected status.

During complex emergencies, combatants often intentionally target civilians for displacement, injury, and death. Many fighters also engage in systematic abuse of human rights, including torture, sexual abuse, and rape as a weapon of war. Those same fighters often intentionally destroy health facilities. Given the nature of some of the fighting and its impact on civilians, large numbers of people have been displaced by some of these conflicts, as noted previously. Sometimes they choose to flee, but sometimes they are forced to flee.[8]

Unfortunately, these are not the only characteristics of CHEs. The disruption of society often leads to food shortages. Besides the loss of some health facilities, it is also common that the publicly supported health system may break down entirely, as it did, for example, during the civil war in Liberia. Damage may also be done to water supply and sanitation systems.[4] In El Salvador, for example, the shortage of safe drinking water for the poor was a significant health threat.[15] One should also note that many factions in civil conflicts have used landmines, and their health effects on individuals can be devastating.[15]

It is important to understand that the migration of large numbers of people, some of whom will live in camps, also produces a number of problems. Migrants carry diseases with them, sometimes into areas that did not previously have those diseases. For example, when Ethiopian refugees who were living in Sudan returned home, they brought malaria from Sudan. Diseases can also spread faster among refugee populations than they would normally, given the large number of people living in crowded conditions, often without appropriate hygiene and sanitation.

In addition, large numbers of migrants, sometimes suddenly, need care from health systems that were weak before and that may be almost nonexistent after suffering the effects of civil conflict.

▶ The Health Burden of Natural Disasters

Although there are very few data available on the morbidity and disability associated with natural disasters, it has been estimated that from 1998 to 2007, about 250 million people each year were affected by climate-related disasters alone.[16] In 2015, natural disasters caused a total of 22,765 deaths, and 110.3 million were affected globally. There was a anomalous decrease in the mortality associated with disasters in 2016, when 8,733 people were killed. This is despite the fact that the number of people affected by natural disasters in 2016 increased to 564 million.[17]

The direct and indirect health effects of natural disasters depend on the type of disaster. Earthquakes, volcanoes, tsunamis, and floods impact human health in different ways. Earthquakes can kill many people quickly. In addition, they can cause a substantial number of injuries in a very short period of time. In the longer term, earthquake survivors face increased risks of permanent orthopedic disabilities, mental health problems, and possibly an increase in the rates of heart disease and other chronic disease. The indirect effect of earthquakes on health depends on the severity and location of the earthquake and the extent to which it damages infrastructure and forces people out of their homes.[12]

In the popular imagination, people are thought to die from the lava flows of volcanoes. In fact, this is rarely the case. About 90 percent of the deaths from volcanoes are due to mud and ash or from floods on denuded hillsides affected by the volcano.[12] In addition, volcanic eruptions can harm health by displacing people, rendering water supplies unsafe, and causing mental health problems among the affected population.[12]

Tsunamis take most of their victims immediately by drowning and cause relatively few injuries, compared to the number of deaths.[12] In storms and flooding, most fatalities occur from drowning and few deaths result from trauma or wind-blown objects. These flood-related events generally lead to an increase in diarrheal disease, respiratory infections, and skin diseases. Most of these problems that relate to natural disasters are relatively short lived, except for drought-related famine. Epidemics do not often spring up as a result of them, except in drought-related famine and when health systems are completely destroyed for long periods of time.

There are few data on the distribution by age and sex of morbidity, disability, and death related to natural disasters. It appears, however, that being very old, very young, or very sick makes one more vulnerable to disasters in which one has to flee for survival. These groups were disproportionately affected by the 1970 tidal wave in Bangladesh and the 2004 tsunami in Asia. Whether men or women suffer the effects of a natural disaster may depend on when and where it occurs and may be most related to the kind of work that men or women are doing. Women, however, face considerable risks in the aftermath of natural disasters if housing has been harmed and people are living in camps, as will be discussed further.[12]

▶ The Health Effects of Complex Humanitarian Emergencies

The burden of illness, disability, and death related to CHEs is large and probably underestimated, given the difficulties of collecting such data. Some of the effects of these CHEs are direct. It has been estimated, for example, that between 320,000 and 420,000 people are killed each year as a direct result of CHEs.[8] In addition, it is estimated that between 500,000 and 1 million deaths resulted from trauma during the genocide in Rwanda in 1994.[8] It is thought that about 4 percent to 13 percent of the deaths during CHEs in northern Iraq, Somalia, and the Democratic Republic of Congo were the direct result of trauma.

Other illness, disability, and death, however, come about as an indirect result of the emergencies. These stem from malnutrition, the lack of safe water and sanitation, shortages of food, and breakdowns in health services. They are exacerbated by the crowded and difficult circumstances in which people have to live when they are displaced. One estimate, for example, suggested that almost 1.7 million more people died in a 22-month period of conflict in the Democratic Republic of Congo than would have died in a normal 22-month period in that country.[8] Damage to health continues even after a conflict ends.[18]

The burden of deaths related to wars is hard to estimate. One estimate suggests that about 200,000 people died in war in 2001 in low- and middle-income countries. Just over 10 percent of these deaths occurred in the South Asia region. Almost 70 percent of these deaths, however, took place in sub-Saharan Africa.[19] Other estimates suggest that between 1975

and 1989 more than 5 million people died in civil conflicts.[20] Since 2011, there has been an increase in deaths related to CHEs, with some of the most severely affected countries being Libya, Syria, and Yemen.[17]

The data on the breakdown of deaths by age in CHEs suggest that child mortality rates early in the CHE are two to three times that of adults, but they slowly decline over time to match the rest of the population. The data on deaths by gender are limited.[21] About 20 percent of the nonfatal injuries in the Bosnian conflict were among children. Almost 50 percent of the deaths in the Democratic Republic of Congo were among women and children younger than 15 years of age.[8] In European conflicts, the overwhelming majority of those who died have been men between 19 and 50 years of age.[8] In the Syrian conflict, men have also died disproportionately.[22]

Causes of Death in CHEs

In the early stages of dealing with large numbers of displaced people in CHEs, most deaths occur from diarrheal diseases, respiratory infections, measles, or malaria.[8,23] Generally, diarrheal diseases are the most common cause of death in refugee situations. Major epidemics of cholera have occurred in refugee camps in Malawi, Nepal, and Bangladesh, among others, and the case fatality rates from cholera have ranged from 3 percent to 30 percent in these settings. Dysentery, which refers to severe diarrhea caused by an infection in the intestine, has also commonly occurred in such situations over the last 20 years, including in camps in Malawi, Nepal, Bangladesh, and Tanzania. The case fatality rate for dysentery has been highest among the very old and very young, for whom it reaches about 10 percent.[8,23] In one of the most significant humanitarian crises in the last few decades, tens of thousands of Rwandan refugees poured into the Democratic Republic of Congo during the genocide in Rwanda. Between July and August 1994, 90 percent of the deaths among the refugees in Goma, Democratic Republic of Congo, were from cholera spread by the contamination of a lake from which the refugees got their water.[8,23]

Measles has also been a major killer in camps for displaced persons. This is especially true for populations that are malnourished and have not been immunized against measles. The risk of a child dying of measles is increased substantially if the child is vitamin A deficient, as would be the case for many refugees. Up to 30 percent of the children who get measles in these situations may die from it.[23]

Malaria is also a significant contributor to death in refugee camps. This is especially the case when refugees move from countries in which there is relatively little malaria to places in which it is endemic. The risk of malaria in such cases is highest in sub-Saharan Africa and a few parts of Asia.[8,23] Acute respiratory infections are also major causes of death in refugee camps. This is to be expected because the camps are crowded, housing is inadequate, and refugees could remain in the camps for many years. Although less common than the problems noted previously, there have also been outbreaks of meningitis in some refugee camps in areas in which that disease is prevalent, such as Malawi, Ethiopia, and Burundi. These outbreaks have generally been contained by mass immunization, as it became clear that there was a risk of epidemic.[4] However, an outbreak in Sudan in 1999 led to almost 2,400 deaths.[8] Outbreaks of hepatitis E have occurred in Somalia, Ethiopia, and Kenya. These led to high case fatality rates among pregnant women in particular.[4]

The populations that are affected by CHEs are generally poor and not well nourished, and nutritional issues are always of grave concern during CHEs, when there may also be problems of food scarcity. In addition, the relationship of infection and malnutrition also poses risks to displaced populations. In CHEs in sub-Saharan Africa, the rates of acute protein-energy malnutrition during at least the early period of a CHE have been very high, particularly among young children. Reported rates of such malnutrition varied from around 12 percent among internally displaced Liberians to as high as 80 percent among internally displaced Somalis.[4,8] During CHEs in Bosnia and Tajikistan, the elderly were the group that was the worst affected by acute protein-energy malnutrition.[8]

The underlying nutritional status of refugees or internally displaced people is often poor, and micronutrient deficiencies can also be very important in CHEs. Vitamin A deficiency can be very important among these populations, given their low stores of vitamin A; the fact that some of the diseases most prevalent in camps, such as measles, further deplete their stores of vitamin A; and the fact that food rations in camps have historically been deficient in vitamin A. There have also been epidemics of pellagra, which is a deficiency of niacin that causes diarrhea, dermatitis, and mental disorders. One such case affected more than 18,000 Mozambican refugees in Malawi, whose rations in the camp were deficient in niacin. Scurvy, from a lack of vitamin C, has also occurred in a number of settings, such as Ethiopia, Somalia, and Sudan. Iron deficiency anemia has also been a problem in some camps and affects primarily women of childbearing age and young children. It appears that women and children who are in the camps without a male adult are at particular risk of not getting enough food in camps and of suffering acute protein-energy malnutrition and micronutrient deficiencies.[23]

Violence Against Women in CHEs

The security conditions during CHEs put women at considerable risk of sexual violence. Rape may be used as a weapon of war. In addition, the chaos and economic distresses of conflict situations place women at risk of sexual violence and sometimes force them to trade sex for food or money, what many call "survival sex." Such women are often very young.

The data on sexual violence against women during CHEs are quite incomplete. Some recent data suggest that the rates of violence against women are very high in these circumstances. A survey carried out in East Timor indicated that 23 percent of the women surveyed after the crisis there reported that they had been sexually assaulted. Fifteen percent of the women in Kosovo who were surveyed reported sexual violence against them during the conflict period. It is estimated that between 50,000 and 64,000 women in Sierra Leone were sexually assaulted during the conflict there, and 25 percent of Azerbaijani women reported sexual violence against them during a 3-month period in 2000.[24] Rohingya women also report widespread sexual assault by Myanmar's military.[25]

Mental Health

Those who study CHEs agree that they are associated with a range of social and psychological shocks to affected people due to changes in their way of living, their loss of livelihoods, damaged social networks, and physical and mental harm to them, their families, and their friends. Nonetheless, there is considerable disagreement among those working with CHEs about the validity of defining the impact on people affected by CHEs through the framework of a Western medical model of mental health.[26,27]

Some studies have focused on post-traumatic stress disorder (PTSD) and have shown rates of prevalence for PTSD among adults that ranged from 4.6 percent among Burmese refugees in Thailand to 37.2 percent among Cambodian refugees in Thailand. By comparison, the rate of PTSD is about 1 percent in the population of the United States. Similar studies showed rates of depression in Bosnian refugees of 39 percent, Burmese refugees of almost 42 percent, and Cambodian refugees of almost 68 percent. In contrast, one estimate of the baseline rate of depression in the U.S. population is 6.4 percent.[28]

Other studies have looked at the mental health impacts of CHEs on children and the extent to which they suffer from both post-traumatic stress and depression. The studies that have been done on such populations have been small ones that cannot be used to draw major conclusions on this question. However, they suggest that children who have been through conflict situations do suffer from high rates of both PTSD and depression. A survey of 170 adolescent Cambodian refugees, for example, indicated that almost 27 percent of them suffered from PTSD. A survey of 147 Bosnian children refugees suggested that almost 26 percent of them suffered from depression.[29]

It should be noted, however, that a number of those involved with the mental health impacts of CHEs believe that the stress placed by some on PTSD is not valid. Rather, they believe that although a small minority of those affected may need psychotropic medication, the most important issue is to help people as rapidly as possible to rebuild their lives and their social networks. This requires a variety of forms of social assistance and help in reuniting families, finding families a place to live, rebuilding social networks, and restoring livelihoods.[26,27] The Inter-Agency Standing Committee of the World Health Organization (WHO) has issued guidelines for planning, establishing, and coordinating integrated responses, across sectors, for mental health and psychosocial well-being in emergencies. The core principles of these guidelines are shown in **TABLE 16-5**.

▶ Addressing the Health Effects of Natural Disasters

The health effects of rapid-onset natural disasters occur in phases, starting with the immediate impact of the event and then continuing for some time until displaced people can be resettled. It is very important that the health situation be assessed immediately after the disaster has occurred. This assessment will set the basis for the initial relief effort. At the same time, care must begin for those injured in the disaster. Once the immediate trauma cases are taken care of, relief workers and health service providers can turn their attention to other injured people who are in need of early care and treatment. This would include urgent psychological problems. In the earliest stages of the

TABLE 16-5 Guidelines on Mental Health and Psychosocial Support in Emergency Settings

Human Rights and Equity
Ensure equity and nondiscrimination in the provision of support services to all affected populations, with a special focus on at-risk populations.

Participation
Promote the participation of the affected population in assistance and reconstruction efforts to improve program quality, equity, and sustainability.

Do No Harm
Reduce the risk of harm to humanitarian workers through recommended techniques, such as the use of *coordination groups,* the integration of *local knowledge* into interventions, *flexibility* and project *transparency, cultural sensitivity,* knowledge of *current research* in emergency response techniques, and an *understanding* of universal human rights, power relations, and participatory approaches.

Building on Available Resources and Capacities
To improve sustainability, use existing mental health services by building on local capacities, supporting self-help practices, and fortifying available resources.

Integrated Support Systems
Integrate activities and programs into a broader structure (i.e., general health services or community support mechanisms) to enable programs to have a more extensive reach, improve sustainability, and reduce stigmatization.

Multilayered Supports
In order to access the majority of the affected population, provide four categories of response: basic services and security, community and family support, focused nonspecialized support, and specialized services.

Data from Inter-Agency Standing Committee (IASC). (2007). *IASC guidelines on mental health and psychosocial support in emergency settings.* Geneva, Switzerland: Author.

disaster, some important public health functions also need to be carried out, including the establishment of continuous disease surveillance among the affected populations and provision of water, shelter, and food.[12]

Many countries do not have the resources needed to cope with the health impacts of a disaster, and they will depend on assistance from other countries to address their health problems. Unfortunately, there have been many instances when such help was poorly coordinated and did not effectively match the conditions on the ground. It has become clear over time, however, that to be most helpful in addressing the impact of natural disasters, external assistance will have to do the following[12]:

- Include all of the external partners
- Be based on a cooperative relationship among the partners
- Have partners working in ways that are complementary to each other
- Be evidence based and transparent
- Involve the affected communities

In some respects, it is easier to predict places that are at risk of natural disasters than it is to predict where CHEs will occur. There are certain countries that are vulnerable to earthquakes, volcanoes, hurricanes, typhoons, and flooding during major rains. In this light, much can be done to prepare for natural disasters and to reduce their health impact. Disaster preparedness plans can be formulated in the following way[12]:

- Identify vulnerabilities
- Develop scenarios of what might happen and their likelihood
- Outline the role that different actors will play in the event of an emergency
- Train first responders and managers to deal with such emergencies

It is also possible when constructing water systems and hospitals, for example, to take measures that will make them less vulnerable to damage during natural disasters.

Given the way that the health impacts of natural disasters unfurl, what would be the most cost-effective ways for external partners to help address the disaster? There are at least several lessons that have emerged on this front. First, although many countries send search-and-rescue teams to assist the victims of natural disasters, the efforts of such teams are not cost-effective. Most people who are freed from the rubble of an earthquake, for example, are saved by people in their own community immediately after the event. By the time foreign search-and-rescue teams arrive, most victims of falling rubble will already have been saved or will be dead. There may be an important humanitarian and foreign policy rationale for external search-and-rescue teams. However, they will generally save few lives at very high cost per life saved.[12]

It is also common that countries will send field hospitals to disaster areas. The cost of each hospital is about $1 million, and they generally arrive 2 to 5 days after the initial event. Unfortunately, by the time they arrive, they are of little value in addressing the most urgent trauma cases. It appears to be more cost-effective to have fewer field hospitals but to have a few that will remain in place for some time, in addition to building some temporary but durable buildings that can also serve as hospitals.[12]

Countries send different kinds of goods to disaster-affected places. Unfortunately, these goods can be inappropriate to the needs of the problem. This has often been the case, for example, for drugs. Better results occur when the affected country clearly indicates what it needs and other countries send only those goods. Large camps of tents are often established after natural disasters. This is generally also not a cost-effective approach to helping the affected community to rebuild. Providing cash or building materials to affected families allows them to rebuild as quickly as possible, in a manner in line with their own preferences. The lack of income, even beyond the cost of rebuilding their home, can be a major impediment to the reconstruction of affected areas. Although it must be managed carefully to avoid abuse, cash assistance to families appears to be a cost-effective way of helping communities rebuild.[12]

▶ Addressing the Health Effects of Complex Humanitarian Emergencies

It is difficult to take measures that can prevent complex humanitarian emergencies from occurring and harming human health because these emergencies so often relate to civil conflict. Thus, the key to avoiding such problems lies in the political realm and in the avoidance of conflict, rather than by taking measures that are directly health related. As some have said, "Primary prevention in such circumstances, therefore, means stopping the violence."[4(p300)]

However, if such conflicts continue to occur, are there measures of secondary prevention that can be taken to detect health-related problems as early as possible and take actions to mitigate them? To a large extent, the early warning systems that exist for natural disasters do not exist for political disasters. Although some groups do carry out analyses of political vulnerability in countries, corruption, and the risk of political instability, these analyses are not used to prepare contingency plans for civil conflict.

Given the extent of conflict, however, it would be prudent if organizations, countries, and international bodies would cooperatively establish contingency plans for areas of likely conflict. It would also be prudent to stage near such areas the materials needed to address displacement and health problems that would occur if conflict breaks out. This would be similar to what is done for disaster preparedness in some places, such as those regularly exposed to hurricanes.[4]

As noted earlier in the chapter, the following are characteristics of CHEs:

- Potentially massive displacement of people
- The likelihood that these displaced people will live in camps for some time
- The need in those camps for adequate shelter, safe water, sanitation, and food
- The importance of security in the camps, especially for women
- The need to address early in the crisis the potentially worst health threats, which are malnutrition, diarrhea, measles, pneumonia, and malaria
- The need to avoid other epidemic diseases, such as cholera and meningitis
- The need as one moves away from the emergency phase of a CHE to deal with longer-term mental health issues, primary health care, TB, and some noncommunicable diseases

Some of the most important measures that can be taken to address these points are discussed briefly hereafter. It is important to keep in mind that the aim of these efforts is to establish a safe and healthy environment, treat urgent health problems and prevent epidemics, and then to address less urgent needs and establish a basis for longer-term health services among the displaced people.[8]

Assessment and Surveillance

As with natural disasters, among the first things that need to be done during the emergency phase of a CHE is to carry out an assessment of the displaced population and establish a system for disease surveillance. Such an assessment would try to immediately gather information on the number of people who are displaced, their age and sex, their ethnic and social backgrounds, and their state of health and nutrition. Although it is difficult to get this information in the chaotic moments of an emergency, it is impossible to rationally plan services for displaced people without this information.

There are a number of health indicators that guide services in CHEs, and a surveillance system needs to be established at the start of the emergency phase of a CHE. Given the difficulties of the emergency, the surveillance system must be simple but still give a robust sense of the health of the affected community. Given the importance of nutrition and the likelihood that a large part of the population will be undernourished, it is essential that the weight for height of all children younger than 5 years of age be checked.[4] It is also important to have surveillance for diseases that cause epidemics among displaced persons, such as measles, cholera, and meningitis.

In general, the daily crude mortality rate is used as an indicator of the health of the affected group; one goal is to keep that rate below 1 death per 10,000 persons in the population per day. Where the daily rate is twice the normal rate, it signifies that a public health emergency is occurring. Say, for example, that the baseline crude mortality rate for sub-Saharan Africa is 0.44/10,000 per day. Thus, if the rate in an affected population were to get to 0.88/10,000 per day, it would signal a public health emergency that would require urgent attention. For children younger than 5 years, say that the crude mortality rate for sub-Saharan Africa is 1.14/10,000 per day. The goal in a public health emergency, therefore, would be to keep that rate below about 2.0/10,000 per day.[29] Death rates in a large camp are not always easy to obtain. Sometimes people have resorted to innovative ways of getting such data, such as daily reports by gravediggers.

A Safe and Healthy Environment

It is critical in camps and other situations with large numbers of displaced people that efforts be made to ensure that environmental and personal hygiene are maintained. This will be the key to avoiding the potentially serious effect of diarrheal disease. It is recommended that 15 liters of water per person per day should be provided, people should not have to walk more than 500 meters to a water source, and people should not have to wait more than 30 minutes to get their water when they get to a source. Of the 15 liters per day that are recommended, about 2.5 to 3 liters are considered the minimum essential for drinking and food. Another 2 to 6 liters are needed for personal hygiene, and the remainder is needed for cooking.[30]

Providing appropriate sanitation in situations of displaced people is also very challenging. Ideally, every family would have their own toilet. This, however, is certainly impossible in the acute phase of an emergency. The goal instead is one toilet for every 20 people. These should be segregated by gender to provide the most safety to women. They should not be more than 50 meters from dwellings, but must be carefully situated to avoid contamination of water sources.[30]

Many of the displaced people will be poor people with little education and, often, poor hygiene practices. It is very important in these circumstances that efforts be made to make the community aware of the importance of good hygiene and to see that soap is available to and used by all families.

Of course, people will also need shelter. The long-term goal is to help them return as quickly as possible to their homes. In the short term, if possible, the goal is to have families be sheltered temporarily with other families. Nonetheless, it is obvious from the tables shown earlier that many displaced people do end up living in camps, often for very long periods of time. When shelter is needed, the goal is to provide 3.5 square meters of covered area per person, with due attention paid in the construction of the shelter to the safety of women. Whenever possible, local and culturally appropriate building materials should be used. In the short run, the aim is to get people into covered areas. When the emergency phase has passed, the need to enhance some of the structures can be prioritized.[31]

Food

It is suggested that each adult in a camp should get at least 2,100 kilocalories of energy from food per day.[32] Food rations should be distributed by family unit, but special care has to be taken, as noted earlier, to ensure that female-headed households and children without their families get their rations. Vitamin A should be given to all children, and the most severely malnourished children may also need urgent nutrition supplementation.[32]

Disease Control

As also suggested earlier, "The primary goals of humanitarian response to disasters are to 1) prevent and reduce excess morbidity and mortality, and 2) promote a return to normalcy."[29] Along these lines, the control of communicable diseases is one of the first priorities in the emergency phase of a disaster, especially a complex humanitarian emergency.

An important priority in the emergency phase of a CHE is to prevent an epidemic of measles. This starts with vaccinating all children from 6 months to 15 years of age. Another important priority is to ensure that children up to 5 years of age get vitamin A. Systems also need to be put in place so that other epidemics that sometimes occur in these situations, such as meningitis and cholera, can be detected and then urgently addressed. Other priorities will include the proper management of diarrhea in children and the appropriate diagnosis and treatment for malaria, in zones where it is prevalent. Of course, health education and hygiene promotion must take place continuously to try to help families prevent the onset of these diseases in the first place.[29]

Unfortunately, preventing the outbreak of communicable diseases is not the only effort that needs to be taken in the emergency phase of a CHE. Measures need to be in place to handle injuries and trauma—first to stabilize people and then to refer them to where they can receive the additional medical help they need. There will almost certainly be pregnant women among the displaced people, and there will be an immediate need for some reproductive health services. This will generally have to focus on the provision of a minimum package of care that would include safe delivery kits, precautions against the transmission of HIV, and transport and referral in the case of complications of pregnancy.[4,29-33]

The care of noncommunicable diseases will be a lower priority in emergency situations than addressing communicable diseases. However, some psychiatric problems will require urgent attention and will need to be treated as effectively as possible with counseling, the continuation of medicines people were taking, and the provision of new medications, if needed. As the emergency recedes, greater attention can be paid to long-term treatment, counseling, and psychosocial support for dealing with mental health problems and the many disruptions that people have faced in their lives.[28] At that time, one can also turn additional attention to ensuring the appropriate medication of people with other noncommunicable diseases.

▶ Coordination of International Emergency Responses

Although the coordination of responses to complex emergencies is difficult and has had gaps in the past, coordination has improved over the past 2 decades. The Office for the Coordination of Humanitarian Affairs (OCHA) is the UN body responsible for strengthening the coordination of UN responses to humanitarian emergencies. OCHA executes this mandate through an Interagency Standing Committee. The full members of that committee are those UN agencies most involved in emergencies and include the Food and Agriculture Organization (FAO), the International Office of Migration (IOM), the United Nations Development Programme (UNDP), the United

Nations High Commissioner for Refugees (UNHCR), the World Food Programme (WFP), UNICEF, and WHO. The Inter-Agency Standing Committee (IASC) is headed by the Emergency Relief Coordinator. Nongovernmental organizations (NGOs) of importance to an effort, including the International Committee of the Red Cross, the International Federation of Red Cross and Red Crescent Societies, and the World Bank, have a standing invitation to the committee.[34]

In 2005, the United Nations implemented a number of reforms aimed at improving the coordination of responses to complex emergencies. The reforms are based on four measures[35]:

- Improved humanitarian leadership through the appointment of a humanitarian coordinator for each emergency
- Enhanced coordination of humanitarian action through the cluster approach, described below
- The promotion of faster, more predictable, and equitable funding through improved humanitarian financing, such as the Central Emergency Response Fund (CERF)
- The creation of more effective partnerships among all humanitarian actors, through the principles of partnership implemented in 2007

The cluster approach is based on the idea of organizations working closely together with other organizations involved in the same sector of activity. A number of clusters have been established at the global level, headed by the relevant UN agency. Clusters are also to be established within countries facing emergencies. The cluster lead is generally the responsible UN agency and is to be appointed by the humanitarian coordinator. There are clusters, for example, for[35,36]:

- Emergency shelter
- Food security
- Health
- Water, sanitation, and hygiene

A wide range of actors are involved in dealing with complex emergencies. Besides the UN agencies, a number of bilateral agencies are involved. A substantial number of NGOs are also involved in emergency responses, and among the most active are Doctors Without Borders (MSF), World Vision, Save the Children, and the International Rescue Committee. It is also important to note that the military forces from a number of countries are often involved in responses to CHEs.

A number of NGOs have also come together in the past decades to create common standards and guiding principles for humanitarian action, notably through the Sphere Project and its handbook. The Sphere Handbook presents a number of minimum standards for humanitarian action. These are technical and quantitative, such as how much water people need per day and how many toilets are needed in a given population. The handbook also articulates core standards and protection principles. The core standards are[37]:

- A people-centered humanitarian response
- Coordination and collaboration
- Assessment
- Design and response
- Performance, transparency, and learning
- Aid-worker performance

These standards guide the process of humanitarian response. The protection principles are as follows[38]:

- Avoid exposing people to further harm as a result of your actions
- Ensure people's access to impartial assistance, in proportion to need and without discrimination
- Protect people from physical and psychological harm arising from violence and coercion
- Assist people to claim their rights, access available remedies, and recover from the effects of abuse

These principles clarify how humanitarian actors should respect the rights of people affected by disaster or armed conflict. Together, these core standards and principles have improved quality and accountability in humanitarian responses. It is important that humanitarian actors operate based on these common standards and principles in order to provide the best assistance possible while respecting the rights and dignity of those affected.

▶ Case Studies

Case studies follow on three CHEs of importance. One concerns the genocide in Rwanda and the plight of Rwandan refugees in Goma, or what is now the Democratic Republic of Congo. A second concerns an earthquake in Haiti in 2010. The comments on Haiti largely follow a chronological account of the work done by Doctors Without Borders in the 6 months following the earthquake. The last case is about the civil war in Syria.

The Rwanda Refugee Crisis

In mid-July 1994, nearly 1 million Hutus fled Rwanda for fear of reprisals from the new Tutsi-led government. The border town of Goma, in what is now the

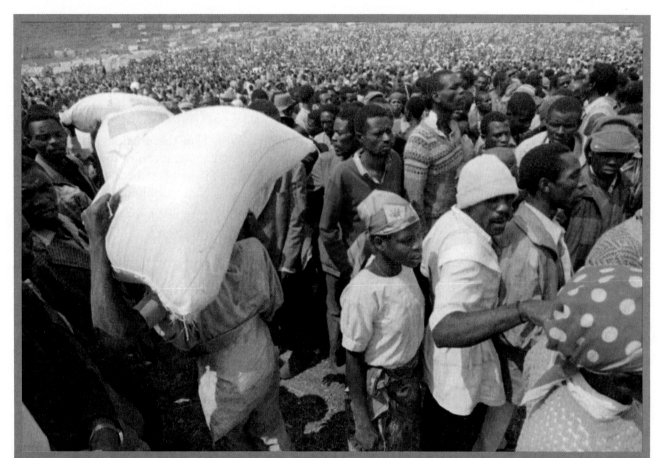

PHOTO 16-1 In 1994, when the civil war broke out in Rwanda, nearly 1 million people fled Rwanda for neighboring Zaire (now the Democratic Republic of the Congo), as shown here. Overnight, there was a need for Zaire, itself a very poor country, to accommodate a continuing stream of refugees. Can individual countries, especially low-income ones, effectively prepare for the arrival of refugees from a neighboring country in conflict? How could the international community help countries receiving refugees deal with so many refugees in such a short period of time?
© Michel Euler/AP/Shutterstock.

Democratic Republic of Congo, situated in the North Kivu region, became the entry point for the majority of the refugees. Many of them settled around Lake Kivu.[39]

Almost 50,000 people died in the first month after the start of the influx, largely as a result of an epidemic of cholera, which was followed by an epidemic of bacillary dysentery. In the first 17 days of the emergency, the average crude mortality rate of Rwandans was 28.1–44.9 per 10,000 per day, compared to the 0.6 per 10,000 per day in prewar conditions inside Rwanda. This crude mortality rate is the highest by a considerable margin over the rate found in any previous CHE. In addition, in Goma, diarrheal disease affected young children and adults alike, whereas normally young children are much more severely affected than adults.[39]

Humanitarian assessments began in the first week of August, 3 weeks after the initial flow of refugees. Rapid surveys conducted in the three refugee camps of Katale, Kibumba, and Mugunga indicated that diarrheal disease contributed to 90 percent of deaths; food

shortages were prevalent, especially among female-headed households; and acute malnutrition afflicted up to 23 percent of the refugees. In early August, a meningitis epidemic arose.[39]

The circumstances were complicated by the large numbers of people who fled to Goma in such a short period of time. In addition, the lake represented an easy source of water, but also one from which disease could readily be spread. The soil around Goma was very rocky, which made it very difficult to construct an appropriate number of latrines. In addition, although Hutu leaders were given control over the distribution of relief, these resources were not shared equitably.[39]

By early August, the response of the international community was beginning to be more effective, under the coordination of the United Nations High Commissioner for Refugees (UNHCR). A disease surveillance network was established. An information system was set up for the camps. Five to 10 liters of safe water per day per person was distributed. Measles immunization was carried out, vitamin A supplements were distributed, and disease problems were attacked using standard protocols.[39]

Despite the exceptional efforts made by many people to deal with the crisis, the events in Goma highlighted a number of shortcomings of the response. First, there was a general lack of preparedness for dealing with this type of emergency, despite the well-known political instability of Rwanda at that time. Second, the medical teams on the ground did not have the physical infrastructure or the experience needed for a task of this magnitude. Many of these staff, for example, were not as knowledgeable about oral rehydration as they needed to be, even though this is fundamental to treating diarrheal disease. Third, the work of the military forces that joined the effort was not integrated into the planning of the other efforts.[39]

Although the Goma crisis was exceptional in many ways, it does suggest a number of lessons for enhancing the response to CHEs in the future, including the following needs:

- Establishing early warning systems for CHEs
- Preparing in advance for CHEs
- Strengthening the existing nongovernmental groups with capability to respond to CHEs

Haiti's 2010 Earthquake[40]

In January 2010, Haiti experienced an earthquake that was centered about 15 miles southwest of Port-au-Prince, the capital city, and measured 7.0 on the Richter scale. Given the magnitude of the earthquake, the poor quality of construction in Haiti, and the exceptionally poor living conditions of many people there, the earthquake caused major devastation. In addition, the country's already weak health system, with only a limited number of trained personnel, was ill equipped to handle the overwhelming health needs stemming from the earthquake. Moreover, with 60 percent of existing health facilities destroyed and 10 percent of medical staff either killed or absent from the country, Haiti was in dire need of external assistance to address the health needs of its people.

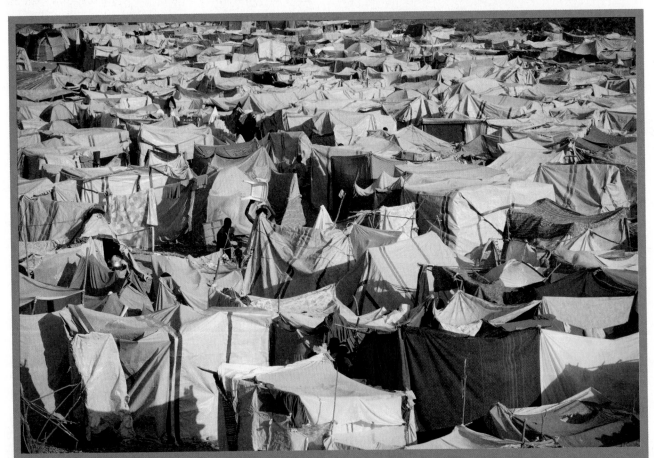

PHOTO 16-2 Haiti suffered an enormous loss of infrastructure from an earthquake in 2010. More than 100,000 people are thought to have died as a result of the earthquake, as well. These are the makeshift homes in a camp in the capital for internally displaced people. What measures could very resource-poor countries like Haiti take on their own and with their partners to avoid such destruction and to be better able to cope with emergencies when they do occur?

© Claudiad/E+/Getty Images.

Doctors Without Borders played a key role in the relief effort. The timeliness and scale of its response was strengthened by the fact that it had already been providing health services in Haiti for 19 years prior to the earthquake. MSF's response to the earthquake provides an informative example of the chronology and focus of health efforts after natural disasters in low-income countries. The actions taken by MSF are also a good reflection of how such external assistance moves through different phases, starting with the acute phase of the emergency and then leading over time toward efforts at reconstruction, rehabilitation, and development.

Providing emergency medical services was the first priority for MSF after the earthquake. In order to perform life-saving surgeries and wound care for people injured by the earthquake, MSF created new emergency facilities. These facilities were needed because so many existing ones had been damaged and because there were so many injured survivors. In addition, MSF sent in more surgical supplies and increased the number of personnel on the ground, which reached 3,500 at its highest point. An inflatable hospital was even constructed, which provided 100 beds and 3 operating theaters. Creating sanitary conditions suitable for performing surgery was one challenge faced in this stage of the emergency response. In total, MSF provided emergency medical care to over 173,000 patients in the 5 months following the earthquake, performing over 11,000 surgeries. The nature of emergency care for earthquake-related injuries soon shifted with time, from lifesaving, often including amputation of limbs, to treating infected wounds.

Provision of emergency obstetric care was also a priority, which is crucial to saving maternal lives. Because MSF's own maternity hospital was demolished, the organization provided support to the Ministry of Health's maternity hospital by providing personnel and critical medicines. MSF helped to deliver 3,752 babies in all its facilities in the first 5 months after the earthquake, spending 4 million euros on maternal health services during this period.

To address the effects of the disaster on mental health, psychological care was integrated with emergency care for trauma patients. Soon after, outreach programs in communities were initiated, reflecting the importance of mental health care both immediately and later in relief efforts. Group counseling sessions and individual consultations were aimed primarily at reducing the anxiety that comes with losing a loved one, coping with injury and poor living conditions, and the fear of an aftershock. MSF delivered psychological care to over 80,000 Haitians in the first 5 months after the earthquake. Even so, due to the lack of healthcare professionals and community-based workers trained in mental health issues, provision of mental health care remains a great challenge in Haiti.

Providing primary health care was also a priority for MSF, which was addressed by setting up additional primary health clinics. In the weeks following the earthquake, 400 to 500 people visited each clinic daily (6 months after the earthquake, about 70 people visited daily). In addition to providing basic checkups, which allowed MSF to monitor common health problems in the area, primary health clinics enabled MSF to screen for disease epidemics. Services provided included ante- and postnatal care, vaccinations, infection treatment, and referrals to mental health services or a hospital.

The delivery of health services consumed the majority of MSF's efforts in Haiti after the earthquake. However, additional efforts were needed as quickly as possible to address the health threats posed by a lack of water, sanitation, and shelter. Thus, MSF set up sanitation areas in camps surrounding Port-au-Prince, each composed of a latrine, shower, and wash area. In addition to the creation of a waste disposal system, good hygiene was promoted through the distribution of 35,000 hygiene kits that included soap, toothpaste, and a toothbrush. As of May 2010, MSF was distributing about 1,270 cubic meters of water per day by water trucks, in partnership with other organizations.

At the same time, MSF attempted to improve living conditions for the displaced by distributing tents for shelter and nonfood household items, such as cooking materials and sheets. Almost 27,000 tents were distributed, which are supposed to last about 6 months.

MSF also expanded its mobile clinics, which included bringing care to communities and seeking out patients. Mobile clinics are commonly used by MSF. However, the number of such clinics was not expanded immediately because the organization's personnel were already overburdened by the number of patients coming on their own immediately following the disaster to other MSF-supported healthcare facilities.

As MSF tried to carry out this work, particularly during the immediate response to the earthquake, it confronted the challenge of obtaining landing spots for planes carrying urgently needed medical supplies and personnel. With planes often diverted to the neighboring Dominican Republic, supplies had to be brought to their destination by car, which took an additional 36 hours.

By the second month after the disaster, medical needs shifted from emergency care to longer-term care, with an emphasis on recovery and rehabilitation. In addition, hospitals and primary care clinics started to treat conditions not inflicted by the earthquake, which amounted to about half of the cases treated by MSF by early June 2010. During this stage of the response, violence-related injuries and pediatric issues were especially common. Hospitals also had to respond more frequently to conditions such as road traffic accidents, burn injuries, sexually transmitted infections, and illnesses such as TB, HIV, and respiratory infections.

By the third month after the earthquake, MSF was able to replace many of its international workers, who had flown to Haiti for emergency relief, with Haitian workers. By June 2010, the ratio of Haitian to international workers had returned to 10 to 1, the standard before the earthquake.

MSF spent about 53 million euros in Haiti in the first 5 months following the earthquake, with 11 million euros spent on surgical and postoperative care and 8.5 million euros spent on providing shelter.

Despite health improvements in Haiti made possible by MSF, the organization faced some major challenges in the aftermath of the earthquake:

- Proper shelter for earthquake victims remained an issue, because reconstruction was slow and the makeshift tents started to deteriorate.
- MSF faced the task of rebuilding medical facilities that were destroyed in the earthquake, in addition to replacing temporary facilities with permanent ones.
- Because Haiti is subject to natural disasters, including hurricanes, a serious hurricane could dramatically complicate the already weak infrastructure in Haiti and create additional health problems.

Health Care in the Syrian Civil War

In March 2011, demonstrations began in the Syrian city of Daraa, protesting the government of Bashar al-Assad and its security forces. Amid a wave of uprisings across the Arab world, protests spread in Syria, as did a harsh government crackdown. Clashes between Assad's government and various rebel forces escalated into a civil war while the involvement of foreign militaries also prolonged the conflict. The conflict is still ongoing.[41]

The Syrian civil war has caused unprecedented displacement while devastating the country's population and infrastructure. Over half of Syrians have fled their homes: 6.6 million people are internally displaced and 5.6 million Syrians have become refugees in Turkey, Lebanon, Jordan, Europe, and beyond.[42] One study estimates that, from 2011 to 2016, the conflict caused 143,630 deaths directly.[43] Men have been more likely to be killed than women: from 2010 to 2015, Syrian women's life expectancy fell 4.8 years

to 73.5, while men's fell 10.7 years to 63.3.[44] Over the course of the war, civilian deaths have risen, in part due to the use of devastating weaponry such as barrel bombs and aerial bombardment.[45] As the proportion of civilian deaths increased, so did the proportion of deaths among children: children composed 9 percent of all civilian deaths in 2011, 19 percent in 2013, and 23 percent in 2016.[43]

The war has damaged the country's healthcare system, destroying more than half of Syrian hospitals, primary health centers, and clinics. Hospitals that do operate often face electricity cuts or cannot obtain sufficient supplies. Many medical personnel have also fled Syria.[46] In 2010, Aleppo had approximately 1 doctor for every 800 residents. However, by 2015 the city only had 1 doctor for every 7,000 residents.[47]

There are international conventions that require **medical neutrality** in conflict, meaning that medical personnel not engaged in acts harmful to the enemy should be respected and protected. However, this has not been the case in Syria: medical facilities and workers have been intentionally targeted. Physicians for Human Rights (PHR) has documented 687 deaths of medical personnel and 329 attacks on medical facilities, mostly in the northern governorates of Aleppo and Idlib. PHR estimates that the Syrian government committed 90 percent of these attacks.[47] A study by the Syrian American Medical Society (SAMS) also documented 200 attacks on medical facilities in northern Syria in just 2016.[48] The effect of a single attack can be great: in September 2017, an airstrike on a hospital forced it to close due to structural damage. That hospital had been providing care to 16,000 patients a month.[49] With so much destroyed, millions of people within Syria have very limited or no access to health care or must travel considerable distances to receive care, such as over 4 hours in northeast Syria.[49] It is important to also note that the Syrian government, pro-government forces, and armed opposition groups have restricted humanitarian aid delivery.[50]

A lack of primary health care has led to the outbreak of infectious diseases. While in 2009, 99 percent of Syrians were covered by measles, polio, and DTP vaccinations, in 2016 coverage rates fell to 63 percent, 57 percent, and 51 percent, respectively.[51] A polio outbreak occurred in 2013, leading to over 30 cases and spreading throughout the country and to Iraq. This was the first outbreak of polio in the Middle East in 15 years. At first, humanitarian organizations faced significant obstruction from the Syrian government in their vaccination campaigns, as they have throughout the conflict. However, the government eventually granted access to non-government-controlled areas, and the organizations were able to conduct several mass vaccinations. Another polio outbreak occurred in 2017 in Raqqa and Deir Ez-Zor but, with increased surveillance mechanisms, was quickly contained.[52] In 2017, a measles outbreak reached all 14 governorates and affected thousands of children.[51]

Weakened healthcare infrastructure has led to excess morbidity and mortality related to trauma, childbirth, and noncommunicable diseases. Without access to timely trauma care, up to one-third of people who are injured in conflict may suffer life-changing disabilities, and many die who would survive if they received appropriate and timely care. Without emergency obstetric care, pregnant women are also at increased risk: the maternal mortality ratio, which had been steadily declining, increased by 39 percent from 2010 to 2015 because of the war. Without access to treatment, Syrians with chronic diseases also face increased death and disability. For instance, 60 percent of Syrians with diabetes are at risk due to limited supplies of insulin.[53]

In the short term, efforts to improve health in Syria should continue to prioritize immunization, particularly in non-government-controlled areas, to prevent further outbreaks. It is also imperative to continue providing treatment for the many Syrians with noncommunicable diseases, such as diabetes or heart disease. Wherever possible, and despite the dangers, it is also necessary to expand emergency trauma and emergency obstetric care. Should the war end, Syria will have an enormous task rebuilding both its health system and health-related infrastructure such as water and sanitation systems.

▶ Future Challenges in Meeting the Health Needs of Complex Humanitarian Emergencies and Natural Disasters

A number of critical challenges confront efforts to address the health effects of natural disasters and CHEs. One such challenge for the future is how to prevent these from having such negative health impacts. It is difficult in resource-poor settings, many of which are poorly governed, to focus attention on the prevention of disasters and their impacts. Nonetheless, through better mitigation measures, such as water control, better building standards, greater education of the community about how to deal with disasters, and having a disaster preparedness plan for which people are trained, it should be possible, even for very poor countries, to reduce deaths from natural

disasters. If these steps are coupled with the development of standard approaches for dealing with health issues when they do arise and the forward staging of medicines, equipment, and materials near disaster-prone areas, it should be possible to reduce deaths from natural disasters, even in very low-income settings. Bangladesh, which is subject to annual flooding, has reduced the annual deaths from such floods, for example, with a series of the previously mentioned measures.[54]

There has been considerable progress among the international community in the establishment of common standards and protocols for responses to disasters. In fact, a code of conduct has been developed for use by the International Red Cross and Red Crescent Societies and NGOs to guide their work in emergencies. The core principles of this code are shown in **TABLE 16-6**. There remains, however, the need to enhance further the coordination of responses. Ideally, the organizations involved in responding to natural disasters and CHEs will do the following[55]:

- Subscribe to a common set of norms, such as the Sphere Project
- Have common protocols for dealing with key issues
- Train their staff to work with those protocols
- Work in close conjunction with the affected communities and local governments

In addition, it is important that responses to disasters focus on cost-effective approaches to the provision of healthcare services in emergencies. We have already seen that search-and-rescue assistance from abroad is not cost effective. The same is true for most field hospitals. Moreover, many agencies have provided health services in emergencies that did not focus on immediate needs and could have waited. Morbidity and mortality can be prevented and reduced more quickly if the agencies involved in disaster relief carefully set priorities for action that would be based on the principle of cost-effectiveness analysis, taking appropriate account of concerns for social justice and equity.[12,55,56]

The continued refinement of indicators that can be used to measure performance of services in disasters will be helpful to gauging the performance of local and international relief efforts.[56]

▶ Main Messages

Natural disasters and CHEs are important causes of illness, death, and disability. They affect large numbers of people, have a huge economic impact, and have aftereffects that can go on for some time. Their biggest relative

TABLE 16-6 The Code of Conduct: Principles of Conduct for the International Red Cross and Red Crescent Movement and NGOs in Disaster Response Programs

The humanitarian imperative comes first.

Aid is given regardless of the race, creed, or nationality of the recipients and without adverse distinction of any kind. Aid priorities are calculated on the basis of need alone.

Aid will not be used to further a particular political or religious standpoint.

We shall endeavor not to act as instruments of government foreign policy.

We shall respect culture and custom.

We shall attempt to build disaster response on local capacities.

Ways shall be found to involve program beneficiaries in the management of relief aid.

Relief aid must strive to reduce future vulnerabilities to disaster as well as meeting basic needs.

We hold ourselves accountable to both those we seek to assist and those from whom we accept resources.

In our information, publicity, and advertising activities, we shall recognize disaster victims as dignified humans, not hopeless objects.

Modified from the International Federation of Red Cross and Red Crescent Societies. (n.d.). *The code of conduct.* Retrieved from http://www.ifrc.org/en/publications-and-reports/code-of-conduct/

impact is on the poor, who are generally more vulnerable to the effects of these disasters than are better-off people. Some of these disasters are caused by humans. Some are slow onset and some are rapid onset.

Natural disasters, such as droughts, famines, hurricanes, typhoons, cyclones, and heavy rains, have important health impacts. Earthquakes and volcanoes are also natural disasters with large potential effects on health. It appears that the number of natural disasters is increasing but the number of deaths from them is decreasing. More than 90 percent of deaths from natural disasters occur in low- and middle-income countries. Climate change could increase the type and severity of natural disasters.

Some deaths are a direct result of natural disasters. However, the impact of those disasters on water supply and sanitation systems, health services, and availability of food can also, indirectly, lead to many more deaths. There are also special health problems associated with living in camps, which sometimes happen to those who survive natural disasters that displace many people from their homes.

In the late 1990s, there were about 40 CHEs each year. There are probably more than 25 million refugees in the world and more than 40 million internally displaced people. Overall, CHEs are associated with considerably larger health impacts than natural disasters. In addition, they may have an acute phase when large numbers of people flee, and they generally go on for long periods of time.

CHEs have increasingly been linked to civil conflict. Like natural disasters, they also have direct and indirect impacts on health. They not only take lives directly through war-related trauma but also lead to the destruction of infrastructure. The health effects of some of these conflicts have been dramatic, sometimes because civilians have been targeted by combatants. Women are especially vulnerable in CHEs to sexual violence.

In the emergency phase of a CHE, when large numbers of displaced persons are coming into camps, a number of health risks have to be addressed. Among the most important are diarrhea, measles, malaria, and pneumonia. Malnutrition is also of exceptional importance. Cholera epidemics can also arise and kill large numbers of people quickly.

Countries at risk can take a number of measures to mitigate vulnerability to damage from natural disasters. This could include preparing a disaster plan, building seawalls and levees, and requiring, for example, that buildings in earthquake-prone areas be earthquake proof. It might also be cost-effective to strengthen other infrastructure, such as water supply systems, so that they can withstand significant threats.

Addressing the health impacts of a natural disaster requires that the health situation be assessed quickly and that urgent cases be handled immediately. Less urgent problems can be handled in the following days, weeks, and months. Long-term support for those psychologically affected by the disaster will also need to be provided in the medium and long term.

The health situation of a CHE also needs to be assessed quickly and continuously. Early attention in dealing with large numbers of displaced people must focus on the environment, shelter, water, and food. The next step is the prevention of disease outbreaks, and their treatment if they do occur. Particular attention must be paid to malnutrition, measles, pneumonia, and malaria. Some immediate attention will also have to be paid to a minimum package of reproductive health services and the avoidance of HIV. As the acute phase of the emergency subsides, more attention can be paid to TB, overall primary health care, noncommunicable diseases, and longer-term mental health issues.

There has been some important progress in the coordination and standardization of measures to address CHEs and natural disasters. However, there are still gaps in the preparation and training of staff in some organizations. In addition, there has been inadequate attention to the cost-effectiveness of interventions. There is now enough information about the lessons of CHEs and natural disasters that the priority actions that are needed should be clear, and organizations active in relief work need to concentrate their efforts on what will prevent the most deaths, disability, and morbidity, at least cost, with due attention to equity and social justice.

Study Questions

1. How does the annual burden of disease from natural disasters and complex humanitarian emergencies compare with other causes of illness, death, and disability?

2. What is a disaster? A natural disaster? A complex humanitarian emergency?

3. What is an internally displaced person? A refugee? An asylum-seeker? What are the differences between them?

4. What have been some of the most significant natural disasters in the last decade? How many deaths were associated with them? How did people die? How did deaths vary for different types of disasters by age and sex?

5. What countries in sub-Saharan Africa have been the largest sources of displaced people? What countries in sub-Saharan Africa have received the largest numbers of refugees?

6. What countries in Asia or the Middle East have been the largest sources of displaced people? What countries in Asia or the Middle East have received the largest numbers of refugees?

7. In the early stages of a complex humanitarian emergency, what are likely to be the most significant health concerns for the refugees? How do those health concerns change over time? Who are the most affected by malnutrition, measles, pneumonia, and cholera?

8. In what ways are women especially vulnerable during complex humanitarian emergencies? What problems do they face as a consequence of these vulnerabilities?

9. What are key steps that can be taken to reduce the vulnerability of certain places to the potential health threats of natural disasters?

10. What are key steps that need to be taken within the first few days of people fleeing to a refugee camp? How do those concerns change over time?

11. How can one try to ensure that relief agencies work together around a common framework and that they focus on the most cost-effective activities?

References

1. National Highway Traffic Safety Administration. (n.d.). *Glossary*. Retrieved from http://www.nhtsa.dot.gov/people/injury/ems/emstraumasystem03/glossary.htm

2. Boutros-Ghali, B. (1995). Concluding Statement of the UN Congress on Public International Law: Towards the Twenty-First Century: International Law as a Language for International Relations, March 13–17, 1995, New York.

3. Burkholder, B. T., & Toole, M. J. (1995). Evolution of complex disasters. *The Lancet, 346*, 1012–1015.

4. Toole, M. J., & Waldman, R. J. (1997). The public health aspects of complex emergencies and refugee situations. *Annual Review of Public Health, 18*, 283–312.

5. United Nations High Commissioner for Refugees. (2001). *The 1951 convention relating to the status of refugees and its 1967 protocol*. Retrieved from http://www.unhcr.org/4ec262df9.html

6. UNHCR. (n.d.). *Asylum-seekers*. Retrieved from http://www.unhcr.org/en-us/asylum-seekers.html

7. Brookings Institute. (2008). *Protecting internally displaced persons: A manual for law and policymakers*. Retrieved from http://www.unhcr.org/50f955599.html/

8. Brennan, R. J., & Nandy, R. (2001). Complex humanitarian emergencies: A major global health challenge. *Emergency Medicine (Fremantle), 13*(2), 147–156.

9. Last, J. M. (2001). *A dictionary of epidemiology* (4th ed., p. 47). New York, NY: Oxford University Press.

10. UCLA School of Public Health. (n.d.). *Definitions*. Retrieved from http://www.ph.ucla.edu/epi/bioter/anthapha_def_a.html

11. Centre for Research on the Epidemiology of Disasters. (2017). *Annual disaster statistical review 2016: The numbers and trends*. Retrieved from https://reliefweb.int/report/world/annual-disaster-statistical-review-2016-numbers-and-trends

12. de Ville de Goyet, C., Zapata Marti, R., & Osorio, C. (2006). Natural disaster mitigation and relief. In D. T. Jamison, J. G. Breman, A. R. Measham, et al. (Eds.), *Disease control priorities in developing countries* (2nd ed., pp. 1147–1152). New York, NY: Oxford University Press.

13. UNHCR. (n.d.). *Figures at a glance*. Retrieved from http://www.unhcr.org/uk/figures-at-a-glance.html

14. Global Humanitarian Assistance. (2018). *Global humanitarian assistance report 2018*. Retrieved from http://devinit.org/wp-content/uploads/2018/06/GHA-Report-2018.pdf

15. Hansch, S., & Burkholder, B. (1996). When chaos reigns. *Harvard International Review, 18*(4), 10–14.

16. Ganeshan, S., & Diamond, W. (2009). *Forecasting the numbers of people affected annually by natural disasters up to 2015*. Oxford, UK: Oxfam.

17. Guha-Sapir, D., Hoyois, P., Wallemacq, P., & Below, R. (2016). *Annual disaster statistical review 2016*. Brussels, Belgium: Centre for Research on the Epidemiology of Disasters (CRED), Institute of Health and Society (IRSS), and Université Catholique de Louvain. Retrieved from https://www.emdat.be/sites/default/files/adsr_2016.pdf

18. Ghobarah, H. A., & Huth P., & Russett, B. (2004). The postwar public health effects of civil conflict. *Social Science & Medicine, 59*(4), 869-884.

19. Lopez, A. D., Mathers, C. D., & Murray, C. J. L. (2006). The burden of disease and mortality by condition: Data, methods, and results for 2001. In A. D. Lopez, C. D. Mathers, M. Ezzati, D. T. Jamison, C. J. L. Murray (Eds.), *Global burden of disease and risk factors* (pp. 45–93). New York, NY: Oxford University Press.

20. Zwi, A. B., & Ugalde, A. (1991). Political violence in the third world: A public health issue. *Health Policy and Planning, 6*, 203–217.

21. Personal communication, R. J. Waldman to R. Skolnik, March 2007.

22. Zannad, F., Zavala, D. E., Zeeb, H., Zhang, H., Zonies, D., Zuhlke, L. J. (2016). Global, regional, and national life expectancy, all-cause mortality, and cause-specific mortality for 249 causes of death, 1980–2015: A systematic analysis for the Global Burden of Disease Study 2015. *The Lancet, 388*, 1459–1544.

23. Waldman, R. J. (2001). Prioritising health care in complex emergencies. *The Lancet, 357*(9266), 1427–1429.

24. Marsh, M., Purdin, S., & Navani, S. (2006). Addressing sexual violence in humanitarian emergencies. *Global Public Health, 1*(2), 133–146.

25. United Nations, Human Rights Council. (2018). *Report of the Independent International Fact-Finding Mission on Myanmar*, A/HRC/39/64. Retrieved from https://www.ohchr.org/EN/NewsEvents/Pages/DisplayNews.aspx?NewsID=23575&LangID=E

26. Ager, A. (2002). Psychosocial needs in complex emergencies. *The Lancet, 360*, s43–s44.

27. Almedom, A., & Summerfield, D. (2004). Mental well-being in settings of "complex emergency": An overview. *Journal of Biosocial Science, 36*, 381–388.

28. Mollica, R. F., Cardozo, B. L., Osofsky, H. J., Raphael, B., Ager, A., & Salama, P. (2004). Mental health in complex emergencies. *The Lancet, 364*(9450), 2058–2067.

29. The Sphere Project. (2011). *The Sphere handbook* (4th Ed., p. 829). Geneva, Switzerland: Author.

30. The Sphere Project. (2011). Minimum standards in water supply, sanitation and hygiene protection. In *The Sphere handbook 2011: Humanitarian charter and minimum standards in disaster response* (pp. 79–138). Geneva, Swizterland: Author.

31. The Sphere Project. (2011). Minimum standards in shelter, settlement and non-food items. In *The Sphere handbook 2011: Humanitarian charter and minimum standards in disaster response* (pp. 239–286). Geneva, Swizterland: Author.

32. The Sphere Project. (2011). Minimum standards in food security and nutrition. In *The Sphere handbook 2011: Humanitarian charter and minimum standards in disaster response* (pp. 139–238). Geneva, Swizterland: Author.

33. Krasue, S. K., Meyers, J. L., & Friedlander, E. (2006). Improving the availability of emergency obstetric care in conflict-affected settings. *Global Public Health, 1*(3), 229–248.

34. UNHCR. (2001). *Coordination in complex emergencies*. Retrieved from http://www.unhcr.org/en-us/partners/partners/3ba88e7c6/coordination-complex-emergencies.html

35. Humphries, V. (2013). Improving humanitarian coordination: Common challenges and lessons learned from the cluster approach. *Journal of Humanitarian Assistance*. Retrieved from https://sites.tufts.edu/jha/archives/1976

36. Interagency Standing Committee (IASC). (2006). *Guidance note on using the cluster approach to strengthen humanitarian response*. Retrieved from https://www.humanitarianresponse.info/sites/www.humanitarianresponse.info/files/documents/files/IASC%20Guidance%20Note%20on%20using%20the%20Cluster%20Approach%20to%20Strengthen%20Humanitarian%20Response%20%28November%202006%29.pdf

37. The Sphere Project. (2011). Core standards. In *The Sphere handbook 2011: Humanitarian charter and minimum standards in disaster response* (pp. 55–73). Geneva, Switzerland: Author.

38. The Sphere Project. (2011). Core standards. In *The Sphere handbook 2011: Humanitarian charter and minimum standards in disaster response* (pp. 33–48). Geneva, Swizterland: Author.

39. Goma Epidemiology Group. (1995). Public health impact of Rwandan refugee crisis: What happened in Goma, Zaire, in July 1994? *The Lancet, 345*(8946), 339–344.

40. Médicins Sans Frontières. (2010). *Emergency response after the Haiti earthquake: Choices, obstacles, activities and finance.* Retrieved from https://www.msf.org/emergency-response -after-haiti-earthquake-choices-obstacles-and-finance

41. The Associated Press. (2018, March 15). Timeline of the Syrian conflict as it enters 8th year. *AP News.* Retrieved from https:// www.apnews.com/792a0bd7dd6a4006a78287f170165408

42. UNHCR. (2018). *Syria emergency.* Retrieved from http:// www.unhcr.org/en-us/syria-emergency.html

43. Guha-Sapir, D., Schlüter, B., Rodriguez-Llanes, J. M., Lillywhite, L., & Hicks M.H.-R. (2017). Patterns of civilian and child deaths due to war-related violence in Syria: A comparative analysis from the Violation Documentation Center dataset, 2011–2016. *The Lancet Global Health.* doi: 10.1016/S2214-109X(17)30469-2

44. Institute for Health Metrics and Evaluation. (n.d.). *Global health data exchange.* Retrieved from http://ghdx.healthdata .org/

45. Mowafi, H., & Leaning, J. (2018). Documenting deaths in the Syrian war. *The Lancet, 6*(1), 14–15. doi: 10.1016/S2214-109X(17)30457-6

46. World Health Organization. (2018). *Seven years of Syria's health tragedy.* Retrieved from http://www.who.int /mediacentre/news/releases/2018/seven-years-syria/en/

47. Physicians for Human Rights. (2015). *Aleppo abandoned: A case study on health care in Syria.* Retrieved from https:// s3.amazonaws.com/PHR_Reports/aleppo-abandoned.pdf

48. Haar, R. J., Risko C. B., Singh, S., Rayes, D., Albalk, A., Ainajar, M., . . . Rubenstein, L. S. (2018). Determining the scope of attacks on health in four governorates of Syria in 2016: Results of a field surveillance program. *PLOS Medicine, 15*(4). doi: 10.1371/journal.pmed.1002559

49. World Health Organization. (2018). *Syrian Arab Republic: Annual report 2017.* Cairo, Egypt: WHO Regional Office for the Eastern Mediterranean.

50. Human Rights Watch. (2018). *Syria: Events of 2017.* Retrieved from https://www.hrw.org/world-report/2018 /country-chapters/syria

51. World Health Organization. (2017). *Syrian Arab Republic: Annual report 2016.* Retrieved from http://www.who.int /hac/crises/syr/sitreps/syria_annual-report-2016.pdf

52. World Health Organization. (2018). *Situation reports on the polio outbreak in Syria.* Retrieved from http://www.emro .who.int/syr/syria-infocus/situation-reports-on-the-polio -outbreak-in-syria.html

53. World Health Organization. (2016). *WHO helps diabetes patients in Syria.* Retrieved from http://www.who.int/news -room/feature-stories/detail/who-helps-diabetes-patients -in-syria

54. ICDDR, B Centre for Health and Population Research. (2004). Documenting effects of the July–August floods of 2004 and ICDDR, B's response. *Health and Science Bulletin, 2*(3), 1–6.

55. The Sphere Project. (2004). *The Sphere handbook 2004: Humanitarian charter and minimum standards in disaster response.* Geneva, Switzerland: Oxfam.

56. Spiegel, P., Sheik, M., Gotway-Crawford, C., & Salama, P. (2002). Health programmes and policies associated with decreased mortality in displaced people in postemergency phase camps: A retrospective study. *The Lancet, 360*(9349), 1927–1934.

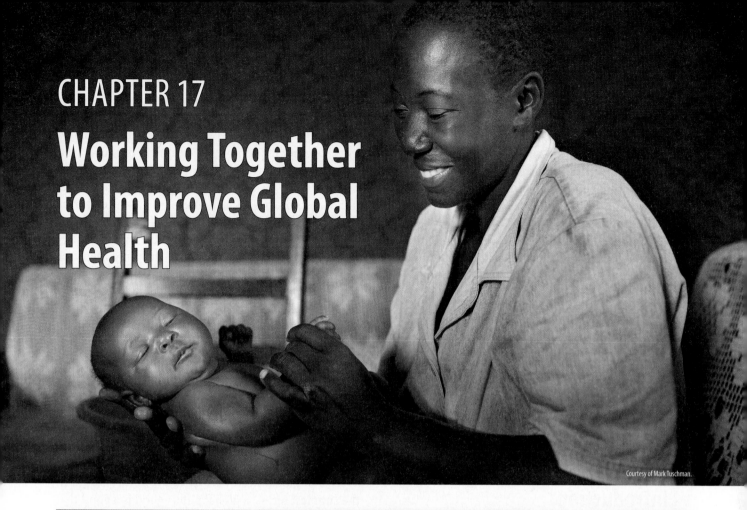
Courtesy of Mark Tuschman.

CHAPTER 17
Working Together to Improve Global Health

LEARNING OBJECTIVES

By the end of this chapter, the reader will be able to do the following:

- Discuss the value of cooperation in addressing global health problems
- Discuss the most important types of cooperative action in global health
- Describe the major organizational actors in global health and the focuses of their global health efforts
- Discuss the rationale for the creation of public–private partnerships for health
- Outline the key challenges to enhancing cooperative action in global health

▶ Vignettes

The world came close to eradicating polio in 2004. However, in 2005, polio spread from northern Nigeria to a number of other African countries, due to the unwillingness of some people in northern Nigeria to immunize their children against polio. By July 2005, polio cases had moved from Africa to Saudi Arabia and Indonesia and then began appearing in Angola, which had not had a case of polio since 2001. By September 2005, cases appeared in Somalia, which had also been free of polio for several years.[1] Stopping new cases of polio and preventing it from spreading from one country to another requires a coordinated global effort.

In 2017, about 10 million people became ill with tuberculosis (TB), and 1.6 million died from it.[2] In fact, TB is one of the leading causes of adult deaths in low-income countries. Despite the importance of TB, however, few new TB drugs have been developed since the 1960s.[3] TB is a disease that largely affects poor people in low- and middle-income countries. These people have little money to spend on drugs, and there is minimal economic incentive for pharmaceutical companies to develop new TB treatments. Can actors in global health work together to encourage the development of new drugs for TB and other neglected diseases? What would they have to do to encourage public and private sector investment in such drugs? What would they have to do to assure investors who develop such drugs that there will be a market for them?

Vaccines are among the most cost-effective investments in health. The basic vaccines for children in low- and middle-income countries have been against six diseases: diphtheria, pertussis, tetanus, TB, measles, and polio. There are also other vaccines that are cost-effective in these countries, including the vaccines for hepatitis B and for *Haemophilus influenza* type B. Yet, throughout the 1990s there were important gaps in coverage of the six basic vaccines in the poorest countries. In addition, the rate of coverage of those vaccines was going down in some countries.[4] Moreover, although the hepatitis B vaccine began to be widely used in high-income countries in the 1980s, almost 20 years later it was still rarely used in low- and middle-income countries. The main reasons behind these gaps included limited money for immunization, a lack of the infrastructure needed to carry out effective immunization programs, and a lack of political interest in immunization. Could key global health actors work together to address gaps in vaccine coverage?

▸ Introduction

This chapter focuses on how different actors work together to enhance global health. First, it discusses the importance of such cooperation. The chapter then reviews the key organizational actors in global health activities. The chapter continues by examining the roles of different types of organizations in cooperation. The chapter then outlines how the global health agenda is set and how it has evolved historically. The chapter concludes with a number of case studies and an assessment of some of the future challenges to cooperative action in global health.

▸ Cooperating to Improve Global Health[5,6]

There are a number of reasons why different actors cooperate in global health activities and why such cooperation is in everyone's interest. First is the value of cooperating to create consensus around and advocate on behalf of different health causes. Although health is an extremely important issue for both individuals and societies, it does not always receive the political, economic, and financial support that it should. A good example of this is the lack of attention given to nutrition in many countries, despite the poor nutritional status of their people. The impact of advocacy efforts is likely to be much greater if numerous

actors, across organizations and across countries, work together to promote important health causes. This has been evident in the field of HIV/AIDS, for example, where AIDS activists worldwide have been able to work together to promote the treatment of people who are HIV-positive with antiretroviral drugs.

The need to share knowledge and to set global standards for health activities are additional reasons for cooperation in the global health field. It has become clear from trials of different antimalarial drugs, for example, that some drug regimens for malaria are more effective than others. This knowledge is especially important because some malaria parasites are resistant to what has been standard treatment. If lessons like this are to be shared globally, then it is important that technical standards be developed and disseminated by an organization that countries believe is technically sound and internationally representative. As you will read later, helping to define and promulgate such standards is one of the main functions of the World Health Organization (WHO).

Another important reason for cooperation to achieve global health aims is the fact that many aspects of global health are **global public goods**. In the simplest terms, a global public good is a good that benefits everyone, such as clean air or the eradication of polio. WHO described global public goods in economic terms:

> Public goods are defined as goods and services that are "non-rival" and "non-excludable." In other words, no one can be excluded from their benefits and their consumption by one person does not diminish consumption by another. . . . Because the benefits of a public good are available to everyone (no one can be excluded), there are diminishing incentives for private sector provision. Consumption by one individual or group does not reduce availability for others, so a price is difficult to set in a market context (non-rivalry).[7]

WHO sees a number of areas in health as global public goods, including, for example, information and knowledge, the control of communicable diseases, and international rules for the control of such diseases.[7,8]

Because of the nature of global public goods, it is only through cooperative efforts that the world can ensure that a sufficient amount of these goods is produced and shared. Individual countries, for example, may not have an interest in reducing pollution generated within their borders that causes health problems in adjacent countries, and it is only through collective action that countries will be able to address such problems. A similar issue arises with respect to efforts to reduce the burden of communicable diseases. Individual countries may have little incentive to take the measures needed to effectively address some communicable diseases, despite the fact that the spread of these diseases does not respect national boundaries. Efforts to deal with them, therefore, require cooperative efforts across countries.

The surveillance of disease also has many aspects of a global public good and requires cooperation among many actors to be successful. It is important for all countries to work together to monitor the presence of diseases and to fashion approaches to dealing with them. Surveillance by individual countries, for example, is not sufficient to stem the spread of disease *across* countries. The global effort to address the severe acute respiratory syndrome (SARS) problem in 2003 is an excellent example of the need for close collaboration among countries on surveillance.[9] The fact that Ebola spread so extensively in West Africa in 2014 and 2015 may indicate what happens when early cooperative action does not take place.

Cooperation to achieve better global health outcomes can also assist in financing health efforts in poorer countries. There are multiple motivations for this aid. In one case, wealthier countries may contribute out of humanitarian concern for the well-being of less fortunate people. Richer countries may also wish to assist in addressing these problems because of enlightened self-interest. In an age of travel and extensive contact among people of different countries, governments may be concerned that the health problems of low- and middle-income countries will endanger their own people if not properly tackled. Many low-income countries, for example, have high burdens of TB but may not have the financial, technical, or institutional resources needed to combat TB effectively. Yet, TB can endanger both their own populations and those of other countries. Thus, it is in everyone's interest for high-income countries to provide financial and technical assistance to low- and middle-income countries to deal effectively with diseases such as TB.

▶ Key Actors in Global Health

The number of actors in the global health arena has grown exponentially. Some of these are international organizations with a global reach. Others are organizations that work globally but are based in individual countries. Some are public organizations. A number are private and for-profit, whereas others are private but operate on a not-for-profit basis. Foundations are also actively involved in global health activities. Increasingly, there are also organizations that bring the public and private sectors together to work cooperatively on a global health problem. The next section discusses some of the most important organizations that are involved in global health and examples of how they operate in that field.

There are so many actors in global health that it is necessary to think in terms of the types of organizations they represent and the kinds of roles they play. **TABLE 17-1** lists a sample of the types of organizations involved in global health and selected organizations representing those types.

It is also important to consider the activities in which these organizations engage. They could,

---

TABLE 17-1 Selected Organizational Actors in Global Health by Type of Organization

United Nations Agencies	National Scientific Organizations
UNAIDS	Canadian Institutes of Health Research
United Nations Development Programme (UNDP)	Institute of Tropical Medicine, Antwerp, Belgium
United Nations Population Fund (UNFPA)	National Health and Medical Research Council, Australia
United Nations Children's Fund (UNICEF)	U.S. National Institutes of Health
World Health Organization (WHO)	

International Health Programs	Nongovernmental Organizations
Gavi, The Vaccine Alliance	BRAC
The Global Fund to Fight AIDS, TB, and Malaria	CARE
	Catholic Relief Services
	Doctors Without Borders (MSF)
	Oxfam
	Partners in Health
	Save the Children

(continues)

TABLE 17-1 Selected Organizational Actors in Global Health by Type of Organization *(continued)*

Multilateral Development Banks African Development Bank Asian Development Bank Inter-American Development Bank The World Bank	**Advocacy Organizations** Global Health Council The ONE Campaign RESULTS
Bilateral Development Agencies Danish International Development Agency (DANIDA) Department for International Development of the United Kingdom (DFID) Irish Aid Norwegian Agency for Development Cooperation (NORAD) U.S. Agency for International Development (USAID)	**Technical Organizations** International Union Against TB and Lung Disease KNCV—The Dutch Tuberculosis Foundation U.S. Centers for Disease Control and Prevention
Foundations The Aga Khan Foundation The Bill & Melinda Gates Foundation The Clinton Foundation The Rockefeller Foundation The Wellcome Trust	**Consulting Firms** Abt Associates FHI 360 JSI PSI
WHO-Related Partnerships Roll Back Malaria Stop TB Special Programme for Research and Training in Tropical Diseases (TDR)	**University-Affiliated Programs** Department of Global Health and Development, London School of Hygiene and Tropical Medicine Harvard Global Health Institute, Harvard University Institute for Health Metrics and Evaluation, University of Washington Institute for Global Health and Infectious Diseases, University of North Carolina
Public–Private Partnerships for Health/Product **Development Partnerships** Global Alliance for TB Drug Development International AIDS Vaccine Initiative Malaria Vaccine Initiative	**Think Tanks** Center for Global Development Results for Development Institute Center for Strategic and International Studies
Human Rights Organizations Amnesty International Human Rights Watch Physicians for Human Rights	

for example, participate in generating and sharing knowledge. They could engage in advocacy. They might be involved in the setting of technical standards or the provision of technical assistance. In addition, they might provide financing for health efforts. Generally, these organizations work along a continuum, engaging in one or more of the listed activities, but often specializing in only a few of them. When reviewing Table 17-1, readers should also be aware that some of the organizations could be placed into more than one category. The Center

for Global Development, for example, does important advocacy work, as well as research on global health policy and practice.

Because of the enormity of the topic, this chapter can be only introductory. It is meant to provide an overview of the main types of actors in global health. It is largely descriptive and outlines the stated aims of the organizations that it covers. This chapter does not look critically at these organizations. Students interested in a more critical view may consult the extensive literature that is available on each of these organizations.[10-12]

Agencies of the United Nations

A number of United Nations (UN) agencies work on health and focus on a specific set of public health concerns. Among the most important are WHO, the United Nations Children's Fund (UNICEF), the United Nations Population Fund (UNFPA), and the United Nations Development Programme (UNDP). This section examines the three UN agencies most involved in health: WHO, UNICEF, and UNAIDS.

World Health Organization

The World Health Organization was established in 1948 and is the United Nations agency responsible for health.[13] The headquarters of WHO is located in Geneva, Switzerland, and WHO employs about 7,000 people, including experts on many health topics. The World Health Organization has offices located in each region of the world, with special responsibility for work within that geographic area, as shown in **TABLE 17-2**. In addition, WHO has 150 field offices in different countries, regions, territories, and areas.[14]

The objective of WHO is to promote "the attainment by all peoples of the highest possible level of health."[13] In pursuit of this goal, WHO largely focuses its attention on the following:

- Advocacy and consensus building for various health causes, such as HIV/AIDS, TB, and non-communicable diseases.
- Generating and sharing health knowledge across countries through studies, reports, conferences, and other forums. The publication of the *World Health Report* on a different topic of global health importance each year is an example of this work.
- Carrying out selected critical public health functions within an international forum, such as the surveillance of epidemics, including influenza, or the outbreak of other potentially dangerous diseases, such as Ebola.
- Setting global standards on key health matters, such as appropriate regimens for drug therapy for leprosy, TB, and HIV/AIDS. This also includes, for example, WHO certification of quality standards for the manufacturing of vaccines and pharmaceuticals.
- Leading the development of international agreements and conventions, such as the Framework Convention on Tobacco Control and the International Health Regulations.
- The provision of technical assistance to its member states, such as helping China to contain the outbreak of SARS, or assistance to countries in managing their child vaccine programs.
- Playing a critical role in a number of cooperative efforts, such as Stop TB, Roll Back Malaria, and the Special Programme for Research and Training in Tropical Diseases Program.

WHO is primarily a technical agency that engages in advocacy and the generation and sharing of knowledge. It also plays critical roles in the setting of technical standards and norms. Although WHO does have relatively small country budgets to assist in the financing of selected health projects in low- and middle-income countries, it is not a financing agency.

WHO is governed through its annual World Health Assembly, which sets policy, reviews and approves the budget, and appoints the director-general of the organization. Voting power at the WHO Health Assembly is based on the principle of one country, one vote. The overall budget of WHO comes from membership assessments and from voluntary contributions. The latter are mostly from better-off countries, but the private sector and foundations also contribute to WHO.

Historically, WHO has helped lead some of the world's most important cooperative efforts in health, including the Health for All program[15] that began with the Declaration of Alma Ata on primary health care. WHO also led the world's smallpox eradication campaign, has played a major role in efforts to expand the coverage of immunization for children in low- and middle-income countries, and is one of the leaders of the world's global polio eradication initiative. More recently, WHO has been instrumental in helping to address issues of tobacco control and in helping to advance the agenda of universal health coverage.

TABLE 17-2 WHO Regional Offices

Regional Office	Location
The Americas	Washington, DC, USA
Europe	Copenhagen, Denmark
Eastern Mediterranean	Cairo, Egypt
Africa	Brazzaville, Congo
South-East Asia	Delhi, India
Western Pacific	Manila, Philippines

Data from World Health Organization. (n.d.). *About WHO: WHO people and offices*. Retrieved from http://www.who.int/about/structure/en/

WHO also leads the global surveillance of disease and has played an active role in work on avian flu, H1N1 influenza, and SARS, among other emerging and re-emerging diseases.

In its own words, the priority action areas for WHO are the following[16]:

- Health for all
- Health emergencies
- Women, children, and adolescents
- The health impacts of climate and environmental change

There is extensive literature on WHO for those who are interested in understanding it in greater detail.

UNICEF

The United Nations Children's Fund was established in 1946 by the United Nations to respond to the effects of World War II on children in Europe and China. UNICEF is headquartered in New York but has offices in 190 countries.[17] The main function of UNICEF is to enhance the health and well-being of children. In these efforts, UNICEF has been deeply involved in the promotion of family planning, antenatal care, safe motherhood practices, and responses to complex emergencies.

UNICEF has an executive board of 36 members who guide all UNICEF work and administration under the leadership of the executive director. All of UNICEF's funding is from voluntary contributions. Governments provide about 41 percent of funding, almost 30 percent comes from within the UN system, and another almost 13 percent comes from intergovernmental agencies. The remainder comes largely from 36 national committees, consisting of private entities and millions of individuals.[18] These national committees are nongovernmental organizations (NGOs) that advocate for children, sell UNICEF products, and raise funds through several well-known campaigns, such as Check Out for Children in grocery stores, Change for Good on airplanes, and Trick or Treat for UNICEF on Halloween.[19]

UNICEF is involved in a wide range of activities in support of its mission, including advocacy, knowledge generation and knowledge sharing, and the financing of investments in health. In addition, UNICEF works closely with other development partners such as WHO and the World Bank to help raise the health status of poor women and children globally. UNICEF has carried out significant programs in a number of areas. Traditionally, it has been involved in critical ways in nutrition and early childhood development issues, in which it has

generally been considered the world's leader. Immunization and child survival have also been areas of deep UNICEF involvement. In addition, UNICEF has been a major supporter of primary education, especially for poor girls in low- and middle-income countries. More recently, UNICEF has paid particular attention to child protection, child rights, and HIV/AIDS. UNICEF is also deeply involved in emergency relief work.[20]

UNICEF now has a number of focus areas[20]:

- Child protection and inclusion
- Child survival
- Education
- Children in complex emergencies
- Gender
- Innovation for children

The UNICEF operating budget for 2018 was about $2.4 billion.[18]

UNAIDS

In 1996, six agencies joined forces to launch UNAIDS—the Joint United Nations Program on HIV/AIDS. Today, as shown in **TABLE 17-3**, UNAIDS has 11 cosponsors.[21] UNAIDS spent $215 million on its activities in 2018.[22]

UNAIDS is based in Geneva, Switzerland, has offices in many countries in which it is involved, and is guided by a program-coordinating board that consists of 22 representatives from country governments, its cosponsors, and 5 NGOs. UNAIDS is the global agency with primary responsibility for dealing with HIV/AIDS. UNAIDS monitors and evaluates the epidemic and the world's response to it. It also advocates on key HIV/AIDS issues and engages civil society, the

TABLE 17-3 UNAIDS Cosponsors

- International Labor Organization
- Office of the United Nations High Commissioner for Refugees
- UNICEF
- United Nations Development Programme
- United Nations Educational, Scientific, and Cultural Organization
- United Nations Population Fund
- United Nations Office on Drugs and Crime
- UN Women
- World Bank
- World Food Program
- World Health Organization

Data from UNAIDS. (n.d.). *UNAIDS cosponsors*. Retrieved from http://www.unaids.org/en /aboutunaids/unaidscosponsors/

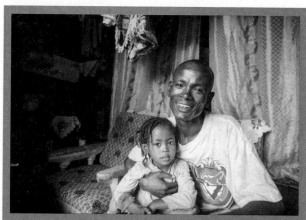

PHOTO 17-1 Although about 50 percent of people requiring treatment for HIV/AIDS still lack it, in the last 15 years many countries have made exceptional progress in providing antiretroviral therapy to those who are HIV-positive. Progress at the country level has been greatly enhanced by cooperative efforts, such as those on the part of WHO, UNAIDS, the Global Fund, and the U.S. PEPFAR program. This photo shows an HIV-positive man in Ethiopia and his child. When he found out he was positive, he initially hid and considered suicide. His life has been dramatically altered for the better through antiretroviral therapy. What additional efforts will it take to provide access to appropriate therapy for all who need it? Are there risks in the present political environment globally that the necessary funds for these efforts will not be available?

Photo courtesy of The Global Fund, photo by John Rae.

private sector, and development partners in the fight against HIV/AIDS. In addition, UNAIDS generates and shares knowledge, sets standards, and mobilizes resources. UNAIDS focuses its attention on the regions of the world most affected by HIV/AIDS, particularly sub-Saharan Africa.[23]

Another important emphasis of the work of UNAIDS is to assist countries in developing and implementing national AIDS plans. Technical experts from UNAIDS also help countries build their technical and institutional capacity and mobilize resources to fight against HIV/AIDS. UNAIDS, for example, assists countries in preparing applications for funding from the Global Fund to Fight AIDS, TB, and Malaria, which is discussed further later.[23]

UNAIDS is engaged in a range of HIV/AIDS activities. First, UNAIDS works with countries to strengthen their surveillance of the epidemic. Second, UNAIDS continues to put an important emphasis on prevention of HIV. Third, UNAIDS is also increasingly involved in efforts to increase the number of HIV-positive people worldwide who are treated with antiretroviral therapy. UNAIDS has a particular concern for the extent to which the epidemic affects females and with reducing TB/HIV co-infection.[24]

In addition, UNAIDS cooperates with others in the search for technologies, such as microbicides and vaccines, that might help halt the epidemic.

Multilateral Development Banks

There are a number of development banks that lend or grant money to low- and middle-income countries and economies in transition to help promote their economic and social development. These banks are owned by all of their member countries and are referred to as "multilateral." These institutions have some characteristics of real banks; however, these banks do not function to earn money through their lending operations. Rather, their main focus is to serve as a financial intermediary. Essentially, they channel financial resources from high-income countries, through bond sales and grants, to help finance development activities in low- and middle-income countries and countries that are making the transition to more open, market-based economies. All of these banks are involved in work on health, to some degree, but those most involved are the African Development Bank, the Asian Development Bank, the Inter-American Development Bank, and the World Bank.

Among the multilateral development banks, the World Bank is the largest, has the broadest scope of activities, and is the most involved in health.[25] The World Bank is located in Washington, DC, and is owned by 187 member countries. The World Bank has about 10,000 staff that work in Washington and in a large number of other country offices.[26,27]

The stated aim of the World Bank is to assist countries in improving the lives of their people and reducing poverty. It seeks to do this by helping them to strengthen the management of their economy and to finance investments in selected areas, including agriculture, transport, private sector development, health, and education. The World Bank lends money at reduced rates to countries with per capita incomes below a certain point, lends money interest free to the poorest countries, and also provides grants to some countries for certain issues that affect the poor, such as HIV/AIDS. The World Bank also has relatively generous time periods for repayment of these loans.

The World Bank supports a wide range of efforts in the health sector. It advocates on behalf of important causes, generates and disseminates information and knowledge about key health issues, provides technical assistance to countries, and finances specific investments in health and related work in nutrition and family planning. The World Bank focuses its health work largely on the links between health and poverty. It pays considerable attention to health financing, the development of health systems, and universal coverage. The World Bank has also emphasized investments in nutrition, maternal and child health, family planning, HIV/AIDS, malaria, and TB. More recently, it has supported global efforts in preventing and responding to pandemics.[28]

The World Bank is also a partner in a number of global health initiatives, including Gavi, The Vaccine Alliance; Stop TB; Roll Back Malaria; and UNAIDS. In addition, the World Bank has provided financing to other initiatives, such as the International AIDS Vaccine Initiative (IAVI). From 2013 to 2017, the World Bank lent almost $12 billion for health, nutrition, and population efforts. This was about 6 percent of total World Bank lending over that period.[29] Until the advent of the Bill & Melinda Gates Foundation and the Global Fund to Fight AIDS, TB, and Malaria, the World Bank was, for many years, the largest provider of development financing for health. Those interested in a more analytical and critical assessment of the World Bank's work both generally and in health can consult extensive literature on those subjects.

Bilateral Agencies

Another set of organizations that are very actively involved in global health includes bilateral agencies. These are mostly the development assistance agencies of high-income countries that work directly with low- and middle-income countries to help them enhance the health of their people. Some of the bilateral development agencies that are most involved in the health sector are shown in **TABLE 17-4**.

USAID is the development assistance agency of the U.S. federal government. USAID seeks to promote U.S. foreign policy goals by advancing economic and social development all over the world. USAID works with other governments and with universities, businesses, international agencies, and NGOs to support

its development assistance efforts. In the health field, USAID engages in a wide variety of activities, including advocacy for global health, the generation and sharing of knowledge, and the financing of health investments.

USAID is headquartered in Washington, DC, and has regional field offices for sub-Saharan Africa, Asia, Latin America and the Caribbean, Europe and Eurasia, the Middle East, and Afghanistan and Pakistan. In addition to these geographic bureaus, USAID has functional bureaus for, among other things, economic growth, education, and the environment; food security; global health; and democracy, conflict, and humanitarian assistance. USAID has offices in many countries, especially poorer countries in Africa, Asia, and Latin America.[30]

USAID's Bureau for Global Health aims to improve health services and enhance the health status of poor and disadvantaged people, particularly in poorer countries. USAID focuses its health work on building sustainable and resilient health systems; maternal and child health; communicable diseases and pandemic preparedness; family planning and reproductive health; and nutrition.[31] For these purposes, USAID provides grants and technical expertise to other governments, NGOs, and the private sector. In supporting the development of health in other countries, USAID collaborates with other development assistance agencies.[31]

In the 1970s and 1980s, USAID helped support research to develop a number of interventions that are key to saving the lives of poor children in low- and middle-income countries, including oral rehydration therapy, vitamin A supplementation, and immunizations. USAID has also been very supportive of efforts to address malaria, TB, HIV/AIDS, and, more recently, neglected tropical diseases. Traditionally, USAID has also been very involved in supporting family planning. Those interested can consult an extensive literature on the work and impact of USAID.

Foundations

Global health is an area in which foundations have been involved for almost a century. Many of the largest foundations support global health efforts, including, for example, the Ford, Hewlitt, MacArthur, Packard, and Soros Foundations. The Rockefeller Foundation has been among the foundations most involved in global health. The Wellcome Trust has also been engaged in global health activities, primarily through support for scientific research, for more than 70 years. More recently, the UN Foundation was established with a focus on health. The Clinton

TABLE 17-4 Selected Bilateral Development Assistance Agencies Involved in Global Health

Danish International Development Agency
Department for International Development of the United Kingdom
KFW (Germany)
Norwegian Agency for Development Cooperation
United States Agency for International Development

Foundation and the Bill & Melinda Gates Foundation have also become major actors in the global health arena. This section comments briefly on the health work of the Rockefeller and Gates Foundations and the Wellcome Trust.

The Rockefeller Foundation

The Rockefeller Foundation is based in New York City and has offices in Bangkok, Thailand, and Nairobi, Kenya. The foundation aims to "promote the wellbeing of humanity throughout the world."[32] To do so, it seeks to advance the development of more equitable and effective health systems. It also focuses on advancing a more nourishing and sustainable food system, promoting innovation in the use of clean energy, expanding job opportunities for U.S. workers, and creating more resilient cities.[33] In the health field, the foundation seeks to enhance attention to planetary health and the health risks of insults to planetary health.[34] It also aims to promote the development of more affordable, higher quality, and more equitable health systems.[35] The foundation also supports global disease surveillance efforts.[36]

The Rockefeller Foundation has focused considerable attention on the development of knowledge and technology that can be applied to addressing the conditions that most affect the health of the poor globally. The Rockefeller Foundation was instrumental in establishing the first schools of public health in the United States and was also deeply involved in the development of a vaccine against yellow fever. The Rockefeller Foundation does finance a small number of activities in health every year. However, its strength as an organization has been the way in which it uses a relatively small amount of money to invest in the generation of knowledge that can make an important difference to the health of the poor globally.

Over parts of the last 2 decades, the Rockefeller Foundation focused its attention on health in three areas. First, the foundation established the framework for developing partnerships between the public and private sectors to meet key health needs that had been neglected. In line with this work, the foundation was instrumental in establishing the first and then a number of additional public–private partnerships for health, including the International AIDS Vaccine Initiative, the International Partnership on Microbicides, and the Global Alliance for TB Drug Development. Second, it tried to help better understand the impact of HIV/AIDS on families and how they might deal with those impacts. Third, the foundation has helped to strengthen the production, deployment, and empowerment of key human resources needed

for delivering health services in poor countries. The foundation has also supported improvements in disease surveillance.[36]

The Wellcome Trust

The Wellcome Trust was founded in London in 1936 with the vision of improving human and animal health through research. Its philosophy is to "improve health for everyone by helping great ideas to thrive."[37] The Wellcome Trust is the second largest charitable foundation in the world, behind the Bill & Melinda Gates Foundation. The trust has an endowment of £25.9 billion, and in 2017–2018, its chartable grants were over £723 million.[38]

The trust has a number of focus areas. The first is to support biomedical research globally to help understand health and disease. The second is to improve health by supporting the development of new diagnostic tests, drugs, medical devices, and ways of changing people's health-related behaviors. The third is to engage the public to try to create more enlightened and broader public involvement in science and health. The last is to influence science and health policy.[39]

Although a majority of the independent researchers funded by the Wellcome Trust conduct their work in the United Kingdom, the foundation also funds programs in other countries.[40] Research is conducted at either independent institutions or institutes created by the foundation. The foundation is particularly well known for sequencing one-third of the human genome, which has significantly enhanced our understanding of the genes associated with disease. In addition, research funded by the Wellcome Trust has uncovered genetic links to cancer and diabetes, paving the way for future treatments.

The foundation supports activities in more than 100 countries. About 24 percent of current funding is for activities outside the United Kingdom. About 9 percent of current funding supports activities in low- and middle-income countries. The foundation focuses its international initiatives mainly in sub-Saharan Africa, South Asia, and central Europe.[41]

The Wellcome Trust has a strong track record in research for antimalarial drugs. In the early 1990s, scientists developed and tested the drug artemisinin in Vietnam and Thailand, which significantly decreased malaria mortality and the incidence of malaria. This drug is now the standard treatment for malaria, when used in combination with other antimalarial drugs.

In addition to funding biomedical research, the Wellcome Trust seeks to improve research facilities and broaden the base for scientific endeavors in low-income countries.[42] For example, the foundation invested £28 million from 2008 to 2009 in the African Institutions Initiative, which funds over 50 scientific institutions in 18 African countries.[43] In addition, the foundation invested £10 million in improving Kenya's and Malawi's research and health policymaking institutions in partnership with the United Kingdom Department for International Development and the International Development Research Centre, Canada.[44] In doing so, the goal of the Wellcome Trust has been to improve the capacity of low-income countries to do research and make informed health policy decisions.[44]

The Bill & Melinda Gates Foundation

One of the most substantial changes in the key actors involved in global health has been the advent of the Bill & Melinda Gates Foundation. The Gates Foundation is based in the United States in Seattle, Washington.

The foundation focuses on issues that can be addressed globally[45]:

- Its Global Health Division aims to reduce health inequities.
- The Global Development Division focuses on improving access to health services and the delivery of high-impact health products and services.
- The Global Growth & Opportunity Division seeks to create and disseminate market-based solutions to inclusive and sustainable economic growth.
- The U.S. Division works to improve secondary and post-secondary education in the United States and to support vulnerable families in Washington state.
- The Global Policy and Advocacy Division seeks to build partnerships that can promote policies that advance work in the focus areas of the foundation.

The foundation has a number of specific focus areas in global health. The first is to help more young people globally to "survive and thrive." The second is to "empower the poorest, especially women and girls." The third is to combat communicable diseases. The last is to "inspire people to take action to change the world."[46]

To enhance the health of women and children, the foundation supports efforts in nutrition that focus on proven approaches to young child nutrition, the nutrition of adolescent girls and women, and strengthening food systems. The foundation also provides major support in addressing communicable diseases. These efforts focus on increasing progress toward eradicating malaria, reducing HIV infections and increasing the health of those living with HIV/AIDS, improving

vaccine coverage, and eradicating polio. The foundation also places major emphasis on helping families get the information they need to make informed choices about family planning and to better access modern family planning methods.[46]

The foundation has paid particular attention to supporting the spread of known technologies for improving health, such as immunization, to the places where they are most needed. It has also focused on encouraging the development of new technologies that can meet the most important health needs of the poor globally. The foundation seeks to meet these aims by working with partners to deliver proven tools, including vaccines, drugs, and diagnostics. It also seeks to enable the discovery of affordable, reliable, and innovative solutions to key global health problems for those who need them most.[45] To advance these aims further, the foundation recently established the Bill & Melinda Gates Medical Research Institute.[47]

In addition to the substantial funding that the foundation has provided for scientific discovery, the foundation has been a supporter of an array of global health organizations, programs, and projects. The foundation has been a major supporter, for example, of public–private partnerships for health since their inception, and has funded, among others, IAVI, the Human Hookworm Vaccine Initiative, and the International Partnership on Microbicides. The foundation has provided considerable funding for reproductive health issues as well, such as a $60 million grant to Johns Hopkins University for improving reproductive health globally. The foundation has also supported major efforts in nutrition, with a focus on breast-feeding, micronutrients, and bio-fortification. The foundation was an early supporter of efforts to save newborn lives, partly through funding efforts by Save the Children. In addition, the Gates Foundation has been a major and continuous financier of Gavi and the Global Fund. The foundation has also financed a major program to address HIV/AIDS in India.[48]

At the end of 2017, the foundation had an endowment of almost $51 billion. It had provided $46 billion in grants since its inception. In 2017, the foundation gave grants worth $4.7 billion, and provided $1.7 billion for efforts under its global health division, which was spent in these key areas[49]:

- HIV/AIDS: 18%
- Malaria: 15%
- Diarrhea and enteric diseases: 12%
- Pneumonia: 10%
- Discovery and translational sciences: 8%
- Neglected tropical diseases: 7%

Other Key National Research Funders

There are a number of organizations whose primary function is to carry out and fund research, some of which focuses on issues in global health. Although it is a foundation, the Wellcome Trust fits into this category. Funding research is also central to the work of the Gates Foundation. The Howard Hughes Medical Research Institute in the United States and the Institut Pasteur in France are also foundations that are deeply involved in medical research. However, many of the organizations focused on conducting and funding research are supported by national governments. The largest of these is the U.S. National Institutes of Health (NIH). Others include the National Health and Medical Research Council of Australia, the Canadian Institutes of Health Research, the Chinese Academy of Medical Sciences, the South African Medical Council, and the Medical Research Council of the United Kingdom. Some comments follow on the work in global health of the U.S. National Institutes of Health.

The U.S. National Institutes of Health[50]

The National Institutes of Health, part of the U.S. Department of Health and Human Services, is the primary federal agency for conducting and supporting medical research to improve human health. NIH fulfills its mission by performing biomedical and behavioral research in its own laboratories, supporting research conducted by scientists at major academic and research institutions in the United States and around the world, supporting the training of research investigators, and fostering communication of medical and health sciences information.

Research in global health is an integral part of the NIH agenda and one of five priorities for the institutes. As part of these efforts, the Fogarty International Center at NIH seeks to do the following[51]:

- Build research capacity to meet present and evolving global health needs
- Stimulate innovation in technologies that can address global health problems
- Support research and research training in implementation science
- Strengthen research on prevention and control of communicable and noncommunicable diseases
- Build and strengthen partnerships to advance global health research

NIH-funded research, conducted both in the United States and in other countries, has yielded numerous discoveries with global health impact. For example, NIH has supported studies that have aided efforts to address HIV/AIDS. These have included research on the effectiveness of male circumcision in the prevention of HIV transmission, simplified HIV combination antiretroviral therapies, and the use of nevirapine for prevention of mother-to-child transmission. During the 2009 H1N1 pandemic, NIH scientists played a crucial role in understanding the epidemiology of the H1N1 virus, which led to recommendations that influenza vaccination be targeted at young-to-middle-aged adults. NIH-supported studies conducted in Tanzania and South Africa demonstrated that unless drug treatment for tuberculosis is properly administered, tuberculosis can evolve rapidly to become resistant to available drugs. Another NIH-funded study conducted in Nigeria identified three genes that contribute to high fatality rates and insensitivity to treatment of breast cancer in African women compared with Caucasian women. NIH has also assisted in the development of a new rotavirus vaccine that India has adopted.[52]

NIH has also provided substantial support to scientific institutions in low- and middle-income countries that have emerged as research hubs in their own region. For example, in 1983, NIH began funding GHESKIO, a Haitian nongovernmental organization dedicated to clinical service, research, and training in HIV/AIDS and related diseases. In leading Haiti's response to the HIV/AIDS epidemic, GHESKIO is making significant contributions to the understanding of clinical presentation, epidemiology, and transmission of AIDS in that country, as well as in implementation of evidence-based models of care.

Similarly, NIH has supported the International Centre for Diarrhoeal Disease Research, Bangladesh (ICDDR,B) for more than 4 decades. ICDDR,B is a pioneer nonprofit organization that conducts research and is credited with, among other things, developing oral rehydration therapy, which has been used to treat millions of young children with diarrheal disease. In addition, the center has trained more than 20,000 researchers over the past 20 years.

Through the NIH Visiting Program, more than 2,000 foreign scientists conduct research and receive research training every year at NIH.[53] The institutes also support training programs for scientists from low- and middle-income countries to conduct health research relevant to their countries, primarily through collaborative programs between research institutions in the United States and abroad.

Those wanting a more critical look at research funding for global health can consult the extensive literature on the conduct and financing of research to address the burden of disease in low- and middle-income countries. There is also a Global Forum for Health Research that pays particular attention to this matter.

Nongovernmental Organizations

There are thousands of NGOs in the world today that have as one of their primary aims the improvement of the health of poor people in low- and middle-income countries. Most of these organizations raise money from private sources or receive grants from governments or global health partnerships that they help to invest in activities that address important health issues, such as improving the availability of clean water, strengthening nutrition and immunization programs, or enhancing programs for the treatment of TB and HIV/AIDS. Some of the organizations are small and focus their attention on only a limited number of activities. Other organizations are very large, comprehensive in the topics they cover, and global in their reach. Some NGOs are completely secular, whereas others are faith based. Some of the most important NGOs that operate internationally on health are listed in **TABLE 17-5**.

Some additional comments are provided in the following sections on BRAC and Doctors Without Borders, two of the most important international

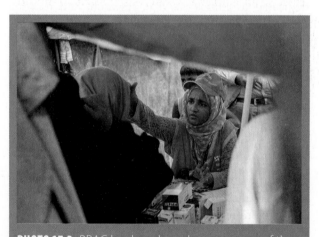

PHOTO 17-2 BRAC has long been known as one of the most effective, efficient, and self-critical NGOs in the world. It has played a major role in social development in Bangladesh and in the last decade has become involved in health and development work in other countries as well. BRAC is also deeply involved in helping Bangladesh address the Rohingya refugee crisis. This photo shows a BRAC community health worker providing services in one of the refugee camps. How much are NGOs involved in health in different settings? How effective are they, both in absolute terms and compared to government-provided services? What measures might be taken in these settings to enable them to maximize their health impact at least cost?

Photo courtesy of BRAC.

TABLE 17-5 Selected Nongovernmental Organizations Involved in Global Health
BRAC
CARE
Catholic Relief Services
Doctors Without Borders (MSF)
Partners in Health
Save the Children

NGOs that work on health globally. These are just a few examples of the many large NGOs that are involved in health efforts in low- and middle-income countries.

BRAC

BRAC was founded in Bangladesh in 1972. It is the largest NGO in the world involved in international development work, reaching 135 million people through its staff and volunteers. With the mission "to empower people and communities in situations of poverty, illiteracy, disease, and social injustice," BRAC is currently working in 10 countries in Asia and Africa, including Afghanistan, Bangladesh, Liberia, Myanmar, Nepal, the Philippines, Sierra Leone, South Sudan, Tanzania, and Uganda.[54,55]

BRAC was originally responsible for relief projects for refugees in rural northeastern Bangladesh but eventually turned its focus toward long-term development work. Its most established programs are in Bangladesh; however, the organization launched international initiatives in Asia in 2002 and in Africa in 2006.[55]

Broadly speaking, BRAC works in the areas of human rights and social empowerment, education and health, economic empowerment and enterprise development, livelihood training, climate change and environmental sustainability, food security, and disaster preparedness.[56] In all its initiatives, women and children are the priority. BRAC is especially well known internationally for its work in reducing infant and child mortality through the spread of oral rehydration therapy, as well as the effectiveness of its community-based approach in other health areas, such as family planning and nutrition.

The main goals of BRAC's health initiatives are to improve maternal, neonatal, and child health and decrease vulnerability to communicable and noncommunicable diseases, paying particular attention to nutrition and family planning. BRAC has also developed an eye care program. BRAC seeks to universalize access to a package of community-based basic health services that are affordable and of high quality.

In addition, BRAC is also deeply involved in addressing the social determinants of health through its work in economic empowerment, water, sanitation, and education.[57]

The core of BRAC's health programs in Bangladesh is a community-based approach to primary health care, called "Essential Health Care (EHC)." Trained healthcare workers, *shasthya shebika*, are the force behind BRAC's Essential Health Care program, which combines promotive, preventive, and basic curative services. These workers are locally recruited women who deliver door-to-door health services in rural areas. They provide health education for families and disseminate health and nutrition messages through health forums, household visits, and community meetings. In collaboration with the Bangladeshi government, BRAC's *shasthya shebika* work in the areas of immunization, family planning, and basic pregnancy-related care. These workers also provide basic curative care for childhood pneumonia. The *shasthya shebika* are volunteers who get trained by BRAC and earn an income from health work through the selling of drugs and basic health commodities to their patient population.

BRAC is also deeply involved in work on TB, malaria, and nutrition. BRAC heads a consortium of local NGOs that work with the government in promoting TB messages in the community, identifying suspected TB cases, referring patients for testing, and helping to ensure they complete their treatment. BRAC's TB work covers a population of almost 93 million people.[58] For malaria, BRAC's frontline workers provide health education, identification of cases, treatment of simple cases, and referral of complicated cases. They also promote the use of insecticide-treated bednets. BRAC's malaria efforts were associated with a 90 percent reduction in malaria deaths in Bangladesh between 2008 and 2013.[59]

BRAC has long been involved in and known for its work on nutrition, which aims at promoting early and exclusive breastfeeding, community-based treatment of acute and moderate malnutrition, the promotion of nutrition in adolescent girls, and nutrition counseling services for pregnant and lactating women. Much of this work is based on home visits by BRAC workers.[60] BRAC also makes and promotes the use of micronutrient powders to reduce anemia and other micronutrient deficiencies. These are sold to most families who can afford them and provided free to families who cannot.[60]

Given the evolving burden of disease, BRAC community health workers are increasingly involved in promoting healthy lifestyles, monitoring their patient population for hypertension and diabetes,

and referring those people with suspected problems. They also provide follow-up to patients who are under treatment.[61] BRAC's community-based health workers also now carry out vision screening, provision of eyeglasses where appropriate, and referral for those who need it.[62]

BRAC's business model is largely based on raising money from earnings in a variety of social enterprises to help cover the costs of its programs that do not earn revenue. The revenue-earning activities include its microfinance program, as well as its social enterprises, which create jobs for poor people in local communities and provide production or marketing support for the enterprises of its microfinance clients. BRAC's social enterprises sell handicrafts, dairy products, agricultural products, and printing supplies, among other goods. Some enterprises produce a commodity that will aid in improving the health of the community, such as iodized salt in Bangladesh.[63]

The scope of BRAC's health work in Bangladesh is enormous and impactful. In 2016, almost 4 million adolescent girls and women received nutritional counseling, about 14 million women and married adolescents received counseling on family planning, and 2.7 million women received maternity services. In addition, BRAC distributed 47 million micronutrient sachets to about 1 million children, aiming to reduce anemia by 33 percent. BRAC also performed almost 30,000 cataract surgeries and provided about 170,000 people with eyeglasses. BRAC achieved 95 percent cure rates in its TB program, and BRAC alone carried out about 65 percent of the TB and malaria screening for all of Bangladesh.[64] BRAC's total expenditures in 2016 were about $990 million.[65]

Doctors Without Borders

Doctors Without Borders is usually referred to by its French name, Médicins Sans Frontières, or by the abbreviation of that name, MSF. Doctors Without Borders was founded in 1971 and has an international office in Geneva, Switzerland. It is an umbrella organization made up of affiliated groups in 21 countries. The groups located in Belgium, France, Holland, Spain, and Switzerland carry out health work in more than 70 countries.[66]

Doctors Without Borders is best known for its work in humanitarian crises. It has often been involved in the provision of health services following natural disasters, such as earthquakes and hurricanes, or those humanitarian emergencies related to war and famine.[67] MSF, for example, assisted Nicaragua after an earthquake, Ethiopia during a famine, and Somalia after a war. MSF has also been extensively engaged in health services for refugees and displaced people. In addition, when health services have been severely weakened due to war or conflict, MSF often helps to provide health services temporarily, while trying to help rebuild health system capacity. One example of this was in Liberia after its civil war.

MSF is also involved in a range of nutrition and disease control efforts and efforts to increase access to essential medicines. MSF has also become very involved with prevention, care, and treatment for HIV/AIDS. In this work, MSF has helped to mobilize international support for antiretroviral therapy in poor countries and has become a leader in trying to lower the price of those drugs.[67] MSF was also deeply involved in the 2014–2015 Ebola outbreak in West Africa, where for some time it provided a very substantial share of assistance to the affected countries.[68]

MSF is well known for its commitment to political independence, medical ethics, and human rights. Related to this, MSF has increasingly sought to become a voice in international health policy arenas for the disenfranchised.

Advocacy Organizations

A number of organizations focus their efforts on advocating on behalf of global health issues. Generally, these organizations carry out research and policy studies and then use these and evidence generated by others to carry out advocacy activities for key stakeholders, including the public at large, funding agencies, and national legislatures and governments. Many of these organizations are membership organizations, in whole or in part. Some of these organizations may be aligned with a specific issue, such as the many organizations of this type that focus on HIV/AIDS. These include, for example, the International HIV/AIDS Alliance and the AIDS Vaccine Advocacy Coalition. Others may work on a cluster of issues, such as communicable diseases. Other advocacy organizations, however, address a broader range of global health topics. Examples of the better-known advocacy organizations that address a range of issues are ONE and RESULTS.

Think Tanks and Universities

A number of organizations focus at least part of their efforts on generating knowledge about key issues in global health. Among the best known of these is the Center for Global Development, based in Washington, DC. The center has a number of staff that are experts in various global health topics. The Center carries out an extensive research program on global health, publishes widely on global health matters, and hosts a wide array of seminars to disseminate the information that it has generated and to highlight important findings by others. The Results for Development Institute, also in Washington, DC, is another think tank that is actively involved in research on policy and program issues in global health. It carried out important work, for example, on the long-term financing of HIV/AIDS in a number of countries. It also focuses important attention on universal health coverage and on innovative approaches to addressing key global health issues. The Center for Strategic and International Studies, also in Washington, DC, has also become involved in a number of ways in global health policy matters, often related to the role of the United States in global health.

As interest in global health has spread and financing for global health has increased, many universities throughout the world have become more involved in teaching, research, and practice on global health issues. Many universities with a public health school, and even some without, have created centers or institutes that bring researchers together from different parts of the university to work on global health. Yale University, for example, has the Yale Institute for Global Health, under which it organizes many of its activities in global health. Harvard University has the Harvard Institute for Global Health, which is meant to play an important role in enabling Harvard's work on education and research in global health. The University of Toronto has the Centre for Global Health Research. Many universities also carry out considerable technical assistance for the design, monitoring, and evaluation of global health programs and projects; some universities have established what are essentially consulting firms to engage in this work.

Consulting Firms

A wide array of consulting firms engage in global health work, either as the main focus of their work or as an important part of their activities. Some of these firms are for-profit, such as Abt Associates. Others, however, operate on a not-for-profit basis, such as FHI 360, MSH, JSI, and PSI. Some of the firms may have a broad range of expertise and be able to work, for example, on key management, economic, financing, or policy issues, as well as on critical health programs, such as maternal and child health or the control of communicable diseases. Others, however, have a particular area of expertise, such as supply chain management, nutrition, behavior change communication, or social marketing. Low- and middle-income countries some-times hire these firms directly; however, an important part of such services provided to low-income countries will be financed by development assistance agencies such as the World Bank, USAID, or DFID. In fact, a substantial share of the development assistance from some agencies, such as USAID, is channeled through consulting firms. The staff of a consulting firm are often quite involved in policy work and in program design, monitoring, and evaluation.

Specialized Technical Organizations

A number of specialized governmental and nongovernmental technical organizations are important actors in global health. Perhaps the best known of these is the U.S. Centers for Disease Control and Prevention (CDC), based in Atlanta, Georgia. The CDC is part of the U.S. Department of Health and Human Services. The CDC describes its mission as follows:

> CDC works 24/7 to protect America from health, safety and security threats, both foreign and in the U.S. Whether diseases start at home or abroad, are chronic or acute, curable or preventable, human error or deliberate attack, CDC fights disease and supports communities and citizens to do the same.[69]

The CDC is deeply involved in helping the United States and other countries to plan and carry out disease prevention, surveillance, and control across a broad range of disease conditions. CDC staff, for example, collaborate with many countries in work on communicable disease control programs, such as those for HIV/AIDS, TB, and malaria. In addition, CDC staff are often called upon to assist WHO and individual countries to identify disease threats and address them. This could be for outbreaks of dengue, the Ebola virus, the plague, or other diseases of national and international importance. The CDC has a team of field epidemiologists that are at the forefront of such work, and it also provides extensive laboratory services to its collaborators. The CDC has also been very involved in technical assistance to build capacity in low- and middle-income countries for improved disease surveillance, prevention, and control, including the strengthening of laboratories.

Two other specialized technical organizations of importance are nongovernmental and work on TB. KNCV is the Dutch TB foundation and is based in The Hague, the seat of government of the Netherlands.[70] KNCV aims to help address TB both in the Netherlands and in low- and middle-income countries by providing technical assistance in the development and implementation of TB control programs. The International Union Against Tuberculosis and Lung Disease (IUATLD), which is based in Paris, France, is a membership organization that is also deeply involved in TB control efforts.[71] The union has a number of regional offices and works not only on TB but also on lung health more broadly. Both KNCV and the union have staff with high levels of expertise in all aspects of TB control. Both have been deeply involved in helping many countries to address TB more effectively and efficiently and to build national capacity for addressing TB in the future.

Partnerships Related to WHO

Some global health problems affect a large number of people in a substantial number of countries. The costs of addressing these problems are great, and the skills needed to combat them are significant. Many resource-poor countries cannot tackle these problems without assistance, and no individual development partner can provide enough assistance to help deal effectively with the scale of these problems. Therefore, a number of organizations have decided to work together to help address some of the most important burdens of disease. Some of the partnerships that have ensued are closely related to WHO, as noted in **TABLE 17-6**. Two of the most important such partnerships are Stop TB and Roll Back Malaria.

Stop TB

The Global Partnership to Stop TB was established in 2001 and has the following aims:

- Ensure that every TB patient has access to effective diagnosis, treatment, and cure
- Stop transmission of TB
- Reduce the inequitable social and economic toll of TB
- Develop and implement new preventive, diagnostic, and therapeutic tools and strategies to stop TB

Stop TB works with 1,500 partners in 100 countries. It carries out its work through seven working

TABLE 17-6 Selected WHO-Related Partnerships for Global Health

Global Polio Eradication Initiative
Lymphatic Filariasis Control Program
Roll Back Malaria
Stop TB
Tropical Disease Research Program

groups that focus on TB diagnosis and treatment; research and development for new TB diagnostics, drugs, and vaccines; and addressing drug-resistant TB and HIV-associated TB.[72] Stop TB is essentially an advocacy agency, an organization that enables better global efforts on TB through the exchange of ideas across partners and by enhancing the environment for TB work globally and locally.

The partnership also leads a number of initiatives related to TB, in addition to substantial advocacy on TB. One effort is a grant program to encourage civil society involvement in TB. Stop TB also oversees the Global Drug Facility, which assists countries in procuring high-quality TB medicines at the best possible prices.[73]

RBM Partnership to End Malaria

The RBM Partnership to End Malaria was founded as the "Roll Back Malaria" partnership in 1998 by WHO, UNDP, UNICEF, and the World Bank to advocate for malaria control, to promote the development of better and more coordinated approaches and technologies for malaria containment, and to help finance and spread appropriate malaria control and treatment.[74] The partnership has expanded since then to include over 500 public and private actors in a number of countries, who are organized into 8 constituencies. The partnership is housed at WHO in Geneva, Switzerland. Roll Back Malaria's vision is "a world free from the burden of malaria."[75] Its mission "is to support malaria-affected countries and galvanize global action across all sectors to end malaria for good."[75] The Partnership to End Malaria also carries out part of its efforts through working groups on case management, malaria in pregnancy, monitoring and evaluation, multisectoral action, social change, and vector control.[76]

Other Partnerships and Special Programs

In the mid- and late 1990s, a number of global health actors expressed concern about gaps in addressing health issues that affected the poor in low- and middle-income countries. One was the need to strengthen immunization programs for children and for pregnant women. The second was the need to make more rapid progress against HIV/AIDS, TB, and malaria. To address immunization more effectively, the Global Alliance for Vaccines and Immunisation (GAVI), now called Gavi, The Vaccine Alliance, was established. The Global Fund to Fight AIDS, TB, and Malaria, referred to as the Global Fund, was established to make more rapid progress against HIV, TB, and malaria.

Gavi

Gavi is a partnership among public and private sector organizations that was established in 2000.[4] The founding partners of Gavi included WHO, UNICEF, and the World Bank. Gavi is based in Geneva, Switzerland. The Bill & Melinda Gates Foundation created a major grant to help establish Gavi and provide for its operations. Gavi is financed today by grants from governments, private sector organizations, and foundations. Some of its work is also financed by "innovative financing mechanisms" such as the International Financing Facility for Immunization.[77]

Gavi seeks to help low- and middle-income countries "accelerate equitable uptake and coverage of vaccines"; improve the effectiveness and efficiency of vaccine programs within strengthened health systems; "enhance the sustainability of national vaccine programs"; and "shape markets for vaccines and other immunization products."[78]

Gavi has tried to improve global health work through two innovative approaches. The first is to tie its financing to the achievement of goals that are agreed to by the countries with which Gavi is working. The second is to work closely with countries to develop plans to sustain the investments that are being supported. Gavi is an organization that advocates for the importance of immunization, provides technical

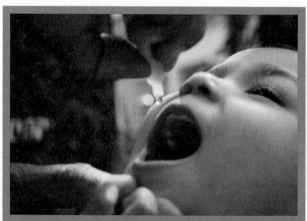

PHOTO 17-3 The creation of Gavi, The Vaccine Alliance, has spurred substantial increases in access to childhood vaccines and a related decline in morbidity and mortality from those diseases. This photo shows a young child getting polio vaccine. This is part of not only a national effort but also a global effort to eradicate polio. What were the forces that led to the creation of Gavi, The Vaccine Alliance? What have been the keys to Gavi's impact? What lessons does Gavi suggest for other areas of cooperation in global health?
© Ramesh Lalwani/Moment/Getty Images.

assistance to countries to enhance their immunization efforts, and finances those efforts. Gavi also works internationally to try to ensure that vaccine markets are developing in a way that can get high-quality vaccines in the numbers needed at affordable prices to low- and middle-income countries.

By 2017, Gavi had supported the immunization of almost 700 million children, averting, according to Gavi's estimates, more than 10 million deaths. Between 2016 and 2020, Gavi aims to support the vaccination of an additional 300 million children, which is projected to avert an additional 5–6 million deaths.[78]

The Global Fund

The Global Fund to Fight AIDS, TB, and Malaria was established in 2002 and is based in Geneva, Switzerland.[79] The driving force behind the establishment of the fund was increasing global concern about HIV/AIDS and an increasing recognition among development partners that measures to address the HIV/AIDS epidemic had been insufficient. Interest in establishing the Global Fund was also heightened by the growing attention to global health more generally and a special concern for the burden of HIV/AIDS, TB, and malaria in Africa.[80]

The Global Fund is a partnership of the public and private sectors; WHO, UNAIDS, and the World Bank are also key partners. The Global Fund is governed by a board of directors that represents governments, international organizations, civil society, and communities affected by HIV/AIDS, TB, and malaria. The fund is financed by grants that come largely from high-income country governments but also from the private, foundation, and philanthropy sectors, including the Bill & Melinda Gates Foundation.

The Global Fund is primarily a financing agency, but it also engages in advocacy and policy work for global health and the three diseases on which it focuses. The main aim of the fund is to finance proposed investments in these diseases, with an emphasis on HIV/AIDS and Africa. It has had a particular interest in helping to scale up programs for antiretroviral therapy against HIV/AIDS. The fund has taken innovative approaches to a number of aspects of development assistance for health, including the following[79]:

- It is strictly a financing mechanism and not a technical or implementing agency.
- It seeks to raise funds for investments that will be supplemental to other funding already available.

- It tries to work on the basis of a national plan that is developed by a group representing diverse national interests.
- It evaluates proposals through an independent review process.
- It tries to operate in a performance-based manner by supporting investments that are meeting their targets and reducing or eliminating support for programs that are not meeting their aims.

The Global Fund also assists countries in enhancing the effectiveness and efficiency of their procurement of equipment, materials, supplies, and drugs related to their programs for HIV/AIDS, TB, and malaria. This work focuses on helping countries to improve the planning of procurement, sharing information on prices, maintaining quality assurance standards, and helping them engage in lower-cost purchasing through a pooled procurement mechanism.[81]

The Global Fund raises and invests each year about $4 billion in projects in about 100 countries. The Global Fund has disbursed more than $38 billion since its founding.[82]

Public–Private Partnerships

As interest in global health rose in the mid-1990s, many of the actors in this field increasingly believed that the mechanisms for developing, manufacturing, and distributing new vaccines, drugs, diagnostics, and medical devices needed to alleviate key global health problems were not sufficient. They noted with growing concern, for example, that the vaccine for TB was more than 75 years old and that no new TB drugs had been developed for decades. They saw insufficient attention to the development of vaccines against HIV and malaria in both the public and the private sectors, with fewer firms willing to engage in vaccine development. They also understood that private pharmaceutical firms did not see a profitable market in the development of low-cost diagnostics, vaccines, drugs, or medical devices that could address the major killers of the poor globally. They knew that without changes in the way the market for these products worked that private sector firms would remain on the sidelines.

In the face of these issues, the Rockefeller Foundation encouraged key global health actors to think creatively about how they could spur the more rapid development of products that could attack global health problems in a low-cost but effective way. One idea that emerged from this was the notion of

TABLE 17-7 Selected Public–Private Partnerships for Public Health

TB Alliance
International AIDS Vaccine Initiative
International Partnership for Microbicides
Malaria Vaccine Initiative
Medicines for Malaria Venture

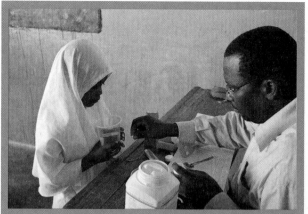

PHOTO 17-4 This photo shows a young girl being given preventive therapy against schistosomiasis in Zanzibar. A range of public and private actors have come together to try to reduce the burden of neglected tropical diseases (NTDs). This cooperation began with drug donations for the program against onchocerciasis and has continued to grow since then. Important progress against a number of NTDs can be attributed to the cooperation of these actors. Are there lessons from cooperation on NTDs that can be applied to other areas of global health work?
Courtesy of The Schistosomiasis Control Initiative, Imperial College London.

organizations that would combine the strengths of public and private organizations in a common quest for better health. They would also seek broader sources of financing for these health ventures; try to tackle intellectual property issues that constrained the availability of affordable diagnostics, drugs, medical devices, and vaccines in poor countries; and see how they could encourage more private sector involvement in the search for these products. In some respects, they were conceived of as venture capital firms that would have a social goal rather than a goal that was mostly aimed at maximizing profit. Today, there is a wide array of public–private partnerships for health. The aim of many of these is to develop new products, and these are often called product development partnerships. Some of the most important of such partnerships are noted in **TABLE 17-7**. Additional information is provided about the TB Alliance in the case studies section of this chapter.

Pharmaceutical Firms

International pharmaceutical firms have been engaged for several decades in partnerships to try to improve global health at low cost. This has generally been done in one of three ways. First, some firms donate drugs to global health programs. Novartis, for example, donates leprosy drugs to the Global Alliance to Eliminate Leprosy, and today no country needs to purchase such drugs.[83] Pfizer donates an antibiotic, azithromycin, to the efforts of the International Trachoma Initiative to reduce trachoma-related blindness.[84] Merck donates ivermectin to the Onchocerciasis Control Program, which has been successful in reducing river blindness in Africa.[85] These are only some of the many donation efforts now under way.

In addition, a number of drug companies have agreed to sell antiretroviral drugs for HIV/AIDS at greatly discounted prices to low- and middle-income countries affected by the HIV/AIDS epidemic. Some of the drug companies also sponsor programs to address diseases such as HIV/AIDS in particular countries, such as Merck's support for the national

HIV/AIDS control program in Botswana.[86] In addition, companies, such as Novartis, are beginning to sell medicines to fight noncommunicable diseases at substantial discounts in selected low- and middle-income countries.[87]

The role of the major drug companies in global health is a subject of considerable controversy. There is a concern among some members of the global health community, for example, that the patenting of drugs by branded drug manufacturers raises the price of drugs beyond what people in low- and middle-income countries can afford. Some people also believe that the major manufacturers should be far more generous than they have been in offering their drugs at reduced prices in low- and middle-income countries. Others have expressed concern that these manufacturers have not been open enough in licensing their products to other companies in a way that would reduce their prices in low- and middle-income countries. The role of pharmaceutical firms in global health is very important, complicated, and controversial and goes considerably beyond the scope of this text.

▶ Trends in Global Health Efforts

The notion of cooperating to improve health globally is not a new one. Rather, different countries have realized for more than 100 years that many health problems could not be solved by individual countries and had to be addressed through collective action across countries.

In the ensuing period, in fact, many actors have cooperated in a variety of health activities. This section examines how the themes of those efforts have varied over time. The threat of cholera, for example, led to the first international conference on health in 1851.[11] Numerous international conferences on health followed, and by 1903, the International Commission on Epidemics was created.[11] In 1909, the International Office of Public Hygiene was set up in Paris, followed by the establishment of the League of Nations Health Office in 1920 in Geneva, Switzerland. The International Sanitary Bureau was set up in 1924. The Rockefeller Foundation assisted in financing and providing technical support to the League of Nations Health Office. The early international organizations for health focused their efforts on the surveillance of disease, the provision of global standards for drugs and vaccines, and selected technical advice to countries on key health matters, including medical education.[11]

International efforts in health took a substantial leap forward with the establishment of the United Nations agencies after World War II, including WHO and UNICEF. In the more than 60 years since there have been a number of areas of focus for international cooperation on health, as noted hereafter.[5,11,88] Following the establishment of WHO, efforts at international cooperation in health shifted to focus on helping to build capacity for global public health efforts, for health systems development in countries that were newly independent, and in working together to fight disease. Perhaps the greatest single effort at global cooperation in health began in 1966 with the start of the global program to eradicate smallpox. During this period of intensive attention to specific diseases, WHO also led work to combat malaria and other communicable diseases of special importance for the poor, such as leprosy,[89] lymphatic filariasis,[90] and onchocerciasis.[88,91]

Historically, another important area of focus for global cooperation has been family planning. Much of the early work on family planning was led by the United States. Over time, the focus on family planning shifted from one that was centered almost exclusively on limiting family size to an approach that centered much more on reproductive health. This shift was encouraged by and reflected in a series of global conferences on family planning, safe motherhood, reproductive health, and women starting in 1974 in Bucharest, Romania.[92] The 1987 conference on women in Nairobi, Kenya, for example, was used to launch the Safe Motherhood Initiative.[88]

In 1978, the world launched a major effort when it produced the Alma Ata declaration on primary health care, as mentioned earlier. This declaration noted that health was a fundamental human right and that countries had the obligation to ensure that all people had access to appropriate primary health care. The Alma Ata declaration heralded a new global focus on primary health care and on the health needs of the poor. It also led to much greater attention to the needs for health systems that could deliver primary care and to the importance of taking a community-based approach to the health needs of poor people. The Alma Ata Declaration was linked to the world's efforts to achieve what was called globally "Health for all by the Year 2000."[93]

An immense amount of attention has also been paid to child survival. Early efforts were focused on what were called the GOBI interventions: growth monitoring, oral rehydration, breastfeeding, and immunization. UNICEF was the leader of this effort. USAID has also been instrumentally involved in child survival activities, which ultimately became an important focus for the World Bank, WHO, and a variety of bilateral organizations.[5]

As the world moved into the late 1980s and early 1990s, considerable concern arose that despite more than 30 years of global efforts to improve the health of the poor, the unfinished agenda remained very large. Many of those working on health believed that some of the weaknesses stemmed from an approach to health that was too disjointed and that needed to be better grounded in a more systemic view of health that would focus on trying to improve health services more broadly. This led to considerable work being done on health sector reform. At the same time, the 1993 *World Development Report* of the World Bank articulated the need to take an approach to decision making on health investments that would be grounded in cost-effectiveness analysis.[94] This framework for analysis soon became the foundation for actions of a number of key actors in global health.

At about the same time, much greater attention began to be paid, even in low-income countries, to the role of the private sector in health. Development partners also created new ways of working together cooperatively within individual countries. Increasingly, for example, development partners would cooperate and jointly help countries to develop and finance investments in health. In much of the work done prior to this period, many development partners worked individually with a country, often leading to a lack of coordination across that country's health sector efforts.

Toward the mid-1990s, the global health community began to pay considerably more attention to HIV/AIDS, as well as to other major killers of the poor in resource-poor countries, including malaria and TB. Particular attention has been paid since then to reducing the cost of AIDS drugs and getting more people treated, raising case finding and cure rates for TB, and strengthening malaria control programs through the use of insecticide-treated bednets, intermittent treatment of pregnant women, more rapid and confirmed diagnosis, and greater use of artemisinin-based combination therapy. More recently, attention has also been given to intermittent treatment of infants and seasonal mass chemoprevention in selected areas. There has also been an enormous increase in cooperation through the many health partnerships that have been formed, as noted earlier in the chapter.

In addition, there has been a renewed emphasis on some of the topics noted previously, greater interest in others, and considerable attention paid to how countries and their partners work together to enhance health. Driven partly by the Millennium and Sustainable Development Goals, greater attention is now being paid, for example, to nutrition and maternal health. Considerable effort is being expended to complete polio eradication, which has proven to be more difficult than planned, and attention to measles, and the possibility of its eradication has also grown. Much greater attention is being paid than previously to the neglected tropical diseases and how they can be addressed in more coherent ways. There is growing concern about drug-resistant TB and the need to ensure that tools exist to diagnose it more rapidly and treat it more effectively. In fact, there is also much greater focus than ever on the development of new diagnostics, drugs, and vaccines that can address the most important burdens of disease of poor people in resource-poor countries. At the same time, substantial efforts are being directed to helping countries to develop more effective and efficient health systems that can provide universal coverage of key health services in more effective and efficient ways and afford more financial protection to their people from the costs of health care. In many respects, in fact, the "quest for universal health coverage" has become the organizing principle for all work in global health.

Much attention is also being paid to how development partners and countries can work together to achieve these aims, particularly in low-income countries. Increasing focus has been placed on ensuring that development assistance for health is harmonized and aligned with development partners working together on a common platform in each country and ensuring that the processes they use follow the processes of the countries with which they are working. There is also an emphasis on how countries can more effectively and efficiently achieve, measure, and report transparently on the intended results from their investments in health, through mechanisms such as results-based financing. Important attention is also being paid to how the investments needed to improve health in low- and middle-income countries, particularly among the poor, can be financed, especially in times of global economic distress. One of these initiatives for addressing this issue, UNITAID, is discussed further in the case studies section of this chapter.

▶ Setting the Global Health Agenda

As we think about how different actors cooperate in global health activities and the themes on which they focus, it is important to consider how global health policies get established. This section comments briefly on how the overall global health agenda and the agenda for particular global health topics are set. This is another topic that is quite complicated and often the subject of controversy that readers may wish to explore further.

One important activity in setting global health priorities is the World Health Assembly of the World Health Organization.[95] Once each year, ministers of health of WHO member countries meet in Geneva, Switzerland, to consider important global health matters and resolutions proclaiming their interest in and commitment to addressing key health issues. The World Health Assembly has been the foundation for some of the most important global health efforts undertaken, such as the smallpox eradication campaign.

Some important developments in global health have been encouraged by writings, advocacy efforts, and program activities of WHO, multilateral or bilateral development assistance agencies, and some of the important NGOs involved in health. The *1993 World Development Report* of the World Bank focused on health and was widely read and debated around the world. This document set the basis for the next generation of World Bank–assisted health projects in many countries and for important work done by other development organizations and countries in health, as well. Given the importance of World Bank assistance for health to so many countries, the approaches suggested in the *1993 World Development Report* had a major impact on the world's thinking about and acting on health in low- and middle-income countries.

Movement in the policy agenda for global health can also follow significant investments by development partners. This has clearly been the case, for example, as a result of the substantial funds that the Bill & Melinda Gates Foundation has provided to selected global health activities. As noted earlier, the Gates Foundation has focused considerable attention on improving and disseminating technology for improving the health of the poor, as well as selected investments in key health problems, such as HIV/AIDS. The investments the Gates Foundation has made, for example, in immunization and malaria have considerably raised the world's attention to these matters and placed them more firmly on the global health agenda.

Popular action, often led by NGOs or other advocates for health, can also influence the setting of the global health agenda. In the late 1990s, for example, Professor Jeff Sachs, then of Harvard University, began to be actively involved in speaking and writing about the importance of health to economic and social development. His work attracted attention to health issues and led to considerable international engagement and action on the health of poor people globally. At around the same time, some important NGOs, such as Doctors Without Borders, became major advocates for AIDS treatment and the reduction of the prices of AIDS drugs. Their advocacy work and efforts to treat people with antiretroviral drugs, and the efforts of people within the affected countries, attracted considerable attention to these topics and had a major impact on the way the world approached them.

Another good example of how an NGO affected the global health agenda is the impact of Partners in Health, an NGO based in Boston, Massachusetts, in the United States, on the global agenda for TB and for HIV/AIDS. Largely led by the work of Dr. Paul Farmer and Dr. Jim Kim of Harvard University, Partners in Health tried to develop in Peru and Haiti a model of how one could treat drug-resistant TB and then HIV/AIDS at an acceptable cost and in a sustainable way. At the time, the prevailing opinion globally was that drugs for these conditions were so expensive that they could not be used in resource-poor settings. The work of Partners in Health helped to shift global efforts toward finding ways to make treatment affordable for all people.[96]

In other respects, one can think of efforts to set the global health agenda as a kind of ongoing meeting around a negotiating table at which important actors in global health are sitting. The organizations most involved in such discussions will generally be WHO, UNICEF, and the World Bank. Selected bilateral development agencies will also participate, such as USAID, the Department for International Development of the United Kingdom, and the Norwegian Development Agency. Australia plays a unique role in parts of Asia in the Pacific. The Global Fund has been increasingly involved in policy discussions as its portfolio has grown, as has UNAIDS as HIV/AIDS has become more important. The Gates Foundation, the Rockefeller Foundation, and selected NGOs might also participate in setting the agenda. Some other NGOs, such as MSF, may not be present, but through advocacy they do bring their interests to the policy-setting group.

The way in which the agenda is set for specific health topics will be similar to the manner described here but will usually also include actors who have particular interests in the topic at hand. WHO and the World Bank will almost always be involved. The key bilateral agencies will also participate. In addition, the agencies working with the topic under discussion and groups representing people affected by particular conditions increasingly have inputs into these discussions. Today, in fact, it would be rare if these stakeholders were not at the policy-making table. If TB is being discussed, for example, then the key NGOs working globally with TB will be involved, as will the TB programs from representative countries. If leprosy is being discussed, then the leprosy programs of some countries, NGOs working in leprosy, and groups of people affected by leprosy are all likely to be involved.

▶ Case Studies

This section contains three case studies that explore some of the concepts discussed in this chapter. The first describes a public–private partnership for developing new TB drugs, the TB Alliance. The second is about the innovative financing mechanism UNITAID. The last is a historical examination of the Onchocerciasis Control Program, one of the early efforts at cooperation to successfully attack a health problem of enormous impact in parts of Africa.

The TB Alliance

The TB Alliance was created in 2000 as the Global Alliance for TB Drug Development, with the mission to accelerate the discovery, development, and delivery of faster-acting and affordable drugs to fight tuberculosis. Its main office is located in New York City, but research is conducted in public and private laboratories around the world.[97]

The TB Alliance is a not-for-profit product development partnership among governments, nongovernmental organizations, professional organizations, academia, foundations, and pharmaceutical and biotechnology companies that have pledged to work together to accomplish this mission. The TB Alliance comprises the largest effort in history for TB drug development, and the partnership has led to the largest portfolio of TB drug candidates to date.[98] The TB Alliance is funded by governments, government-supported research bodies, and the Bill & Melinda Gates Foundation.[99]

The TB Alliance aims to enable the development of a universal regimen for all forms of TB that will be short, simple, and accessible. In doing so, the partnership hopes to increase cure rates overall by improving patient adherence to treatment and lowering toxic side effects. The long-run vision of the alliance is to "have a transformative impact on the disease by introducing an ultra-short, simple, and affordable TB regimen that works in virtually all people with tuberculosis. This requires a multi-drug regimen comprised entirely of new drugs. Such a regimen would unify the treatment of all current forms of TB under one cure."[100] Currently, the alliance is involved with phase 1 trials of two regimens, phase 3 trials of three regimens, and phase 4 trials on the pediatric regimen the TB Alliance was involved in developing.[98]

A main concern of the TB Alliance is that treatment for TB, once developed, must be widely available and affordable, especially in low-income countries. To accomplish this goal, the partnership works toward patent and marketing arrangements that will allow any new TB drugs to be sold at affordable prices in low-income countries. It is also working with drug regulatory authorities to ensure that future drugs will get early approval in the countries in which they are to be sold.[98] In addition, the TB Alliance is collaborating with others to ensure that any future TB drugs can be manufactured at the lowest possible cost.[101]

Innovative Financing Mechanisms for Global Health: UNITAID

Over the last three decades, there has been significant growth in international development assistance for health. Nonetheless, there remains a substantial gap between the available financing and the estimated financial needs for meeting the Sustainable Development Goals (SDGs).

Besides being insufficient in amount, conventional development financing for health has a number of shortcomings. First, most countries can allocate such assistance only on a year-to-year basis, which makes it difficult for recipient countries to plan how to use the assistance in the soundest way. Second, this type of assistance may not provide the incentives needed to achieve desired outcomes in the most effective and efficient manner. This relates to the fact that development assistance for health has typically financed health inputs, such as drugs, medical equipment, clinics, training, and technical advice, rather than finance outputs and measurable results on the ground, such as vaccine coverage for childhood diseases or reduction in malaria morbidity and mortality from the use of bednets. There has also been a concern that getting financial assistance from multiple sources can lead to wasteful spending and inefficient duplication of systems for procurement, financial management, and reporting.[102]

In this light, discussion began in 2004 to develop innovative financing mechanisms for development assistance in health that could increase the amount of funding available and be more predictable and stable than traditional development assistance for health. Such discussions have centered on financial mechanisms that include levies on currency transactions, a voluntary rebate by businesses on their value-added taxes for the use of international development, and other kinds of voluntary consumer contributions. One such effort that has been put into place is UNITAID.[102]

In 2006, Brazil, Chile, France, Norway, and the United Kingdom collaborated to develop an international drug purchase facility, called UNITAID. Officially launched in September 2006, UNITAID was established to scale up access to HIV/AIDS, TB, and malaria treatment for people in low-income countries. UNITAID now has the support of its founders plus Mauritius, Madagascar, South Korea, and the Bill & Melinda Gates Foundation. UNITAID is housed at WHO.[103]

UNITAID is largely financed by a new source of funding: a tax on the purchase of airline tickets in nine countries. Since its inception, UNITAID has raised almost $3 billion to support its efforts.

The overarching goal of UNITAID is to enable better access to health products that can enhance global health in equitable ways. Its aim is to support the development of "innovative medicines, diagnostic tools and public health techniques and link them quickly, and at affordable prices, to those most in need."[104] UNITAID's strategic objectives are to achieve the above by doing the following[104]:

- Promoting innovation by connecting innovators and the people who can most benefit from their products
- Overcoming barriers to and enhancing access to health products where they are most needed
- Helping countries to scale up the adoption and use of the interventions they support

UNITAID focuses its support on four areas[105]:

- HIV, including diagnosis, prevention, treatment and co-infection
- Malaria, including diagnosis, prevention, treatment, and vector control
- TB, including diagnosis, prevention, treatment, and drug resistance
- Market issues, including market analysis and quality assurance

UNITAID calls for proposals, and an independent review committee assesses the proposals to select those that UNITAID believes are worthy of support. The criteria for such support include the potential for having a global impact, being innovative and scalable, targeting low- and middle-income countries, being led by a group with a proven track record, and having a "lean" budget.[106] A small number of examples of UNITAID support would include the development and launching in partnership with the TB Alliance and others of TB drugs specifically adapted for children, the creation of the Medicines Patent Pool to promote voluntary licensing of HIV drugs, and efforts with Stop TB and WHO to launch Xpert, a new diagnostic for TB.[107]

Onchocerciasis

The case study that follows deals with the effort to eliminate onchocerciasis in Africa, which has seen some important successes. More detailed information on this case is available in *Case Studies in Global Health: Millions Saved.*[108]

Background

Onchocerciasis, or river blindness, is a pernicious disease afflicting approximately 26 million people worldwide. More than 99 percent of its victims are in sub-Saharan Africa.[109] Historically, in the most endemic areas, over one-third of the adult population was blind, and infection often approached 90 percent.[110] In 11 West African countries in 1974, nearly 2.5 million of the area's 30 million inhabitants

were infected with onchocerciasis, and approximately 100,000 were blind. The remaining 19 endemic countries in Central and East Africa were home to 60 million people at risk of the disease.

The Intervention

Onchocerciasis is caused by a worm called *Onchocerca volvulus*, which enters its human victim through the bite of an infected blackfly. The flies breed in fast-moving waters in fertile riverside regions. Once inside a human, the tiny worm grows to a length of 1 to 2 feet and produces millions of microscopic offspring called microfilariae. The constant movement of the microfilariae through the infected person's skin causes torturous itching, lesions, muscle pain, and, in severe cases, blindness. Fertile land is often abandoned for fear of the disease.

Early efforts to control the disease proved ineffective because blackflies cover long distances and cross national borders, rendering unilateral efforts ineffective. An international conference in Tunisia in 1968 concluded that onchocerciasis could not be controlled without regional collaboration and long-term funding of at least 20 years to break the life cycle of the worm. World Bank President Robert McNamara's tour of drought-stricken West Africa in 1972 served as a catalyst to progress. Moved by seeing communities where nearly all the adults were blind and were led by children, McNamara decided to spearhead an international effort against onchocerciasis.[111]

The Onchocerciasis Control Program (OCP), the World Bank's first large-scale health program, was launched in 1974 in conjunction with WHO, the UN Food and Agriculture Organization (FAO), and UNDP. The program included a significant research budget and set out to eliminate onchocerciasis in 7, and eventually in 11, West African countries.[111] Breeding grounds of blackflies were sprayed with larvicide, and the spraying program was able to persist even through regional conflicts and coups. In the 1980s, a Merck drug called ivermectin was included as a powerful new weapon against the disease, a single dose of which could effectively paralyze the tiny worms for up to a full year.[112] The drug proved popular because it quickly reduced uncomfortable symptoms and provided protection against other parasites. Merck donated ivermectin, and Dr. William Foege of the Carter Center managed its distribution.

The African Programme for Onchocerciasis Control (APOC) was established in 1995 as a broad international partnership to control the disease throughout Africa and to carry onchocerciasis control to 19 countries in East and Central Africa. These were countries in which long distances and thick forests made spraying difficult. APOC pioneered a system of community-directed treatment (ComDT) with ivermectin to ensure local participation, reach remote villages, and maintain distribution of the drug after donor funding expired in 2010.[113] ComDT workers are often the only health personnel to reach distant villages, and their access could be used for other health interventions in the future.

The Impact

By 2002, OCP halted transmission of onchocerciasis in 11 West African countries, preventing 600,000 cases of blindness, and protecting 18 million children born in the OCP area from the risk of the disease. About 25 million hectares of arable land—enough to feed an additional 17 million people—are now safe for resettlement.[114] APOC is expanding this success to Central and East Africa, where 40,000 cases of blindness are expected to be prevented each year.

Costs and Benefits

OCP operated with an annual cost of less than $1 per protected person. Total commitments from 22 donors amounted to $560 million. The annual return on investment, due mainly to increased agricultural output, was 20 percent, and it is estimated that $3.7 billion will be generated from improved labor and agricultural productivity.[115] APOC coverage cost even less, at just 11 cents per person. The economic rate of return for the program has been estimated at 17 percent for the years 1996 to 2017, and it is estimated that 27 healthy life days will be added per dollar invested.[116]

Lessons Learned

Success in controlling onchocerciasis could not have been attained without a genuinely shared vision among all partners in the program. Commitment among the African governments was critical to coordinating a regional effort across national borders. Long-term commitments from donors, along with Merck's decision to donate ivermectin indefinitely, were essential elements for the program's sustainability. The participation of a wide range of organizations, such as multilateral institutions, private companies, and local NGOs, allowed for a cost-effective and efficient intervention. The ComDT framework, by emphasizing local ownership and participation, proved a cost-effective and self-sustaining means of delivering drugs to remote populations. The onchocerciasis program proved that effective aid programs, implemented with transparency and accountability, can deliver lasting results.

▶ Future Challenges to Cooperation in Global Health

There are a number of challenges to effective collaborative action in global health. First, the types of health conditions that the world faces are evolving, with an increasing burden of noncommunicable diseases, even in low- and middle-income countries. Second, there have been and will continue to be emerging and re-emerging infectious diseases that could challenge the ability of both countries and the global community to respond effectively, as Ebola virus has done in 2014, 2015, and 2018. The global community needs to align its assistance with changing burdens of disease and has to be ready, through collaborative efforts, to carry out surveillance, prevention, and treatment of any diseases that emerge or re-emerge.

In addition, it will be very important for development partners to work together to help countries strengthen their health systems, as well as to try to combat individual diseases. If countries are to be able to meet their most important health needs in a sustainable manner in the future, then they must have health systems that work. In most low-income countries, this will require better management, more appropriate forms of organization, sounder systems for key public health functions, better-trained staff at all levels, and a consistent manner of providing financing for health system needs and for financial protection of the population from the costs of health care. It will also require a central focus on the quality of care and of all key services. Achieving health system strengthening may not be as attractive politically as working together to fight a specific disease or health problem. Yet, in the long run, a systems approach must be taken to developing health services, and different global health actors will have to work together to achieve this.

Another set of future challenges concerns the need to ensure that actors in global health work together to address the knowledge gaps that prevent sufficient progress against health conditions that cause people to be sick too often and to die prematurely, especially poor people in low-income countries. There will continue to be an important need, for example, for increasing our knowledge of the basic science concerning many diseases, including HIV/AIDS, TB, and malaria. It will not be possible to develop preventive or therapeutic vaccines for these diseases or better treatment for them without significant improvements in scientific knowledge.

There will also be a need for operational research—increasingly called "implementation science"—so that we can learn more about what approaches are effective and efficient. What is the most cost-effective way, for example, to ensure that people take all of their drugs for HIV/AIDS or TB? How should a health system in a low- or middle-income country be organized to ensure that it can operate in a cost-efficient way, while paying sufficient attention to the poor? These questions can only be answered through the generation and sharing of knowledge and experience globally, a process dependent upon cooperation and coordination.

The factors that have encouraged the development of public–private partnerships for health will also continue to challenge the global health community. There are many such partnerships now, and it will be very important to learn as quickly as possible which aspects of these partnerships encourage product development in effective and efficient ways and which ones do not. It is also necessary to continue to encourage the development of new and innovative approaches to enabling the development of new diagnostics, vaccines, and therapies that will be affordable in low- and middle-income countries. If any of the public–private partnerships are successful in developing new products, then it will be essential that efforts turn to ensuring that they are used quickly where they are most needed.

The financial needs for addressing global health concerns are very considerable and will continue to have a prominent place on the global health agenda. The multilateral development banks, bilateral aid agencies, and special programs such as Gavi and the Global Fund need continuous financing. In addition, some of the important initiatives that have been started, such as the considerable push for treatment against HIV/AIDS, cannot be sustained in at least the lowest-resource settings without many years of additional financing by high-income countries, foundations, the private sector, and their partners. There are many risks that donors will develop aid fatigue and not have the political will necessary to continue financing global health efforts at the level needed. These risks have heightened recently, in light of growing populism in some countries.

It will be important that any development financing for health be as effective as possible. Although the topic of development effectiveness is considerably beyond the scope of this text, **TABLE 17-8** summarizes some of the factors most closely associated with the success of development assistance in health.

There are also a number of important challenges to the way that actors in global health cooperate to assist

TABLE 17-8 Factors Associated with Positive Outcomes in Development Assistance

- Strong leadership in the host government and in the development partner agencies
- Close collaboration among governments, donors, and nongovernmental organizations in the design and implementation of the program
- Household and community participation in the design, implementation, and monitoring of programs
- Simple and flexible technologies and approaches that can be adapted to local conditions and do not require complex skills to operate and maintain
- Approaches that help to strengthen health systems, especially human resources for health
- Consistent, predictable funding

Modified from Hecht R. M., & Shah, R. (2006). Recent trends and innovations in development assistance in health. In D. T. Jamison, J. G. Breman, A. R. Measham, et al. (Eds.), *Disease control priorities in developing countries* (2nd ed., p. 246). Washington, DC, and New York, NY: The World Bank and Oxford University Press.

countries in investing in the health sector. In recent years, development assistance agencies have increasingly tried to cooperate closely in their aid work in specific countries. However, there are always tendencies in development agencies to act independently rather than in coordination with other agencies and to focus too much on process issues, such as how they work with others. In the last 3 decades, the number of organizations that work on global health has greatly increased. Although we should expect these tensions to continue, it is important if development assistance in health is to be effective that agencies work increasingly in a cooperative fashion and focus on the content of their efforts.

Finally, it will be very important that good leadership in the global health field continues. Different agencies will need to work together in ways that address the challenges noted earlier. New groups and organizations need to join the community of global health actors to continue to inspire innovative and efficient methods of addressing and financing global health needs.

▶ Main Messages

It is very important that key actors work together to address global health problems because they may have effects that go beyond one country, they may be expensive to deal with, and they may require technical and managerial resources larger than some lower-income countries can bring to bear on their own.

In addition, it is very important that there be global standards in some health fields, and these standards need to be broadly developed and widely accepted. Good examples of areas in which it is imperative that different actors work together globally include efforts to carry out disease surveillance, the global fight for polio eradication, and the standards for some disease control programs, such as TB.

There are many actors in global health; among the most actively involved are WHO, UNICEF, UNAIDS, and the World Bank. Most high-income countries have development assistance organizations, such as USAID, AusAID, and DFID, and they often play important roles in global health. The Global Fund and Gavi are also prominent global health actors. A number of foundations are also deeply involved in global health work, and the Bill & Melinda Gates Foundation has become a major actor in global health since the late 1990s. NGOs such as BRAC are deeply involved in health efforts, both in their own country, and also in many others. Many international NGOs are also very engaged in global health activities; Doctors Without Borders is among the best known of these. Organizations like these play one of several roles, alone or in combination, including advocacy, knowledge generation, technical assistance, financing, or program development and implementation.

Public–private partnerships for health have been created specifically to deal with problems concerning the development of diagnostics, drugs, and vaccines for a number of health conditions. These organizations include, among others, the International AIDS Vaccine Initiative, the International Partnership on Microbicides, and the TB Alliance. Essentially, they try to combine the skills and financing of public and private sector organizations in order to advocate for specific health issues; develop new vaccines, diagnostics, or drugs; and ensure that what they develop will be appropriate to the health needs of poor countries and affordable to them, as well. Some other organizations, which can best be thought of as international partnerships, such as Gavi and the Global Fund, have been established to try to dramatically increase the pace of immunizing children and pregnant women and combating HIV/AIDS, TB, and malaria.

The global health community is likely to face many challenges that will continue to require collective action by global health actors. Some of the key challenges will include filling key gaps in knowledge and encouraging public and private sector organizations to develop the diagnostics, vaccines, and drugs needed to address the most important global health issues. They will also include the need for organizations to work together to strengthen health systems, to combat individual diseases, to be ready to address emerging diseases, and to try to ensure that critical global health needs have adequate financing.

Study Questions

1. What are the most important organizations that work on global health issues?
2. What functions do these organizations play?
3. Why is it important that different actors cooperate to address global health concerns?
4. Name some of the most important successes of cooperative action on global health.
5. What were some of the key factors that led to those successes?
6. What are the lessons of these successes for future global health efforts?
7. What are some of the future challenges that demand continued or strengthened collaboration in global public health?
8. What is a public–private partnership for health, and why might it be valuable?
9. Why is cooperative action needed to address problems like onchocerciasis and Guinea worm?
10. How might the world raise the money needed to further address problems like HIV and the need for drug treatment against AIDS?

References

1. UNICEF. (2004, June 22). *Polio experts warn of largest epidemic in recent years, as polio hits Darfur: Epidemiologists "alarmed" by continuing spread of virus.* Retrieved from http://www.unicef.org/media/media_21872.html
2. World Health Organization. (2018). *Global tuberculosis report 2018.* Retrieved from http://www.who.int/tb/publications/global_report/en/
3. TB Alliance. (n.d.) *Inadequate treatment.* Retrieved from https://www.tballiance.org/why-new-tb-drugs/inadequate-treatment.
4. The Gavi Alliance. (n.d.). Homepage. Retrieved from http://www.Gavialliance.org

5. Merson, M. H., Black, R. E., & Mills, A. J. (Eds.). (2001). *International public health: Diseases, programs, systems, and policies.* Gaithersburg, MD: Aspen.

6. Lele, U., Ridker, R., & Upadhyay, J. (2005). *Health system capacities in developing countries and global health initiatives on communicable diseases.* Retrieved from http://www.eldis .org/document/A16303

7. Ress, M. A. (2013). *Global public goods, transnational public goods: Some definitions.* Knowledge Ecology International. Retrieved from https://www.keionline.org/book/global publicgoodstransnationalpublicgoodssomedefinitions

8. Woodward, W., & Smith, R. D. (n.d.). *Global public good and health: Concepts and issues.* World Health Organization. Retrieved from http://www.who.int/trade/distance_learning /gpgh/gpgh1/en/index1.html

9. Heymann, D. L., & Rodier, G. (2004). Global surveillance, national surveillance, and SARS. *Emerging Infectious Diseases, 10*(2), 173–175.

10. Walt, G. (2001). Global cooperation in international public health. In M. H. Merson, R. E. Black, & A. J. Mills (Eds.), *International public health* (pp. 667–672). Gaithersburg, MD: Aspen.

11. Basch, P. (2001). *Textbook of international health* (2nd ed., pp. 486–509). New York, NY: Oxford University Press.

12. Kickbusch, I., & Buse, K. (2001). Global influences and global responses: International health at the turn of the twenty-first century. In M. H. Merson, R. E. Black, & A. J. Mills (Eds.), *International public health* (pp. 701–733). Gaithersburg, MD: Aspen.

13. World Health Organization. (1946). *Constitution of the World Health Organization.* Retrieved from http://apps.who .int/gb/DGNP/pdf_files/constitution-en.pdf

14. World Health Organization. (n.d.). *About WHO: WHO people and offices.* Retrieved from http://www.who.int /about/structure/en/

15. Mahler, H. (1988). Health for all—all for health. *World Health, 9,* 3-4. World Health Organization. Retrieved from https://apps.who.int/iris/handle/10665/50724.

16. World Health Organization. (n.d.). *WHO priorities.* Retrieved from http://www.who.int/dg/priorities/en/

17. UNICEF. (2012). *Structure and contact information: How UNICEF works.* Retrieved from http://www.unicef.org /about/structure/

18. The UNICEF Transparency Portal. (2018). *Distribution of programme funds.* Retrieved from http://open.unicef.org

19. UNICEF. (2003). *Support UNICEF.* Retrieved from http:// www.unicef.org/support/14884.html

20. UNICEF. (n.d.). *What we do.* Retrieved from http://www .unicef.org/whatwedo/

21. UNAIDS. (n.d.). *Cosponsors.* Retrieved from http://www .unaids.org/en/aboutunaids/unaidscosponsors

22. UNAIDS. (n.d.). *Transparency portal: UNAIDS spending in 2018.* Retrieved from https://open.unaids.org/?utm _source=unaids-site-design&utm_medium=display&utm _campaign=en-HP_ads

23. UNAIDS. (2014). *Gap report.* Retrieved from http:// www.unaids.org/sites/default/files/media_asset/UNAIDS _Gap_report_en.pdf

24. UNAIDS. (n.d.). *Goals.* Retrieved from http://www.unaids .org/en/targetsandcommitments/

25. The World Bank. (2007). *Healthy development: The World Bank strategy for health, nutrition, and population results.* Retrieved from http://www-wds.worldbank.org/external /default/WDSContentServer/WDSP/IB/2007/09/21 /000310607_20070921140425/Rendered/PDF/409280 PAPER0He101OFFICIAL0USE0ONLY1.pdf.

26. Bretton Woods Project. (2009). *Bank's $100 billion annual lending plan.* Retrieved from http://www .brettonwoodsproject.org/art-565290

27. The World Bank. (2006). *Working for a world free of poverty.* Retrieved from http://siteresources.worldbank.org /EXTABOUTUS/Resources/wbgroupbrochure-en.pdf

28. The World Bank. (2018). *Health: Overview.* Retrieved from http://www.worldbank.org/en/topic/health/overview#3

29. The World Bank. (2018). *Annual report, 2017 lending data.* Retrieved from http://pubdocs.worldbank.org/en /715821506096225983/AR17-FY17-Lending-Data.pdf

30. USAID. (2018). *Who we are: Organization.* Retrieved from www.usaid.gov/who-we-are/organization

31. USAID. (2018). *What we do: Global health.* Retrieved from https://www.usaid.gov/what-we-do/global-health

32. The Rockefeller Foundation. (n.d.). Homepage. Retrieved from https://www.rockefellerfoundation.org

33. The Rockefeller Foundation. (n.d.). *Our work.* Retrieved from https://www.rockefellerfoundation.org/our-work/

34. The Rockefeller Foundation. (n.d.). *Planetary health.* Retrieved from https://www.rockefellerfoundation.org/our-work /initiatives/planetary-health/

35. The Rockefeller Foundation. (n.d.). *Transforming health systems.* Retrieved from https://www.rockefeller foundation.org/our-work/initiatives/transforming -health-systems/

36. The Rockefeller Foundation. (n.d.). *Disease surveillance networks.* Retrieved from https://www.rockefellerfoundation .org/our-work/initiatives/disease-surveillance-network

37. Wellcome. (n.d.). *Our strategy.* Retrieved from https:// wellcome.ac.uk/about-us/our-strategy

38. Wellcome. (n.d.). *Investments.* Retrieved from https:// wellcome.ac.uk/about-us/investments

39. Wellcome. (n.d.). *What we do.* Retrieved from https:// wellcome.ac.uk/what-we-do

40. Wellcome Trust. (n.d.) *Current grant portfolio and 2014/2015 grant funding data.* Retrieved from https://wellcome.ac.uk /sites/default/files/wtp060206.pdf

41. Wellcome. (n.d.). *Funding.* Retrieved from https://wellcome .ac.uk/funding/grant-funding-data-2016-2017

42. Wellcome Trust. (n.d.). *Improving health through the best research.* Retrieved from https://wellcome.ac.uk/sites/default /files/science-strategy-improving-health-through-best- research.pdf

43. Wellcome Trust. (2009). *2009 annual report and financial statements.* Retrieved from https://wellcome.ac.uk/sites /default/files/wtx057901.pdf

44. Wellcome Trust. (2012). *Wellcome Trust response to the House of Commons Science and Technology Committee: Science and International Development.* Retrieved from https://wellcome .ac.uk/sites/default/files/wtvm054041.pdf

45. Bill & Melinda Gates Foundation. (n.d.). *What we do.* Retrieved from https://www.gatesfoundation.org/What -We-Do

46. Bill & Melinda Gates Foundation. (n.d.). Homepage. Retrieved from https://www.gatesfoundation.org/

47. Bill & Melinda Gates Foundation. (n.d.) *Bill & Melinda Gates Medical Research Institute*. Retrieved from https://www.gatesmri.org/.

48. Bill & Melinda Gates Foundation. (n.d.). *Recently awarded grants*. Retrieved from http://www.gatesfoundation.org/How-We-Work

49. Bill & Melinda Gates Foundation. (n.d.). *Who we are: Annual report 2017*. Retrieved from https://www.gatesfoundation.org/Who-We-Are/Resources-and-Media/Annual-Reports/Annual-Report-2017

50. The section on NIH is based on a draft of this section provided by the Fogarty International of Center of NIH and in a series of personal communications with the Fogarty International Center in October 2010 and March 2015.

51. U.S. National Institutes of Health. (n.d.). *Strategic plan of the Fogarty International Center at NIH*. Retrieved from http://www.fic.nih.gov/about/pages/strategic-plan.aspx

52. U.S. National Institutes of Health. (2013). *Results of the ROTAVAC rotavirus vaccine study in India*. Retrieved from http://www.nih.gov/news/health/may2013/niaid-14.htm

53. U.S. National Institutes of Health. (n.d.) *Visiting Scientists*. Retrieved from https://www.ors.od.nih.gov/pes/dis/Visiting Scientists/Pages/AboutNIHVisitingProgram.aspx

54. BRAC. (n.d.). *Who we are: Mission & vision*. Retrieved from http://www.brac.net/content/who-we-are-mission-vision

55. BRAC. (n.d.) *Where we work*. Retrieved from http://www.brac.net/where-we-work

56. BRAC. (n.d.). *What we do*. Retrieved from http://www.brac.net/what-we-do

57. BRAC. (n.d.). *Health, nutrition and population: Integrated healthcare for everyone*. Retrieved from http://www.brac.net/program/health-nutrition-and-population/

58. BRAC. (2016). *Tuberculosis control programme*. Retrieved from http://www.brac.net/health-nutrition-population/item/868-tuberculosis-control-programme

59. BRAC. (2016). Malaria control programme. Retrieved from http://www.brac.net/health-nutrition-population/item/869-malaria-control-programme

60. BRAC. (2016). *Nutrition activities*. Retrieved from http://www.brac.net/health-nutrition-population/item/870-nutrition

61. BRAC. (2016). *Non-communicable disease (NCD) programme*. Retrieved from http://www.brac.net/health-nutrition-population/item/872-non-communicable-disease-ncd-programme

62. BRAC. (2016). *Eye care interventions*. Retrieved from http://www.brac.net/health-nutrition-population/item/871-eye-care-interventions

63. BRAC. (n.d.). *Annual report 2017*. retrieved from http://www.brac.net/publications/annual-report/2017/

64. BRAC. (n.d.). *Annual report 2017*. Retrieved from http://www.brac.net/sites/default/files/annual-report/2017/BRAC-AR-2017e.pdf

65. BRAC. (n.d.). *At a glance*. Retrieved from http://www.brac.net/partnership

66. Doctors Without Borders. (n.d.). *Who we are: Around the world*. Retrieved from https://www.doctorswithoutborders.org/who-we-are/how-we-work/how-were-structured/around-world

67. Doctors Without Borders. (n.d.). *About us*. Retrieved from https://www.doctorswithoutborders.ca/content/about-us

68. Doctors Without Borders. (n.d.). *Medical issues: Ebola*. Retrieved from http://www.doctorswithoutborders.org/our-work/medical-issues/ebola

69. Centers for Disease Control and Prevention. (n.d.). *Mission, role, and pledge*. Retrieved from https://www.cdc.gov/about/organization/mission.htm

70. KNCV. (n.d.). *Who we are*. Retrieved from https://www.kncvtbc.org/en/who-we-are/

71. International Union Against Tuberculosis and Lung Disease. (n.d.). *The Union: From evidence to public health action*. Retrieved from http://www.theunion.org/who-we-are

72. Stop TB Partnership. (n.d.). *About us*. Retrieved from http://stoptb.org/about/

73. Stop TB Partnership. (n.d.). *Our work*. Retrieved from http://stoptb.org/about/

74. RBM Partnership to End Malaria. (n.d.). *About us*. Retrieved from http://www.rollbackmalaria.org/

75. RBM Partnership to End Malaria. (n.d.). *Vision*. Retrieved from https://endmalaria.org/about-us/vision

76. RBM Partnership to End Malaria. (n.d.). *What we do*. Retrieved from https://endmalaria.org/our-work/what-we-do

77. Gavi. (n.d.). *Investing in Gavi*. Retrieved from https://www.gavi.org/funding/

78. Gavi. (n.d.). *Gavi's strategy*. Retrieved from https://www.gavi.org/about/strategy/

79. The Global Fund. (n.d.). Homepage. Retrieved from http://www.theglobalfund.org/en

80. The Global Fund. (n.d.). *Overview*. Retrieved from https://www.theglobalfund.org/en/overview/

81. The Global Fund. (n.d.). *Use strategy*. Retrieved from https://www.theglobalfund.org/en/strategy/

82. The Global Fund. (n.d.). *Financials*. Retrieved from https://www.theglobalfund.org/en/financials/

83. International Federation of Pharmaceutical Manufacturers & Associations. (2017). *Pharma supports "Reaching a Billion—ending Neglected Tropical Diseases Gateway to UHC" report and call to actions*. Retrieved from https://www.ifpma.org/resource-centre/pharma-supports-reaching-a-billion-ending-neglected-tropical-diseases-gateway-to-uhc-report-and-call-to-action/

84. International Trachoma Initiative. (n.d.). *The International Trachoma Initiative manages Pfizer's donation of the antibiotic needed to treat trachoma*. Retrieved from http://www.trachoma.org/fighting-trachoma-zithromax

85. Benton, B. (2001). The onchocerciasis (river blindness) programs: Visionary partnerships. *Findings, 174*. Retrieved from http://www-wds.worldbank.org/external/default/WDSContentServer/WDSP/IB/2010/05/31/000334955_20100531073551/Rendered/PDF/547850BRI0Box31740Jan0200101PUBLIC1.pdf

86. African Comprehensive HIV/AIDS Partnerships (ACHAP). (n.d.). Homepage. Retrieved from http://www.achap.org

87. Novartis. (2016). *Novartis Access 2016 one year report: Capturing first learnings*. Retrieved from https://www.novartis.com/sites/www.novartis.com/files/novartis-access-report-2016.pdf

88. Whaley, R. F., & Hashim, T. J. (1994). *A textbook of world health: A practical guide to global health care*. New York, NY: Parthenon.

89. World Health Organization. (2018). *Leprosy: Key facts.* Retrieved from http://www.who.int/mediacentre/factsheets/fs101/en

90. World Health Organization. (2018). *Lymphatic filariasis: Key facts.* Retrieved from http://www.who.int/mediacentre/factsheets/fs102/en

91. World Health Organization. (n.d.). *Onchocerciasis.* Retrieved from http://www.who.int/topics/onchocerciasis/en

92. Bruce, F. C. (2002). Highlights from the national summit on safe motherhood: Investing in the health of women. *Maternal and Child Health Journal, 6*(1), 67–69.

93. World Health Organization. (1978). *Declaration of Alma-Ata.* International Conference on Primary Health Care. Alma-Ata, USSR: Author.

94. The World Bank. (1993). *World development report 1993.* New York, NY: The World Bank, Oxford University Press.

95. World Health Organization. (2005). *Fifty-eighth World Health Assembly.* Retrieved from http://www.who.int/mediacentre/multimedia/2005/wha58/en/

96. Kidder, T. (2003). *Mountains beyond mountains.* New York, NY: Random House.

97. TB Alliance. (n.d.). *Our mission.* Retrieved from https://www.tballiance.org/about/mission

98. TB Alliance. (n.d.). *Our pipeline.* Retrieved from https://www.tballiance.org/portfolio

99. TB Alliance. (n.d.) *About. Donors.* Retrieved from https://www.tballiance.org/about/donors.

100. TB Alliance. (n.d.) *Scientific vision.* Retrieved from https://www.tballiance.org/rd/scientific-vision

101. TB Alliance. (n.d.). *Developing new regimens.* Retrieved from https://www.tballiance.org/rd/developing-new-regimens

102. Hecht, R., Palriwala, A., & Rao, A. (2010). *Innovative financing for global health: A moment for expanded U.S. engagement?* Washington, DC: Center for Strategic and International Studies. Retrieved from http://csis.org/files/publication/100316_Hecht_InnovativeFinancing_Web.pdf

103. UNITAID. (2018). *Accelerating innovation in global health.* Retrieved from http://unitaid.org/assets/factsheet-about-unitaid-en.pdf

104. UNITAID. (n.d.) *About us: Strategy.* Retrieved from https://unitaid.org/about-us/strategy/#en

105. UNITAID. (n.d.). *Core investment areas.* Retrieved from https://unitaid.org/core-investment-areas/#en

106. UNITAID. (n.d.). *Apply for funding.* Retrieved from https://unitaid.org/apply-for-funding/#en

107. UNITAID. (n.d.). *Our impact.* Retrieved from https://unitaid.org/impact/#en

108. Levine, R., & What Works Working Group. (2007). *Case studies in global health: Millions saved.* Sudbury, MA: Jones and Bartlett.

109. World Health Organization. (2017). *Onchocerciasis. Epidemiology.* Retrieved from https://www.who.int/onchocerciasis/epidemiology/en/

110. Laolu, A. (2003). Victory over river blindness. *Africa Recovery, 17*(1), 6.

111. Benton, B., Bump, J., Seketeli, A., & Liese, B. (2002). Partnership and promise: Evolution of the African river blindness campaigns. *Annals of Tropical Medicine and Parasitology, 96*(Suppl. 1), S5–S14.

112. Mectizan Donation Program and the Task Force for Global Health. (2012). *Mectizan Donation Program celebrates 25 years of partnership and progress.* Retrieved from https://mectizan.org/news-resources/mectizan-donation-program-celebrates-25-years/

113. Amazigo, U., Brieger, W., Katabarwa, M., Akogun, O., Ntep, M., Boatin, B., . . . Sékétéli, A. (2002). The challenges of community-directed treatment with ivermectin (CDTI) within the African Programme for Onchocerciasis Control (APOC). *Annals of Tropical Medicine and Parasitology, 96*(1), S41–S58.

114. The World Bank. (2012). *Pushing back neglected tropical diseases in Africa.* Retrieved from http://www.worldbank.org/en/news/feature/2012/11/17/pushing-back-neglected-tropical-diseases-in-africa

115. Hopkins, D., & Richards, F. (1997). Visionary campaign: Eliminating river blindness. In E. Bernstein (Ed.), *Medical and health annual* (pp. 8–23). Chicago, IL: Encyclopaedia Britannica.

116. Benton, B. (1998). Economic impact of onchocerciasis control through the African Programme for Onchocerciasis Control: An overview. *Annals of Tropical Medicine and Parasitology, 92*(Suppl. 1), S33–S39.

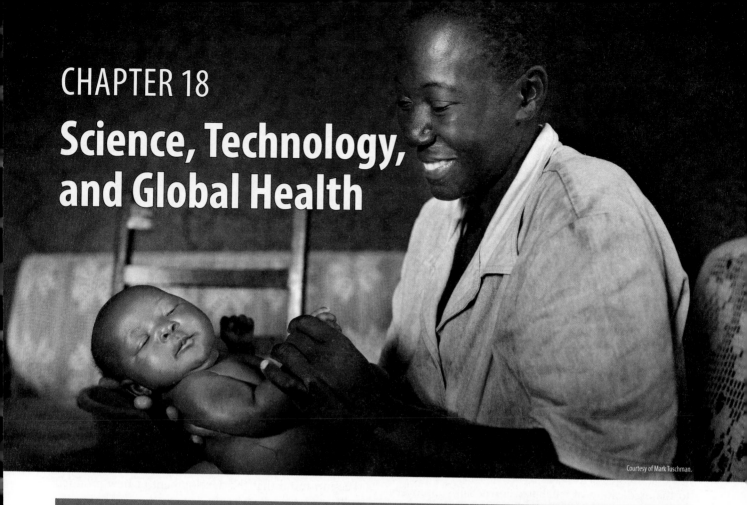

CHAPTER 18
Science, Technology, and Global Health

Courtesy of Mark Tuschman.

LEARNING OBJECTIVES

By the end of this chapter, the reader will be able to do the following:

- Articulate the needs for diagnostics, vaccines, and drugs to address high-burden diseases that affect the poor in low- and middle-income countries
- Assess the extent to which existing products meet those needs
- Note the potential of science and technology to develop new products to address high-burden diseases
- State some of the key constraints to investments in such products
- Indicate mechanisms to overcome these constraints and encourage the development and uptake of new diagnostics, vaccines, and drugs
- Outline lessons for future efforts from selected cases of new product development

▶ Vignettes

Juan lived in the highlands of Peru. He had tuberculosis (TB) and was being treated at a local TB clinic. He had to take four drugs for the first 2 months of his treatment and two drugs for 4 months after that. Juan felt better within weeks of starting his drugs but struggled to take the remaining pills because there were so many to take and he had to take them for so long.

Wezi lived in South Africa, where about 19 percent of the adults are HIV-positive.[1] Despite intensifying efforts to reduce the spread of new HIV infections in South Africa, the number of these infections is still large. In fact, the latest estimates suggest there were about 270,000 new infections in 2017 and that about 7.2 million people in South Africa are now living with HIV/AIDS.[2] Some people believe that stopping the transmission of HIV in countries like South Africa will depend on the discovery of a safe, effective, and affordable HIV vaccine.

Mei-Ling was 4 years old and lived in the west of China. Like so many children in her region, Mei-Ling was infected with hookworms. The community had a deworming program, and every 6 months Mei-Ling was given medicine to get rid of the worms. This medicine was generally safe and effective. However, it had to be given twice a year, and there was some indication that the hookworms were becoming resistant to it.

David was 7 years old and lived in the eastern part of Kenya. He had a high fever and chills, and his mother took him to the local health clinic. The nurse there examined David, decided he had malaria, and prescribed antimalarial medicine. This was the third time in a year that David had malaria. A safe, effective, and affordable malaria vaccine would have prevented him from getting malaria, being sick so often, missing so much school, and spending so much money on medical care.

▶ Introduction

Scientific and technological progress has contributed substantially to improvements in human health. Such progress has included, for example, new and more effective diagnostics for a range of diseases; vaccines for a number of potential killers; a variety of drugs, such as penicillin; and safer and more effective family planning devices.

In fact, some scientific and technological discoveries have been of exceptional importance to public health. The discovery of the smallpox vaccine led to the first important efforts at vaccination and ultimately to the eradication of smallpox. Jonas Salk's discovery of the polio vaccine began to eliminate the scourge of polio from many societies, and his work was advanced further by Albert Sabin's work on the oral polio vaccine. It is difficult to imagine living in a world without antibiotics but they emerged only just before World War II.

The enhancement of medical devices has also had an important impact on public health. The invention of the bifurcated needle was instrumental in enhancing the effectiveness of the smallpox eradication campaign. The intraocular lens for cataracts has provided a very low-cost tool for improving visual acuity.

The purpose of this chapter is to examine how science and technology could assist in speeding up the development and dissemination of new products that could address the largest burdens of disease in low- and middle-income countries. First, the chapter examines the characteristics that such products need to possess if they are to have the desired impact. Next, the chapter reviews the extent to which some existing diagnostics, vaccines, and drugs have those traits. The chapter then discusses the potential of science and technology to develop products in selected areas of importance and reviews constraints to product development. Several case studies illustrate the key concepts of the chapter.

As you read this chapter, it is very important that you keep several things in mind. First, you should remember that very substantial gains in health could be obtained from the effective implementation of existing technologies. There are a number of low-cost but highly effective interventions that are well known but not used widely enough:

- Reducing maternal disability and deaths through better identification of complications, speedy transport to the hospital, and appropriate emergency obstetric care
- Reducing neonatal deaths by training birth attendants in resuscitation, keeping the baby warm, and providing antibiotics for infection
- Reducing young child deaths by expanding vaccination coverage with the six basic antigens and Hib, rotavirus, and pneumococcal vaccines
- Reducing infant morbidity and mortality by promoting exclusive breastfeeding for 6 months
- Reducing morbidity and mortality from TB by expanding case finding and cure rates
- Better controlling hypertension to reduce the risk of stroke

In addition, we must remember that better hygiene practices, such as handwashing with soap, do not require the development of any new products but could substantially improve health.

As you read this chapter, it is also important to keep in mind that the development of new products will not be a quick fix. Rather, while supporting the continued search for scientific and technical progress, it is critical to continue to focus on the underlying sources of ill health in low- and middle-income countries. These include, among other things, poverty, the lack of education, the lack of political interest in the health of the poor, and the place of some minority groups and women in society. Enhancing basic infrastructure, water, and sanitation will also be critical in many settings to sustainable improvements in health.[3]

Finally, you should note that this chapter focuses on a narrow range of the scientific and technological matters that concern global health. It looks largely at new product development, the constraints to it, and what might be done to speed up the process. It does not examine research or operational research. Nor does it focus on the dissemination of existing technologies.

▶ The Need for New Products

As we think about the characteristics of diagnostics, drugs, vaccines, and medical devices that could most effectively and efficiently address the critical health problems of low- and middle-income countries, we need to keep several points in mind. First, the most important target groups for these products are poor people. Their financial resources are limited, and the countries in which they live, particularly low-income countries, generally spend little per capita on health. Second, the quality of care in many countries is low and injection safety is often poor. Third, many low- and middle-income countries have health systems that are poorly organized and cannot effectively manage logistics. In addition, transport and storage of goods is weak, and the supply of electricity for keeping goods cool is often limited.

In this light, what are some of the ideal characteristics of diagnostics, drugs, vaccines, and medical delivery devices to help address the most critical burdens of disease in low- and middle-income countries? The most important of these characteristics are shown in **TABLE 18-1**.

As you can see in the table, it is important that diagnostics be specific, sensitive, easy to use, and noninvasive. Ideally, diagnostic tests could be done quickly by relatively untrained workers and would rapidly produce easy-to-read results. They would also be easy to transport, heat stable, inexpensive, and not require refrigeration.

Much the same would be true for the ideal drugs. These drugs would be safe, effective, inexpensive, and have a long shelf life. They could also be used for many years without becoming susceptible to resistance. In addition, the number of pills that patients would have to take would be limited, and patients would not have to take them for very long.

Vaccines to meet the most important health needs in low- and middle-income countries would also be safe, effective, and inexpensive. They would be easy to transport and store, would be heat stable, and would not require refrigeration. The ideal vaccines would be an inexpensive combination of many antigens, and only one dose would confer lifelong immunity against a number of diseases. It would also be ideal if

TABLE 18-1 Some Ideal Characteristics of Diagnostics, Vaccines, Drugs, and Delivery Devices

Diagnostics: Affordable; specific and sensitive; provide quick and easy-to-interpret results; easy to store and transport; heat stable

Vaccines: Affordable; safe and effective; require few doses; confer lifelong immunity; easy to transport and store; heat stable

Drugs: Affordable; safe and effective; not easy for pathogens to become resistant to; require small doses over a limited period; easy to store and transport; heat stable

Delivery devices: Affordable; safe and effective; not invasive; easy to transport and store; heat stable

therapeutic vaccines, which are vaccines that can be used to treat diseases rather than prevent them, could be developed for some diseases.

The present state of key products does not meet the ideals noted here. Until recently, for example, a child receiving full coverage of the six basic antigens in many countries would require six contacts with the health system to get all of these vaccines.[4]

Could vaccines be developed that combine required antigens in such a way that only a few contacts would be needed between the health system and patients to fully vaccinate a child? The pentavalent vaccine is a step in this direction.[5]

There is a cultural preference in many societies for injections, despite problems with injection safety. Could vaccines be delivered in noninvasive ways, such as sprays, air injectors, and skin patches, that would be safe, effective, heat stable, easy to transport, not very costly, and culturally acceptable?

There is a vaccine for tuberculosis and drugs that are effective against TB. However, the effectiveness of the TB vaccine against adult pulmonary TB is variable.[6] In addition, the drugs that are used to treat TB require a large pill burden, and TB bacteria are increasingly becoming resistant to some of them.[7] What is needed to develop new drugs for TB that could make treatment shorter and easier? Is it possible to develop a safe TB vaccine that could be effective against all forms of TB?

Artemisinin-based combination therapy is effective against malaria that is resistant to chloroquine, although resistance to artemisinin is already growing. However, the cost per treatment with this drug, even at globally negotiated prices, has been about 10 times the cost per treatment with chloroquine for children and 20 times the cost for adults.[8] The search for a malaria vaccine has gone on for many years, and there has been some progress in developing and testing a vaccine. However, there is only one vaccine, RTS,S, that has shown any efficacy in reducing the burden of malaria in young children, when combined with other interventions, and it is now being carefully piloted in a number of countries.[9] What would it take to develop additional low-cost and highly effective malaria drugs? What can encourage the development of a safe and even more effective malaria vaccine?

Drugs for HIV/AIDS can control the virus for most people but cannot cure them. In addition, many people develop resistance to those drugs, and some of the drugs have important side effects. Moreover, there is still no preventive or therapeutic vaccine for HIV/AIDS. How can the world encourage the development of safer and more effective HIV/AIDS drugs, an HIV/AIDS vaccine, and mechanisms, such as microbicides, by which women could protect themselves better from the risk of HIV?

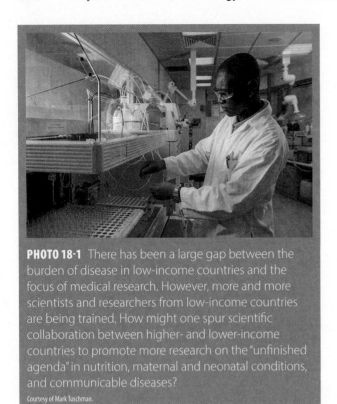

PHOTO 18-1 There has been a large gap between the burden of disease in low-income countries and the focus of medical research. However, more and more scientists and researchers from low-income countries are being trained. How might one spur scientific collaboration between higher- and lower-income countries to promote more research on the "unfinished agenda" in nutrition, maternal and neonatal conditions, and communicable diseases?
Courtesy of Mark Tuschman.

The scientific and technological gaps indicated previously also apply to some of the neglected diseases. Despite the ubiquity of hookworm, there is no vaccine for this parasite, the drug used to treat it has to be administered regularly, and resistance to it is increasing. Can a safe, effective, easy-to-use, affordable vaccine be developed for hookworm and some of the other "wormy" diseases?

▶ The Potential of Science and Technology

Scientific progress has led to a number of areas in which science could be harnessed to address some of the gaps noted in the previous section and to improve human health. Four such areas, as examples, are noted in this section.

Sequencing the genomes of important pathogens will help scientists better understand why they cause disease, how they develop resistance, and what drugs can best fight them, while reducing the onset of resistance. The genomes have been sequenced for more than 30,000 microbial species.[10] The speed with which the SARS virus was sequenced is an indication of the speed with which this can be done, if sufficient priority is given to this work.[11] The sequencing of the mosquito genome may allow scientists to engineer mosquitoes so that they cannot carry malaria and other diseases, such as lymphatic filariasis.[12] Scientists have already sequenced the genome of 16 species

of *Anopheles* mosquito, including the *Anopheles stephensi* mosquito, a key vector of malaria throughout the Indian subcontinent.[13] This research has provided new insights into mosquito biology and mosquito–parasite interactions, which have important implications for the prevention of malaria transmission.[14]

Improvements in information technology, chemistry, and robotics, as well as in genetic and molecular epidemiology, will also facilitate the development of new and better drugs. These tools will allow scientists to understand better the nature of disease. They will also enable scientists to more quickly try different chemical compounds to address those pathogens.[15]

In addition, a number of technologies exist that can assist in the design and manufacture of new and improved vaccines.[15] The use of recombinant DNA technology, for example, helped an Indian vaccine company reduce the cost of the hepatitis B vaccine from about $8 to 50 cents.[12] DNA technology should also be very helpful to the development of drugs.[12]

Genetic modification of plants is a controversial subject because, among other things, there are concerns over the environmental and health risks associated with it. Yet, it is possible to engineer plants that can carry higher levels of certain nutrients, such as vitamin A, while being very resistant to disease.[12] In addition, plants can be modified genetically so that they can produce edible vaccines. However, while research on this front has provided proof of the concept, no such vaccine is very far along in development.[16]

There is an increasing understanding of the promise of science and technology for improving global health. In one study, the views of 28 experts were sought about the biotechnologies that could help improve health in low- and middle-income countries in the following 5 to 10 years.[17] In particular, these scientists were polled about how these potential biotechnologies could[17]:

- Improve health
- Be affordable and appropriate in low- and middle-income countries
- Have an ability to address the most pressing health needs
- Be developed in the next 5 to 10 years
- Advance knowledge
- Yield important indirect benefits

They were also asked how they would use science and technology to achieve these aims. As the highest priority, these scientists would use biotechnology to develop new diagnostics, vaccines, and drugs, in that order. They would use technology to improve the environment, including water and sanitation.

The scientists also put a premium on the development of products that can help empower women to protect themselves against sexually transmitted diseases, including HIV, such as microbicides.[17]

In fact, the Grand Challenges initiative aims to engage the world's most innovative researchers in defining and addressing critical research and operational challenges in global health. The Bill & Melinda Gates Foundation launched the initiative in 2003, in conjunction with the Canadian Institute for Health Research, the Foundation for the U.S. National Institutes of Health, and the Wellcome Trust. This effort has now grown into a family of initiatives, supported largely by the Gates Foundation, Canada, and USAID. To date, these programs have awarded 2,390 grants in 90 countries.[18] The list of members of the Grand Challenges initiative is shown in **TABLE 18-2**.

TABLE 18-2 The Grand Challenges Initiatives

Grand Challenges
Grand Challenges is a family of initiatives that aims to foster innovation to solve key global health and development problems.

Grand Challenges Explorations
The Bill & Melinda Gates Foundation launched this initiative to engage more innovators to get more quickly involved in trying to address high-risk, high-reward ideas.

Grand Challenges Canada
The government of Canada established this effort in 2010. It aims to promote integrated innovation in low- and middle-income countries and Canada.

Grand Challenges for Development
The U.S. Agency for International Development (USAID) and partners established Grand Challenges for Development in 2011. This effort seeks to create and support sustainable solutions for a variety of development challenges.

Grand Challenges Brazil
Grand Challenges Brazil, launched in 2012, is a partnership among the Ministry of Health of Brazil, its National Council on Research (CNPq), and the Bill & Melinda Gates Foundation. It aims to catalyze innovative health research within Brazil.

Grand Challenges India
Grand Challenges India is a partnership set up in 2013 among the Department of Biotechnology in India, the Indian Biotechnology Industry Research Assistance Council (BIRAC), and the Bill & Melinda Gates Foundation. It seeks to catalyze innovative health research within India.

Grand Challenges South Africa
Grand Challenges South Africa is a partnership among the South African Medical Research Council, the Department of Science and Technology of the Republic of South Africa, and the Bill & Melinda Gates Foundation. It aims to catalyze innovative health research within South Africa.

Grand Challenges Africa
This effort was established in 2015 by the African Academy of Sciences (AAS) and the New Partnership for Africa's Development (NEPAD), with the support of the Wellcome Trust, the Bill & Melinda Gates Foundation, and the United Kingdom's Department for International Development (DFID). Grand Challenges Africa is a partnership framework to launch joint challenges for scientific innovation in health in Africa.

Grand Challenges China
Grand Challenges China was launched in 2015 and is a partnership between the National Natural Science Foundation of China (NSFC) and the Bill & Melinda Gates Foundation. It seeks to catalyze innovative health research within China.

Grand Challenges Korea
Grand Challenges Korea was established and is funded by the Korean Ministry of Foreign Affairs. It is a partnership framework for collaboration across the global Grand Challenges network.

Modified from Grand Challenges. (n.d.). *Grand Challenges*. Retrieved from https://grandchallenges.org/initiatives

Grand Challenges began by focusing on scientific innovation to increase access to diagnostics, drugs, and vaccines that could help address the needs of poor people in low- and middle-income countries. **TABLE 18-3** indicates some of the specific areas of involvement supported earlier by Grand Challenges. Today, this family of initiatives supports innovation in a number of fields, including the diagnosis and control of a range of diseases, reproductive health, nutrition, agricultural development, child welfare, and education.[18] **TABLE 18-4** indicates the thematic areas of some recent Grand Challenges grants that are related to global health.

▶ Constraints to Applying Science and Technology to Global Health Problems

Given the strengths of existing scientific knowledge, why is it that some of the products that could make an important difference to the health of the poor globally have not been developed? Beyond the inherent scientific difficulties in some of these efforts, such as the development of HIV and malaria vaccines, there are several common constraints to the development of these desired products. First, much of the research and development on new diagnostics, vaccines, drugs, and delivery devices is carried out in the for-profit sector, and that sector has historically believed it could not make a sufficient return from products oriented toward low- and middle-income countries. These firms see the market for their goods in low- and middle-income countries as a small one. They also doubt the ability of governments and individuals in low-income countries to pay prices for their products that would give them a sufficient return on their capital. As evidence of this, for example, they pointed earlier to the slow uptake in low- and middle-income countries of the vaccines against *Haemophilus influenzae* type b (Hib) and hepatitis B.

TABLE 18-3 Selected Goals of Grand Challenges in Global Health
Improve Vaccines
▪ Create effective single-dose vaccines that can be used soon after birth.
▪ Prepare vaccines that do not require refrigeration.
▪ Develop needle-free delivery systems.
Create New Vaccines
▪ Devise reliable tests in model systems to evaluate live attenuated vaccines.
▪ Solve how to design antigens for effective, protective immunity.
▪ Learn which immunological responses provide protective immunity.
Control Insect Vectors
▪ Develop a genetic strategy to deplete or incapacitate a disease-transmitting insect population.
▪ Develop a chemical strategy to deplete or incapacitate a disease-transmitting insect population.
Improve Nutrition
▪ Create a full range of optimal, bioavailable nutrients in a single staple plant species.
Limit Drug Resistance
▪ Discover drugs and delivery systems that minimize the likelihood of drug-resistant microorganisms.
Cure Infection
▪ Create therapies that can cure latent infection.
▪ Create immunological methods that can cure chronic infections.
Measure Health Status
▪ Develop technologies that permit quantitative assessment of population health status.
▪ Develop technologies that allow assessment of multiple conditions and pathogens at the point of care.

Data from Grand Challenges. (n.d.). *About Grand Challenges*. Retrieved from http://www.grandchallenges.org/Pages/BrowseByGoal.aspx

TABLE 18-4 Thematic Areas of Selected Recent Grand Challenges Grants for Global Health

Agricultural programs

Antigen design, vaccines, vaccine model systems, vaccine manufacturing

Cell phone applications

Diagnostics, diagnostic systems, point-of-care diagnostics

Drug resistance, drug-resistance burden

Family planning, contraceptive discovery, contraceptive technologies, the next-generation condom

Global mental health, maternal mental health

Growth, birth, and development

HIV infection

Human and animal health

Hypertension

Malaria analytics, drugs, transmission, and eradication

Mosquito control

Nutrition

Pneumonia

Poliovirus eradication

Putting women and girls at the center of development

Sanitation technologies, reinvent the toilet

Saving lives at birth

TB biomarkers, latency, treatment

Based on data from Grand Challenges. (n.d.). *Explore awarded grants.* Retrieved from https://grandchallenges.org/#/list

Moreover, the costs of research and development on new products can be very high, some suggesting as high as $800 million, to bring a new drug from research to market. Given these costs, profit-making firms will invariably want to use their capital to develop, for example, a potential blockbuster drug against high cholesterol that can be sold in high-income countries, rather than a drug for low-income countries on which the firm believes it will not be able to recoup its investment.[19]

In addition, vaccine markets have some particular constraints to entry. Vaccine development requires a considerable amount of upstream investment, the cost of developing vaccine candidates is very high, and governmental regulations may also reduce the potential for sufficient profit from vaccines to attract firms to this market. In addition, the number of firms engaged in vaccine production worldwide is small and production capacity is limited. The development of vaccines for low- and middle-income country markets has also been complicated by the fact that, until recently, vaccine manufacturers often had to produce formulations of vaccines for some low- and middle-income countries that were different from the relatively expensive combination vaccines that were used in other countries. Moreover, pharmaceutical companies can generally earn a higher return on money invested in the development of drugs than money invested in developing vaccines.[20]

Another constraint to greater focus on the health conditions of low- and middle-income countries until recently has been insufficient attention to them by some of the major national research institutions. The basic research that is conducted at places like the U.S. National Institutes of Health often sets a foundation for product development later by the for-profit manufacturers. The greater the attention that national research institutes in high-income countries pay to the high-burden problems of low- and middle-income countries, the greater the likelihood that new products for them will eventually be developed.

Some of these constraints are reflected in the extent to which drugs have been developed to address diseases that most affect poor people in low- and middle-income countries. A study of drugs that were approved for marketing showed that between 1975 and 1999, for example, 1,393 new chemicals were approved, but only about 3 percent were relevant to infectious and parasitic diseases that are the most significant burdens of disease in low-income countries. The same study looked at the number of new drugs approved for every million DALYs and found that two to three times more drugs were produced for every million DALYs attributable to diseases of high-income countries, rather than diseases of low- and middle-income countries.[19] Over the same period, only about 1 percent of the drugs approved concerned neglected tropical diseases, and only about 0.2 percent concerned TB.[21] Moreover, about 90 percent of expenditure on research and development on health has been oriented toward the diseases of the high-income countries, and only about 10 percent toward the diseases of the low- and middle-income countries.[22,23] The Global Forum for Health Research called this the "10/90 gap."[23]

▶ Enhancing New Product Development

We have seen that gaps in the development of diagnostics, drugs, vaccines, and medical devices that serve the needs of low- and middle-income countries reflect market failures. In general, the public sector tries to reduce its risks by waiting for such products to be developed by the private sector. However, the private sector generally believes that it is too risky to produce products that are expensive to develop and for which an adequate return on investment cannot be assured. Is it possible to change the market for these products? Can one reduce the cost of product research and development to the point where the private for-profit sector might be interested in such products? What other steps can be taken to speed product development?

Push Mechanisms

A number of steps could encourage a larger share of research and development to focus on the needs of low- and middle-income countries. Some of these are shown in **FIGURE 18-1**, which depicts push and pull mechanisms and where in the product development cycle they have the most impact.

One type of effort is called "push mechanisms." These refer to mechanisms meant to encourage product development by reducing the risks and costs of investments.[20] Push mechanisms could include the following[20]:

- Direct financing: government financing or carrying out of research activities needed to develop a product.
- Performing or facilitating clinical trials: This could include government measures to make it easier to carry out clinical trials for the product and to help with the ethical issues involved in such trials.
- Tax credits for research and development: Governments can lower the cost to firms of research and development by giving them credits against their taxes for certain investments.

These push mechanisms operate on the early stages of product development. Such mechanisms have been used successfully before. In addition, they can reduce risk and thereby encourage investment in product development. The disadvantage of push mechanisms, however, is that there is no guarantee that they will lead to the development of a desired product. In addition, even if a product is developed, it

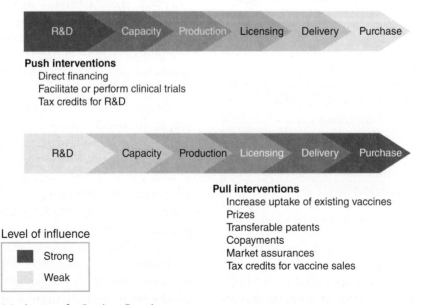

FIGURE 18-1 Push/Pull Mechanism for Product Development

Modified from Glass, S. N., Batson, A., & Levine, R. (2008). *Issues paper: Accelerating new vaccines.* Geneva, Switzerland: Global Alliance for Vaccines and Immunizations.

may not be the best one, and product developers will then not produce what might have been better candidates. Furthermore, when the money is spent on push mechanisms, it is gone, whether or not a product has been developed.[20]

Some of the direct financing and facilitation of clinical trials could be done through programs like the U.S. National Institutes of Health or similar institutes in other countries. Additional money could also be channeled, for example, to the Special Program for Research and Training in Tropical Diseases (TDR), which is sponsored by the World Health Organization (WHO), UNICEF, the United Nations Development Programme, and the World Bank.[24] Some of the financing of the Bill & Melinda Gates Foundation, like that for Grand Challenges, is meant to push new product development.

In conjunction with these efforts, it is important to strengthen the links between researchers in low- and middle-income countries and those in high-income counties. The links can also be enhanced among researchers in low- and middle-income countries. The aim of these efforts would be to attract more research money to institutions within the low- and middle-income countries that are engaged in research and development on the most important burdens of disease in such countries. A number of low- and middle-income countries, especially India, China, Brazil, South Africa, Mexico, Indonesia, and Cuba, already have the ability to carry out basic research and to develop products that emanate from that research. Additional funding might deepen and speed their research, as Grand Challenges intends to do.[18,25]

It is also important to comment on some aspects of governmental regulation of pharmaceutical and vaccine development. Regulation is necessary, but it is also an important part of the costs of research and development. By arranging to speed drug approvals and harmonize approval processes across countries, the costs of research and development can be reduced to provide some incentives to manufacturers. Granting fast-track approval for generic AIDS drugs, for example, has encouraged the development of such drugs.[21]

Pull Mechanisms

A number of mechanisms are intended to help ensure that a future return is provided to those who do develop new products. These are called pull mechanisms.[20,22] The following are some of the most important pull mechanisms[20]:

- Increasing the uptake of existing vaccines: Using public funds to increase the use of vaccines that have not been taken up sufficiently.
- Prizes: Offering monetary rewards to those firms that develop desired products.
- Transferable patents: In exchange for the development of the desired product, providing the manufacturer with the right to extend a patent on another one of its products or patents in markets in high-income countries.
- Copayments: Governments can provide the manufacturer with a payment for every product sold.
- Market assurances: The public sector can promise to buy the products if they are produced.
- Tax credits for vaccine sales: Governments can offer tax credits for products that are sold.

From the point of view of the public sector, pull mechanisms have the advantage of providing funds only when desired products have been developed. However, governments and the private sector have to agree early on what such arrangements would be for any product, and neither party might be satisfied with these arrangements when products do emerge.[20] There has been little experience until recently with financing mechanisms that are meant to exert a pull on new product development and use, but the Advance Market Commitments and the International Finance Facility for Immunisation are now in place and are discussed later in the chapter.

A mechanism that has been used for vaccines for some time and more recently for AIDS drugs is called *tiered pricing*. This is an arrangement by which a firm charges different prices in different markets. The idea behind tiered pricing is that a firm can charge enough to make a profit in high-income markets to offset the fact that the products will not make a profit in low- and middle-income markets. The profits from one market could cross-subsidize the sales at reduced prices in other markets. This is being practiced now for some drugs for which there is a global market. However, tiered pricing is not likely to work effectively for products that are needed exclusively in low- and middle-income countries because the basis for cross-subsidizing will not exist.[21]

In addition, considerable hope has been put until recently into the role that public–private partnerships can play in encouraging the development of the diagnostics, drugs, vaccines, and medical devices that could have a significant impact on the health of the poor in low- and middle-income countries. As indicated earlier, many of these efforts are organized around the search for new products for particular diseases, such as HIV, TB, and malaria. These public–private partnerships are also referred to as product development partnerships (PDPs) and are organized on a not-for-profit basis. They aim to attract private, public, and philanthropic funds to invest in needed research and development, tapping the strengths of the private sector in product development as they do so. There are now PDPs for a number of vaccines and drugs, including, for example, TB and malaria. The PDP arena, however, has changed recently with the establishment by the Gates Foundation of its own medical research institute.[26]

Meeting product development goals will probably require a combination of these efforts. First, they can start with a greater focus by research institutions in high-income countries on the problems of low- and middle-income countries. They can also promote greater networking of research institutions in low- and middle-income countries. This can help encourage product development, with other push mechanisms. At the same time, it will be important to change the market and perceptions of the market for needed products through pull mechanisms that can ensure that money will be available for products if they are developed. Third, the public and private sectors can collaborate with each other, bringing complementary skills and financing to the partnership.

▶ Case Studies

This section contains a number of case studies that highlight some of the different approaches to harnessing science and technology to enhance new product development and improve health outcomes. Mobile technology and telemedicine are increasingly used in health work in many countries, and this section begins with a case study on each of those topics. This is followed by case studies that touch on the development of new diagnostics for TB and a device intended to reduce the risk of maternal hemorrhage. The next case study discusses cooperative efforts to develop a meningitis vaccine for Africa. The last cases concern innovative financing mechanisms that are intended to provide a pull on new product development and diffusion: the advance market commitments (AMC) and the International Finance Facility for Immunisation (IFFIm).

mHealth: Using Mobile Technology to Improve the Health of the Poor in Poor Countries

What Is mHealth?

mHealth, or mobile health, is commonly defined as medical and public health practice supported by mobile devices, such as mobile phones, patient monitoring devices, personal digital assistants (PDAs), and other wireless devices that can transmit text messages, photos, and data at the touch of a button. TABLE 18-5 lists the different categories of mobile health technologies, potential applications, and selected examples of mHealth programs. mHealth is a rapidly growing area in the development of health technology and is a component of eHealth, or the delivery of health care by electronic means.[27] More than 90 percent of the world is now covered by a mobile network, and as a result, the overwhelming majority of WHO member countries have mHealth programs. The largest expansion of mHealth has occurred in the Asia-Pacific region due to more extensive mobile data networks. mHealth has seen the largest barriers in Africa, due largely to limited infrastructure, but great progress has been made there, as programs such as SIMpill and Child Count+ demonstrate. Within low- and middle-income countries, mHealth has been more commonly adopted in healthcare areas related to maternal and child health, HIV/AIDS, and primary care.[28] There is hope that mHealth can offer cost-effective programs and interventions to support the performance of health workers and disseminate health education information, especially in places where health systems face significant challenges of human and physical resources.[29]

What Is the Scope of mHealth?

In 2009, the World Health Organization conducted the second global survey of mHealth technologies and used a classification system based on six categories to describe the scope of mHealth initiatives globally.[27]

Although there are many programs that fall within these categories, there is substantial innovation in mHealth, and there is greater diversity of mHealth than these categories capture. For example, applications have been developed that allow mHealth to help support the diagnostic process, while other applications act as attachments to traditional medical tools such as the stethoscope.[30]

TABLE 18-5 WHO Classification of mHealth Technologies		
Technology Category	**Applications**	**Example Programs**
Communication: Individuals to health services	Health call centers; emergency toll-free telephone services	Healthline (Bangladesh); Ligne Verte toll-free hotline (Democratic Republic of the Congo)
Communication: Health services to individuals	Appointment reminders; medication reminders; health promotion	On Cue Compliance (South Africa); SIMpill (South Africa)
General consultations	Telemedicine	Mobile Doctors Network (Ghana); Aceh Behar Midwives with Mobile Phone project (Indonesia)
Emergency communication	Referrals; transports	Dial 1298 for Ambulance (India)
Monitoring & surveillance	Mobile surveys; patient reminders	Episurveyor (Senegal); Cam e-WARN (Cambodia)
Health information access	Patient records; population data	Child Count+ (Malawi, Uganda); OpenMRS (many countries)

Data from World Health Organization. (2014). *mHealth: New horizons for health through mobile technologies: Second global survey on eHealth*. Retrieved from https://www.who.int/goe/publications/goe_mhealth_web.pdf; Unite for Sight. (2013). *mHealth technology in global health*. Retrieved from http://www.uniteforsight.org/global-health-university/mhealth#_ftn27

Communication: Individuals to Health Services

One of the most common mHealth initiatives has been the creation of health call centers that allow individuals to call in or text health questions and receive immediate answers. These help lines have been developed with the goal of increasing access to health advice and information, while overcoming potential barriers, such as shortage of healthcare professionals and the costs of service provision and transportation. For example, a medical hotline called Healthline in Bangladesh received more than 3.5 million calls in its first 3 years of operation from individuals seeking answers from a licensed health professional. Similarly, an initiative called the Ligne Verte (Green Line) toll-free hotline was introduced in the Democratic Republic of the Congo to provide confidential family planning information and to refer patients to nearby clinics that offer contraception services. Each call cost the equivalent of $0.36. The most successful of these healthcare centers in meeting their stated aims have been operated by for-profit organizations that partner with mobile network operators. As a result, health call centers may not be as accessible to the poor as desired.[27]

Communication: Health Services to Individuals

One of the greatest challenges in many health systems is patient compliance. A 2007 pilot study in South Africa demonstrated that when a mobile application technology, SIMpill, was introduced, patient compliance could jump to over 90 percent in areas previously recording 22 percent to 60 percent compliance. This application is a medication container that communicates with a patient's mobile phone to remind the patient about the timing of the next medication dose. Repeated or missed dosages are brought to the attention of healthcare workers, who then follow up with the patient and arrange for an in-person visit.[31]

General Consultations

Telemedicine initiatives have also been widespread and can help improve the quality of care for rural populations by creating more opportunities for interaction with qualified medical professionals in urban settings. Many pilot telemedicine programs have been successful, including a program in Taiwan that had an 85 percent accuracy rate in the remote diagnosis of soft tissue injuries. Other telemedicine programs have attempted to enhance the referral process by facilitating communication among physicians. The Mobile Doctors Network (MDNet) in Ghana was launched in 2008 and was the first program in Africa to provide free mobile-to-mobile voice and text services to all physicians in Ghana. It has been successful in enhancing physician connectivity, the frequency of consultations, the success rate of diagnosis and treatment for populations with limited access to specialized care, the time needed for referral, and the patient's recovery experience.[27] The start-up costs for telemedicine projects can be minimal if telecommunications providers are incentivized to donate the infrastructure and resources such as SIM cards, but the cost-effectiveness of these types of efforts is still being investigated.

Emergency Communication

In emergency situations, a rapid response can be the difference between life and death. Although emergency response systems in high-income countries are well established, those in low- and middle-income countries are often limited or nonexistent.[31] Nonetheless, mHealth offers applications that at low cost can capitalize on the mobile network coverage that does exist in these low-resource settings. On a national scale, for example, nationwide alert systems can be implemented through these networks. After the 2010 Haitian earthquake, three mHealth organizations—Ushahidi, FrontlineSMS, and SamaSource—created a logistics map using short message service (SMS) alerts for missing people or immediate humanitarian needs that was widely used by aid organizations throughout Haiti. Unfortunately, these types of programs have only been evaluated in a limited manner.[31]

Monitoring and Surveillance

An array of mHealth technologies has been used for health monitoring and surveillance. Senegal piloted a program called Episurveyor that indicated that only 55 percent of the country's health districts were systematically using partograms, graphical tools that monitor the trajectory of labor in a pregnant woman. Based on the information from this survey, Senegal's Ministry of Health was able to increase the distribution of partograms and institute initiatives that encouraged midwives to use them. A follow-up survey demonstrated that this intervention led to an average increase of 28 percent in partogram use in the applicable regions.[27]

This pilot effort was part of a larger mHealth program funded by the UN Foundation and Vodafone Foundation Technology Partnership.[27]

Access to Health Information

Electronic medical records have become a gold standard for health systems. In low- and middle-income countries, electronic records have been implemented slowly, but the introduction of mHealth can help reduce the burden on health workers and health facilities by allowing easier access to information and its sharing. For example, OpenMRS allows frontline health workers to access information from a patient's health record using a mobile device and then add information to the health record after a consultation. ChildCount+ has been very successful in sub-Saharan Africa in enhancing the efforts of community health workers. The program offers an integrated system that links individual patient records with population data in order to improve follow-up services and better understand a community's needs.[31] It is important to note, however, that the literature on the outcomes and cost-effectiveness of health information applications is still limited.

The Need for Evaluation

It is important to know whether the investments in time and resources in mHealth have been both impactful and cost-effective and if they are good candidates for scaling up. Despite extensive innovation in the development of mobile health technologies, evaluation of the effectiveness of these technologies has been limited, as repeatedly noted. Although some uses of mHealth appear to be successful and others appear to be promising, only a small share of all mHealth activities in low- and middle-income countries have been subjected to high-quality, rigorous evaluation. Thus, there are still very few examples of proven impact at large scale of mHealth programs.[32]

Looking Forward

As evidence from well-planned evaluations grows, it is likely that there will be a transition from experimentation with different technologies to strategic implementation of the technologies known to be cost-effective. Moreover, as the application of mHealth continues to advance, it is clear that other issues will also need to be addressed more fully, including data privacy and ways to integrate various applications. Overall, there is hope that mHealth will offer cost-effective solutions to improving health outcomes and access to health information in low- and middle-income countries. However, it is important to note that this hope has not yet been realized at scale in ways that are based on rigorous evaluation and evidence of cost-effectiveness.[33]

New Diagnostics for TB: Xpert MTB/RIF

Although the overwhelming majority of TB deaths could be prevented with early diagnosis and proper treatment, diagnosis of TB has faced substantial challenges.[34] First, the traditional standard for diagnosing pulmonary TB, microscopic examination of sputum samples from a TB suspect, is estimated to correctly diagnose only about 20 percent to 60 percent of adults who have TB.[35] Second, sputum microscopy cannot be used to diagnose TB in young children, because they cannot produce sputum samples. In addition, substantial training is required for consistently accurate diagnosis of extrapulmonary TB, and even skilled clinicians experience significant variability in their results.[36] Finally, the diagnosis of multidrug-resistant TB (MDR-TB) has required that samples be cultured, which can be done only in select laboratories and takes substantial time to produce results.

In light of this situation, the global TB community has long sought improved tools for diagnosing TB, and progress has been made in this direction. In 2006, the Foundation for Innovative New Diagnostics (FIND) partnered with Cepheid Inc. and the University of Medicine and Dentistry of New Jersey to try to develop an enhanced diagnostic tool for TB.[36] They sought to use existing technology to improve the sensitivity and specificity of TB detection—especially in difficult cases involving drug resistance and coinfection with HIV—all while automating the process to reduce interuser variability.

From this collaboration came the Xpert TB test. In just 2 hours, Xpert detects the presence of mycobacterium tuberculosis by amplifying and analyzing genetic material in the sputum sample.[34] Furthermore, the technology detects resistance to the first-line drug rifampicin (RIF), which can serve as a good proxy for MDR-TB.[37] Moreover, the Xpert MTB/RIF system offers high sensitivity and specificity compared to sputum smear microscopy, with rates of 98 percent to 100 percent and 100 percent, respectively, in individuals without HIV co-infection.[38] In addition, clinical trials have shown that the system detects TB in individuals co-infected with HIV with a sensitivity of 70 percent, rather than the 50 percent sensitivity offered by conventional sputum smear microscopy.[39]

FIND and the manufacturer have negotiated prices for use in low- and middle-income countries, with Xpert costing $17,000 for the permanent equipment and $9.98 for each test cartridge, instead of the standard price of $16.86.[40] This concessional pricing is possible because organizations including the President's Emergency Plan for AIDS Relief (PEPFAR), USAID, UNITAID, and the Bill & Melinda Gates Foundation provided financial support and negotiated a discount on each cartridge. Although the automation of Xpert means workers will no longer need to spend time examining sputum by microscopy, Xpert does require annual maintenance and is still more expensive than traditional techniques.[41] It is expected that diagnosing a case of TB will now cost $61, about 55 percent more than when using traditional methods.[42] The most recent assessments have shown Xpert to be "generally cost-effective."[43(pxiv)]

WHO now recommends the use of Xpert as the initial diagnostic test for any child or adult suspected of having TB.[37] The use of Xpert technology has increased steadily. However, recent studies suggest that the test is still substantially underutilized.[44]

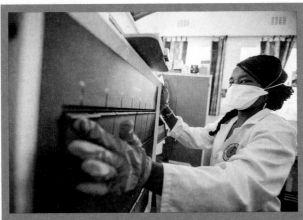

PHOTO 18-2 There is little incentive for the private sector to invest in diagnostics for TB, because most people with TB are poor and live in low- and lower middle-income countries. However, a number of not-for-profit organizations, like the Foundation for Innovative New Diagnostics, are working on better diagnostics for some of the communicable diseases such as TB. This photo shows the Xpert machine, which provides a diagnostic test that WHO has recommended for the diagnosis of drug-susceptible TB and TB that is resistant to rifampicin. What steps could the global community take to further incentivize for-profit and not-for-profit companies to invest more money in the development of new diagnostics for the "unfinished agenda" of communicable diseases?
Courtesy of The Global Fund, photo by John Rae.

The development of the Xpert MTB/RIF test owes its success to collaboration across disciplines and organizations. Researchers developed a working technology to improve the efficiency of a common laboratory technique, and a team at the University of Medicine and Dentistry of New Jersey applied the technology to analyze TB in sputum samples.[45] FIND aided in negotiations between funding organizations and Cepheid Inc. to reduce the price per cartridge for resource-poor countries. By bringing advanced diagnostics at reduced costs to resource-poor settings, Xpert should improve care for TB patients throughout the world. In addition, this important development has set a foundation for additional efforts in the search for better TB diagnostics.

Saving Women's Lives: The Non-pneumatic Anti-shock Garment

Postpartum hemorrhages are the largest cause of maternal death worldwide.[46] Especially in resource-poor settings, healthcare workers may lack the training to manage labor appropriately, which can lead to improper uterine muscle tone and subsequent hemorrhage. However, a multitude of other factors also contribute to postpartum hemorrhages (PPH). Ruptured uteruses, vaginal lacerations, and retained placentas are other common causes of PPH that are difficult to manage in resource-poor settings.[46] These problems are particularly troublesome in cases of delayed care, and reducing the rate of blood loss can have a significant effect on the clinical outcome. Thus, there is an important need for treatment of shock and prevention of blood loss among women giving birth.[47] Anti-shock garments—which inflate to compress the abdomen to prevent blood loss—were developed decades ago, but their price and complexity have been barriers for adoption in low-resource settings where they might be particularly helpful.[48,49]

The non-pneumatic anti-shock garment (NASG) is based on technology from the United States National Aeronautics and Space Administration (NASA). The product was developed by PATH, the University of California, San Francisco (UCSF) Safe Motherhood Program,[50] Pathfinder International, and the Blue Fuzion Group.[51] Rubber belts with Velcro are tightened around a mother's abdomen to reduce bleeding while the woman is transported to a care provider as quickly as possible. The garment acts to both treat shock and shift blood toward critical organs, stabilizing the mother's condition during delays in care. When WHO originally recommended the NASG for patients with PPH, at $170 per device, the technology

was thought to be too expensive for resource-poor countries.[46,51] PATH, a global health organization based in the United States, worked to make manufacturing more cost-effective, which reduced the price to just $54 for each reusable garment.[49] The NASG has been validated in clinical trials analyzed by the UCSF Safe Motherhood Initiative in Egypt, Nigeria, Zambia, Zimbabwe, and India.[52]

The NASG reduces bleeding by 50 percent and could reduce maternal morbidity and mortality due to hemorrhage.[47] Indeed, in a trial in Egypt, mortality was reduced by 20 percent and morbidity by 160 percent when the NASG was applied upon obstetric hemorrhage until time of care.[53] Delays in care happen often in low-resource settings, and the rate of bleeding of a woman who has just delivered can mean the difference between life and death. The device is composed of just rubber and Velcro attachments, so it can be employed in a variety of low-resource settings with minimal need for technical expertise and training.[46]

This promising garment suggests that some existing technologies can be of great use in resource-poor settings after a limited number of simplifying modifications. Inflatable pressure suits were first developed to prevent blood loss during surgery, but they were designed for use only by trained surgeons in the operating room.[48] By developing a non-pneumatic version, UCSF researchers made it easier for untrained personnel to use and also economical for resource-poor countries to purchase. PATH further enhanced the technology by optimizing manufacturing to minimize costs. This simple garment appears likely to be able to buy precious time, in cost-effective ways, for dying mothers seeking treatment.

However, it will be important to see the extent to which the technology is adopted and over what period of time. A review was conducted in 2016 of the uptake of the device in Ethiopia, India, Nigeria, and Zimbabwe—all countries of exceptional importance to the numbers of women who suffer maternal mortality. This study suggested that there was considerable variance in the time and scale of uptake across the countries, with Ethiopia having the most rapid uptake.[54]

Addressing Meningitis in Africa[55]
The Problem

Until recently, there was an outbreak of meningitis A every 5 to 14 years across a belt in Africa stretching from Senegal to Ethiopia. These epidemics were caused by the *Neisseria meningitidis* serogroup A bacterium.

This infection is exceptionally virulent. Without treatment, the case fatality rate can reach 80 percent. Even with treatment, 5 percent to 10 percent of the infected still die. Major epidemics have infected as many as 1 out of every 100 people, and the worst epidemic to date infected 250,000 people and led to 25,000 deaths.

Moreover, until the development of the new vaccine, regional governments sought to address the epidemics with a polysaccharide vaccine and antibiotics. These were partly effective. However, this vaccine was costly, conferred immunity only for 2 to 3 years, and provided little protection to young children. Thus, the economic and social costs of these meningitis epidemics were exceptionally high for the affected countries. On average, for example, families lost about a month of work when a family member fell ill with meningitis.

Taking Action

Deeply concerned about these epidemics, leaders of the health sector in Africa requested that WHO assist in enabling the development of a more effective conjugate vaccine against meningitis A. Such a vaccine had been highly effective in eliminating meningitis A in western Europe. After a feasibility study, WHO joined with the NGO PATH to create the Meningitis Vaccine Project (MVP) to develop the new vaccine. The Bill & Melinda Gates Foundation provided $70 million to launch the initiative. MVP then embraced other partners, including the U.S. Food and Drug Administration; the Serum Institute of India; a Dutch biotech company, SynCo; and the U.K. National Institute for Biological Standards and Control.

During the early stages of the partnership, the leadership of MVP sought the views of African health leaders about the profile of the desired vaccine, the price they thought they could pay for it, and the likely demand for the vaccine.

In 2005, much earlier than one would normally expect for the development of a new vaccine, a candidate vaccine was ready for testing. The vaccine turned out to be safe and much more effective than the polysaccharide vaccine. WHO gave fast-track approval to the vaccine in 2010, which was produced by the Serum Institute of India and named "MenAfriVac."

About 25 million doses of the vaccine would be needed yearly for 10 years. In addition, African leaders had stressed the importance of keeping the price of the vaccine below $1 per dose. The Serum Institute of India ultimately set $0.40 per dose as the initial cost of the vaccine, with increases to be set for inflation.

African governments, led by Burkina Faso, rolled out the vaccine in 2010. They were assisted in this effort by WHO and its regional office for Africa and Gavi, the Vaccine Alliance. Governments wishing to participate in the program had to commit to financing half the operational costs of the program. Vaccination was phased in across the hardest-hit countries, with special attention to difficult-to-reach groups, such as nomadic and refugee groups. By 2014, 214 million people in 15 countries were vaccinated.

Impact

The vaccination program had dramatic effects. Burkina Faso, for example, reported no cases of meningitis A in the 2013 epidemic season. The same was true in target areas of Chad. There was also a 94 percent difference in meningitis infections between targeted and non-targeted areas in Chad that year. It has been estimated that the vaccine will avert 142,000 deaths and almost 300,000 disabilities over its first 10 years of use. So far, it has also shown itself to be safe.

Costs of the Program

The vaccine was developed for $70 million, which is substantially below the average cost to develop a vaccine of around $350 million. It has been estimated that the vaccine between 2010 and 2013 cost almost $100 per DALY averted, which would make it a very good "buy."

Keys to Success

The evaluation of the program suggests a number of factors set the foundation for its success. The following factors were among the most important:

- Commitment of African leaders
- The development of a creative public–private partnership
- Technological innovation
- Developing the vaccine to meet local needs and ability to pay
- Funding from the Bill & Melinda Gates Foundation
- Financial and operational support from Gavi

Future Challenges

Despite the important successes to date, the program faces a number of potential challenges. First, it is not yet known for how long the vaccine will confer immunity. This, of course, could have an important bearing on the cost-effectiveness of the vaccine. Second is the risk that other meningitis strains will fill the void left by the elimination of meningitis A. The third would be the prospect of developing an even more heat-stable, affordable vaccine that could target all of the strains affecting Africa.

Advance Market Commitments

The advance market commitment (AMC) is a financing mechanism that aims to encourage investment in the development and manufacturing of vaccines that can be sold at affordable prices in low-income countries. The AMC was devised in 2005 and further refined from 2006 to 2009. It started in 2009 and is housed at Gavi.[56]

The need for a financing mechanism such as the AMC is based on the problem discussed earlier—the unwillingness of vaccine manufacturers to invest in newer vaccines that meet the needs of low-income countries because the manufacturers believe that the market for such vaccines will not be profitable. The high risks and high cost of such an investment ultimately leave suppliers with little incentive to produce. What's more, even if a manufacturer did find reason to supply vaccines, these vaccines would be unaffordable for people in low-income countries at the prices at which they would have to be sold for the manufacturers to make a profit on them.

The AMC can best be thought of as a fund that will make financing available to vaccine manufacturers under certain circumstances they agree to with the AMC management. To erase uncertainties about the market for vaccines and provide an incentive to vaccine manufacturers to produce the needed quantities of the desired vaccines, a pool of money from donors guarantees that the manufacturer will receive a set price per dose produced, provided that the manufacturers will supply a predetermined quantity of vaccines for a certain amount of time at the agreed price.

In addition, manufacturers participating in the scheme must meet certain technical criteria for vaccine quality and safety predetermined by WHO. The AMC ensures that no single supplier receives all of the funding for a particular vaccine, thereby avoiding the possibility of a monopoly and problems of supply if a sole manufacturer could not meet its production commitments.

The first AMC pilot program for a vaccine against pneumococcal disease was adopted by a group of core donors including Italy, the United Kingdom, Canada, Norway, the Russian Federation, and the Gates Foundation and became fully operational in 2009. The decision to invest in a pneumococcal vaccine for the pilot program was made by a diverse group of experts in epidemiology and vaccine manufacturing.[56] Gavi pledged to contribute $1.3 billion to this effort through 2015, with the hope of making the vaccine available to nearly 60 countries by this time.[56]

Participating manufacturers must commit to supplying a share of the 200 million doses required over 10 years. Those manufacturers must sell the vaccine at or below the predetermined price of $3.50 a dose, to ensure that the vaccine is affordable in low-income countries. Gavi and the participating country, as part of their normal cofinancing arrangements, will cover the $3.50 cost. In addition, each participating manufacturer will receive a share of the $1.5 billion AMC fund, in proportion to the supply commitment. A manufacturer, for example, who supplied 20 million doses would receive one-tenth of the AMC funding, or $150 million.[57]

Setting an appropriate price for the pneumococcal vaccine and subsidy for manufacturers was a major challenge in devising the pilot program. This is largely due to suppliers keeping information about manufacturing costs confidential. To overcome this obstacle, outside consultants helped to assess the cost of manufacturing. The fact that the two main multinational suppliers of the pneumococcal vaccine and several emerging suppliers from India all expressed interest in participating in the AMC suggests that they find the AMC price, plus the payment of AMC funds, to be reasonably remunerative.

The large number of donor and technical organizations that worked together with Gavi and low- and middle-income country partners to develop the AMC and launch the pilot is a testimony to the widespread interest in this innovative mechanism. In addition to the donors mentioned earlier, who committed $1.5 billion to the AMC, the World Bank is providing its financial services, WHO is responsible for technical matters related to the AMC, and UNICEF is leading vaccine procurement efforts.[58]

International Finance Facility for Immunisation

The International Finance Facility for Immunisation (IFFIm) is a financing mechanism that seeks "to rapidly accelerate the availability and predictability of funds for immunization." IFFIm funds are used by Gavi to accomplish its mission of "reducing the number of vaccine-preventable deaths and illnesses among children under 5."[59] IFFIm was originally launched in 2006 as a charity by the government of the United Kingdom but now includes Australia, France, Italy, the Netherlands, Norway, South Africa, Spain, and Sweden.[60] Brazil has signaled its intent to contribute to the IFFIm as well.[61]

The IFFIm was created to address the lack of secure funding for immunization in low-income countries. Another issue the IFFIm seeks to address is that donors usually provide financing on a year-to-year basis, making it hard for recipient governments to plan their budgets for programs that receive assistance, such as immunization programs. The IFFIm is meant to help ensure longer-term and more predictable financing for vaccine programs.

To ensure a reliable stream of funding for Gavi, donor countries have pledged $6.5 billion over 25 years to the facility. IFFIm sells bonds to raise this money in the capital markets of high-income countries. This makes the money available immediately, without having to wait for year-to-year financing from donor governments. The donor countries repay the bonds over time, based on their initial pledges. The fact that the IFFIm is backed by the promises of these countries allows it to maintain a good credit rating and to sell bonds at rates that are acceptable to the donor countries that have to honor the bonds.[61]

Gavi is using IFFIm funds to purchase and deliver vaccines in countries that receive its support, in addition to working with health services to strengthen immunization programs. With funding from the IFFIm, Gavi has introduced a pentavalent vaccine, which immunizes against diphtheria, pertussis, tetanus, hepatitis B, and Hib in a single vaccine.[62] In fact, the IFFIm enabled Gavi to double its spending between 2006 and 2009. By 2014, the IFFIm had provided Gavi, for example, with $191 million to purchase stockpiles of polio vaccines for use in outbreaks, more than $1 billion for the pentavalent vaccine, and about $100 million for pneumococcal vaccine.[63] An independent evaluation of the IFFIm estimated that the facility had helped Gavi save more than 2.1 million lives between 2006 and 2011.[61]

With secure funding, Gavi hopes to deliver reliable aid to countries for the long term, enabling these countries to plan and implement immunization programs more effectively. In addition, having more secure and longer-term funding allows Gavi to purchase vaccines in bulk and at lower prices than would otherwise be possible. Thus, the IFFIm hopes to enable the purchase of more vaccines with the same amount of money.

▶ Main Messages

Science and technology have the potential to make major contributions to the development of diagnostics, vaccines, drugs, and medical devices that can help address the burdens of disease in low- and middle-income countries. Progress in scientific areas like the sequencing of genes, information technology, chemistry, robotics, and biotechnology can help, for example, to engineer mosquitoes that will not carry disease, discover new drugs much more rapidly than before, and develop less expensive and more effective vaccines.

In a more ideal world, diagnostics, vaccines, drugs, and medical devices would be appropriate to the needs of the health conditions that cause the largest burden of disease in low- and middle-income countries. They would also be appropriate to the ability of countries to manage their health systems. If these were the case, they would be affordable to low-income patients and countries that are unable to spend much on health. They would also be heat stable, not require refrigeration, and be easy to store and transport. The number of pills needed to cure a disease would be few and require a short course of therapy. Ideal vaccines would be a combination of many of the vaccines that exist today, so that children would need fewer vaccinations to be fully covered. Given the risks of injections being unsafe, the delivery devices for vaccines would increasingly rely on noninvasive means, such as nasal sprays, skin patches, or, perhaps, vaccines that are edible.

Unfortunately, the needed advances are unlikely to come about on their own. This is largely a reflection of the fact that the for-profit sector has historically been a major developer of diagnostics, vaccines, and drugs but does not believe that the market for these products in low- and middle-income countries is sufficient to give it an adequate return on its investment. In addition, the public sector is risk averse and would prefer to purchase a product developed by the private sector rather than to try to develop these products itself. The failure of the market is reflected, for example, in the very small number of drugs that have been developed over the last 30 years to address the main burdens of disease among the poor in low- and middle-income countries. Moreover, vaccine development is constrained by the need for substantial investments and limited capacity in an industry with a very small number of producers.

Overcoming these market failures and encouraging the development of the desired products will probably require a series of measures. Some of these can be push mechanisms that are meant to lower the cost of research and development for the private sector. These could include, for example, direct financing of research by the government, the facilitation of clinical trials by the government, or governments offering tax credits for research and development. Push mechanisms do lower the cost of research and development, but they provide no certainty that the desired product will be produced.

Another set of efforts could focus on pull mechanisms, which are intended to help assure a satisfactory return to investors in the event that a product is produced. These mechanisms could include funding mechanisms to increase the uptake of existing vaccines, prizes, transferable patents, copayments, market assurances, and tax credits for vaccine sales. Pull mechanisms have the advantage of providing funding only when the desired product is available. However, they have the disadvantage of having to be negotiated far in advance of product availability, and parties may not be satisfied with the terms of their agreement at the time in the future when the products are available.

A mechanism already in use for vaccines and for AIDS drugs is tiered pricing. This is an arrangement in which products are sold at different prices in different markets, with the principle being that the price of sales in high-income country markets will help defray the cost of the products in low- and middle-income country markets. However, these arrangements have generally been put in place only when products were established; efforts are now under way to try to put them in place at the early stages of a product's life.

Considerable hope for new product development is being placed in public–private product development partnerships, such as the TB Alliance, the Medicines for Malaria Venture, and the Human Hookworm Vaccine Initiative. The aim of these ventures is to bring the strengths of the public and private sectors together in complementary ways that can spur the development of new products. A number of innovative financing mechanisms have also been developed to spur product development and use. In its case studies, the chapter suggests some steps that can be taken both to develop products that are needed and to see that they are widely used once they are developed.

Study Questions

1. What are some of the ideal properties that diagnostics, vaccines, and drugs should have to be most appropriate to the health and health system needs of low- and middle-income countries?

2. To what extent do some of the available vaccines for the six basic antigens and the vaccination schedule for them meet the ideal?

3. What health conditions and risk factors deserve additional attention from science and technology? Why have you chosen those conditions and risk factors?

4. What are some of the specific gaps in diagnostics, drugs, vaccines, and other medical equipment that could most improve global health if filled?

5. What have been some of the major constraints to the development of drugs and vaccines that could better meet health needs in low- and middle-income countries?

6. What steps can be taken to overcome those constraints? What are the roles in this of publicly supported research? What are the roles of public–private partnerships for health?

7. Why has only 10 percent of all research expenditure worldwide focused on the diseases that most affect the poor in low- and middle-income countries? What is the 10/90 research gap?

8. What push and pull mechanisms could most help to encourage the development of new diagnostics, drugs, and vaccines?

9. What lessons does the case study on Xpert suggest for the discovery of diagnostics, drugs, and vaccines?

10. If you were in charge of the Bill & Melinda Gates Foundation, how would you spend money on research and development of new products for global health? Why?

References

1. The World Bank. (n.d). *Data: Prevalence of HIV, total (% of population ages 15–49).* Retrieved from https://data.worldbank.org/indicator/SH.DYN.AIDS.ZS

2. Avert. (n.d.). *HIV and AIDS in South Africa.* Retrieved from https://www.avert.org/professionals/hiv-around-world/sub-saharan-africa/south-africa

3. Birn, A. E. (2005). Gates's grandest challenge: Transcending technology as public health ideology. *The Lancet, 366*(9484), 514–519.

4. UNICEF. (2010). *Facts for life* (4th ed.). Retrieved from https://www.unicef.org/publications/files/Facts_for_Life_EN_010810.pdf

5. Gavi. (n.d.). *Pentavalent vaccine support.* Retrieved from https://www.gavi.org/support/nvs/pentavalent/

6. Centers for Disease Control and Prevention. (n.d.). *BCG vaccine.* Retrieved from http://www.cdc.gov/tb/publications/factsheets/prevention/BCG.htm

7. Global Alliance for TB Drug Development. (2006, May 24). *New TB drugs urgently needed to replace treatment from the 1960s. Second Gates grant to TB Alliance quadruples initial support.* Retrieved from http://www.tballiance.org/downloads/pressreleases/PR_GatesGrant_5-23-06.pdf

8. Institute of Medicine Committee on the Economics of Antimalarial Drugs; Arrow, K. J., Panosian, C., & Gelband, H.

(Eds.). (2004). The cost and cost-effectiveness of antimalarial drugs. In *Saving lives, buying time: Economics of malaria drugs in an age of resistance* (pp. 61–78). Washington, DC: National Academies Press. Retrieved from http://www.ncbi.nlm.nih.gov/books/NBK215621/

9. MVI. (n.d.). *RTS,S.* Retrieved from https://www.malariavaccine.org/malaria-and-vaccines/first-generation-vaccine/rtss

10. Land, M., Hauser, L., Jun, S. R., Nookaew, I., Leuze, M. R., Ahn, T. H., . . . Ussery, D. W. (2015). Insights from 20 years of bacterial genome sequencing. *Functional & Integrative Genomics, 15*(2), 141–161. doi: 10.1007/s10142-015-0433-4

11. World Health Organization. (2002). *Genomics and world health: A report of the Advisory Committee on Health Research.* Retrieved from http://whqlibdoc.who.int/hq/2002/a74580.pdf

12. Weatherall, D., Greenwood, B., Chee, H. L., & Wasi, P. (2006). Science and technology for disease control: Past, present, and future. In D. T. Jamison, J. G. Breman, A. R. Measham, et al. (Eds.), *Disease control priorities in developing countries* (2nd ed., pp. 119–137). New York, NY: Oxford University Press.

13. University of Notre Dame. (2014, November 27). Genomes of malaria-carrying mosquitoes sequenced. *ScienceDaily.* Retrieved from https://www.sciencedaily.com/releases/2014/11/141127212323.htm

14. Jiang, X., Peery, A., Brantley Hall, A., Sharma, A., Chen, X. G., Waterhouse, R. M., . . . Tu, Z. (2014). Genome analysis of a major urban malaria vector mosquito, *Anopheles stephensi. Genome Biology, 15*(9). Retrieved from http://genomebiology.com/2014/15/9/459

15. Fauci, A. S. (2001). Infectious diseases: Considerations for the 21st century. *Clinical Infectious Diseases, 32*(5), 675–685.

16. Spilde, I. (2012). Edible vaccines can be grown everywhere. *ScienceNordic.* Retrieved from http://sciencenordic.com/edible-vaccines-can-be-grown-everywhere

17. Daar, A. S., Thorsteinsdottir, H., Martin, D. K., Smith, A. C., Nast, S., & Singer, P. A. (2002). Top ten biotechnologies for improving health in developing countries. *Nature Genetics, 32*(2), 229–232.

18. Grand Challenges. (n.d.). *Explore awarded grants.* Retrieved from https://grandchallenges.org/#/map

19. Mahmoud, A., Danzon, P. M., Barton, J. H., & Mugerwa, R. D. (2006). Product development priorities. In D. T. Jamison, J. G. Breman, A. R. Measham, et al. (Eds.), *Disease control priorities in developing countries* (2nd ed., pp. 139–155). New York, NY: Oxford University Press.

20. Glass, S. N., Batson, A., & Levine, R. (2006). *Issues paper: Accelerating new vaccines.* Geneva, Switzerland: Global Alliance for Vaccines and Immunisation.

21. Trouiller, P., Torreele, E., Olliaro, P., White, N., Foster, S., Wirth, D., & Pécoul, B. (2001). Drugs for neglected diseases: A failure of the market and a public health failure? *Tropical Medicine and International Health, 6*(11), 945–951.

22. Bloom, B. R., Michaud, C. M., LaMontagne, J. R., & Simonsen, L. (2006). Priorities for global research and development interventions. In D. T. Jamison, J. G. Breman, A. R. Measham, et al. (Eds.), *Disease control priorities in developing countries.* (2nd ed., pp. 103–118). New York, NY: Oxford University Press.

23. International Policy Network. (2004). *Diseases of Poverty and the 10/90 Gap.* Retrieved from https://www.who.int/intellectualproperty/submissions/InternationalPolicyNetwork.pdf

24. World Health Organization. (2014). *TDR: About us.* Retrieved from http://www.who.int/tdr/about/en/

25. Morel, C. M., Acharya, T., Broun, D., Dangi, A., Elias, C., Ganguly, N. K., . . . Yun, M. (2005). Health innovation networks to help developing countries address neglected diseases. *Science, 309*(5733), 401–404.

26. Bill & Melinda Gates Research Institute. (n.d.). *Bill & Melinda Gates Medical Research Institute.* Retrieved from https://www.gatesmri.org/

27. World Health Organization. (2011). *mHealth: New horizons for health through mobile technologies: Second global survey on eHealth.* Geneva, Switzerland: Author.

28. Lewis, T., Synowiec, C., Lagomarsino, G., & Schweitzer, J. (2012). E-health in low- and middle-income countries: Findings from the Center for Health Market Innovations. *Bulletin of the World Health Organization, 90,* 332–340. doi: 10.2471/BLT.11.099

29. Kallander, K. (2013). Mobile health (mHealth) approaches and lessons for increased performance and retention of community health workers in low- and middle-income countries: A review. *Journal of Medical Internet Research, 15*(1), e17. doi: 10.2196/jmir.2130

30. Mossman, K., McGahan, A., Mitchell, W., & Bhattacharyya, O. (2014). Evaluating high-tech health approaches in low-income countries. *Stanford Social Innovation Review.* Retrieved from http://www.ssireview.org/blog/entry/evaluating_high_tech_health_approaches_in_low_income_countries

31. Unite for Sight. (2013). *mHealth technology in global health.* Retrieved from http://www.uniteforsight.org/global-health-university/mhealth

32. Colaci, D., Chaudhri, S., & Vasan, A. (2016). mHealth interventions in low-income countries to address maternal health: A systematic review. *Annals of Global Health, 82*(5), 922–935.

33. Hurt, K., Walker, R. J, Campbell, J. A., & Egede, L. E. (2016). mHealth interventions in low and middle-income countries: A systematic review. *Global Journal of Health Science, 8*(9), 183–193. doi: 10.5539/gjhs.v8n9p183

34. World Health Organization. (2018). *Tuberculosis. Key Facts.* Retrieved from https://www.who.int/news-room/fact-sheets/detail/tuberculosis

35. Steingart, K. R., Ng, V., Henry, M., Hopewell, P. C., Ramsay, A., Cunningham, J., Urbanczik, R., . . . Pai, M. (2006). Sputum processing methods to improve the sensitivity of smear microscopy for tuberculosis: A systematic review. *The Lancet Infectious Diseases, 6*(10), 664–674. doi: 10.1016/S1473-3099(06)70602-8

36. World Health Organization. (2010). *Frequently asked questions on Xpert MTB/RIF assay.* Retrieved from http://www.who.int/tb/laboratory/xpert_faqs.pdf

37. World Health Organization. (2016). Tuberculosis diagnostics: Automated real-time DNA amplification test for rapid and simultaneous detection of TB and Rifampicin resistance: Xpert MTB/RIF assay. Retrieved from https://www.who.int/tb/publications/factsheet_xpert.pdf?ua=1

38. Blakemore, R., Story, E., Helb, D., Kop, J., Banada, P., Owens, M. R., . . . Alland, D. (2010). Evaluation of the analytical performance of the Xpert MTB/RIF assay. *Journal of Clinical Microbiology, 48*(7), 2495–2501. doi: 10.1128/jcm.00128-10

39. Theron, G., Peter, J., van Zyl-Smit, R., Mishra, H., Streicher, E., Murray, S., . . . Dheda, K. (2011). Evaluation of the Xpert MTB/RIF assay for the diagnosis of pulmonary tuberculosis in a high HIV prevalence setting. *American Journal of*

Respiratory and Critical Care Medicine, 184(1), 132–140. doi: 10.1164/rccm.201101-0056OC

40. Piatek, A. S., Van Cleeff, M., Alexander, H., Coggin, W. L., Rehr, M., Van Kampen, S., . . . Mukadi, Y. (2013). GeneXpert for TB diagnosis: Planned and purposeful implementation. *Global Health: Science and Practice, 1*(1), 18–23. doi: 10.9745/ghsp-d-12-00004

41. Schito, M., Peter, T. F., Cavanaugh, S., Piatek, A. S., Young, G. J., Alexander, H., et al. (2012). Opportunities and challenges for cost-efficient implementation of new point-of-care diagnostics for HIV and tuberculosis. *Journal of Infectious Diseases, 205*(Suppl. 2), S169–S180. doi: 10.1093/infdis/jis044

42. Meyer-Rath, G., Schnippel, K., Long, L., MacLeod, W., Sanne, I., Stevens, W., . . . Dowdy, D. W. (2012). The impact and cost of scaling up GeneXpert MTB/RIF in South Africa. *PLoS One, 7*(5), e36966. doi: 10.1371/journal.pone.0036966

43. World Health Organization. (2013). *Using the Xpert MTB/RIF assay to detect pulmonary and extrapulmonary tuberculosis and rifampicin resistance in adults and children. Expert Group Meeting Report 2013*. Geneva, Switzerland: Author.

44. Cazabom, D., Tripti Pande, T., Kirk, S., Van Gemert, W., Sohn, H., Denkinger, C., . . . Pai, M. (2018). Market penetration of Xpert MTB/RIF in high tuberculosis burden countries: A trend analysis from 2014–2016. *Gates Open Research*. Retrieved from https://gatesopenresearch.org/articles/2-35/v2

45. Helb, D., Jones, M., Story, E., Boehme, C., Wallace, E., Ho, K., . . . Alland, D. (2010). Rapid detection of mycobacterium tuberculosis and rifampin resistance by use of on-demand, near-patient technology. *Journal of Clinical Microbiology, 48*(1), 229–237. doi: 10.1128/jcm.01463-09

46. Mourad-Youssif, M., Ojengbede, O., Meyer, C., Fathalla, M., Morhason-Bello, I., Galadanci, H., . . . Miller, S. (2010). Can the non-pneumatic anti-shock garment (NASG) reduce adverse maternal outcomes from postpartum hemorrhage? Evidence from Egypt and Nigeria. *Reproductive Health, 7*(1), 24.

47. Miller, S., Martin, H. B., & Morris, J. L. Anti-shock garment in postpartum haemorrhage. *Best Practice & Research Clinical Obstetrics & Gynaecology, 22*(6), 1057–1074. doi: 10.1016/j.bpobgyn.2008.08.008

48. Vahedi, M., Ayuyao, A., Parsa, M., & Freeman, H. (1995). Pneumatic antishock garment-associated compartment syndrome in uninjured lower extremities. *Journal of Trauma, 384*(4), 616–618.

49. World Health Organization. (2011). *Non-pneumatic anti-shock garment*. Retrieved from http://www.who.int/medical_devices/innovation/new_emerging_tech_30.pdf

50. ZOEX NIASG. (n.d.). *Zoex non-inflatable anti-shock garment*. Retrieved from http://www.zoexniasg.com/

51. PATH. (n.d.). *Postpartum hemorrhage kills more new mothers than any other cause, but antishock garments can save lives*. Retrieved from http://www.path.org/projects/antishock-garment.php

52. Bixby Center for Global Reproductive Health. (n.d.). *Preganancy and childbirth*. Retrieved from http://bixbycenter.ucsf.edu/research/safe_motherhood.html

53. Sutherland, T., Downing, J., Miller, S., Bishai, D. M., Butrick, E., Fathalla, M. M., . . . Kahn, J. G. (2013). Use of the non-pneumatic anti-shock garment (NASG) for life-threatening obstetric hemorrhage: A cost-effectiveness analysis in Egypt and Nigeria. *PLoS One, 8*(4), e62282. doi: 10.1371/journal.pone.0062282

54. Jordan, K., Butrick, E., Yamey, G., & Miller, S. (2016). Barriers and facilitators to scaling up the non-pneumatic anti-shock garment for treating obstetric hemorrhage: A qualitative study. *PLoS One, 11*(3), e0150739. doi: 10.1371/journal.pone.0150739

55. This case is based on Glassman, A., Temin, M., & the Millions Saved Team and Advisory Group. (2016). Beginning of the end: Eliminating meningitis A across Africa's meningitis belt. In A. Glassman, M. Temin, & the Millions Saved Team and Advisory Group (Eds.), *Millions Saved* (pp. 13–22). Washington, DC: Center for Global Development. Those interested in a more complete account of the case and additional references will want to read the case in *Millions Saved*.

56. Cernuschi, T., et. al. (2011). Advance market commitment for pneumococcal vaccines: putting theory into practice. *Bulletin of the World Health Organization, 89*, 913–918. doi: 10.2471/BLT.11.087700

57. Gavi. (n.d.). *How the pneumococcal AMC works*. Retrieved from https://www.gavi.org/funding/pneumococcal-amc/how-the-pneumococcal-amc-works/

58. Gavi. (n.d.). *Pneumococcal AMC*. Retrieved from http://www.gavi.org/funding/pneumococcal-amc/

59. IFFIm. (n.d.). *Homepage*. Retrieved from http://www.iff-immunisation.org

60. IFFIm. (n.d.). *Overview*. Retrieved from http://www.iffim.org/about/overview/

61. Gavi. (n.d.). *International finance facility for immunisation*. Retrieved from https://www.gavi.org/funding/iffim/

62. IFFIm. (2013). *The International Finance Facility for Immunisation (IFFIm)*. Retrieved from http://www.iffim.org/Library/Publications/Factsheets/The-International-Finance-Facility-for-Immunisation-(IFFIm)--Brochure/

63. IFFIm. (n.d.). *Results*. Retrieved from http://www.iffim.org/funding-gavi/results/

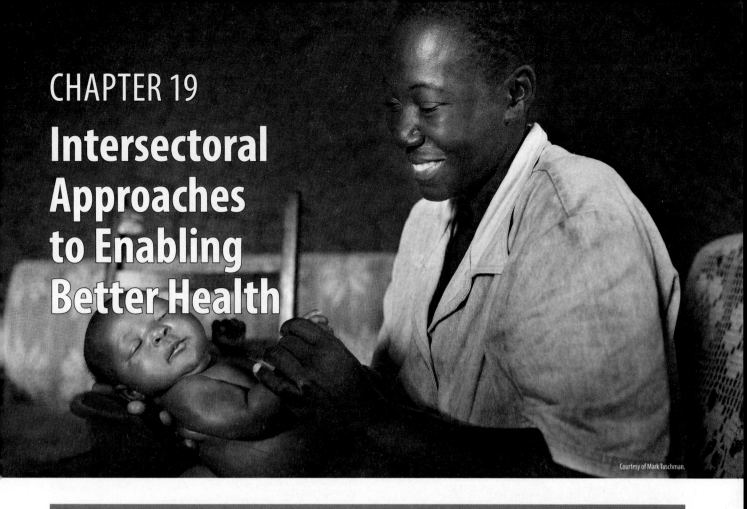

CHAPTER 19

Intersectoral Approaches to Enabling Better Health

Courtesy of Mark Tuschman.

LEARNING OBJECTIVES

By the end of this chapter, the reader will be able to do the following:

- Take a more holistic view of the factors that determine health and the range of measures across agencies that are needed to ensure better health
- Articulate the value of health impact assessments and how they are conducted
- Speak about a "health in all" perspective for government policymaking
- Note the most important policy measures that countries can take to address health through intersectoral approaches

▶ Vignettes

Juan is a 4-year-old boy in Guatemala. Juan is stunted—he is much too short for his age. It is also likely that Juan's full cognitive potential will never be realized because he has been undernourished for so long. Why has Juan failed to get sufficient nourishment? Is it because his family is poor, uneducated, or from a minority ethnic group? Is it because his family lacks access to safe water and sanitation and he frequently gets infections? Is it because of inappropriate economic and agricultural policies by the government? Or is it some combination of these factors? In any case, can the ministry of health alone adequately address the problem of undernutrition for children like Juan?

Shahnaz is a 24-year-old woman in Pakistan. She has been sick for some time with coughing, night sweats, and weight loss. She fears that she has tuberculosis (TB). However, she will not seek treatment for her illness for fear of being forced from her home by her husband's family if she *is* found to have TB. The crowded conditions in which she lives put her at risk for contracting TB. Gender norms in her country mitigate against her seeking and receiving appropriate care for TB. Can the ministry of health alone address these issues in the short or medium term? Or, will it need to work in tandem with agencies such as the ministry of education and the women's development program to help address issues related to Shahnaz's illness and her inability to seek care in a timely manner?

Josef is a heavy smoker of tobacco. He is aware of the health risks of smoking. However, he has smoked for many years, he does not feel like quitting, and he doubts, in any case, that he could quit. The ministry of health can provide information about the risks of smoking, counsel those who smoke to help them quit, and provide smoking cessation patches to smokers who say they wish to stop smoking. However, will these measures be enough to help those who currently smoke quit smoking? Will they be enough to keep young people from taking up smoking? Or, are there measures that must be taken outside of the ministry of health to make a more substantial dent in the number of smokers now and in the future?

▶ Reviewing the Determinants of Health

Key Definition

This chapter focuses on the importance of taking a broad view of health and on the role of "intersectoral approaches" to improving health. Such approaches can be defined in the following way:

Actions undertaken by sectors outside the health sector, possibly, but not necessarily, in collaboration with the health sector, on health or health equity outcomes or on the determinants of health or health equity.[1]

The Determinants of Health

Any effort to consider how intersectoral approaches can improve population health needs to start by examining what causes people to get sick, become disabled, and die and why these conditions exist. Let's begin this chapter by quickly reviewing the determinants of health and the key risk factors for health.

As you know, one's health is determined by a range of factors, as largely reflected in **FIGURE 19-1**.

Genetics and sex are intrinsic factors that are central to one's well-being. The growth and development of a child in utero, from conception to birth, also has an important impact on later health and well-being.

In addition, a range of nonintrinsic factors directly relate to one's health. Among other factors, these include the following:

- Cultural practices
- Child rearing and child caring behaviors
- Environmental and occupational factors, such as access to safe water and sanitation or the circumstances in which one is employed
- Personal health behaviors, such as those concerning nutrition, tobacco and alcohol use, and sexual practices

There is also a range of factors that exert a more indirect—but important—influence on health. Among other factors, these might include the following:

- Level of income
- Level of education

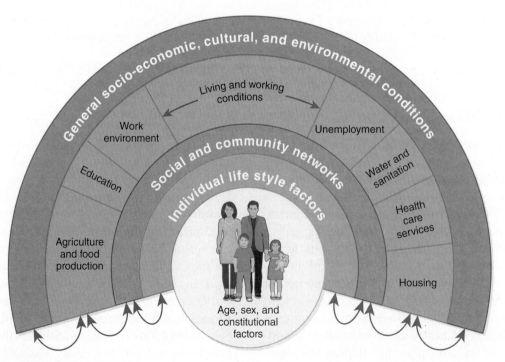

FIGURE 19-1 Key Determinants of Health

Reproduced from Dahlgren, G., & Whitehead, M. (1991). *Policies and strategies to promote social equity in health.* Stockholm, Sweden: Institute for Futures Studies. http://www.iffs.se/media/1326/20080109110739filmZ8UVQv2wQFShMRF6cuT.pdf

- Stigma and discrimination
- Gender norms

Government policies and programs and how they are implemented also exert an important influence on the health of individuals and communities. Does the government promote high-quality schooling for its children, including its female children? Does the government promote access to safe water and sanitation? Does the government seek to promote a fair society in which everyone has equal opportunities to live and thrive?

At the broadest level of thinking about the determinants of health, one can consider what the World Health Organization (WHO) calls the "social determinants of health." The WHO definition of social determinants of health is as follows:

The conditions in which people are born, grow, work, live, and age, and the wider set

of forces and systems shaping the conditions of daily life. These forces and systems include economic policies and systems, development agendas, social norms, social policies, and political systems.[2]

In any case, it is clear that one must think broadly when considering the determinants of health, moving from the most direct influences on health to the broader social forces that have a profound impact on health.

Risk Factors

As we think about why people are healthy or not, we also need to take into account the most important risk factors for illness, disability, and death. **TABLE 19-1** highlights the 10 most important risk factors for disability-adjusted life years (DALYs) in low-income, lower middle-income, upper middle-income, and high-income countries.[3]

TABLE 19-1 Top 10 Risk Factors for DALYs in 2016

Rank	Low-Income Countries	Lower Middle-Income Countries	Upper Middle-Income Countries	High-Income Countries
1	Low birthweight and short gestation	Low birthweight and short gestation	High blood pressure	Smoking
2	Child growth failure	High blood pressure	Smoking	High blood pressure
3	Household air pollution	High fasting plasma glucose	High body mass index	High body mass index
4	Unsafe water	Ambient particulate matter	High fasting plasma glucose	High fasting plasma glucose
5	Unsafe sex	Smoking	Alcohol use	Alcohol use
6	Unsafe sanitation	Child growth failure	High total cholesterol	High total cholesterol
7	No access to handwashing facility	High body mass index	Ambient particulate matter	Low whole grains
8	High blood pressure	Household air pollution	High sodium	Drug use
9	Ambient particulate matter	High total cholesterol	Low whole grains	Impaired kidney function
10	High fasting plasma glucose	Unsafe water	Low fruit	Low fruit

Data from Institute of Health Metrics and Evaluation (IHME). (n.d.). GBD Compare: Viz Hub. Retrieved from https://vizhub.healthdata.org/gbd-compare/

As shown in the table, some of the most important attributable risk factors for DALYs include the following:

- Undernutrition
- Other dietary risks
- High fasting plasma glucose
- High body mass index
- Unsafe sex
- Tobacco use
- Alcohol use
- Lack of safe water and sanitation
- Air pollution

As one thinks about risk factors and how they might be addressed, it is useful to categorize those risk factors. One of a number of ways to do this is as follows[4]:

- *Intrinsic risk factors, such as age, sex, and genetic makeup:* These cannot be modified but have an important relationship with well-being.
- *Diseases as risk factors for other diseases*: Some diseases are risk factors for other diseases, such as diabetes for cardiovascular disease.
- *Behavioral and environmental risk factors*: Some of the important behavioral risk factors include diet, physical activity, tobacco smoking, and excessive alcohol use. Some of the important environmental risk factors include household air pollution, unsafe water, and unsafe sanitation. The circumstances under which people live and work also may be related to environmental risk factors.

The Burden of Behavioral and Environmental Risk Factors

As shown in **TABLE 19-2**, DCP3 estimates of the global burden of disease included data on the proportion of deaths attributable to behavioral and environmental risk factors for the three groups of diseases listed in the table.[5]

As we can see in the table, 20 percent to 30 percent of all deaths in 2015 are estimated to have been attributable to behavioral and environmental risk factors. This is a substantial proportion of all deaths, and addressing these risk factors successfully would lead to a significant improvement in health in a range of settings.

It is important to remember that the determinants of health and risk factors may be linked to one or more health conditions in a variety of different ways. A single risk factor could be associated with a number of different health conditions. Outdoor air pollution, for example, is linked to chronic obstructive pulmonary disease, asthma, heart disease, and lung cancer. In addition, several risk factors can overlap and interact. This is the case, for example, with some of the risk factors for cardiovascular disease, such as tobacco smoking, high body mass index, and low physical activity. Those interested may wish to explore further the "pathways" for the influence of different determinants and risk factors for different health conditions.[4]

TABLE 19-2 Magnitude of the Impact of Top Environmental and Behavioral Risk Factors on Major Causes of Death

	Number of Deaths Globally in 2015	Proportion of Deaths Attributable to Behavioral or Environmental Risks	Top Risk Factors
Communicable, maternal, perinatal, and nutritional conditions	12 million	30%	Unsafe water, sanitation, and handwashing; maternal and child nutritional risks; unsafe sex; air pollution; tobacco smoke
Noncommunicable diseases	40 million	24%	Dietary risks; tobacco smoke; air pollution; alcohol and drug use; low physical activity; occupational hazards
Injuries	5 million	20%	Alcohol and drug use

Watkins, D. A., Nugent, R., Saxenian, H., Yamey, G., Danforth, K., González-Pier, E., . . . Jamison, D. T. (2018). Intersectoral policy priorities for health. In D. T. Jamison, H. Gelband, S. Horton, et al. (Eds.), *Disease control priorities: Improving health and reducing poverty* (3rd ed., Vol. 09, pp. 23–42). Washington, DC: The World Bank.

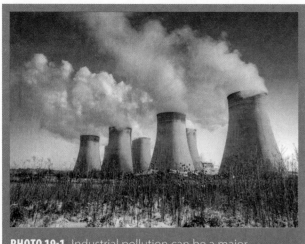

PHOTO 19-1 Industrial pollution can be a major public health hazard. What measures can be taken to reduce the public health impact of industries that are major sources of pollution? What agencies must be responsible for leading these efforts?
© Bill Brooks/Moment/Getty Images.

The Role of Intersectoral Approaches in Addressing the Determinants of Health and Health Risk Factors

Let's now ask ourselves the following:

■ What is the extent to which the determinants of health and critical risk factors can be addressed by actions within the health sector?

■ What is the extent to which they can be addressed only through actions by agencies outside the health sector or by those agencies in collaboration with the health sector?

Intrinsic Risk Factors and Risk Factors Related to Fetal Development

Intrinsic risk factors cannot be changed, except perhaps by highly scientific, technological, or medical means that are generally within the purview of the health system. If a person is born with a genetic disorder, it would normally fall upon the health system to diagnose and treat that disorder, if possible. There would be little or no role in diagnosis and treatment from agencies outside the health sector.

The factors that relate to the development of a healthy newborn are complex. They include, among many other things, the nutritional, educational, and income status of the mother; whether or not the mother smokes tobacco or engages in the abuse of other substances; and the access of the mother to prenatal care and a delivery attended by a skilled healthcare provider. Clearly, the ministry of health is responsible for prenatal care and skilled attendance at delivery. However, the other factors noted depend exclusively or largely on other agencies. Policies of the ministry of agriculture have a strong influence on nutritional status. Educational status will depend to a large degree on the ministry of education. Policies and programs related to tobacco use and substance abuse will depend not only on the ministry of health but also on the ministry of finance and law enforcement agencies, among others.

Diseases as Risk Factors for Other Diseases

We generally assume that the health sector would be the main, if not sole, actor in dealing with diseases that are risk factors for other diseases, such as diabetes as a risk factor for cardiovascular disease, human papilloma virus (HPV) as a risk factor for cervical cancer, or hepatitis B as a risk factor for liver cancer.

However, the diseases that are risk factors for other diseases also have risk factors themselves. Some of these underlying risk factors are social and behavioral in nature. Solutions to these issues typically do involve the ministry of health. Nonetheless, there is often an important role for intersectoral approaches in addressing the underlying risk factors of the diseases that are risk factors for other diseases.

Several key risk factors for diabetes, for example, relate to nutrition (such as "undernutrition, other dietary risks, high-fasting plasma glucose, and high body mass index").[3] These can be most comprehensively addressed with support from outside the health sector. Appropriate infant and child feeding practices depend on the level of education of the caregivers and their ability to buy healthy foods for their children. These relate largely to policies on education, agriculture, and a range of social matters. Moreover, the price of foods and their availability, for both children and adults, also relate to government economic and agricultural policies. In addition, a person's health depends on access to safe water and sanitation, which relates mostly to infrastructure policies and programs. A person's ability to get enough physical activity depends partly on access to recreational facilities and the extent to which people see them as safe. These generally fall under the purview of urban planners and law enforcement agencies.

Unsafe sex is a risk factor for HPV, a sexually transmitted infection (STI) that is a risk factor for cervical cancer. Unsafe sex is also a risk factor for human immunodeficiency virus (HIV), which, in turn, is a risk factor for a number of diseases, such as TB. The health sector *can* implement health promotion activities that encourage monogamous sexual relationships, the use of a condom to promote safer sex, medical male circumcision, and testing and treatment for STIs, including HIV/AIDS. However, some aspects of unsafe sex can only be addressed outside the ministry of health. The ability of a woman to negotiate safe sex practices relates to her level of education and income and her social standing, which are strongly linked to societal gender norms. In addition, there is evidence that the longer girls stay in school, the later their sexual debut, the more social autonomy they have, and the fewer risks they face of becoming infected with HIV.[6,7] These factors are determined largely by matters *outside* of the health sector, such as policies that promote gender equality and girls' education. Once again, effectively addressing key risk factors requires a combination of efforts within *and* outside the health sector.

Social and Behavioral Risk Factors

Many social and behavioral risk factors also must be addressed by going beyond the health sector, as one can see in the examples discussed next.

Tobacco use is a leading risk factor for death and disability across the world for cardiovascular disease and cancer. The health ministry *can* engage in health promotion to discourage tobacco use. The health ministry *can* also provide counseling services for patients and prescribe nicotine replacement therapy. However, there is considerable evidence that the best way to reduce the uptake and consumption of tobacco is through taxation of tobacco, which is usually controlled by the ministry of finance.[8,9] Other measures to reduce the consumption of tobacco, such as banning advertising and sales to minors and reducing hours for sales of tobacco, are led by agencies outside the health sector, such as law enforcement.[8,9] Thus, while the health sector can help address tobacco consumption, the most effective measures to address it are controlled outside the health sector.

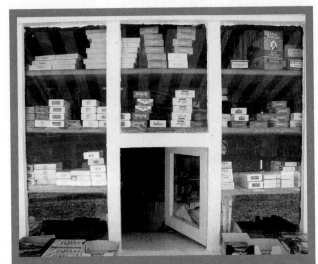

PHOTO 19-2 This kiosk in Greece sells cigarettes. The single best way to reduce consumption of tobacco is to levy very high taxes on cigarettes. Which ministries would have to be involved in decisions about such taxes? Which ministries would need to be involved in discussions of other parts of a package to reduce consumption, including prohibiting sales to minors, banning advertising, and putting warning labels on cigarette packages?
© Steve Outram/Photographer's Choice RF/Getty Images.

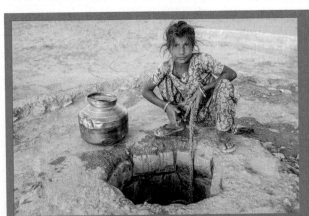 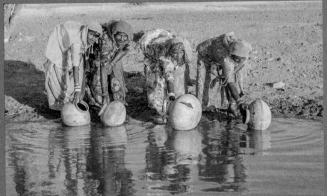

PHOTO 19-3 & 19-4 Many people in the world, like those shown in these photos from Rajasthan state, India, continue to get their water from uncovered wells or open sources, like lakes and rivers. This contributes to the large and sometimes deadly burden of diarrheal disease. The ministry of health can promote safer use of water, better sanitation, and handwashing with soap. However, it is usually not responsible for making investments in water and sanitation. What kind of cooperation across ministries must a government promote if it is to improve access to safe water and sanitation? What ministry is likely to be in charge of such investments?
© Hadynyah/E+/Getty Images.

The lack of safe water and sanitation and poor hygiene practices are major risk factors for ill health, especially in low-income countries. The health ministry *can* encourage the use of safe water and the sanitary disposal of human waste. It *can* promote handwashing with soap before eating and after defecating. However, ministries of urban or rural development or of civil works are generally in charge of water and sanitation infrastructure, and they must play a central role in ensuring better access to these important investments.

Air pollution generally relates to a range of factors, almost all of which are *outside* the direct control of the ministry of health. These include industrial policies and regulation of pollutants, such as coal and lead. The amount of air pollution also depends on policies that encourage the use of more efficient stoves and clean fuels, especially by the poor—and this, too, is beyond the ministry of health. Policies set outside of the health ministry about the use of vehicles will also have an important bearing on air pollution.

One can see in these examples the importance of intersectoral approaches to addressing key determinants of health and health risk factors.

▶ Policy and Program Approaches to Addressing Intersectoral Issues

The "Whole of Government" or "Health in All Policies" Approach

There are several ways in which countries can organize themselves to address health issues that require an intersectoral approach.[10] One such approach is called "health in all policies" or a "whole of government" approach. In this case, all ministries in a government are required to account for the health implications of their policies, plans, and programs. To varying degrees, Cuba, England, New Zealand, and Norway take such an approach to improving the health of their populations. The central government of these countries asks *all* government agencies to work together to maximize the health of their people and/or to reduce inequities in health.[1(p7)]

Achieving a successful "health in all policies" approach, however, may require more organizational and management capacity than may be available in some low- and middle-income countries.[10] Nonetheless, most of these countries could seek opportunities to work across sectors on specific health issues that require an intersectoral approach. The government, for example, might choose to address some of the biggest risks, such as tobacco, with an intersectoral approach.

A coordinating committee could then oversee that effort.[11] The ministry of health could engage in health awareness activities about tobacco; the ministry of commerce could limit advertising, sales to minors, and sales hours; the ministry of agriculture could promote alternative crops for tobacco farmers; and the ministry of finance could oversee the raising of taxes on tobacco.

A number of countries have taken this type of approach to addressing critical issues in health or health disparities:

- Uganda established intersectoral committees with representatives from multiple ministries to deal with the health (and other needs) of internally displaced people during a period of conflict in the north of the country.[1(p25)]
- In India, the Sonagachi Project took an intersectoral approach to trying to prevent infection of commercial sex workers with HIV. The project included a number of interventions aimed at enhancing the self-confidence of sex workers, their income earning ability, and their ability to negotiate safe sex. These encompassed, for example, literacy and cultural programs, training in political activism and advocacy, and microcredit schemes for the sex workers.[1(p34)]
- The municipality of Cotacachi in Ecuador created an intersectoral health council that engaged the local offices of the ministries of health and education and was associated with the elimination of maternal and child deaths and a dramatic decline in illiteracy.[1(p33)]

Health Impact Assessments

Governments also might gain a better understanding of the intersectoral actions needed to address some health issues by carrying out a **health impact assessment**.[12] A health impact assessment has been defined by WHO as follows:

> A combination of procedures, methods and tools by which a policy, program or project may be judged as to its potential effects on the health of a population, and the distribution of those effects within the population.[12]

Alternatively, the U.S. National Academies of Sciences, Engineering, and Medicine have defined health impact assessment in this way:

> A structured process that uses scientific data, professional expertise, and stakeholder input to identify and evaluate public health consequences of proposals and suggests actions that could be taken to minimize adverse health impacts and optimize beneficial ones.[13(p3)]

The purpose of the health impact assessment is to examine the health consequences of activities across a range of economic sectors. The findings of health impact assessments should provide policy makers with the information they need to maximize the positive effects of investments and minimize the negative effects.

The most effective health impact assessments do the following[14]:

- Bring together and take account of the views of a wide range of stakeholders
- Take a broad perspective, looking at social, economic, and environmental issues, among other factors
- Examine *whose* health is likely to be affected by the investment that is being assessed
- Provide policy makers with data-driven recommendations about how to minimize the adverse effects of the proposed investment and maximize its health gains

Let's examine briefly why health impact assessments can be so valuable. Investments in roads, for example, might produce substantial economic benefits. At the same time, the construction of the road and the road itself might be associated with pooling water and an increase in mosquito-borne diseases or an increase in traffic injuries. The use of fertilizer and pesticides can produce larger crop yields, which can help address undernutrition and improve young child health.

However, if not used properly, these chemicals might lead to poisonings among some of the people who handle them. New manufacturing plants can create job opportunities and other economic benefits, but if not regulated carefully, they might also lead to increased air pollution or toxic industrial waste. If health impact assessments are carried out during the planning of investments like those noted above, governments can identify potential health risks of the investment and propose measures for preventing or mitigating them.

Putting Together an Intersectoral Policy Package

A recent study examined the importance of intersectoral approaches to addressing environmental, social, and behavioral risk factors and how they might be structured in different country settings.[4] That study concluded that intersectoral policies could usefully be divided into four categories: taxes and subsidies, regulation and related enforcement mechanisms, policies related to the built environment, and policies concerning the provision of information. The study identified 79 intersectoral policies to be of greatest priority.[4] The study further concluded that about half of those policies, as summarized in **TABLE 19-3**, should be adopted at an early stage, even in low-income and lower middle-income countries.

The study also highlighted that those countries that have been able to make the most progress in

TABLE 19-3 Recommended Intersectoral Policies		
Key Health Risk	**Policy Instruments**	**Key Ministries to Engage**
Air pollution	■ Fiscal measures and regulations to reduce carbon emissions	■ Finance
	■ Subsidies and regulations to support cleaner household fuels	■ Energy ■ Transport
	■ Building and strengthening affordable public transportation systems in urban areas	■ Statistical services
	■ Implementing national monitoring systems that track all sources of air pollution	
Tobacco smoke	■ Large excise taxes on tobacco products	■ Finance ■ Law enforcement
	■ Bans on smoking in public places and on advertising, promotion, and sponsorship, with adequate enforcement	■ Industry ■ Agriculture ■ Sports
	■ Warning labels and plain packaging on tobacco products	■ Education

Dietary risks	■ Fortification of food products with iron and folic acid	■ Agriculture
		■ Industry
	■ Iodization of salt products	■ Education
	■ Bans on trans fats and replacement with polyunsaturated fats	
	■ Actions to reduce salt in manufactured food products and discourage discretionary use	
	■ Product taxes on sugar-sweetened beverages	
	■ Actions to discourage consumption of unhealthy foods, including restrictions on marketing to children and sales in schools	
Injuries	■ Excise taxes on alcohol products	■ Finance
		■ Transport
	■ Restrictions on access to retail alcohol	■ Industry
		■ Environment
	■ Regulations on drunk driving, including enforcement of blood alcohol concentration limits	■ Planning
	■ Legislation and enforcement of personal transport safety measures, including seatbelts in vehicles, and helmets for motorcycle users	
	■ Setting and enforcement of speed limits on roads	
	■ Adoption of and strict control over selective bans on highly hazardous pesticides	
Other environmental risks	■ National standards for safe drinking water and sanitation within and outside of households	■ Public works
		■ Environment
	■ Legislation and enforcement of standards for hazardous waste disposal	■ Industry
		■ Agriculture
	■ Actions to reduce human exposure to lead, including bans on leaded fuels and phase-out of lead-based consumer products	■ Food and drug administration
	■ Reduction and eventual phase-out of subtherapeutic antibiotic use in agriculture	

Watkins, D. A., Nugent, R., Saxenian, H., Yamey, G., Danforth, K., González-Pier, E., . . . Jamison, D. T. (2018). Intersectoral policy priorities for health. In D. T. Jamison, H. Gelband, S. Horton, et al. (Eds.), *Disease control priorities: Improving health and reducing poverty* (3rd ed., pp. 23–42). Washington, DC: The World Bank.

reducing air pollution and road traffic injuries took an intersectoral approach.[4]

The study also focuses attention on the exceptional importance of the ministry of finance in helping to lead and to address health risks. That ministry, for example, would deal with taxes on tobacco and alcohol. That ministry also might levy taxes on sugar or sugary beverages or on highly polluting processes, such as vehicular emissions. In addition, the ministry of finance could limit subsidies that are detrimental to health, such as those encouraging the production of unhealthy food or fossil fuels.[4]

▶ Main Messages

An important part of the burden of disease can only be addressed effectively through intersectoral approaches—actions by agencies outside the health sector alone or in combination with the health sector. This stems from the fact that an important share of the determinants of health and health risk factors concern matters outside of the health sector, such as economic and social policies, education, the lack of access to safe water and sanitation, and the economic costs of engaging in certain behaviors, such as tobacco smoking.

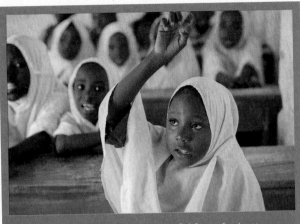

PHOTO 19-5 Education is a powerful force for better health and overall development. The education of females is especially important. How do you think that the education of these young girls in Nigeria will be linked to their better health and the better health of their own families?

Courtesy of Mark Tuschman.

One way to engage in intersectoral action in health would be for a government to take a "health in all" or "whole of government" approach. In this case, all government agencies work together to examine the health impact of their work and how their agencies can be involved in enhancing health. However, this may require a level of governance that is beyond that of many countries. Nonetheless, countries with less administrative capacity can encourage agencies to work together on selected

health issues of the greatest consequence, such as tobacco use.

Another valuable approach to identifying and mitigating health issues related to different economic and social endeavors is the health impact assessment. This is a review, carried out with the participation of a wide range of stakeholders, of the potential health impact of investments, who will be affected, and how health risks from the investment can be eliminated, mitigated, or otherwise addressed. The information gained from a health impact assessment can help guide intersectoral action in health.

There are a wide range of intersectoral actions that are essential in addressing an important share of the determinants of health. An important study recently suggested that low- and middle-income countries should prioritize a package of such efforts, including, for example, intersectoral measures to address air pollution and other environmental risks, tobacco smoking, dietary risks, and injuries. The study further highlighted the importance of ministries of finance to these efforts, including through the use of fiscal policy tools, such as tobacco taxes and taxes on sweetened beverages.[4]

Successfully addressing an important share of the burden of disease in today's low- and middle-income countries requires a holistic approach to identify the determinants of disease, disability, and death. It also requires a holistic approach to identify the efforts that need to be taken to address key health issues by the ministry of health, by that ministry in collaboration with other agencies, and by other agencies alone.

Note

This chapter is based, to an important extent, on Watkins, D. A., Nugent, R., Saxenian, H., Yamey, G., Danforth, K., González-Pier, E., . . . Jamison, D. T. (2018). Intersectoral policy priorities for health. In D. T.

Jamison, H. Gelband, S. Horton, et al. (Eds.), *Disease control priorities: Improving health and reducing poverty* (3rd ed., pp. 23–42) Washington, DC: The World Bank.

References

1. Public Health Agency of Canada and World Health Organization. (2008). *Health equity through intersectoral action: An analysis of 18 country case studies.* Retrieved from http://www.who.int/social_determinants/resources/health_equity_isa_2008_en.pdf
2. World Health Organization. (n.d.). *Social determinants of health.* Retrieved from http://www.who.int/social_determinants/sdh_definition/en/
3. Institute of Health Metrics and Evaluation (IHME). (n.d.). GBD Compare: Viz Hub. Retrieved from https://vizhub.healthdata.org/gbd-compare/
4. Watkins, D. A., Nugent, R., Saxenian, H., Yamey, G., Danforth, K., González-Pier, E., . . . Jamison, D. T. (2018). Intersectoral policy priorities for health. In D. T. Jamison, H. Gelband, S. Horton, et al. (Eds.), *Disease control priorities:*

Improving health and reducing poverty (3rd ed., pp. 23–42) Washington, DC: The World Bank.
5. GBD 2015 Risk Factors Collaborators. (2016). Global, regional, and national comparative risk assessment of 79 behavioural, environmental and occupational, and metabolic risks or clusters of risks, 1990–2015: A systematic analysis for the Global Burden of Disease Study 2015. *The Lancet, 388*(10053),1659–1724.
6. Baird, S., Chirwa, E., McIntosh, C., & Özler, B. (2010). The short-term impacts of a schooling conditional cash transfer program on the sexual behavior of young women. *Health Economics, 19,* 55–68. doi:10.1002/hec.1569
7. Jukes, M., Simmons, S., & Bundy, D. (2008). Education and vulnerability: The role of schools in protecting young women and girls from HIV in Southern Africa. *AIDS, 22*(4), S41–S46.

8. Jha, P., Chaloupka, F. J., Moore J., Gajalakshmi, V., Gupta, P. C., Peck, R., . . . Musgrove, P. (2006). Tobacco addiction. In D. T. Jamison, J. G. Breman, A. R. Measham, et al. (Eds.), *Disease control priorities in developing countries* (2nd ed., pp. 869–885). New York, NY: Oxford University Press.

9. Jha, P., MacLennan, M., Yurekli, A., Ramasundarahettige, C., Palipudi, K., et al. Global hazards of tobacco and the benefits of smoking cessation and tobacco tax. In Gelband, G., Jha, P., Sankaranarayanan, R., & Horton, S. (Eds.), *Disease control priorities*, Vol. 3: *Cancer* (3rd ed.). Washington, DC: The World Bank.

10. Khayatzadeh-Mahani, A., Sedoghi, Z., Mehrolhassani, M. H., & Yazdi-Feyzabadi, V. (2016). How health in all policies are developed and implemented in a developing country? A case study of a HiAP initiative in Iran. *Health Promotion International, 31*(4), 769–781. doi: 10.1093/heapro/dav062

11. World Health Organization. (2011). *Intersectoral action on health: A path for policy-makers to implement effective and sustainable action on health.* Retrieved from http://www.who.int/kobe_centre/publications/intersectoral _action_health2011/en/

12. World Health Organization. (n.d.). *Health impact assessment (HIA): Definitions of HIA.* Retrieved from http://www.who .int/hia/about/defin/en/

13. Committee on Health Impact Assessment, National Research Council. (2011). *Improving health in the United States: The role of health impact assessment.* Washington, DC: National Academies Press.

14. The Pew Charitable Trusts. (n.d.). *Health Impact Project: Health impact assessment.* Retrieved from http://www .pewtrusts.org/en/projects/health-impact-project/health -impact-assessment

Glossary

A

Abortion Premature expulsion or loss of embryo, which may be induced or spontaneous.

Acceptable risk/benefit ratio The balance that needs to be attained for participants in research that maximizes social value and minimizes potential harm.

Adenolymphangitis (ADL) One of the clinical signs of lymphatic filariasis, it involves the recurrent attacks of fever and inflammation of the lymph nodes.

Adolescent A person from 10 to 19 years of age.

Ancillary care Medical care that is provided to research participants but that is not required by the scientific design of the study.

Anemia Low level of hemoglobin in the blood.

Antigen Any substance that can induce an immune response in the body.

Arm In a research study, the comparison group that receives an established treatment, a placebo, or nothing at all.

Asphyxia A condition of severely deficient oxygen supply to the body.

Asylum-seeker A person claiming protection outside of their home country whose request for sanctuary has yet to be processed.

Attack rate The cumulative incidence of infection in a group observed over a period of time during an epidemic.

B

Barrier analysis A study approach that focuses on trying to understand barriers to the adoption of positive health behaviors so that more effective behavior change communication messages and support activities can be developed.

Behavioral approach A component of combination prevention for HIV involving efforts to change people's behavior so they have less risk of becoming infected with HIV.

Behavioral change In health, this refers to changing people's behaviors so they engage in more health-enabling behaviors, such as giving up tobacco consumption or wearing seat belts.

Biomedical approach A component of combination prevention for HIV infection involving interventions such as male medical circumcision, treating sexually transmitted infections, and antiretroviral therapy.

Bipolar disorder A brain disorder, also known as manic-depressive illness, that brings unusual shifts in mood, energy, activity levels, and the ability to carry out day-to-day tasks.

Blood glucose Blood sugar that is transported through the bloodstream to the body cells for energy.

Body mass index Body weight in kilograms divided by height in meters squared.

Brain drain The migration of health personnel in search of a better standard of living and quality of life, higher salaries, access to advanced technology, and more stable political conditions in different places worldwide.

Burden of disease A term used to describe the combination of morbidity, disability, and mortality, usually measured in DALYs in global health work

C

Caesarean delivery (section) The delivery of a fetus by surgical incision through the abdominal wall and uterus.

Cancer Cancer refers to a range of diseases characterized by body cells that divide without stopping and spread to surrounding tissues.

Cardiovascular disease A disease of the heart or blood vessels.

Cascade of care (also called HIV care continuum) A model that outlines the sequential steps or stages of HIV medical care that people living with HIV go through, from initial diagnosis to achieving the goal of viral suppression. There are also cascades of care for dealing with other diseases, such as TB.

Case fatality rate The proportion of cases of a specified condition that are fatal within a specified period of time.

Case management (treatment) and improved care giving An approach to communicable disease control (and for other health conditions) involving a collaborative process of assessment, planning, facilitation, care coordination, evaluation, and advocacy for options and services to meet an individual's and family's comprehensive health needs.

Case surveillance, reporting, and containment An approach to communicable disease control involving identification of cases, epidemiological analysis, and systematic planning to immediately contain each case to eliminate the possibility of further transmission.

Cataract A clouding of the lens of the eye.

CD4 cell count CD4 cells are white blood cells that can serve as an indicator of the health of the immune system; a normal count is between 500 and 1,500 cells/mm^3 of blood.

Child The UN Convention on the rights of the child defines a child as anyone under 18 years of age, unless the laws in their country give them majority status before that age.

Cholesterol A waxy, fat-like substance that is found in all cells of the body.

Chronic disease A disease or condition that lasts a long time, usually a year or more.

Chronic obstructive pulmonary disease (COPD) Chronic lung disease that cause limitations in lung airflow.

Climate change The increase in the earth's average temperature that has been observed and the consequences that might be associated with this rise in temperature.

Communicable diseases (also called infectious diseases) Illnesses that are caused by a particular infectious agent and that spread directly or indirectly from people to people, from animals to animals, from animals to people, or from people to animals.

Complex emergency (also called complex humanitarian emergency) A humanitarian crisis marked by a natural and/or man-made disaster, such as warfare or major civil disturbance, that results in an extensive loss of life, displacement of populations, and overall damage to society. Complex emergencies necessitate international multifaceted assistance.

Conditional cash transfer A payment to families on an agreed-upon time frame, provided that the family engages in agreed-upon nutrition, health, or education behaviors.

Contracting in (health services) One level of government or a public institution contracts with a lower level of government facility, such as a district, a province, or another facility, to deliver services.

Contracting out (health services) A financing agency (government, insurance entity, or development partner), also known as a "purchaser," provides resources to a non-state provider (NSP, such as an NGO or private sector firm), also known as a "contractor," to provide a specified set of services, in a specified location, with specified objectives.

Control (disease control) Reduction of disease incidence, prevalence, morbidity, or mortality to a locally acceptable level.

Cost-effectiveness analysis In health, a tool for comparing the relative cost of two or more investments with the amount of health that can be purchased with those investments.

Cretinism A condition of severely stunted physical and mental growth owing to untreated congenital deficiency of thyroid hormone, usually as a result of iodine deficiency.

Crude mortality rate The proportion of people who die from a population at risk over a specified period of time.

Cultural competence The ability to interact effectively with people of different cultures.

Cultural humility A lifelong process of self-reflection and self-critique whereby the individual not only learns about another's culture but also examines her/his own beliefs and cultural identities.

Cultural relativism The concept that because cultures are unique, they can be evaluated only according to their own standards and values.

Culture A set of rules or standards shared by members of a society that, when acted upon by the members, produce behavior that falls within a range of variation that members consider proper and acceptable.

D

Death rate The number of deaths per 1,000 population in a given year.

Degenerative disease A disease resulting from the continuous deterioration of tissues or organs.

Demographic dividend The growth in an economy when there is a change in the age structure of society from declining fertility and declining mortality. This change leads to a larger share of the population being of working age.

Demographic transition The shift from high fertility and high mortality to low fertility and low mortality.

Depression Clinical depression is a mood disorder in which feelings of sadness, loss, anger, or frustration interfere with activities of everyday life for a significant period.

Determinants of health The range of personal, social, economic, and environmental factors that determine the health status of individuals or populations.

Diabetes Medical illness caused by too little insulin or poor response to insulin.

Diarrhea A condition in which the sufferer has frequent and watery or loose bowel movements.

Disability The temporary or long-term reduction in a person's capacity to function.

Disability-adjusted life year (DALY) A composite measure of premature deaths and losses due to disabilities in a population.

Disaster Any occurrence that causes damage, ecological destruction, loss of human lives, or deterioration of health and health services on a scale sufficient to warrant an extraordinary response from outside the affected community area.

Disease The malfunctioning or maladaptation of biologic and psychophysiological processes in the individual.

Displaced person A person who is forced to leave his or her locality of residence in order to flee from or avoid the effects of war, natural disaster, persecution, or violations of human rights.

Dowry The gift that a bride's family gives to the family of a groom.

Dowry death The murder or suicide of a married woman caused by a dispute over her dowry.

Drug resistance The extent to which infectious and parasitic agents develop an ability to resist drug treatment.

E

Eclampsia A serious, life-threatening condition in late pregnancy in which very high blood pressure can cause a woman to have seizures.

eHealth The delivery of health care by electronic means.

Elderly support ratio The ratio between the number of people who are 15 to 64 years of age, compared with the number who are 65 years of age or older.

Elephantiasis The hardening or thickening of the skin, also known as lymphatic filariasis, caused by an infection transmitted through mosquitoes.

Elimination (of disease) Reduction of case transmission to a predetermined very low level.

Emerging infectious disease A newly discovered disease.

Environment External physical, chemical, and microbiological exposures and processes that impinge upon individuals and groups and are beyond the immediate control of individuals.

Environmental health A set of public health efforts that is concerned with preventing disease, death, and disability by reducing exposure to adverse environmental conditions and promoting behavior change. It focuses on the direct and indirect causes of disease and injuries and taps resources inside and outside the healthcare system to help improve health outcomes.

Epidemiologic transition A shift in the pattern of disease from largely communicable diseases to noncommunicable diseases.

Epidemiology The study of the patterns and causes of disease in specific populations and the application of this information to control health problems.

Equity Fairness.

Eradication (of disease) Reduction to zero globally of the incidence of any infectious disease.

Essential surgery Surgery for conditions that are mainly or extensively treated by surgery (procedures and other surgical care), have a large health burden, and can be successfully treated by a surgical procedure (and other surgical care) that is cost-effective and feasible to promote globally.

Ethnocentrism The evaluation of other cultures according to the standards and customs of one's own culture.

Exclusive breastfeeding (EBF) The practice of giving only breastmilk to an infant for the first 6 months of life.

Extensive drug resistance (XDR) Resistance to any fluoroquinolone, and at least one of three second-line injectable TB-drugs (capreomycin, kanamycin, and amikacin), in addition to multidrug resistance.

F

Fair subject selection The equitable distribution of the benefits and burdens of research through the enrollment of participants in a study.

Fairness of financial contribution The risks each household faces due to the costs of the health system are distributed according to ability to pay rather than to the risk of illness.

Family planning The conscious effort of couples to regulate the number and spacing of births through artificial and natural methods of contraception; connotes conception control to avoid pregnancy and abortion, but also includes efforts of couples to induce pregnancy.

Female genital mutilation (also called female circumcision and female genital cutting) A collective term for various traditional practices that are all related to the cutting of the female genital organs; four different forms and grades are usually distinguished.

Financial protection Financing health care in a way that does not cause people to be denied access to health care or to become impoverished because of their inability to pay for health services.

Folk illnesses Local, cultural interpretations of physical states that people perceive to be illnesses without a physiological cause.

Foodborne (illness) A disease originating from the contamination of food.

Food security A state when people have availability and adequate access at all times to sufficient, safe, nutritious food to maintain a healthy and active life.

G

Gender The behavioral, cultural, or psychological traits typically associated with one sex.

Gestational diabetes or gestational diabetes mellitus Diabetes that develops during pregnancy because of improper regulation of blood sugar; it usually goes away after delivery, but can increase the woman's risk of developing type II diabetes later.

Global health Health problems, issues, and concerns that transcend national boundaries and may best be addressed by cooperative actions.

Global public good Goods or services that benefit everyone and exclude no one.

Governance The actions and means adopted by a society to organize itself in the promotion and protection of its population.

Gram-negative bacteria A form of bacteria that appears red or pink when stained with a purple-colored stain and that can cause many types of infections.

Gross domestic product The total market value of all the goods and services produced within a country during a specified period of time.

Gross national product A measure of the incomes of residents of a country, including income they receive from abroad but subtracting similar payments made to those abroad.

H

Health A state of complete mental, physical, and emotional well-being and not merely the absence of disease or infirmity.

Health-adjusted life expectancy (HALE) A composite health indicator that measures the equivalent number of years in full health that a newborn can expect to live, based on current rates of ill health and mortality.

Health disparities A type of difference in health that is closely linked with social or economic disadvantage.

Health equity The achievement of health and the capability to achieve good health, including the fairness of processes.

Health impact assessment A combination of procedures, methods, and tools by which a policy, program, or project may be judged as to its potential effects on the health of a population, and the distribution of those effects within the population.

Health inequality Differences in health status or in the distribution of health determinants between different population groups.

Health inequity Differences in health that are not only unnecessary and avoidable but also unfair and unjust.

Health literacy The degree to which individuals have the capacity to obtain, process, and understand basic health information and services needed to make appropriate health decisions.

Health maximization The allocation of healthcare resources that ensures the largest possible beneficial impact on health.

Health system The combination of resources, organization, and management that culminates in the delivery of health services to the population.

Hemorrhage (related to pregnancy) Significant and uncontrolled loss of blood, either internally or externally from the body. Antepartum (prenatal) hemorrhage occurs after the 20th week of gestation but before delivery of the baby; postpartum hemorrhage is the loss of 500 ml or more of blood from the genital tract after delivery of the baby; primary postpartum hemorrhage occurs in the first 24 hours after delivery.

Herd immunity When a high enough proportion of a population is immune to an infectious disease, people who cannot get vaccinated, such as very young children or people with immune system issues, are indirectly protected from the spread of disease.

High-risk drinking Drinking 20 grams or more per day of pure alcohol for a woman and 40 grams a day for a man.

Hookworm A parasite that lives in the small intestine of its host, which may be a mammal such as a dog, cat, or human.

Human capital People's ability to be productive and to accumulate the knowledge and skills they need to be productive.

Hydrocele Scrotal swelling, often accompanying lymphatic filariasis.

Hyperglycemia in pregnancy See gestational diabetes.

Hypertension High blood pressure.

I

Illness Represents personal, interpersonal, and cultural reactions to disease or discomfort.

Immunization The process of inducing immunity, usually through vaccination.

Improved care seeking, disease recognition An approach to controlling the spread of communicable disease involving enhancing people's ability to seek health care when they become infected, as well as improving people's ability to correctly recognize particular diseases.

Improved water, sanitation, hygiene A strategy for controlling the spread of communicable disease involving providing safe access to clean water and sanitation, as well as promoting hygienic practices (such as handwashing).

Incidence rate The rate at which new cases of a disease occur in a population.

Infant mortality rate The number of deaths of infants under age 1 per 1,000 live births in a given year.

Informed consent Permission granted by a participant to partake in research after fully understanding the possible risks and benefits.

Inhalation A path of transmission of infectious disease involving the respiration of aerosolized droplets containing the infectious agent (e.g., tuberculosis, influenza, meningitis).

Injuries The result of an act that damages, harms, or hurts; unintentional or intentional damage to the body resulting from acute exposure to thermal, mechanical, electrical, or chemical energy or from the absence of such essentials as heat or oxygen.

Insulin resistance The diminished action of insulin, resulting in an increased amount of glucose in the blood.

Intentional injury An injury resulting from someone trying to do another person harm.

Internally displaced person Someone who is forced to flee his or her home, often due to persecution, war, natural disaster, or violence, but who remains within his or her own country.

Intrauterine growth restriction A condition in which a fetus does not grow properly.

Iodine deficiency disorders A number of possible health problems, such as mental restriction, cretinism, goiter, hypothyroidism, and some developmental abnormalities, that stem from an insufficient amount of iodine.

Ischemic heart disease Also known as coronary heart disease and characterized by a reduced blood supply to the heart.

L

Life expectancy at birth The average number of years a newborn baby could expect to live if current mortality trends were to continue for the rest of the newborn's life.

Life table A representation of the probable years of survivorship of any population. For the Global Burden of Disease Study there is a standard reference life table that takes account of the highest life expectancy at birth globally and is used in calculations of years of life lost due to premature deaths.

Loa loa A parasitic worm passed on to humans from deerflies that causes loiasis.

Low birthweight Birthweight less than 2,500 grams.

Lymphedema Swelling in an arm or a leg due to a buildup of lymph fluid.

M

Malaria A disease of humans caused by blood parasites of the species *Plasmodium falciparum, vivax, ovale, knowlesi*, or *malariae* and transmitted by anopheline mosquitoes.

Malnutrition Various forms of poor nutrition, including underweight, stunting, wasting, and overweight or obesity, as well as micronutrient deficiencies.

Mass chemotherapy A preventive form of mass administration of drug therapy to control infection.

Maternal death The death of a woman while pregnant, during delivery, or within 42 days of delivery, irrespective of the duration and the site of pregnancy. The cause of death is always related to or aggravated by the pregnancy or its management and does not include accidental or incidental causes.

Maternal mortality ratio The number of women who die as a result of pregnancy and childbirth complications per 100,000 live births in a given year.

Measles A highly communicable disease characterized by fever, general malaise, sneezing, nasal congestion, a brassy cough, conjunctivitis, and an eruption over the entire body, caused by the rubeola virus.

Medical neutrality The concept that medical personnel not engaged in acts harmful to the enemy should be respected and protected during a conflict.

Mental health A state of well-being in which every individual realizes his or her own potential, can cope with the normal stresses of life, can work productively and fruitfully, and is able to make a contribution to her or his community.

mHealth Medical and public health practice supported by mobile devices, also known as mobile health.

Microbicide A substance to be applied inside the vagina or rectum to substantially reduce the transmission of sexually transmitted infections (STIs), including HIV.

Mono-resistance Resistance to one first-line anti-TB drug only.

Morbidity Illness.

Mortality Death.

Multidrug resistance (MDR) Resistance to at least both isoniazid and rifampicin (for tuberculosis).

N

Natural disaster A natural event that causes loss of life, damage, and disruption to daily patterns of living. Examples include tornadoes, hurricanes, earthquakes, or floods.

Neonatal mortality rate Number of deaths of children under 28 days of age in a given year per 1,000 live births in that year.

Noncommunicable diseases Illnesses that are not spread by any infectious agent.

Nongovernmental organization A nonprofit group or association organized outside of institutionalized political structures to realize particular social objectives, such as environmental protection, or serve particular constituencies, such as indigenous peoples.

Nontraumatic contact Contact with a certain infectious agent that can cause disease but does not require injury for entry (e.g., anthrax).

O

Obesity (For an adult) Body mass index over 30.

Obstetric fistula An injury in the birth canal that allows leakage from the bladder or rectum into the vagina, leaving a woman permanently incontinent, often leading to isolation and exclusion from the family and community.

Onchocerciasis A neglected tropical disease caused by infection with the parasitic worm *Onchocerca volvulus*.

Symptoms include severe itching, bumps under the skin, and blindness.

One Health The integrative effort of multiple disciplines working locally, nationally, and globally to attain optimal health for people, animals, and the environment.

Out-of-pocket health expenditures A form of private health expenditure when costs are not covered or reimbursed by an insurance program.

Overweight (For an adult) A body mass index between 25 and 30.

P

Pandemic preparedness The ability to effectively deal with a global outbreak of disease.

Panic disorders A mental disorder in which people have attacks of fear that last several minutes or longer.

Parasite An animal or vegetable organism that lives on or in another and derives its nourishment therefrom.

Patterns of resort The manner in which people and families care for illnesses.

Pentavalent vaccine A vaccine that has antigens against five childhood diseases: diphtheria, tetanus, pertussis (whooping cough), hepatitis B, and *Haemophilus influenzae* type b (Hib).

Personal responsibility The idea that outcomes are the result of an individual's own actions or behaviors.

Pertussis A highly contagious bacterial disease that causes uncontrollable, violent coughing.

Planetary Health Planetary health is the health of human civilization and the state of the natural systems on which it depends.

Pneumonia An inflammation, usually caused by infection, involving the alveoli of the lungs.

Point prevalence The proportion of the population that has a condition at a given point in time.

Poliomyelitis (polio) Infantile paralysis, a viral paralytic disease.

Poly-resistance Resistance to more than one first-line anti-TB drug, other than both isoniazid and rifampicin.

Positive rights Rights that obligate the provision of benefits and services, such as by a government, to the rights holder.

Preeclampsia (previously called toxemia) A hypertensive disorder of pregnancy said to exist when a pregnant woman with gestational hypertension develops proteinuria. Originally, edema was considered part of the syndrome of preeclampsia, but presently the former two symptoms are sufficient for a diagnosis of preeclampsia.

Prevalence The number of people suffering from a certain condition over a specific time period.

Primary care The provision of first contact, person-focused, ongoing care over time that meets the health-related needs of people; refers to a hospital only those problems too uncommon to maintain competence; and coordinates care when people receive services at other levels of care.

Primary health care Health care that is essential and socially acceptable, addresses the needs of the community, is based on evidence, is affordable, and is made universally available.

Primary prevention Intervening before health effects occur.

"Priority to the worse off" Allocating health resources on the basis of who is already disadvantaged.

Private health expenditure Health expenditure that comes from sources other than governments.

Prognostic loss At the group level, it is the loss of future health defined as the difference between normal healthy life expectancy, at the time of treatment or onset of disease, and the length and quality of life a person would have without the new intervention being considered. It is often measured as the loss of quality-adjusted life years (QALYs).

Public health The science and art of preventing disease, prolonging life, and promoting physical health and mental health and efficiency through organized community efforts toward a sanitary environment, control of community infections, education in hygiene, and the development of social machinery to ensure capacity in the community to maintain health.

Public health expenditure Health expenditure by any level of government or of a government agency.

Push mechanism Interventions that reduce the risks and costs of investments.

Pull mechanism Interventions that assure a future return in the event that a product is produced.

Q

Quality-adjusted life years (QALYs) A measure of health that is adjusted to reflect the quality of life of a person or group of persons, in which one QALY is the equivalent of one year of life in perfect health.

R

Reemerging infectious disease An existing disease that has increased in incidence or has taken on new forms.

Refugee A person who has fled and is outside of his own country because of fear of persecution.

Replacement fertility The total fertility rate needed for a population to exactly replace itself from one generation to the next, without migration.

Respect for enrolled subjects Under the umbrella of ethical duties researchers have toward participants, this respect includes protecting confidentiality and allowing participants to withdraw from a study.

Responsiveness to the expectations of the population How the system performs relative to non-health aspects, meeting or not meeting a population's expectations of how it should be treated by providers of prevention, care, or non-personal services.

Results-based financing Any program that rewards the delivery of one or more outputs or outcomes by one or more incentives, financial or otherwise, after the principal has verified that the agent has delivered the agreed-upon results.

Rifampicin resistance (RR) Resistance to rifampicin detected using phenotypic or genotypic methods, with or without resistance to other anti-TB drugs. It includes any resistance to rifampicin, in the form of mono-resistance, poly-resistance, MDR, or XDR.

Right to health The highest attainable standard of health is a fundamental right of every human being including access to timely, acceptable, and affordable health care of appropriate quality.

Risk factor An aspect or personal behavior or lifestyle, an environmental exposure, or an inborn or inherited characteristic that, on the basis of epidemiologic evidence, is known to be associated with health-related conditions.

Risk pooling In health insurance, this refers to managing the risk of expensive claims by spreading insurance coverage over the largest number of people possible. It also refers to the sharing of risks among insurance companies.

S

Schizophrenia A chronic, severe, and disabling brain disorder.

Scientifically valid Research that is executed accurately and successfully measures what it intends to measure using the principles of the scientific method.

Secondary care Medical care provided by a specialist or facility upon referral by a primary care physician.

Secondary prevention Screening to identify diseases in the earliest stages, before the onset of signs and symptoms and providing treatment, as appropriate, to prevent any diagnosed conditions from worsening.

Self-efficacy Whether or not people feel that they could actually carry out a particular behavior if they tried.

Sepsis Infection in the blood.

Severe acute malnutrition An extreme form of malnutrition defined by a very low weight-for-height measurement of three z scores below the median WHO growth standards.

Sex Either of the two major forms of individuals that occur in many species and that are distinguished respectively as female or male especially on the basis of their reproductive organs and structures.

Sex-selective abortion The practice of aborting a fetus after a determination, usually by ultrasound but also rarely by amniocentesis or another procedure, that the fetus is an undesired sex, typically female.

Sexual or bloodborne A path of transmission for certain communicable diseases (e.g., HIV, hepatitis) involving contact between blood, semen, vaginal fluid, or anal mucosa.

Sexually transmitted infections (STIs) Diseases, also known as sexually transmitted diseases (STDs), that are commonly transmitted between partners through some form of sexual activity, most commonly vaginal intercourse, oral sex, or anal sex.

Social determinants of health The conditions in which people are born, grow, live, work, and age, all of which have an impact on their health.

Social impact assessment A process for assessing the social impacts of planned interventions or events and for developing strategies for the ongoing monitoring and management of those impacts.

Social media Activities, practices, and behaviors among communities of people who gather online that make it possible to create and easily transmit content in the form of words, pictures, videos, and audios.

Social value The benefits conferred to society.

Society A group of people who occupy a specific locality and share the same cultural traditions.

Soil-transmitted helminths Intestinal worms infecting humans that are transmitted through contaminated soil, including *Ascaris lumbricoides* (sometimes called just "*Ascaris*"), whipworm (*Trichuris trichiura*), and hookworm (*Anclostoma duodenale* and *Necator americanus*).

Stewardship The wide range of functions carried out by governments as they seek to achieve national health policy objectives. The careful and responsible management of something entrusted to one's care.

Stroke Temporary or permanent loss of the blood supply to the brain.

Structural approach A component of combination prevention for HIV that addresses the underlying societal elements that predispose a person to the risk of infection.

Stunting Failure to reach linear growth potential because of inadequate nutrition or poor health; two z-scores below the international reference.

T

Task shifting The rational redistribution of tasks among health workforce teams. Specific tasks are moved, where appropriate, from highly qualified health workers to health workers with shorter training and fewer qualifications in order to make more efficient use of the available human resources for health.

Tertiary care Specialized consultative care, usually on referral from primary or secondary medical care personnel, by specialists working in a center that has personnel and facilities for special investigation and treatment.

Tertiary prevention Managing disease post diagnosis to slow or stop disease progression.

Tetanus A bacterial and often fatal infection that enters the body through a wound or puncture. It is especially important to prevent neonatal tetanus through vaccination of the mother and sterile delivery conditions.

Tiered pricing A financing mechanism under which companies sell medicines at different prices depending on the income level of the country involved.

Total expenditure on health The sum of general government expenditure on health (commonly called public expenditure on health) and private expenditure on health.

Traditional medicine The sum total of the knowledge, skill, and practices based on the theories, beliefs, and experiences indigenous to different cultures used in the maintenance of health as well as in the prevention, diagnosis, improvement, or treatment of physical and mental illness.

Transgender Refers to people whose sense of their gender identity differs from the sex they were assigned at birth.

Traumatic contact A scratch or bite through which certain infectious diseases can be spread (e.g., rabies).

U

Under-5 mortality rate The probability that a newborn baby will die before reaching age 5, expressed as a number per 1,000 live births.

Undernutrition A state of being underweight for one's age, too short for one's age (stunted), dangerously thin for one's height (wasted), or deficient in vitamins and minerals (micronutrient malnutrition).

Underweight Low weight-for-age; two z-scores below the international reference for weight-for-age.

Unintentional injury That subset of injuries for which there is no evidence of predetermined intent.

Universal health coverage Ensuring that all people can use the promotive, preventive, curative, rehabilitative, and palliative health services they need, of sufficient quality to be effective, while also ensuring that the use of these services does not expose the user to financial hardship.

User fees Charges levied at the point of use for any aspect of health services. For example, registration fees, consultation fees, fees for drugs and medical supplies, or charges for any health service rendered, such as outpatient or inpatient care.

Uterine prolapse A condition in which the uterus protrudes into, and sometimes out of, the vagina.

V

Vaccination A biological preparation that improves immunity to a particular disease and typically contains an agent that resembles a disease-causing microorganism.

Vaccine hesitancy The delay in accepting or the unwillingness to accept available vaccines.

Vector-borne (diseases) Diseases transmitted through mosquitoes, sandflies, triatomine bugs, blackflies, ticks, tsetse flies, mites, snails, and lice.

Vector control A method to contain or totally eradicate any insects, rats, mammals, or disease-transmitting animals. Most commonly seen with mosquito control.

Viral load The number of viral particles found in each milliliter of blood.

Vital registration A system by which the government of a country records vital events, including births, deaths, and the causes of death.

Vitamin A deficiency An insufficiency of vitamin A in the body that can cause a number of health problems, such as blindness, and that has an important association with excess morbidity and mortality in young children from a number of health conditions, such as pneumonia and measles.

W

WASH Water, sanitation, and hygiene.

Wasting Weight, measured in kilograms, divided by height in meters squared that is two z-scores below the international reference.

Waterborne (illness) A disease caused by drinking contaminated water.

Western biomedicine A system in which medical doctors and other healthcare professionals (such as nurses, pharmacists, and therapists) treat symptoms and diseases using drugs, radiation, or surgery. Also called allopathic medicine, biomedicine, conventional medicine, mainstream medicine, and orthodox medicine.

Y

Youth The United Nations defines "youth" as a person between the ages of 15 and 24 years.

Z

Zoonoses A disease that can be transmitted to humans from animals.

Z-score A statistical term, meaning the deviation of an individual's value from the median value of a reference population, divided by the standard deviation of the reference population.

Index

Note: Page numbers followed by f or t indicate materials in figures and tables respectively.